The Reticuloendothelial System
A COMPREHENSIVE TREATISE

Volume 8
Pharmacology

The Reticuloendothelial System
A COMPREHENSIVE TREATISE

General Editors:
Herman Friedman, *University of South Florida, Tampa, Florida*
Mario Escobar, *Medical College of Virginia, Richmond, Virginia*
and
Sherwood M. Reichard, *Medical College of Georgia, Augusta, Georgia*

MORPHOLOGY
Edited by Ian Carr and W. T. Daems

BIOCHEMISTRY AND METABOLISM
Edited by Anthony J. Sbarra and Robert R. Strauss

PHYLOGENY AND ONTOGENY
Edited by Nicholas Cohen and M. Michael Sigel

IMMUNOPATHOLOGY
Edited by Noel R. Rose and Benjamin V. Siegel

CANCER
Edited by Ronald B. Herberman and Herman Friedman

IMMUNOLOGY
Edited by Joseph A. Bellanti and Herbert B. Herscowitz

PHYSIOLOGY (In two parts)
Edited by Sherwood M. Reichard and James P. Filkins

PHARMACOLOGY
Edited by John W. Hadden and Andor Szentivanyi

HYPERSENSITIVITY
Edited by S. Michael Phillips and Peter Abramoff

INFECTION
Edited by John P. Utz and Mario R. Escobar

The Reticuloendothelial System
A COMPREHENSIVE TREATISE

Volume 8
Pharmacology

Edited by
JOHN W. HADDEN
and ANDOR SZENTIVANYI

University of South Florida
College of Medicine
Tampa, Florida

SPRINGER SCIENCE+BUSINESS MEDIA, LLC

Library of Congress Cataloging in Publication Data

Main entry under title:

The Reticuloendothelial system.

   Includes bibliographies and indexes.
   Contents: v. 1. Morphology.—v. 2. Biochemistry and metabolism.—[etc.]—v. 8. Pharmacology.
   1. Reticulo-endothelial system—Collected works. 2. Macrophages—Collected works. I. Friedman, Herman, 1931-   . II. Escobar, Mario R. III. Reichard, Sherwood, M. [DNLM: 1. Reticuloendothelial system. WH650 R437]
QP115.R47   591.2′95   79-25933
ISBN 978-1-4615-9408-6   ISBN 978-1-4615-9406-2 (eBook)
DOI 10.1007/978-1-4615-9406-2

© 1985 Springer Science+Business Media New York
Originally published by Plenum Press, New York 1985
Softcover reprint of the hardcover 1st edition 1985

A Division of Plenum Publishing Corporation
233 Spring Street, New York, N.Y. 10013

Contributors

DOLPH O. ADAMS • Department of Pathology, Duke University Medical Center, Durham, North Carolina

JACQUES BENVENISTE • INSERM U-200, Université Paris-Sud, Clamart, France

GORO CHIHARA • National Cancer Center Research Institute, Tsukiji, Chuo-ku, Tokyo, Japan

RONALD G. COFFEY • Department of Pharmacology and Therapeutics, University of South Florida College of Medicine, Tampa, Florida

JACK H. DEAN • Department of Cell Biology, Chemical Industry Institute of Toxicology, Research Triangle Park, North Carolina

M. JANE EHRKE • Department of Experimental Therapeutics and Grace Cancer Drug Center, Roswell Park Memorial Institute, New York State Department of Health, Buffalo, New York

ROBERT M. FAUVE • Unit of Cellular Immunophysiology, Pasteur Institute, Paris, France

KURT B. P. FLEMMING • Institute of Biophysics and Radiation Biology, Albert Ludwig University, Freiburg, Federal Republic of Germany

ARTHUR FLYNN • Department of Molecular and Cellular Biology, Research Division, Cleveland Clinic Foundation, Cleveland, Ohio

JOHN W. HADDEN • Departments of Microbiology, Immunology, and Internal Medicine, University of South Florida College of Medicine, Tampa, Florida

JUNJI HAMURO • Department of Basic Immunological Research, Central Research Laboratories, Ajinomoto Company, Yokohama, Japan

MICHAEL A. KALINER • Allergic Diseases Section, Laboratory of Clinical Investigation, National Institute of Allergy and Infectious Diseases, National Institutes of Health, Bethesda, Maryland

KAZUO KOBAYASHI • Department of Pathology, University of Connecticut Health Center, Farmington, Connecticut

EDGAR LEDERER • Institut de Biochimie, Université Paris-Sud, Orsay, France

STANLEY S. LEFKOWITZ • Department of Microbiology, Texas Tech University Health Science Center, Lubbock, Texas

GENEVIÈVE LEMAIRE • Institut de Biochimie, Université Paris-Sud, Orsay, France

ROBERT F. LEMANSKE, JR. • Departments of Pediatrics and Medicine, University of Wisconsin Medical School, Madison, Wisconsin

ENRICO MIHICH • Department of Experimental Therapeutics and Grace Cancer Drug Center, Roswell Park Memorial Institute, New York State Department of Health, Buffalo, New York

JEAN-FRANÇOIS PETIT • Institut de Biochimie, Université Paris-Sud, Orsay, France

RÉGINE ROUBIN • INSERM U-200, Université Paris-Sud, Clamart, France

JOHN R. SADLIK • Department of Hematology–Oncology, Ohio State University, Columbus, Ohio

THOMAS E. SCHINDLER • Xytronyx, Inc., Chicago, Illinois

RICHARD M. SCHULTZ • Department of Immunology, Lilly Research Laboratories, Indianapolis, Indiana

T. Y. SHEN • Merck Sharp & Dohme Research Laboratories, Rahway, New Jersey

ANDOR SZENTIVANYI • Department of Pharmacology and Therapeutics, University of South Florida College of Medicine, Tampa, Florida

JEAN-PIERRE TENU • Institut de Biochimie, Université Paris-Sud, Orsay, France

JOSEPH F. WILLIAMS • Department of Pharmacology and Therapeutics, University of South Florida College of Medicine, Tampa, Florida

TAKESHI YOSHIDA • Department of Pathology, University of Connecticut Health Center, Farmington, Connecticut

Foreword

This comprehensive treatise on the reticuloendothelial system is a project jointly shared by individual members of the Reticuloendothelial (RE) Society and biomedical scientists in general who are interested in the intricate system of cells and molecular moieties derived from those cells which constitute the RES. It may now be more fashionable in some quarters to consider these cells as part of what is called the mononuclear phagocytic system or the lymphoreticular system. Nevertheless, because of historical developments and current interest in the subject by investigators from many diverse areas, it seems advantageous to present in one comprehensive treatise current information and knowledge concerning basic aspects of the RES, such as morphology, biochemistry, phylogeny and ontogeny, physiology, and pharmacology as well as clinical areas including immunopathology, cancer, infectious diseases, allergy, and hypersensitivity. It is anticipated that, by presenting information concerning these apparently heterogeneous topics under the unifying umbrella of the RES, attention will be focused on the similarities as well as interactions among the cell types constituting the RES from the viewpoint of various disciplines. The treatise editors and their editorial board, consisting predominantly of the editors of individual volumes, are extremely grateful for the enthusiastic cooperation and enormous task undertaken by members of the biomedical community in general and especially by members of the American as well as European and Japanese Reticuloendothelial Societies. The assistance, cooperation, and great support from the editorial staff of Plenum Press are also valued greatly. It is hoped that this unique treatise, the first to offer a fully comprehensive treatment of our knowledge concerning the RES, will provide a unified framework for evaluating what is known and what still has to be investigated in this actively growing field. The various volumes of this treatise provide extensive in-depth and integrated information on classical as well as experimental aspects of the RES. It is expected that these volumes will serve as a major reference for day-to-day examination of various subjects dealing with the RES from many different viewpoints.

Herman Friedman
Mario R. Escobar
Sherwood M. Reichard

Preface

The reticuloendothelial system represents a broad body network composed principally of fixed and mobile cellular components of the monocyte–macrophage series. Its primary functions are the continuous cleansing of bodily fluids to remove particulate matter through phagocytosis and a cooperation with the lymphoid system in responding immunologically and specifically to various antigenic challenges. It is impossible to discuss the reticuloendothelial system without a heavy focus on its intertwinement with its co-partner the immune system, and, in this sense, it is often difficult to dissociate and to define the distinct roles of the two systems in immune responses. Recognizing this problem we embarked on an analysis of the pharmacology of the reticuloendothelial system. Through the many contributions to this volume, it is evident that we found it possible to delineate such a pharmacology and that, in many aspects, it is an immunopharmacology. We also found the field undercultivated scientifically. Many areas have not been developed while others, particularly the immunologic, have received considerable attention. Perhaps the broadest area of ignorance involves the microenvironmental relationships between the endothelial components of this system and macrophages and lymphoid cells. Many studies seem to clarify the individual functions and biochemical processes that pertain to isolated cells in culture, but what is lacking is a clear and detailed picture of how the entire system cooperates to achieve its functions.

Many studies attest to the pharmacologic sensitivity that the isolated cells possess, and these chapters document well this aspect of the pharmacology of the system. Needed are more studies on the organs of the system *in vitro* and *in vivo* and particularly on the interrelationships of the system with the central nervous system. It is notable that, for example, lymphocytes and macrophages bear receptors for adrenergic and cholinergic mediators. Yet in the context of their percolation through bodily fluids they may never see the agonists for these receptors; it is only in residence in the reticuloendothelial system, where the appropriate neural contacts exist, that such interactions of agonist and receptor take place. Much needs to be learned of these relationships and their impact on the function of the system.

Without further elaborating on what is not known, we would like to express our thanks to the contributors for their many fine expositions on what is known about the pharmacology of the reticuloendothelial system. A number of chapters describe the effects of the soluble products of mast cells, lymphocytes, macrophages, and nonspecific inflammation on the functions of the major cellular components of the system, particularly the macrophage. The cyclic nucleotide pharmacology of the actions of many of these products is outlined. The actions of microbial products, immunomodulators, and fungal glycans on cells of the system are described, as are their possible roles in the therapy of disease states in which the reticuloendothelial system participates as a defense mechanism. The immunosuppressive effects of cancer chemotherapy, immunosuppressive agents, abused drugs, and environmental immunotoxicants are also dealt with in great detail. Together these chapters offer a unique and composite picture of the pharmacologic regulation of this system by both endogenous and exogenous products. In conjunction with the other volumes in this series on the reticuloendothelial system, this text contributes a clear picture of the state of scientific understanding of this important system and points the way to many future areas of productive research to increase that understanding.

John W. Hadden
Andor Szentivanyi

Contents

4. Release of Lipid Mediators from Macrophages and Its Pharmacological Modulation

RÉGINE ROUBIN and JACQUES BENVENISTE

5. Lymphokines: Pharmacologic Modulation of Their Production and Action

TAKESHI YOSHIDA and KAZUO KOBAYASHI

6. Effects of Nonspecific Inflammation on the Reticuloendothelial System

ROBERT M. FAUVE

7. The Role of Macrophage-Derived Arachidonic Acid Oxygenation Products in the Modulation of Macrophage and Lymphocyte Function

RICHARD M. SCHULTZ

8. Immunopharmacologic Regulation of the Mononuclear Phagocyte System

THOMAS E. SCHINDLER, JOHN R. SADLIK, and JOHN W. HADDEN

9. Effects of Microbially Derived Products on Mononuclear Phagocytes

GENEVIÈVE LEMAIRE, JEAN-PIERRE TENU, JEAN-FRANÇOIS PETIT, and EDGAR LEDERER

10. Stimulation and Depression of the RES by Pharmacological Agents

Kurt B. P. Flemming

Pharmacokinetic and Pharmacodynamic Parameters Affected by RE Cell Activators

JOSEPH F. WILLIAMS and ANDOR SZENTIVANYI

1. INTRODUCTION

The onset, intensity, and duration of drug effects depend to a large degree on achieving and maintaining an appropriate concentration of the agent at its site of action. The two branches of pharamacology concerned with the study of various factors that influence drug concentration and drug response are pharmacokinetics and pharmacodynamics. Pharmacokinetics embraces investigations of the various factors that affect absorption, distribution, metabolism, and excretion of pharmacologically active agents. Pharmacodynamics is concerned with those biochemical and/or physiological alterations elicited by a compound relative to its concentration, i.e., the dose–response relationship. Inherent within the latter is also the consideration of the mechanism of drug action, i.e., the primary alteration that underlies the sequence of events leading to a demonstrable effect. Pharmacokinetic and pharmacodynamic parameters thus are key considerations in governing the selection and adjustment of drug dosage and dosage schedules. In a therapeutic context, alterations, either positive or negative, of these parameters due to disease processes, genetic factors, age, or prior drug exposure may significantly attentuate or accentuate the therapeutic effectiveness of a particular agent. Indeed, at the two extremes, complete failure to achieve therapeutic effect or frank toxicity may result from inappropriate consideration of the status and interplay between pharmacokinetic and pharmacodynamic parameters.

Within the last few years, it has become increasingly evident that injection of experimental animals with a number of agents, known primarily as immu-

JOSEPH F. WILLIAMS and ANDOR SZENTIVANYI • Department of Pharmacology and Therapeutics, University of South Florida College of Medicine, Tampa, Florida 33612.

nomodulators, causes a decrease in the activity of the hepatic microsomal drug-metabolizing enzyme system responsible for the biotransformation of a wide variety of drugs, other xenobiotics, and certain endogenous compounds, such as steroids, fatty acids, cholesterol, and prostaglandins. This enzyme system plays a pivotal pharmacokinetic role in the activation as well as inactivation of many pharmacological agents.

A possible role of the reticuloendothelial cell system (RES) in altering drug disposition was suggested by Samaras and Dietz (1953). They observed that following injection of animals with trypan blue there was a prolongation of pentobarbital sleep-time, a parameter inversely related to the rate of metabolism of the barbiturate. On the other hand, it was reported that when the sleep-time measurement was determined a few days after trypan blue administration the duration of narcosis was considerably shortened. Samaras and Dietz (1953) interpreted these results to indicate the direct participation of the RES in barbiturate metabolism. They proposed the initial prolongation of sleep-time occurred due to the dye-induced blockade of RES function, resulting in decreased barbiturate metabolism by this cellular system. The subsequent shortening of sleep-time duration was assumed to occur as a result of rebound RES stimulation following elimination of the trypan blue. Other reports indicating effects of RES-active agents on barbiturate sleep-time were those of Wooles and Borzelleca (1964, 1966) and DiCarlo et al. (1965). However, these studies showed that RES stimulation by a variety of compounds increased rather than decreased the duration of barbiturate-induced narcosis.

Wooles and Munson (1971) demonstrated that the functional state of the RES, as measured by phagocytic activity, was not correlated with the effect of RES-active agents to depress barbiturate metabolism. Indeed, they reported a decrease in drug metabolism following administration of compounds that stimulated as well as after those that inhibited phagocytic activity. Barnes and Wooles (1970) and Wooles and Munson (1971) showed that the prolongation of barbiturate sleep-time could be explained by the decrease in the *in vitro* hepatic microsomal drug-metabolizing enzyme activity prepared from animals treated with RES stimulants.

Table 1 lists various RES-active agents that are currently known to cause

TABLE 1. IMMUNOACTIVE AGENTS SHOWN TO AFFECT THE ACTIVITY OF THE HEPATIC MICROSOMAL DRUG-METABOLIZING ENZYME SYSTEM

Glucan	Protein-bound polysaccharide from *Coleolus vesicolor* Quél
Methyl palmitate	Tilorone
Zymosan	Quinacrine
Mycobacterium	Viruses
BCG and BCG-cell wall skeleton	Pyran copolymer
Muramyl dipeptide	Poly(rI:rC)
Cornyebacterium parvum	Interferon (α/β?, γ)
Bordetella pertussis	Colloidal carbon
Endotoxin	Glyceryl trioleate
Lipid A	Statalon
OK432 streptococcal preparation	Thorium dioxide

alteration in drug biotransformation activity. With few exceptions, the ability of these agents to elicit this effect is seen only *in vivo*. Little evidence exists that they exert significant inhibitory influences when added *in vitro* to microsomal preparations used to assay for drug-metabolizing activity. Also, the effect of these agents to inhibit drug-metabolizing activity apparently occurs without evidence of major hepatotoxicity. It should also be mentioned at this point that, although most reports have focused on the effects of the listed agents to decrease drug-metabolizing activity, there is some evidence that certain drug biotransformation reactions, possibly occurring in cells of the RES, may be stimulated by these agents.

This chapter presents a brief review of the effects of the various immunomodulators to alter drug disposition. The primary focus will be on their effects on the hepatic microsomal drug-metabolizing enzyme system that is responsible for the oxidation of a wide variety of agents. A few studies have shown that relatively similar effects also occur in the drug-metabolizing activity of certain extrahepatic tissues (Carlson and Ciaccio, 1975). For each agent we will also discuss the current understanding of the possible mechanisms involved in these effects. Available information relative to the occurrence and significance of altered drug biotransformation after the clinical use of the immunomodulators will be presented. The extreme breadth of the experimental literature concerning these topics encompasses areas of immunology, microbiology, pathology, biochemistry, onocology, as well as pharmacology. Such diversity of informational sources makes it possible that pertinent observations may have been unintentionally omitted from the discussion. However, it is felt the following represents a relatively complete coverage of knowledge in this area at the present time.

2. HEPATIC MICROSOMAL DRUG-METABOLIZING ENZYME SYSTEM

The following will serve as a brief introduction to the salient features of the drug-metabolizing enzyme system.

The liver is the major site where the oxidation, reduction, hydrolysis, and conjugation of foreign compounds occurs. Of these reactions, the oxidation of drugs is of particular interest because of the pivotal role these reactions play in the inactivation or activation of many diverse chemical agents. The hepatic enzyme system responsible for the oxidation of many drugs is located primarily in the smooth endoplasmic reticulum of the hepatic parenchymal cell, the so-called microsomal fraction isolated by differential centrifugation of liver homogenates. Hence, the system is frequently referred to as the hepatic microsomal drug-metabolizing enzyme system. Analogous enzyme activities have been shown to occur in other tissues, e.g., lung, skin, intestine, and kidney, but generally the enzyme activity in these extrahepatic sites is a small fraction of that localized in the liver (Burke and Orrenius, 1979). The extrahepatic metabolism of drugs is, therefore, probably of minor significance with respect to the overall biotransformation rate. However, the intratissue metabolic activity may be important with respect to local drug concentration and, thus, to the intensity of local drug effect or toxicity. Of the various metabolic biotransformation reactions, the effects of RES-active agents on the hepatic microsomal drug oxidation reactions have been the most extensively investigated.

The oxidative drug-metabolizing enzyme system is a multicomponent system, consisting of a flavoprotein reductase, a phospholipid fraction, and a hemoprotein, called cytochrome P-450, which functions as the terminal oxidase. This oxidative enzyme system is also referred to as the mixed-function oxidases or monooxygenases as it requires NADPH and molecular oxygen, and catalyzes the transfer of one atom of molecular oxygen to the substrate, forming hydroxylated intermediates or products, while the second oxygen atom appears in water. A brief scheme of microsomal electron transport is shown in Fig. 1.

As indicated, the primary electron donor is NADPH, and the flavoprotein reductase, NADPH-cytochrome P-450 reductase (referred to as NADPH-cytochrome c reductase in the older literature), catalyzes the electron transfer to cytochrome P-450. Drug–substrate binding occurs with the oxidized form of this hemoprotein. The drug–cytochrome P-450 complex accepts the electrons from NADPH-cytochrome P-450 reductase to form the reduced cytochrome P-450–drug complex. The reduced complex combines with molecular oxygen and, after a second electron transfer to the oxygenated complex, the hydroxylated substrate, water, and oxidized cytochrome P-450 are generated. Unlike most enzyme systems, the cytochrome P-450 drug-metabolizing enzyme system acts on many structurally diverse compounds and catalyzes a wide variety of oxidative reactions, such as aromatic and aliphatic hydroxylation, N- and O-dealkylation, sulfoxidation, N-oxidation, and hydroxylation. This unusually wide substrate specificity has recently been shown to be attributable to the presence of multiple forms of hepatic microsomal cytochrome P-450 (Lu and West, 1980). Further details on the kinetics of the enzyme system can be found in recent review articles (Gander and Mannering, 1980; Omura, 1980; Schenkman *et al.*, 1981).

Hepatic mixed-function oxidase activity is influenced significantly by various hormonal, environmental, and genetic factors (Paine, 1981). In particular, altered rates of cytochrome P-450 synthesis and/or degradation occur subsequent to changes in various hormone levels or in response to drug exposure. A number of pharmacological agents have been shown to increase the cytochrome P-450-dependent enzyme activities and the level of the hemoprotein (Snyder and Remmer, 1979). The increase has been attributed to induced synthesis of the cytochrome since it can be prevented by inhibitors of nucleic acid or protein

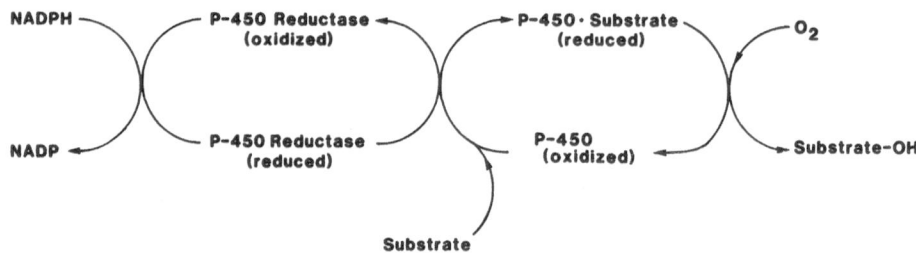

FIGURE 1.   The major components of the hepatic microsomal drug-metabolizing enzyme system.

synthesis, The protein moiety is synthesized on the endoplasmic reticulum and combines with heme, supplied by the mitochondrial heme synthesis system, to form the holocytochrome P-450. On the other hand, the metabolic turnover of cytochrome P-450 appears to involve, in part, the dissociation of heme from the holoenzyme and the metabolism of the dissociated heme to biliverdin through the action of microsomal heme oxygenase, the rate-limiting step in heme catabolism, and subsequently to bilirubin. Presently it is unclear whether the heme and protein moieties of cytochrome P-450 turn over at the same rate. Gasser *et al.* (1982) measured a $t_{\frac{1}{2}}$ of 12.4 hr for the heme moiety and a $t_{\frac{1}{2}}$ of 19.1 hr for the apoprotein moiety of cytochrome P-450b in phenobarbital-induced animals, suggesting coordinated turnover. It is also uncertain whether the protein once dissociated from the heme moiety is able to accept new heme to re-form active holocytochrome P-450.

3. *MYCOBACTERIUM* AND RELATED AGENTS

Early studies reporting the effects of RES-active substances to alter hepatic mixed-function oxidase activity were those in which Freund's complete adjuvant was used to induce a chronic inflammatory condition in certain strains of rats. Adjuvant-induced polyarthritis (AIP) in animals mimics in several aspects the rheumatoid arthritic disease state in man, and has been widely used as an animal model to screen for clinically effective antiarthritic and antiinflammatory agents (Stoerck *et al.*, 1954; Pearson, 1956; Newbould, 1963; Arrigoni-Martelli, 1979). The so-called "adjuvant" is a suspension of heat-killed *Mycobacterium*, usually *M. smegmatis*, *butyricum*, or *tuberculosis*, in an oily vehicle, generally mineral oil. For the induction of AIP, the adjuvant is usually injected into either a footpad or the tail of the rat, other routes of administration being less effective. Use of other species of mycobacteria or other vehicles may result in the development of a less severe disease state. In addition, not all strains of rats are equally susceptible to the effects of the adjuvant, and hamsters, guinea pigs, and mice seem remarkably resistant to the development of AIP.

Quevauviller *et al.* (1968) appear to be the first to note an increased barbiturate sleep-time in rats with AIP. These investigators coined the term *pathopharmacodynamics* to distinguish the difference between this alteration in drug response caused by the production of an experimental disease state from the more common situation where an administered drug modifies the disease state. Morton and Chatfield (1970) reported that the *in vitro* hepatic microsomal *N*-demethylation of *d*-propoxyphene and the levels of microsomal cytochrome P-450 were progressively reduced between 3 and 16 days following injection of adjuvant, reaching approximately 16% of control values by day 16. Injection of the tubercle bacilli in saline solution caused a depression of hepatic enzyme activity of lesser severity and duration. No decrease in hepatic activity was seen if the adjuvant was injected into rat cervical lymph nodes, a route of injection that does not induce AIP, but will cause delayed hypersensitivity to tuberculin. These investigators also showed that the *in vivo* metabolism of acetaminophen was significantly reduced, and that impaired metabolism of phenobarbital was also evident by an increased toxicity of the barbiturate. Adjuvant-induced alterations in the metabolism and/or toxicity of acetylsalicylic acid, phenylbutazone, and indomethacin have also been reported (Perrey *et al.*, 1976; Sofia, 1977). In contrast, Grindel *et al.* (1982) reported an increase in the hepatic clearance, the renal clearance, and the volume of distribution of tolmetin in AIP rats.

A relative dissociation between the occurrence of the AIP disease state and the hepatic dysfunction was demonstrated in a series of studies using arthritogenic and nonarthritogenic, "dummy," adjuvants, as well as use of strains of rats not susceptible to the induction of AIP (Whitehouse, 1973; Whitehouse and Beck, 1973; Beck and Whitehouse, 1973, 1974). Injection of a suspension of *M. tuberculosis* in mineral oil or in saturated normal hydrocarbons containing 12 or more carbon atoms (arthritogenic adjuvants) induces arthritis whereas use of short-chain hydrocarbons or polyunsaturated long-chain hydrocarbons as the vehicles for the *mycobacteria* does not (nonarthritogenic adjuvants) (Whitehouse, 1973). However, considerable prolongation of hexobarbital-induced sleep-time was seen 48 hr after inoculation of animals with either the arthritogenic or the nonarthritogenic adjuvant. Although treatment of animals with either type of adjuvant decreased drug metabolism *in vivo* and *in vitro*, the impairment was more persistent in animals receiving the arthritogenic adjuvants. Beck and Whitehouse (1973) reported that the Buffalo rat, which develops minimal AIP in response to arthritogenic adjuvants, displayed significant changes in drug-metabolizing enzyme activity following adjuvant inoculation. It was further observed that the decrease in hepatic drug-metabolizing activity was apparent within 24 hr after injection whereas adjuvant disease was more protracted in its development (Beck and Whitehouse, 1973; Cawthorne *et al.*, 1976).

In contrast to the impairment of microsomal drug oxidation reactions, it has been reported that administration of Freund's complete adjuvant increases the N-acetylation of sulphadimidine in rats and rabbits (Zidek *et al.*, 1977; du Souich and Courteau, 1981; Zidek and Janku, 1981) and the activity of hepatic alcohol dehydrogenase (Ciaccio and Barbieri, 1979). It has been suggested that the RES represents the main site of drug acetylation (Govier, 1965; Ziedek *et al.*, 1977; Notter and Roland, 1978). Thus, the difference between the effect of adjuvant on oxidation versus acetylation may be related to the different cellular localization of the metabolic reactions. On the other hand, alcohol dehydrogenase is a soluble enzyme located in the cytosol of the hepatocyte (Ciaccio and Barbieri, 1979). Thus, the differential effects on soluble (alcohol dehydrogenase) versus membrane-bound (cytochrome P-450) enzyme activity would tend to indicate that the effect of Freund's adjuvant is not as a general hepatotoxin, and that the alterations in hepatic drug biotransformation reactions represent specific responses to unknown stimuli.

Initial concern for the effects of Freund's adjuvant to depress monooxygenase activity was directed toward the implication of altered pharmacokinetics in pharmaceutical drug development, particularly with respect to antiinflammatory agents. However, with the development of the potential use of bacterial adjuvants as immunomodulators in conjunction with cancer chemotherapeutic agents, a new and clinically relevant implication emerged.

Farquhar *et al.* (1976) emphasized the possible importance of adjuvant-induced impairment of drug-metabolizing activity to the efficacy and toxicity of agents utilized during cancer chemoimmunotherapy. They showed that administration of Bacillus Calmette Guérin (BCG), one of the most extensively investigated immunoadjuvants, caused a sex-related, time-dependent impairment of the rat hepatic microsomal drug-metabolizing enzyme system without the concomitant development of AIP. The effect was greatest in female rats and persisted for as long as 14 days. Intravenous injection of BCG was the most effective route of administration; subcutaneous injection produced erratic responses, and intradermal injection had no perceptible effect on the microsomal drug oxidation system. However, Ruzicka *et al.* (1980) reported that intracutaneous BCG injections in weekly intervals for 4 weeks significantly depressed arylhydrocarbon hydroxylase activity, and *O*-dealkylation of 7-ethoxycoumarin. Interestingly, both Farquhar *et al.* (1976) and Ruzicka *et al.* (1980) noted that levels of cytochrome P-450 did not closely correlate with the alterations in enzyme activities.

Injection of whole *Mycobacterium* organisms apparently is not necessary to produce the decrease in hepatic microsomal drug-oxidation. Beck and Whitehouse (1973) reported that the administration of purified BCG-cell wall skeleton (BCG-CWS) into the footpads of rats, but not mice, decreased the metabolism of cyclophosphamide. In contrast, Hojo and Hashimoto (1977) observed a decrease in aniline hydroxylase and aminopyrine *N*-demethylase activity in microsomal preparations obtained 24 hr after mice were injected intraperitoneally with BCG-CWS twice at 6-hr intervals. The difference between the results obtained in these two investigations appears to be the route of administration. Recent studies (Williams and Szentivanyi, 1982a, 1983a) have shown that intraperitoneal administration of a saline solution of muramyl dipeptide (MDP), the smallest peptidoglycan fragment of the mycobacterial cell wall shown to possess adjuvant activity (Adams *et al.*, 1981), is also effective in decreasing hepatic microsomal drug-metabolizing activity. In the mouse, a significant decrease in 7-ethoxycoumarin *O*-deethylase, but not aniline hydroxylase activity, was seen at MDP doses of 1 and 10 mg/kg. In rats, aniline hydroxylase activity was also decreased, and this species appeared more susceptible to the effect of MDP to decrease 7-ethoxycoumarin *O*-deethylase activity. In both species, the level of cytochrome P-450 was decreased by a dose of 10 mg/kg, but not 1 mg/kg. Williams and Szentivanyi (1983a) also reported that mice injected for 3 days with 10 mg/kg MDP did not have a significant decrease in cytochrome P-450, but 7-ethoxycoumarin *O*-deethylase activity was approximately 30% of control values. This lack of correlation between the effect of MDP on cytochrome P-450 levels and loss of enzyme activity is similar to observations noted above in studies using BCG (Farquhar *et al.*, 1976; Ruzicka *et al.*, 1980). In contrast to these observations, Zidek *et al.* (1983) reported that rats receiving subcutaneous injection of MDP for 21 days did not show any significant loss of drug-oxidation activities.

The mechanism involved in the loss of drug-oxidation activity following administration of mycobacteria or their cellular products has not been extensively investigated. Some investigators have suggested that the effect may be an adaptive alteration of the hepatocyte priorities due to the increased hepatic synthesis of acute-phase proteins elicited by the inflammatory condition. Others implicate the ability of these bacterial agents to induce interferon (IFN), a topic discussed below in Section 7. The possible participation of the RES in the response is suggested by a recent preliminary report of Ishizuki *et al.* (1983). They reported that hepatic nonparenchymal cells isolated from rats injected with Freund's complete adjuvant and then incubated with hepatocytes isolated from a control animal caused a significant decrease in the metabolism of aminopyrine by the control hepatocytes, suggesting the possible involvement of a mediator substance of unknown nature derived from the nonparenchymal cells of the adjuvant-treated animals.

4. *CORYNEBACTERIUM PARVUM*

Analogous with the observations following administration of mycobacteria, initial reports that *Corynebacterium parvum* (CP) vaccine modified hepatic drug-oxidation reactions dealt with the abnormal sensitivity of the CP-treated animals to barbiturate anesthesia (Castro, 1974; Mosedale and Smith, 1975). Subsequently, Soyka *et al.* (1976) showed that from 1 to 14 days following CP treatment (350 μg/mouse) the specific activities of hepatic microsomal *N*-demethylase, aniline hydroxylase, and *p*-nitroanisole *O*-demethylase activities were significantly decreased. The decrease in enzyme activities paralleled the development of hepatosplenomegaly in the CP-treated animals. A clear dose-dependent relationship was not observed, but as little as 22 μg of CP per mouse was shown to significantly decrease each of the above enzyme activities. Schroeder *et al.* (1976) observed a 90% decrease in ethylmorphine *N*-demethylase activity and a 75% reduction in the level of cytochrome P-450 6 days after intravenous administration of 35 mg/kg (200 mg/m^2) CP to rats. However, intravenous injection of 35 mg/m^2 was without effect on any of the above parameters. On the other hand, Macnee and Nimmo-Smith (1978) found that intraperitoneal administration of 35 mg/m^2 to mice did cause a significant decrease in the rate of *O*-demethylation of *p*-nitroanisole, and the level of cytochrome P-450. Besides the difference in the species of animals and the route of administration, these two studies also differ with respect to the time after administration at which the enzyme activities were assessed. Schroeder *et al.* (1976) assayed for enzyme activity at 6 days whereas Macnee and Nimmo-Smith (1978) determined that maximal effect was not seen until 11 days after CP treatment. Macnee and Nimmo-Smith also noted that different strains of mice may show differing responses to the effect of CP on hepatic drug metabolism. Mullen (1981) showed that, although a decrease in murine hepatic cytochrome P-450 was observed in animals sacrificed 7 days after CP, no effect on the *in vivo* pharmacokinetic parameter of phenytoin could be demonstrated. These studies exemplify the present difficulties in evaluating various reports of the effects of immunomodulators on the hepatic monooxygenase system in that variables, such as species, dose, route of administration, time after administration, as well as other aspects of experimental protocol, differ significantly in the various reports and have not been extensively or critically examined.

Involvement of the RES in the manifestation of the effect of CP to decrease hepatic microsomal mixed-function oxidase activity has been suggested (Soyka et al., 1979; Soyka, 1981). Various procedures, such as silica injection, splenectomy, and whole-body uv irradiation (WBI), known to modify macrophage function, abrogated the effects of CP to decrease drug metabolism activity. The effectiveness of these techniques was critically dependent on the treatment schedule employed. Thus, splenectomy or silica injection was effective only if performed prior to CP administration. On the other hand, WBI only blocked the effect of CP on enzyme activity if performed concurrently or 2 hr after CP administration.

5. BORDETELLA PERTUSSIS

Bordetella pertussis (BP) vaccination depresses hepatic microsomal drug metabolism and cytochrome P-450 in both mice and rats (Williams and Szentivanyi, 1975, 1977; Renton and Mannering, 1976b). Inoculation of female mice with 7×10^9 killed BP organisms/mouse caused a significant loss in aniline hydroxylase activity, aminopyrine and ethylmorphine N-demethylase activity, and the level of cytochrome P-450 as determined 5 days after vaccination. The onset and duration of the loss of hepatic drug-metabolizing activity after BP injection were shown to parallel the development of histamine hypersensitivity, a well-characterized effect of BP vaccination in susceptible animals (Williams et al., 1977, 1980a; Szentivanyi and Williams, 1980). The decrease in drug-metabolizing activity and the increased histamine hypersensitivity were evident 24 hr after BP administration and persisted for at least 15 days. Renton (1979) observed that rats pretreated for 24 hr with BP vaccine showed depressed hepatic microsomal phenytoin hydroxylase activity and cytochrome P-450 levels.

The development of hypersensitivity to histamine in animals receiving BP has previously been associated with a heat-lable constitutent of the bacterial cell wall, the so-called histamine-sensitizing factor (HSF) (Munoz, 1963; Munoz and Bergman, 1968). Several lines of investigation indicate that HSF may be identical to the protective antigen and the leukocytosis-promoting factor also obtained from BP (Szentivanyi and Williams, 1980, Wardlaw and Parton, 1983). In a series of experiments, Williams et al. (1980a) demonstrated that the effect of BP to depress cytochrome P-450-dependent reactions was possibly attributable to two separate components of the BP organism. One was heat stable and the other heat labile. Injection of vaccine that had been heated at 80°C for 0.5 hr caused a decrease in drug-oxidation activity within 24 hr, but the activities returned to control values within 3 days. This effect of the heat-treated vaccine was shown to be similar to that seen after injection of E. coli endotoxin, suggesting that the heat-stable component of BP responsible for decreasing drug-metabolizing activity was the lipopolysaccharide (LPS) component. The protracted (15 days) effect of BP vaccine on hepatic drug metabolism was ablated by the heat treatment, but was shown not to be due to heat-labile HSF in that administration of partially purified HSF failed to affect any of the mixed-function oxidase activities, but did cause histamine sensitization. At present the identity of the heat-labile component involved in depressing cytochrome P-450-dependent activities is unknown. In other studies, Williams *et al.* (1981) also demonstrated that the effect of BP to decrease microsomal drug-metabolizing activity was not ablated by splenectomy, in contrast to the effect of splenectomy to block the effect of CP (Soyka *et al.*, 1979). On the other hand, BP vaccine did not produce a sustained depression of aniline hydroxylase, or ethylmorphine *N*-demethylase activity when injected into athymic, nude mice (Williams *et al.*, 1981). An initial (24 hr) depression was observed, but the enzyme activity was equivalent to the control value at 7 days. These results suggest that the initial short-lived decrease is probably due to the endotoxin component of BP vaccine, whereas the second more protracted depression may involve a T-cell-dependent effect of this gram-negative organism.

6. BACTERIAL LIPOPOLYSACCHARIDE

Of all the RES-active agents, the one perhaps most extensively investigated is the LPS (endotoxin) component of the gram-negative bacterial cell wall. Table 2 lists some of the myriad of effects elicited by LPS injection into the rabbit, dog, mouse, rat, man, and other endotoxin-sensitive species. The chemistry, immunochemistry, and biological activity of LPS have recently been reviewed (Bradley, 1979; Luderitz *et al.*, 1982; Westphal *et al.*, 1983). It is now appreciated that practically all of the endotoxic properties of LPS reside in the lipid A component. This fact needs to be stressed because in the studies to be discussed the dosages of LPS used were generally calculated on a dry weight basis. Thus, some of the apparent differences between various studies may be due to use of preparations that differ in lipid A content. Other factors that may explain apparent discrepancies in the various studies are use of LPS obtained by different extraction procedures (e.g., Boivin or Westphal), route of administration, and doses employed. In many cases, comparison between studies is difficult because dosage is not expressed on a body weight basis, but simply as amount per animal.

TABLE 2. ENDOTOXIC REACTIONS ELICITED BY LPS

Pyrogenicity	Macrophage activation
Lethal toxicity in mice	Induction of colony-stimulating factor
Local Shwartzman reaction	Induction of prostaglandin synthesis
Complement activation	Induction of interferon production
Platelet aggregation	Induction of tumor-necrotizing factor
Toxicity enhanced by BCG	Induction of mouse liver pyruvate kinase
Toxicity enhanced by adrenalectomy	Induction of hepatic heme oxygenase activity
Enhanced dermal reactivity to epinephrine	Inhibition of hepatic phosphoenolpyruvate carboxykinase
Induction of nonspecific resistance to infection	Inhibition of hepatic mixed-function oxidase activity
Induction of tolerance to endotoxin	
Adjuvant activity	Inhibition of glucocorticoid induction of tryptophan oxygenase
Mitogenic activity for cells	
Tumor necrotic activity	

Utili *et al.* (1977) reviewed many of the alterations in hepatic function observed following the administration of LPS. These authors stressed that the liver
appears to be an organ at great risk to the endotoxic effects of LPS. In addition, it
has been emphasized that endotoxins of intestinal origin may be important in
the pathogenesis of liver disease (Nolan, 1975, 1979; Liehr and Grun, 1979).

Alterations in drug pharmacokinetics and pharmacodynamics have been
reported to occur following the administration of LPS to experimental animals.
Ladefoged (1978) reported that a significant alteration in the pharmacokinetics of
warfarin was seen in rabbits, but not in pigs, injected 1 hr after at a relatively high
dose (0.5 μg/kg body wt) of endotoxin. A significant increase in the apparent
volume of warfarin distribution and a decreased elimination of the anticoagulant
were observed. However, it was not possible to conclude whether the altered
elimination was due to decreased warfarin metabolism, or secondary to the
hemodynamic alterations accompanying the endotoxic response. Ritschel *et al.*
(1982) observed proportional increases in both the volume of coumarin distribution and the $t_\frac{1}{2}$ in rabbits; total body clearance was consequently unchanged. LPS
has also been shown to enhance the pharmacokinetics and lethality of a number
of antineoplastic agents (Marecki and Bradley, 1973; Marecki *et al.*, 1975; Lu *et al.*,
1981; Sasaki *et al.*, 1982), the toxicity of Δ^9-tetrahydrocannabinol (Martin *et al.*,
1978; Munson *et al.*, 1978), and to alter the pharmacokinetics of a sulfadimidine
(Lapka *et al.*, 1980) and chloroquine (Osifo, 1980). Floersheim and Szeszak (1971)
noted the prolongation of hexobarbital sleep-time following LPS administration
to mice.

Vainio (1973) reported that in rats given a lethal dose (100 mg/kg) of endotoxin there was a progressive decrease over a 6-hr period in the hepatic microsomal drug-metabolizing activity. Gorodischer *et al.* (1976) showed that, at a
dose of 1 mg/kg of *E. coli* endotoxin, limited hepatic pathological abnormalities
(e.g., necrosis, fatty infiltration, or inflammation) were present, but a significant
decrease was seen in microsomal aniline hydroxylase activity, benzpyrene hydroxylase activity, and the level of cytochrome P-450.

The onset, intensity, and duration of the loss of hepatic microsomal drug-
metabolizing activity appear to be dose related and may correlate with the lipid
A content of the LPS preparation. Bissell and Hammaker (1976a,b) found a 30%
loss of cytochrome P-450 in rats injected with 1.5 mg/kg of *S. typhimurium*
endoxtoxin at 9 hr after injection. Williams and Szentivanyi (1983b), using *E. coli*
O26:B6 LPS at a dose of 2 mg/kg, did not find any significant effect at 12 hr
postinjection, but by 24 hr the cytochrome P-450 level was decreased to 40% of
control values. Abernathy *et al.* (1980b) showed a dose-and time-dependent
effect of endotoxin on hexobarbital sleep-time and zoxazolamine paralysis time.
These investigators also showed that two preparations of LPS from *E. coli*
O127:B8 with different lipid A content (Boivin, 15.5%; Westphal, 8.74%), when
compared on a dry weight basis, caused markedly different prolongation of
hexobarbital sleep-time, the Boivin preparation being more active than the Westphal extracted material. However, when dosage was adjusted for lipid A content, the two preparations gave equivalent results. Kasai (1976) and Egawa and
Kasai (1979) reported that intraperitoneal injection of 2–20 μg of the endotoxin

glycolipid from the *S. minnesota* Re mutant caused a marked depression of hepatic microsomal aminopyrine *N*-demethylase activity. This preparation lacks the *O*-specific polysaccharide portion of the endotoxin molecule, but retains the lipid A moiety linked to the core oligosaccharide. Egawa and Kasai (1979) and Yoshida *et al.* (1982) examined five of the degradation products of endotoxin obtained by either alkaline or acidic hydrolysis for their effects on hepatic microsomal drug-metabolizing activity. Lipid A obtained after mild acetic acid hydrolysis of the glycolipid was the most active. Alkali-extracted lipid A and the polysaccharide portion of the endotoxin were inactive. These results suggest that the intact lipid A moiety is required for the effect on hepatic mixed-function oxidase activity.

It is well known that exposure of animals to low doses of endotoxin for a period of a few days leads to the establishment of a refractory state, known as endotoxin tolerance, during which the animal is protected from many of the biological and lethal effects of LPS. In addition, certain strains of mice have been shown to be genetically unresponsive to most of the biological activities of endotoxin. The effect of LPS to affect hepatic cytochrome P-450-dependent activities has been examined in these LPS-tolerant and unresponsive animals (Abernathy *et al.*, 1980a; Williams *et al.*, 1980b; Williams and Szentivanyi, 1982b, 1983c). Abernathy *et al.* (1980a) observed that both acute doses of endotoxin and induction of endotoxin tolerance prolonged hexobarbital sleep-time and zoxazolamine paralysis time in mice, indicating a decreased rate of *in vivo* metabolism of these two agents. However, the decreased rate of drug-metabolizing activity was greater in animals receiving the acute dose than in those made tolerant to LPS. In addition, an acute challenge dose of LPS to the tolerant animals did not cause any additional prolongation of hexobarbital sleep-time beyond that noted in the endotoxin-tolerant mice given no acute LPS. Williams and Szentivanyi (1982b, 1983c) examined the microsomal drug-metabolizing activity and heme oxygenase activity in rats and mice rendered tolerant to LPS. LPS tolerance was produced by the dosing schedule of Nolan and Ali (1973) and the animals were challenged with an acute dose of endotoxin 2 days later. Aniline hydroxylase activity and heme oxygenase activity in the LPS-tolerant animals were not significantly different from the activity of control animals and were not significantly affected by acute challenge with endotoxin. Cytochrome P-450 and ethylmorphine *N*-demethylase activity were significantly lower in the microsomal preparations obtained from the LPS-tolerant animals than for the control preparations. Following an acute dose of endotoxin to the LPS-tolerant animals, cytochrome P-450 levels and ethylmorphine *N*-demethylase activity decreased an additional amount, but the enzyme activities in LPS-tolerant animals were not decreased to as great an extent as those of control animals given the acute dose. These results suggest that animals can be made at least partially tolerant to the effects of LPS to decrease hepatic drug-metabolizing activity. The reason for the difference between the effects of LPS challenge to tolerant animals on aniline hydroxylase activity and ethylmorphine activity is presently unknown, but may be related to possible effects of LPS to decrease different species of cytochrome P-450 involved in catalyzing the metabolism of these two substrates. In contrast to the preceding, Williams *et al.* (1980b) reported that injection of *E. coli* endotoxin into C3H/HeJ mice, a mouse strain reportedly tolerant to most of the biological effects of LPS, caused decreases in microsomal drug-metabolizing activity equivalent to that seen in the LPS-responsive C3H/HeN mouse strain. It is now appreciated that the unresponsiveness of the C3H/HeJ mice to LPS may be limited to certain biological parameters as well as to certain LPS preparations. Thus, the observations of Williams *et al.* (1980b) may simply reflect a biological effect of LPS in which the C3H/HeJ mice do not differ from other strains of mice.

Although it is apparent from the above-reported studies that LPS administration causes a marked alteration in the pharmacokinetics of drug elimination, the mechanism by which the effect is elicited is less well understood. Two issues are of interest in this regard. First is the question whether the effects of LPS on microsomal drug-metabolizing activity are the result of direct interaction of LPS with the hepatic parenchymal cell, or whether these metabolic changes are mediated by products released from other cell types, particularly macrophages, during endotoxemia. It is well known that following LPS injection a considerable array of soluble mediators, including catecholamines, histamine, prostaglandins, as well as products of RES origin, are released *in vivo* into the circulation. Second, the cellular perturbations responsible for the loss of cytochrome P-450 and the related enzyme activities need to be elucidated.

Recent studies have indicated that both the hepatic parenchymal cell as well as the Kupffer cell may be involved in the binding and uptake of LPS (Zlydaszyk and Moon, 1976; Ramadori *et al.*, 1979; Mathison and Ulevitch, 1979; Ruiter *et al.*, 1981; Maitra *et al.*, 1981; Munford *et al.*, 1981; Freudenberg *et al.*, 1982). However, a number of investigations have failed to observe any significant effect of the *in vitro* addition of LPS on the enzyme activity of isolated hepatic parenchymal cells. Thus, liver gluconeogenic and glycogenolytic activities and the glucocorticoid induction of hepatic phosphoenolpyruvate carboxykinase (PEPCK) and tryptophan oxygenase (TO) activities, shown to be markedly affected after the *in vivo* administration of LPS, were unaffected by the *in vitro* addition of LPS to isolated hepatocytes (Filkins and Cornell, 1974; Filkins and Buchanan, 1977; Lowitt *et al.*, 1978, 1979, 1981; McCallum, 1980). Indeed, a primary role for interaction of endotoxin with cells of the RES in eliciting effects in hepatic parenchymal cells was presented by McCallum (1980) and Lowitt *et al.* (1978, 1979, 1981). These studies suggested that the incubation of LPS with preparations of hepatic nonparenchymal cells, for the most part Kupffer cells, resulted in the elaboration of a substance that altered parenchymal cell PEPCK activities (McCallum, 1980) and blocked the induction of TO by dexamethasone (Lowitt *et al.*, 1981). At the present time, a similar involvement of the hepatic nonparenchymal RES cellular fraction in the effect of LPS on hepatic parenchymal drug-metabolizing cell activity is unresolved, but incubation of isolated rat hepatocytes with LPS for as long as 8 hr has been shown not to alter the rate of aniline hydroxylase activity or cytochrome P-450 levels (Williams, unpublished observations).

In vivo evidence for the LPS production of soluble mediator(s) being involved in the decrease in hepatic parenchymal cell mixed-function oxidase activity has been presented (Egawa *et al.*, 1981). Serum derived from lipid A-treated mice when injected into control mice was effective in decreasing cytochrome P-450 levels. The highest activity was found in the serum taken from animals 9 hr after LPS injection. The factor was shown to be stable to heating at 56°C for 30 min, and was considered not to be endotoxin itself or endotoxin-induced IFN (*vid infra*). The identity of this serum factor is unknown, but may be distinct from other LPS-induced mediators, such as glucocorticoid-antagonizing factor, colony-stimulating factor, and tumor-necrosis factor. Studies by Williams and Szentivanyi (1982b, 1983b) also appear to rule out the involvement of catecholamines and prostaglandins. Pretreatment of rats with either α- or β-adrenergic antagonists or with indomethacin, an inhibitor of prostaglandin biosynthesis, did not alter the effect of LPS to decrease cytochrome P-450, aniline hydroxylase activity, and ethylmorphine N-demethylase activity. Interestingly, in the same study the administation of α-adrenergic blockers, such as phenoxybenzamine and phentolamine, prevented the LPS inhibition of the glucocorticoid induction of hepatic TO activity. Bloksma *et al.* (1982) have reported that α-adrenoceptor blocking agents prevent the endotoxin-induced release of tumor-necrosis factor and heat-labile IFN. Thus, the participation of these mediators in the *in vivo* response of LPS to decrease drug-metabolizing activity seems questionable. Preliminary evidence (Williams and Szentivanyi, 1983c) for a macrophage-derived mediator in the effect of endotoxin has been obtained using murine peritoneal macrophages cultured *in vitro* in the presence of LPS. Culture medium from macrophages exposed for 24 hr to 50 μg/ml of LPS when injected to LPS-tolerant mice caused a decrease in aniline hydroxylase activity and cytochrome P-450 level. Injection of medium from macrophages not exposed to endotoxin, but to which LPS was added in an equivalent concentration, was ineffective. Additional experiments are necessary to further characterize this response.

The intracellular alteration elicited by LPS or its mediator(s) appears to involve perturbations in cellular heme and possibly protein metabolism. Gemsa *et al.* (1974) reported that microsomal heme oxygenase activity, the rate-limiting step in heme catabolism, was induced following endotoxin administration. Bissell and Hammaker (1976a,b) showed that the increase in heme oxygenase activity was correlated with the effect of endotoxin to affect the degradation of cytochrome P-450. These workers also showed that endotoxin prevented the allylisopropylacetamide (AIA) induction of δ-aminolevulinic acid (ALA) synthetase, the rate-limiting step in heme biosynthesis. Endotoxin was also shown to cause a 25% decrease in basal ALA synthetase activity and an increase in the heme saturation of hepatic TO (Bissell and Hammaker, 1977). These results are compatible with the hypothesis (Bissell and Hammaker, 1976a,b) that endotoxin causes a dissociation of heme from holocytochrome P-450. The suppression of ALA synthetase, increased heme saturation of TO, and induction of heme oxygenase are the consequence of an increase in the heme concentration in a "free heme" regulatory pool. Williams *et al.* (1979) demonstrated that animals treated with endotoxin and phenobarbital, a known inducer of cytochrome P-450, had significantly less hemoprotein levels than animals receiving the barbiturate alone. It was considered possible that endotoxin might have blocked heme biosynthesis through inhibition of ALA synthetase activity, as shown by Bissell and Hammaker (1976a,b), but not the synthesis of the apoprotein moiety. Correia and Meyer (1975) previously showed that after the concurrent administration of phenobarbital and cobalt, an inhibitor of heme synthesis, the synthesis of the apoprotein moiety induced by phenobarbital could be demonstrated by *in vitro* reconstitution with exogenous heme, yielding holocytochrome P-450. Williams *et al.* (1979), however, could not find any reconstitutable P-450 in animals treated with LPS or with LPS and phenobarbital. Thus, endotoxin may also inhibit the synthesis of the apoprotein or in other ways prevent its ability to bind heme.

7. INTERFERON INDUCERS AND INTERFERON

IFN was discovered in 1957 (Isaacs and Lindenmann, 1957) and has been widely studied for its antiviral activity. Recent reviews of various aspects of IFN production, chemistry, and pharmacokinetics have appeared (Johnson and Baron, 1977; Bocci, 1981; Pollard, 1982, De Maeyer and De Maeyer-Guignard, 1982; Burke, 1982).

Kato *et al.* (1963) were the first to report the alteration of hepatic microsomal drug-metabolizing activity following infection of mice with murine hepatitis virus. An initial increase in the *in vitro* microsomal metabolism of hexobarbital and strychnine was seen 12 hr after infection, but a marked depression of enzyme activity occurred between 48 and 60 hr. They also reported that viral infection potentiated the effect of phenobarbital to induce hexobarbital metabolism. Similar effects of viral infections to alter microsomal drug-oxidation activity have been shown by others (Buynitzky *et al.*, 1977, 1978; Renton, 1981a,b).

Pyran copolymer and poly (rI:rC), both inducers of IFN, were shown to decrease liver microsomal enzyme activity by Morahan *et al.* (1972). A review of the effects of pyran copolymers on hepatic microsomal mixed-function oxidases has recently been published (Barnes, 1980). Renton and Mannering (1976a) and Leeson *et al.* (1976) demonstrated that tilorone, an antiviral agent thought to produce its effect by inducing IFN, also depressed the hepatic cytochrome P-450-dependent monooxygenase system. Subsequently, Renton and Mannering (1976b) examined 12 IFN-inducing agents for their effect to depress cytochrome P-450, ethylmorphine *N*-demethylase activity, and aniline hydroxylase activity. Included were BP, endotoxin, and poly(rI:rC), agents previously shown (*vide supra*) to elicit this response, as well as statalon, quinacrine, Mengo virus, and several other agents. All possessed to varying degrees the ability to suppress the mixed-function oxidase activities and cytochrome P-450 levels. On the other hand, injection of poly(rI) or poly(rC), which do not induce IFN when injected separately, did not depress the microsomal activities. Interestingly, Deloria and Mannering (1982) have reported that if administration of poly(rI) is followed shortly by poly(rC) injection, a depression of the cytochrome P-450 system does occur. The sequential administration of these single-stranded polyribonucleotides has also been shown to result in antiviral activity and increased IFN titers (DeClercq and DeSomer, 1972; Deloria and Mannering, 1982).

Renton and Mannering (1976b) suggested that the alteration in drug-metabolizing enzyme activity may be a general property of all IFN-inducing agents. This proposal has been widely accepted. However, some caution is warranted in using this effect of IFN-inducing agents to implicate IFN *per se*. Barnes *et al.* (1979) and Barnes (1980) noted that whereas pyran copolymers possess considerable antiviral activity, they are weak inducers of IFN. Mannering *et al.* (1980) also remark that although endotoxin is not a very good inducer of IFN, it is a potent depressor of the P-450 systems. Parkinson *et al.* (1982) suggested that the rapid loss of injected IFN from serum relative to the rate of decrease in drug-metabolizing activity may indicate an indirect mechanism of action. Indeed, Renton *et al.* (1978) observed that the addition of poly(rI:rC) or a crude mouse IFN preparation to cultures of mouse hepatocytes resulted in the induction of the cytochrome P-450-dependent monooxygenase system rather than depression of enzyme activity as is seen after *in vivo* administration. Also, Nebert and Friedman (1973) showed that IFN pretreatment of fetal mouse or rat liver cultures resulted in enhanced induction of arylhydrocarbon hydroxylase activity by subsequent exposure to benzanthrane.

Strains of mice that differ genetically in their responsiveness to induction of IFN levels elicited by Newcastle disease virus (NDV) have been used to examine whether IFN titers might be correlated with decreased drug-oxidation activity (Renton, 1981a,b; Singh and Renton, 1981). Animals that posses the high-production allele responded to NDV injection with high circulating IFN titers and a depressed hepatic cytochrome P-450 level and decreased aminopyrine N-demethylase activity. Animals possessing the low-production allele showed no significant effect on NDV injection to either increase IFN levels or decrease mixed-function oxidase activity.

Initial attempts to elicit a decrease in hepatic drug-metabolizing enzyme activity by passive transfer of IFN-containing serum obtained from animals treated with IFN inducers were unsuccessful (Renton and Mannering, 1976a; Renton, 1981b; Singh and Renton, 1981). However, Singh *et al.* (1982) reported that passive transfer of a crude murine IFN-α/β preparation will cause the loss of cytochrome P-450 levels and drug biotransformation activity. Passive transfer of IFN-γ has been shown to significantly decrease cytochrome P-450 and drug-metabolizing levels in microsomal preparations and, in addition, to alter the *in vivo* pharmacokinetics of pharmacological agents (Sonnenfeld *et al.*, 1980; Harned *et al.*, 1982; Smith *et al.*, 1983; Sonnenfield, 1983). Singh *et al.* (1982) and Parkinson *et al.* (1982) have shown that highly purified recombinant human leukocyte IFN when injected into mice caused a decrease in drug-metabolizing activity that correlated with the antiviral activity of the IFN preparation.

Although it appears that depression of hepatic drug-metabolizing activity can be elicited by IFN and IFN inducers, some comparative differences have been noted with respect to the response elicited with specific agents. Alterations in heme catabolism have been shown (el Azhary and Mannering, 1979; el Azhary *et al.*, 1980; Mannering *et al.*, 1980) as discussed in Section 6. Zerkle *et al.* (1980)

reported that quantitative as well as qualitiative differences in the multiple species of cytochrome P-450 proteins, separated on polyacrylamide gels, are found for microsomal preparations obtained from rats given tilorone, poly(rI:rC), or Freund's complete adjuvant. Tilorone did not decrease any of the six separated cytochrome P-450 hemoproteins, poly(rI:rC) decreased three, and Freund's adjuvant decreased another of the molecular weight species distinct from those affected by poly(rI:rC). Thus, although both tilorone and poly(rI:rC) may increase heme turnover (el Azhary *et al.*, 1980), only poly(rI:rC) appears to affect the hemoprotein level, and this effect is specific for certain of the cytochrome P-450 apoprotein species (Zerkle *et al.*, 1980). At present it is unknown whether decreased synthesis or increased degradation of the specific P-450 apoproteins is affected by this inducing agent.

As discussed previously, the role of the RES in the mechanism of action of the various immunoregulators was suggested by the observations of Soyka *et al.* (1979) using CP. Giampietri *et al.* (1981) examined whether interference with the RES in ways shown to block the CP-induced depression of hepatic mixed-function oxidase activity would attenuate the effect of pyran copolymer. However, neither injection of silica nor WBI was effective in preventing the pyran-induced depression of monooxygenase activity. These authors suggested that interaction of pyran and CP with the host immune system need not involve the same processes. Thus, uptake and processing by the RES may be essential for CP, but not for pyran. It should also be recalled that Williams *et al.* (1980b, 1981) demonstrated that splenectomy, another procedure shown to block the effect of CP, did not block the effect of BP, nor was the effect of endotoxin altered in C3H/HeJ mice whose RES is known to be unresponsive to lipopolysaccharides. Thus, it would appear that the apparently similar effects of the various immunomodulators to decrease hepatic monooxygenase activity may result from a very complex phenomenon and that the common modality, if any, is yet to be discovered.

8.   CLINICAL OBSERVATIONS

Pharmacokinetic evaluation of phenytoin and antipyrine has been reported for humans receiving immunotherapy with CP or BCG (Rios *et al.*, 1977; Mullen *et al.*, 1978; Wan *et al.*, 1979; Hamilton *et al.*, 1980). Mullen *et al.* (1978) could not demonstrate a significant alteration in the disposition kinetics of phenytoin in a group of patients who had received five "multiple puncture gun" injections of BCG in each limb or in a group of patients administered 2 mg/m^2 of CP by intravenous infusion over a 3-hr interval. Phenytoin pharmacokinetic parameters were determined in both sets of patients before and 10 days after immunotherapy. In contrast, Rios *et al.* (1977) noted an increase in the antipyrine elimination half-time 5–7 days after patients had received the same dose of CP daily for 10 days. Hamilton *et al.* (1980) reported antipyrine pharmacokinetics to be unaffected by CP pretreatment of patients.

Obviously, the differences in the results of the above studies may be due to certain factors such as the duration of immunotherapy, different pharmacological test substances, etc. It should also be noted that the cancer patients in the study of Wan *et al.* (1979) had significantly lower phenytoin kinetic values than healthy volunteer subjects, suggesting the decrease due to the disease state might have prevented detection of a decrease due to the immunotherapeutic regimen. It is not known whether a similar effect of metastatic disease was observed in the studies using antipyrine.

Effects of influenza vaccination on the *in vivo* disposition of theophylline and aminopyrine by man have been reported by Renton *et al.* (1980) and Kramer and McClain (1981). Renton *et al.* (1980) reported an increase in theophylline half-time from a mean prevaccine value of 3.3 hr to a 24-hr postvaccine value of 7.3 hr; no significant alteration in theophylline apparent volume of distribution was observed. Kramer and McClain (1981) reported a prolonged effect of influenza vaccination on aminopyrine metabolism. A significant decrease in metabolic activity in the vaccinated group occurred between 2 and 7 days post-injection, and was still partially depressed at 21 days. Chang *et al.* (1978) also reported an alteration in the elimination of theophylline occurring during the clinical presence of upper respiratory viral infections in pediatric patients.

9. SUMMARY

At the present time, a unified statement regarding the relative effect of the various immunomodulating agents on drug pharmacokinetics and pharmacodynamics cannot be presented. There appears to be no question that administration of the various agents to experimental animals does result in a decrease in the level of cytochrome P-450 and the associated drug-metabolizing enzyme activities, at least as determined *in vitro* with microsomal preparations. However, there appears to be a question as to what degree this will alter *in vivo* drug pharmacokinetics. In this regard, the study by Mullen (1981) wherein mice given BCG were shown to have normal pharmacokinetic handling of phenytoin despite significantly lower microsomal cytochrome P-450 levels is particularly pertinent. Also pertinent are the observations of Grindel *et al.* (1982), who showed that in rats with AIP the pharmacokinetic evaluation of tolmetin disposition suggested an increase in hepatic clearance, and by inference increased hepatic drug oxidation, at a time when microsomal drug-oxidation activity has previously been shown to be significantly impaired. On the other hand, there are numerous studies documenting altered pharmacokinetics and pharmacodynamics that would be compatible with the depression of hepatic drug oxidation observed in microsomal preparations. Final resolution of these apparently contradictory studies will probably require more extensive and critical experimental studies with particular attention given to the selection of the substrates used to evaluate the *in vivo* pharmacokinetic parameters, the dose and the frequency and route of administration of the immunomodulating agent. In addition, evaluation of other pharmacokinetic parameters, such as protein drug binding, drug volume of distribution, and renal drug clearance, may be important since these factors are important determinants of pharmacokinetic drug elimination.

The common denominator, if it exists, responsible for the effect of the various immunomodulators to reduce hepatic microsomal cytochrome P-450 drug oxidation is still an enigma. The proposal that IFN is the initiating agent seems less tenable in view of the contrasting inhibitory effects seen after *in vivo* IFN administration and the inducing effect reported after the *in vitro* addition of IFN to hepatocyte cell cultures. It is conceivable that IFN induction is a common link between the various agents, but that IFN may cause the generation of the final unknown effector. It is tempting to speculate that further studies of this intriguing area may reveal an important biological interplay between the regulation of hepatic drug-oxidation activity and infection, inflammation, and immunity not previously recognized.

REFERENCES

Abernathy, C. O., Zimmerman, H. J., and Utili, R., 1980a, Effects of endotoxin tolerance on in vivo drug metabolism in mice, *Res. Commun. Chem. Pathol. Pharmacol.* **29**:193.

Abernathy C. O., Zimmerman, H. J., and Utili, R., 1980b, Factors influencing endotoxin (ET) induced inhibition on in vivo drug metabolism in mice, *Gastroenterology* **79**:1000.

Adams, A., Petit, J. F., Lefrancier, P., and Lederer, E., 1981, Muramyl peptides: Chemical structure, biological activity, and mechanism of action, *Mol. Cell. Biochem.* **41**:27.

Arrigoni-Martelli, E., 1979, Screening and assessment of antiinflammatory drugs, *Meth. Find. Exp. Clin. Pharmacol.* **1**:157.

Barnes, D. W., 1980, Effects of anionic polymeric drugs and other immunoactive agents on hepatic microsomal mixed-function oxidases, in: *Anionic Polymeric Drugs* (L. G. Donaruma, R. M. Ottenbrite, and O. Vogl, eds.), pp. 255–275, Wiley, New York.

Barnes, D. W., and Wooles, W. R., 1970, Reticuloendothelial stimulation and drug metabolism, *J. Reticuloendothel. Soc.* **7**:684.

Barnes, D. W., Morahan, P. S., Loveless, S., and Munson, A. E., 1979, The effects of maleic anhydride-divinyl ether (MVE) copolymers on hepatic microsomal mixed-function oxidases and other biologic activities, *J. Pharmacol. Exp. Ther.* **208**:392.

Beck, F. J., and Whitehouse, M. W., 1973, Effect of adjuvant disease in rats on cyclophosphamide and isophosphamide metabolism, *Biochem. Pharmacol.* **22**:2453.

Beck, F. J., and Whitehouse, M. W., 1974, Impaired drug metabolism in rats associated with acute inflammation: A possible assay for anti-injury agents, *Proc. Soc. Exp. Biol. Med.* **145**:135.

Bissell, D. M., and Hammaker, L. E., 1976a, Cytochrome P-450 heme and the regulation of hepatic heme oxygenase activity, *Arch, Biochem. Biophys.* **176**:91.

Bissell, D. M., and Hammaker, L. E., 1976b, Cytochrome P-450 heme and the regulation of δ-aminolevulinic acid synthetase in the liver, *Arch. Biochem. Biophys.* **176**:103.

Bissell, D. M., and Hammaker, L. E., 1977, Effect of endotoxin on tryptophan pyrrolase and delta-aminolevulinate synthetase: Evidence for an endogenous regulatory haem fraction in rat liver, *Biochem. J.* **166**:301.

Bloksma, N., Hofhuis, F., Benaissa-Trouw, B., and Willers, J., 1982, Endotoxin-induced release of tumour necrosis factor and interferon in vivo is inhibited by prior adrenoceptor blockade, *Cancer Immunol. Immunother.* **14**:41.

Bocci, V., 1981, Pharmacokinetic studies of interferons, *Pharmacol. Ther.* **13**:421.

Bradley, S. G., 1979, Cellular and molecular mechanisms of action of bacterial endotoxins, *Annu. Rev. Microbiol.* **33**:67.

Burke, D. C., 1982, The mechanism of interferon production, *Philos. Trans. R. Soc. London Ser. B* **299**:51.

Burke, M. D., and Orrenius, S., 1979, Isolation and comparison of endoplasmic reticulum membranes and their mixed function oxidase activities from mammalian extrahepatic tissues, *Pharmacol. Ther.* **7**:549.

Buynitzky, S. J., Tritz, G. J., and Ragland, W. L., 1977, Correlation of induced drug metabolism with titer of duck hepatitis virus in chickens, *Res. Commun. Chem. Pathol. Pharmacol.* **17**:275.

Buynitzky, S. J., Ware, G. O., and Ragland, W. L. 1978, Effect of viral infection on drug metabolism and pesticide disposition in ducks, *Toxicol. Appl. Pharmacol.* **46**:267.

Carlson, R. P., and Ciaccio, E. I., 1975, Effect of benzo(a)pyrene induction of liver and lung metabolism in adjuvant-diseased rats, *Biochem. Pharmacol.* **24**:1893.

Castro, J. E., 1974, The effect of *Corynebacterium parvum* on the structure and function of the lymphoid system in mice, *Eur. J. Cancer* **10**:115.

Cawthorne, M. A., Palmer, E. D., and Green, J., 1976, Adjuvant-induced arthritis and drug-metabolizing enzymes, *Biochem. Pharmacol.* **25**:2683.

Chang, K. C., Bell, T. D., Lauer, B. A., and Chai, H., 1978, Altered theophylline pharmacokinetics during acute respiratory viral illness, *Lancet* **1**:1132.

Ciaccio, E. I., and Barbieri, E. J., 1979, Effect of adjuvant polyarthritis on liver alcohol dehydrogenase in the rat, *Biochem. Pharmacol.* **28**:943.

Correia, M. A., and Meyer, U. A., 1975, Apocytochrome P-450: Reconstitution of functional cytochrome with hemin in vitro, *Proc. Natl. Acad. Sci. USA* **72**:400.

DeClercq, E., and DeSomer, P., 1972, Mechanism of the antiviral activity resulting from sequential administration of complementary hemopolyribonucleotides to cell cultures, *J. Virol.* **9**:721.

Deloria, L. B., and Mannering, G. J., 1982, Sequential administrations of polyriboinosinic acid and polyribocytidylic acid induce interferon and depress the hepatic cytochrome P-450-dependent monooxygenase system, *Biochem. Biophys. Res. Commun.* **106**:947.

DeMaeyer, E., and De Maeyer-Guignard, J., 1982, Immunomodulating properties of interferons, *Philos. Trans. R. Soc. London Ser. B* **299**:77.

DiCarlo, F. J., Haynes, L. J., Coutinho, C. B., and Phillips, G. F., 1965, Pentobarbital sleeping time and RES stimulation, *J. Reticuloendothel. Soc.* **2**:360.

du Souich, P, and Courteau, H., 1981, Induction of acetylating capacity with complete Freund's adjuvant and hydrocortisone in the rabbit, *Drug Metab. Dispos.* **9**:279.

Egawa, K., and Kasai, N., 1979, Endotoxin glycolipid as a potent depressor of the hepatic drug-metabolizing enzyme systems in mice, *Microbiol. Immunol.* **23**:87.

Egawa, K., Yoshida, M., and Kasai, N., 1981, An endotoxin-induced serum factor that depresses hepatic δ-aminolevulinic acid synthetase activity and cytochrome P-450 levels in mice, *Microbiol. Immunol.* **25**:1091.

el Azhary, R., and Mannering, G. J., 1979, Effects of interferon inducing agents (polyriboinosinic acid·polyribocytidylic acid, tilorone) on hepatic hemoproteins (cytochrome P-450, catalase, tryptophan 2,3-dioxygenase, mitochondrial cytochromes), heme metabolism and cytochrome P-450-linked monooxygenase systems, *Mol. Pharmacol.* **15**:698.

el Azhary, R., Renton, K. W., and Mannering, G. J., 1980, Effect of interferon inducing agents (polyriboinosinic acid·polyribocytidylic acid and tilorone) on the heme turnover of hepatic cytochrome P-450, *Mol. Pharmacol.* **17**:395.

Farquhar, D., Loo, T. L. Gutterman, J. U., Hersh, E. M., and Luna, M. A., 1976, Inhibition of drug-metabolizing enzymes in the rat after Bacillus Calmette-Guerin treatment, *Biochem. Pharmacol.* **25**:1529.

Filkins, J. P., and Buchanan, B. J., 1977, In vivo vs. in·vitro effects of endotoxin on glycogenolysis, gluconeogenesis, and glucose utilization, *Proc. Soc. Exp. Biol. Med.* **155**:216.

Filkins, J. P., and Cornell, R. P., 1974, Depression of hepatic gluconeogenesis and the hypoglycemia of endotoxin shock, *Am. J. Physiol.* **227**:778.

Floersheim, G. L., and Szeszak, J. J., 1971, Poly I·poly C and endotoxins share immuno-suppressive properties and increase the toxicity of α-amanitin and hexobarbital, *Agents Actions* **2**:150.

Freudenberg, M. A., Freudenberg, N., and Galanos, C., 1982, Time course of cellular distribution of endotoxin in liver, lungs and kidneys of rats, *Br. J. Exp. Pathol.* **63**:56.

Gander, J. E., and Mannering, G. J., 1980, Kinetics of hepatic cytochrome P-450-dependent monooxygenase systems, *Pharmacol. Ther.* **10**:191.

Gasser, R., Hauri, H. P., and Meyer, U. A., 1982, The turnover of cytochrome P-450b, *FEBS Lett.* **147**:239.

Gemsa, D., Woo, C. H., Fudenberg, H. H., and Schmid, R., 1974, Stimulation of heme oxygenase in machrophages and liver by endotoxin, *J Clin. Invest.* **53**:647.

Giampietri, A., Puccetti, P., and Contessa, A. R., 1981, Depression of hepatic biotransformations by chemical immunoadjuvants, *Int. J. Immunopharmacol.* **3:**251.

Gorodischer, R., Krasner, J., McDevitt, J. J., Nolan, J. P., and Yaffe, S. J., 1976, Hepatic microsomal drug metabolism after administration of endotoxin in rats, *Biochem. Pharmacol.* **25:**351.

Govier, W. C., 1965, Reticuloendothelial cells as the site of sulfanilamide acetylation in the rabbit, *J. Pharmacol. Exp. Ther.* **150:**305.

Grindel, J. M., Migdalof, B. H., Yorgey, K. A., and Pritchard, J. F., 1982, Pharmacokinetics and metabolism of tolmetin in normal and adjuvant arthritic Lewis rats, *Eur. J. Drug Metab. Pharmacokinet.* **7:**299.

Hamilton, C. W., DeAngelis, R. L., Gall, S. A., Fisher, B., and Whisnant, J. K., 1980, Failure of *Corynebacterium parvum* to inhibit antipyrine metabolism in man, *Cancer Immunol. Immunother.* **8:**157.

Harned, C. L., Nerland, D. E., and Sonnenfeld, G., 1982, Effects of passive transfer and induction of gamma (type II immune) interferon preparations on the metabolism of diphenylhydantoin by murine cytochrome P-450, *J. Interferon Res.* **2:**5.

Hojo, H., and Hashimoto, Y., 1977, Inhibition of drug-metabolizing enzymes in the mouse after treatment with host-mediating antitumor drugs *Toxicol. Lett.* **1:**89.

Isaacs, A., and Lindenmann, J., 1957, Virus interference. I. The interferon, *Proc. R. Soc. London Ser. B* **147:**258.

Ishizuki, S., Furuhata, K., Kaneta, S., and Fujihira, E., 1983, Reduced drug metabolism in isolated hepatocytes from adjuvant arthritic rats, *Res. Commun. Chem. Pathol. Pharmacol.* **39:**261.

Johnson, H. M., and Baron, S., 1977, Evaluation of effects of interferon and interferon inducers on the immune response, *Pharmacol. Ther.* **1:**349.

Kasai, N., 1976, Structure and biological activity of endotoxin, *Jpn. J. Bacteriol.* **31:**44.

Kato, R., Nakamura, Y., and Chiesara, E., 1963, Enhanced phenobarbital induction of liver microsomal drug-metabolizing enzymes in mice infected with murine hepatitus virus, *Biochem. Pharmacol.* **12:**365.

Kramer, P., and McClain, G. J., 1981, Depression of aminopyrine metabolism by influenza vaccination, *N. Engl. J. Med.* **305:**1262.

Ladefoged, O., 1978, Endotoxin-induced changes in the pharmacokinetics of warfarin in rabbits, *Acta Vet. Scand.* **19:**479.

Lapka, R., Langmeierova, M., Vanecek, J., and Raskova, H., 1980, Changes of pharmacokinetics and metabolism of sulfadimidine in endotoxin pretreated rabbits, *Arch. Toxicol. Suppl.* **4:**325.

Leeson, G. A., Biedenback, S. A., Chan, K. Y., Gibson, J. B., and Wright, G. J., 1976, Decrease in the activity of the drug metabolizing enzymes of rat liver following the administration of tilorone hydrochloride, *Drug Metab. Dispos.* **4:**232.

Liehr, H., and Grun, M., 1979, Endotoxins in liver disease, in: *Progress in Liver Diseases*, Volume 6 (H. Popper and F. Schaffner, eds.) pp. 313–362, Grune & Stratton, New York.

Lowitt, S., Williams, J. F., and Szentivanyi, A., 1978, Dexamethasone induction of tryptophan oxygenase activity in vivo and in isolated rat hepatic parenchymal cells: Effect of bacterial endotoxin, *Pharamacologist* **20:**157.

Lowitt, S., Williams, J. F., and Szentivanyi, A., 1979, Endotoxin attenuation of dexamethasone induction of tryptophan oxygenase activity in isolated hepatic parenchymal cells: Dependence upon nonparenchymal cells, *Fed. Proc.* **38:**366.

Lowitt, S., Szentivanyi, A., and Williams, J. F., 1981, Endotoxin inhibition of dexamethasone induction of tryptophan oxygenase in suspension culture of isolated rat parenchymal cells, *Biochem. Pharmacol.* **30:**1999.

Lu, A. Y. H., and West, S. B., 1980, Multiplicity of mammalian microsomal cytochromes P-450, *Pharmacol. Rev.* **31:**277.

Lu, K., Rosenblum, M. G., and Loo, T. L., 1981, Effects of endotoxin on the pharmacology of antineoplastic agents, *Cancer Chemother. Pharmacol.* **5:**227.

Luderitz, O., Galanos, C., and Ritschel, E. T., 1982, Endotoxins of gram-negative bacteria, *Pharmacol. Ther.* **15:**383.

McCallum, R. E., 1980, Mediated inhibition of hepatic gluconeogenesis by endotoxin, in: *Microbiology, 1980* (D. Schlessinger, ed.), pp. 87–90, American Society for microbiology, Washington, DC.

Macnee, C. M., and Nimmo-Smith, R. H., 1978, Effects of *Corynebacterium parvum* vaccine on drug metabolism in the mouse, *Dev. Biol. Stand.* **38**:427.

Maitra, S. K., Rachmilewitz, D., Eberle, D., and Kaplowitz, N., 1981, The hepatocellular uptake and biliary excretion of endotoxin in the rat, *Hepatology* **1**:401.

Mannering, G. J., Renton, K. W., el Azhary, R., and Deloria, L. B., 1980, Effects of interferon-inducing agents on hepatic cytochrome P-450 drug metabolizing systems, *Ann. NY Acad. Sci.* **350**:314.

Marecki, N. M., and Bradley, S. G., 1973, Enhanced toxicity for mice of combinations of bacterial endotoxin with antitumor drugs, *Antimicrob. Agents Chemother.* **3**:599.

Marecki, N. M., Bradley, S. G., Munson, A. E., and Drummond, D. C., 1975, Effect of bacterial lipopolysaccharide, lipid A, and concanavalin A on lethality of 5-fluorouracil for mice, *Toxicol. Appl. Pharmacol.* **31**:83.

Martin, B. R., Montgomery, J., Dewey, W. L., and Harris, L. S., 1978, Alterations in the pharmacokinetics of ^{3}H-Δ^9-tetrahydrocannabinol in mice by bacterial endotoxin, *Drug Metab. Dispos.* **6**:282.

Mathison, J. C., and Ulevitch, R. J., 1979, The clearance, tissue distribution, and cellular localization of intravenously injected lipopolysaccharide in rabbits, *J. Immunol.* **123**:2133.

Morahan, P. S., Regelson, W., and Munson, A. E., 1972, Pyran and polyribonucleotides: Differences in biological activities, *Antimicrob. Agents Chemother.* **2**:16.

Morton, D. M., and Chatfield, D. H., 1970, The effects of adjuvant-induced arthritis on the liver metabolism of drugs in rats, *Biochem. Pharmacol.* **19**:473.

Mosedale, B., and Smith, M. A., 1975, Letter to the editor: *Corynebacterium parvum* and anaesthetics, *Lancet* **1**:168.

Mullen, P. W., 1981, Immuno-enhancement and drug elimination kinetics in vivo, in: *Advances in Immunopharmacology* (J. Hadden, L. Chedid, P. Mullen, and F. Spreafico, eds.), pp. 3–9, Pergamon Press, Elmsford, N.Y.

Mullen, P. W., Thatcher, N., Wan, H. H., and Wilkinson, P. M., 1978, The effect of immunotherapy on phenytoin metabolism in man, *Br. J. Clin. Pharmacol.* **1**:353P.

Munford, R. S., Andersen, J. M., and Dietschy, J. M., 1981, Sites of tissue binding and uptake in vivo of bacterial lipopolysaccharide–high density lipoprotein complexes, *J. Clin. Invest.* **68**:1503.

Munoz, J. J., 1963, Immunological and other biological activities of *Bordetella pertussis* antigens, *Bacteriol. Rev.* **27**:325.

Munoz, J. J., and Bergman, R. K., 1968, Histamine-sensitizing factors from microbial agents with special reference to *Bordetella pertussis*, *Bacteriol. Rev.* **32**:103.

Munson, A. E., Sanders, V. M., Bradley, S. G., Loveless, S. E., and Harris, L. S., 1978, Lethal interaction of bacterial lipopolysaccharide and naturally occurring cannabinoids, *J. Reticuloendothel. Soc.* **24**:647.

Nebert, D. W., and Friedman, R. M., 1973, Stimulation of aryl hydrocarbon hydroxylase induction in cell cultures by interferon, *J. Virol.* **11**:193.

Newbould, B. B., 1963, Chemotherapy of arthritis induced in rats by mycobacterial adjuvant, *Br. J. Pharmacol. Chemother.* **21**:127.

Nolan, J. P., 1975, The role of endotoxin in liver injury, *Gastroenterology* **69**:1346.

Nolan, J. P., 1979, The contribution of gut-derived endotoxins to liver injury, *Yale J. Biol. Med.* **52**:127.

Nolan, J. P., and Ali, M. V., 1973, Endotoxin and the liver. II. Effect of tolerance on carbon tetrachloride-induced injury, *J. Med. (Basel)* **4**:28.

Notter, D., and Roland, E., 1978, Localization des N-acetyl-transferases dans les cellules sinusoidales hepatiques: Influence du zymosan sur l'actylation de la sulfamithazine et de l'isoniazide chez le rat et dans le foie isole perfuse, *C.R. Soc. Biol.* **172**:531.

Omura, T., 1980, Cytochrome P-450 linked mixed function oxidase: Turnover of microsomal components and effects of inducers on the turnover of phospholipids, proteins, and specific enzymes, *Pharmacol. Ther.* **8**:489.

Osifo, N. G., 1980, Chloroquine pharmacokinetics in tissues of pyrogen treated rats and implications for chloroquine related pruritus, *Res. Commun. Chem. Pathol. Pharmacol.* **30**:419.

Paine, A. J., 1981, Hepatic cytochrome P-450, *Essays Biochem.* **17**:85.

Parkinson, A., Lasker, J., Kramer, M. J., Huang, M. T., Thomas, P. E., Ryan, D. E., Reik, L. M.,

Norman, R. L., Levin, W., and Conney, A. H., 1982, Effects of three recombinant human leukocyte interferons on drug metabolism in mice, *Drug Metab. Dispos.* **10**:579.

Pearson, C. M., 1956, Development of arthritis, periarthritis, and periostitis in rats given adjuvants, *Proc. Soc. Exp. Biol. Med.* **91**:95.

Perrey, K., Jonen, H. G., Kahl, G. F., and Jahnchen, E., 1976, Elimination and distribution of phenylbutazone in rats during the course of adjuvant-induced arthritis, *J. Pharmacol. Exp. Ther.* **197**:470.

Pollard, R. B., 1982, Interferons and interferon inducers: Development of clinical usefulness and therapeutic promise, *Drugs* **23**:37.

Quevauviller, A., Chalchat, M. A., Brouilhet, H., and Delbarre, F., 1968, Action des barbituriques chez le rat attient de'une polyarthrite adjuvant, *C.R. Soc. Biol.* **162**:618.

Ramadori, G., Hopf, U., and Meyer zum Buschenfelde, K. H., 1979, Binding sites for endotoxin lipopolysaccharide on the plasma membrane of isolated rabbit hepatocytes, *Acta Hepato-Gastroenterol.* **26**:368.

Renton, K. W., 1979, The deleterious effect of *Bordetella pertussis* vaccine and poly (rI·rC) on the metabolism and disposition of phenytoin, *J. Pharmacol. Exp. Ther.* **208**:267.

Renton, K. W., 1981a, Depression of hepatic cytochrome P-450 dependent mixed function oxidases during infection with encephalomyocarditis virus, *Biochem. Pharmacol.* **30**:2333.

Renton, K. W., 1981b, Effects of interferon inducers and viral infection on the metabolism of drugs, in: *Advances in Immunopharmacology* (J. Hadden, L. Chedid, P. Mullen, and F. Spreafico, eds.), pp. 17–24, Pergamon Press, Elmsford, N.Y.

Renton, K. W., and Mannering, G. J., 1976a, Depression of the hepatic cytochrome P-450 monooxygenase system by administered tilorone (2,7-bis [2-(diethylamino) ethoxy] fluoren-9-one dihydrochloride), *Drug Metab. Dispos.* **4**:223.

Renton, K. W., and Mannering, G. J., 1976b, Depression of hepatic cytochrome P-450-dependent monooxygenase systems with administered interferon inducing agents, *Biochem. Biophys, Res. Commun.* **73**:343.

Renton, K. W., Deloria, L. B., and Mannering, G. J., 1978, Effects of polyriboinosinic acid·polyribocytidylic acid and a mouse interferon preparation on cytochrome P-450-dependent monooxygenase systems in cultures of primary mouse hepatocytes, *Mol. Pharmacol.* **14**:672.

Renton, K. W., Gray, J. D., and Hall, R. I., 1980, Altered theophylline disposition following influenza vaccine, *Can. Med. Assoc. J.* **23**:288.

Rios, A., Farquhar, D., and Loo, T. L., 1977, Effect of immunotherapy with intravenous *C. parvum* on antipyrine metabolism, *Am. Soc. Clin. Oncol.* Abstr. C-332.

Ritschel, W. A., Alcorn, G. J., and Ritschel-Beurlin, G., 1982, Antipyretic and pharmacokinetic evaluation of coumarin in the rabbit after endotoxin administration, *Meth. Find. Exp. Clin. Pharmacol.* **4**:407.

Ruiter, D. J., Van Der Muelen, J., Brouwer, A., Hummel, M. J. R., Mauw, B. J., Van Der Ploeg, J. C. M., and Wisse, E., 1981, Uptake by liver cells of endotoxin following its intravenous injection, *Lab. Invest.* **45**:38.

Ruzicka, T., Goerz, G., Vizethum, W., and Kratka, J., 1980, Effects of intravenous and intracutaneous Bacillus Calmette-Guerin application on the drug-metabolizing system of the liver, *Dermatologia (Mexico City)* **160**:135.

Samaras, S. C., and Dietz, N., Jr., 1953, Physiopathology of detoxification of pentobarbital sodium (Nembutal), *Fed. Proc.* **12**:122.

Sasaka, K., Furusawa, S., and Takayanagi, G., 1982, Drug interaction of antitumor drugs. III. Antitumor activity of tegefur in lipopolysaccharide treated mice, *Jpn. J. Pharmacol.* **32**:1135.

Schenkman, J. B., Sligar, S. G., and Cinti, D. L., 1981, Substrate interaction with cytochrome P-450, *Pharmacol. Ther.* **12**:43.

Schroeder, D. H., Hinton, M. L., Thornburgh, B. A., Nichol, C. A., and Welch, R. M., 1976, Effects of *Corynebacterium parvum* on hepatic drug metabolism in rats, *Fed. Proc.* **35**:407.

Singh, G., and Renton, K. W., 1981, Interferon-mediated depression of cytochrome P-450-dependent drug biotransformation, *Mol. Pharmacol.* **20**:681.

Singh, G., Renton, K. W., and Stebbing, N., 1982, Homogenous interferon from *E. coli* depresses hepatic cytochrome P-450 and drug biotransformation, *Biochem. Biophys. Res. Commun.* **106**:1256.

Smith, P. K., Nerland, D. E., and Sonnenfeld, G., 1983, Effect of interferon on murine cytochrome P-450: Effect of partially purified antigen-specific interferon-gamma, *J. Interferon Res.* **3**:219.

Snyder, R., and Remmer, H., 1979, Classes of hepatic microsomal mixed function oxidase inducers, *Pharmacol. Ther.* **7**:203.

Sofia, R. D., 1977, Alteration of hepatic microsomal enzyme systems and the lethal action of non-steroidal anti-arthritic drugs in acute and chronic models of inflammation, *Agents Actions* **7**:289.

Sonnenfeld, G., 1983, Interactions of the interferon system with cellular metabolism, in: *Clinical Applications of Interferons and Their Inducers* (D. A. Stringfellow, ed.), Dekker, New York.

Sonnenfeld, G., Harned, C. L., Thaniyavarn, S., Huff, T., Mandel, A. D., and Nerland, D. E., 1980, Type II interferon induction and passive transfer depress the murine cytochrome P-450 drug metabolism system, *Antimicrob. Agents Chemother.* **17**:969.

Soyka, L. F., 1981, Immunostimulants and hepatic drug metabolism, in: *Advances in Immunopharmacology* (J. Hadden, L. Chedid, P. Mullen, and F. Spreafico, eds.), pp. 11–15, Pergamon Press, Elmsford, N.Y.

Soyka, L. F., Hunt, W. G., Knight, S. E., and Foster, R. S., Jr., 1976, Decreased liver and lung drug-metabolizing activity in mice treated with *Corynebacterium parvum*, *Cancer Res.* **36**:4425.

Soyka, L. F., Stephens, C. C., MacPherson, B. R., and Foster, R. S., Jr., 1979, Role of mononuclear phagocytes in decreased hepatic drug metabolism following administration of *Corynebacterium parvum*, *Int. J. Immunopharmacol.* **1**:101.

Stoerck, H. C., Bielinski, T. C., and Budzilovich, T., 1954, Chronic polyarthritis in rats injected with spleen in adjuvants, *Am. J. Pathol.* **30**:616.

Szentivanyi, A., and Williams, J. F., 1980, The constitutional basis of atopic disease, in: *Allergic Diseases of Infancy, Childhood, and Adolescence* (C. W. Bierman and D. S. Pearlman, eds.), pp. 173–210, Saunders, Philadelphia.

Utili, R., Abernathy, C. O., and Zimmerman, H. J., 1977, Minireview: Endotoxin effects on the liver, *Life Sci.* **20**:553.

Vainio, H., 1973, Defective drug metabolism in rat liver in endotoxin shock, *Ann. Med. Exp. Biol. Fenn.* **51**:65.

Wan, H. H., Thatcher, N., Mullen, P. W., Smith, G. N., and Wilkinson, P. M., 1979, Lack of effect of immunotherapy with BCG and *Corynebacterium parvum* on hepatic drug hydroxylation in man, *Br. J. Cancer* **39**:441.

Wardlaw, A. C., and Parton, R., 1983, *Bordetella pertussis* toxins, *Pharmacol. Ther.* **19**:1.

Westphal, O., Jann, K., and Himmelspach, 1983, Chemistry and immunochemistry of bacterial lipopolysaccharide as cell wall antigens and endotoxins, *Prog. Allergy* **33**:9.

Whitehouse, M. W., 1973, Abnormal drug metabolism in rats after an inflammatory insult, *Agents Actions* **3**:312.

Whitehouse, M. W., and Beck, F. J., 1973, Impaired drug metabolism in rats with adjuvant-induced arthritis: A brief review, *Drug Metab. Dispos.* **1**:251.

Williams, J. F., and Szentivanyi, A., 1975, Effect of *Bordetella pertussis* vaccine on the drug-metabolizing enzyme system of mouse liver, *Fed. Proc.* **34**: 1001.

Williams, J. F., and Szentivanyi, A., 1977, Depression of hepatic drug-metabolizing enzyme activity by *B. pertussis* vaccination, *Eur. J. Pharmacol.* **43**:281.

Williams, J. F., and Szentivanyi, A., 1982a, Continued studies on the effect of interferon inducers on the hepatic microsomal mixed-function oxidase system of rats and mice, Abstracts, 2nd International Congress for Interferon Research, Miami.

Williams, J. F., and Szentivanyi, A., 1982b, Possible involvement of α-adrenergic mechanisms and reticuloendothelial activation in the effects of bacterial lipopolysaccharide on hepatic enzyme activities, *Fed. Proc.* **41**:1722.

Williams, J. F., and Szentivanyi, A., 1983a, Continued studies on the effect of interferon inducers on the hepatic microsomal mixed-function oxidase system of rats and mice, *Interferon Res.* **3**:219.

Williams, J. F., and Szentivanyi, A., 1983b, Investigation of adrenergic and and prostaglandin influences in the endotoxin alteration of hepatic heme oxygenase, microsomal mixed-function oxidase, and glucocorticoid-induced tryptophan oxygenase activities, *Immunopharmacology* **6**:75.

Williams, J. F., and Szentivanyi, A., 1983c, Effect of endotoxin in endotoxin-tolerant animals on mixed-function oxidase and heme oxygenase activities, *Pharmacologist* **25**:218.

Williams, J. F., Lowitt, S., and Szentivanyi, A., 1977, Depression of hepatic drug-metabolizing activity by *Bordetella pertussis*, *Ann. Allergy* **38**:376.

Williams, J. F., Lowitt, S., and Szentivanyi, A., 1979, Effect of endotoxin and phenobarbital on heme enzymes of rat liver, *Pharmacologist* **21**:232.

Williams, J. F., Lowitt, S., and Szentivanyi, A., 1980a, Involvement of a heat-stable and heat-labile component of *Bordetella pertussis* in the depression of the murine hepatic mixed-function oxidase system, *Biochem. Pharmacol.* **29**:1483.

Williams, J. F., Lowitt, S., and Szentivanyi, A., 1980b, Endotoxin depression of hepatic mixed-function oxidase system in C3H/HeJ and C3H/HeN mice, *Int. J. Immunopharmacol.* **2**:285.

Williams, J. F., Winters, A. L., Lowitt, S., and Szentivanyi, A., 1981, Depression of hepatic mixed-function oxidase activity by *B. pertussis* in splenectomized and athymic nude mice, *Int. J. Immunopharmacol.* **3**:101.

Wooles, W. R., and Borzelleca, J. F., 1964, Prolongation of barbiturate sleeping time in mice by stimulation of the reticuloenodthelial system (RES), *J. Reticuloendothel. Soc.* **1**:354.

Wooles, W. R., and Borzelleca, J. F., 1966, Prolongation of barbiturate sleeping time in mice by stimulation of the reticuloendothelial system (RES), *J. Reticuloendothel. Soc.* **3**:41.

Wooles, W. R., and Munson, A. E., 1971, The effect of stimulants and depressants of reticuloendothelial activity on drug metabolism, *J. Reticuloendothel. Soc.* **9**:108.

Yoshida, M., Egawa, K., and Kasai, N., 1982, Effect of endotoxin and its degradation products on hepatic mixed-function oxidase and heme enzyme systems in mice, *Toxicol. Lett.* **12**:185.

Zerkle, T. B., Wade, A. E., and Ragland, W. L., 1980, Selective depression of hepatic cytochrome P-450 hemoprotein by interferon inducers, *Biochem. Biophys. Res. Commun.* **96**:121.

Zidek, Z., and Janku, I., 1981, Increased acetylation and elimination of sulphadimidine in rats with adjuvant-induced arthritis, *Eur. J. Drug Metab. Pharmacokinet.* **6**:255.

Zidek, Z., Friebova, M., Janku, I., and Elis, J., 1977, Influence of sex and Freund's adjuvant on liver N-acetyltransferase activity and elimination of sulphadimidine in urine of rats, *Biochem. Pharmacol.* **26**:69.

Zidek, Z., Kamenikova, L., Buchar, E., Janku, I., and Masek, K., 1983, Biotransformation of drugs in rats treated with a synthetic muramyl dipeptide, N-acetylmuramyl-L-alanyl-D-isoglutamine (MDP), *Int. J. Immunopharmacol.* **5**:151.

Zlydaszyk, J. C., and Moon, R. J., 1976, Fate of ^{51}Cr-labeled lipopolysaccharide in tissue culture cells and livers of normal mice, *Infect. Immun.* **14**:100.

2

Cyclic Nucleotide Pharmacology of Macrophage Functions

RONALD G. COFFEY and JOHN W. HADDEN

1. INTRODUCTION

Macrophages are critical in the expressions of immune response, especially in the defense against facultative intracellular bacteria and viruses and in the defense against the development of cancer. Historically, studies of the macrophage since the days of Metchnikoff focused on the important role played by this cell in the resistance to infection. With increasing understanding of the immune response, the macrophage was considered the principal cell in the expression of cell-mediated immunity. With the discovery of the role of the thymus and the functions of the T lymphocyte, the macrophage was placed in a role secondary to that of the lymphocyte. Currently, important interrelationships of the two cell populations are being elucidated, and a central role for the macrophage in tumor immunity is emerging.

The importance of cyclic nucleotides in the regulation of the immune response has been realized for a decade [see reviews by Bourne *et al.*, 1974, and in *Immunopharmacology* (Hadden *et al.*, 1977)]. Mitogenic stimulation of lymphocytes is associated with early increases in cGMP[1] and is prevented by cAMP.

---

[1]The abbreviations used are: BCG, *Bacillus Calmette Guerin*; C3, C5, complement, 3rd and 5th components; Con A, concanavalin A; CFU-c, colony forming unit of culture; CSF, colony stimulating factor; cyclic AMP, adenosine 3',5'-monophosphate; cyclic GMP, guanosine 3',5'-monophosphate; ETYA, 5,8,11,14-eicosatetraynoic acid; FMLP, formyl methionyl leucyl phenylalanine; HETE, hydroxyeicosatetraenoic acid; HPETE, hydroperoxyeicosatetraenoic acid; IF, interferon; LAF, lymphocyte activating factor; LIF, leukocyte inhibitory factor; LPS, lipopolysaccharide; MAF, macrophage activating factor; MDP, muramyl dipeptide (N-acetyl-muramyl-L-alanyl-D-isoglutamine); MIF, macrophage inhibitory factor; MMF, macrophage mitogenic factor; MNNG, N-methyl-N'-nitro-N-nitrosoguanidine; PG, prostaglandin; PHA, phytohemagglutinin; PMA, phorbol-12-myristate-13-acetate; PTH, parathyroid hormone; WGA, wheat germ agglutinin.

RONALD G. COFFEY • Department of Phamacology and Therapeutics, University of South Florida College of Medicine, Tampa, Florida 33612.   JOHN W. HADDEN • Departments of Microbiology, Immunology, and Internal Medicine, University of South Florida College of Medicine, Tampa, Florida 33612.

Differentiation of lymphocytes, on the other hand, may be positively linked to cAMP. cAMP is inhibitory to the induction of allergic histamine release from blood basophils and tissue mast cells, whereas agents that augment cGMP enhance mediator release. Similarly, degranulation of platelets and neutrophils is associated with increases in cGMP and is inhibited by increases in cAMP.

The roles of cyclic nucleotides in biological responses of macrophages are, in contrast, less clearly defined. One reason for this is the relatively recent appearance of such research on these cells. Another is the great heterogeneity of the systems studied, ranging from the bone marrow to the mobile blood monocytes, to peritoneal exudate macrophages (either resident or induced by a variety of irritating substances), and to alveolar macrophages. Also, the species have varied, including mouse, rat, rabbit, guinea pig, and man. Macrophages have been studied while adhered to glass or plastic, spread out or rounded up, or in free suspension. Rarely have cyclic nucleotide measurements been made with the intention of comparing these different conditions (Hagmann and Fishman, 1980; Minkin et al., 1977).

Despite this heterogeneity, certain relationships between effector substances and cyclic nucleotides in macrophages have emerged. The effects of over 50 agents on cAMP and cGMP levels are listed in Table 1. Apparent controversies regarding the effects of a substance occur in such a list. As these are sometimes due to different origins of cells, the species and types of cell preparations are indicated.

Macrophages from several sources respond to β-adrenergic agonists such as isoproterenol and epinephrine, and to other well-known adenylate cyclase stimulants including cholera toxin and prostaglandins of the E and A series, with the expected rise in cellular levels of cAMP. Timed studies in the absence of phosphodiesterase inhibitors reveal peak effects of isoproterenol within 1 sec (Welscher and Cruchaud, 1978) to several minutes with other agents. Several agents could not be shown to stimulate cAMP levels in guinea pig peritoneal macrophages unless phosphodiesterase inhibitors were added (Bromberg and Pick, 1981). Activities of both cAMP and cGMP phosphodiesterases have been determined in careful studies (Thompson et al., 1980; Wedner et al., 1979). Important changes in cAMP phosphodiesterase may occur during phagocytosis (Merdrignac et al., 1982; Zendegui and Klein, 1982).

Drugs, hormones, and neurotransmitters that increase cGMP levels in other systems and that are similarly effective in macrophages are ascorbate, carbamylcholine, and serotonin. In most systems these effects require the presence of calcium. A category of cGMP stimulants that do not require calcium includes a series of nitric oxide-generating agents [azide, hydroxylamine, nitrite, nitroprusside, N-methyl-N'-nitro-N-nitrosoguanidine (MNNG)] (Bromberg and Pick, 1980; Rohrer and Atkinson, 1980). Such stimulants differ from the Ca^{2+}-dependent agents in their inability to promote intracellular events in a variety of tissues and are not considered in detail here.

In addition to a myriad of drugs and hormones, macrophages are delicately regulated by such products of the immune system as antibodies, complement, and lymphokines. Macrophages contribute in turn to the regulation of lymphocyte function and development through the digestion and processing of antigen and the secretion of regulatory molecules such as lymphocyte-activating factor (LAF), colony-stimulating factor (CSF), interferon (IFN), and prostaglandins. The basic functions of the macrophages to be discussed with reference to cyclic nucleotides include:

1. Migration and chemotaxis
2. Activation and proliferation
3. Phagocytosis
4. Respiratory burst and degranulation reactions
5. Cytoxicity

This arbitrary separation will serve to facilitate the discussion of effects that frequently involve changes in more than one of these functions. The literature was searched through December 1982 for this review.

2. MACROPHAGE MIGRATION AND CHEMOTAXIS

An important function of macrophages is their ability to move toward sites of antigen–antibody reactions and inflammation. The earliest report of cyclic nucleotide effects in macrophage motility was that of Pick (1972). He demonstrated inhibition of random migration of paraffin oil-induced guinea pig peritoneal macrophages by cAMP and agents that raise its levels such as isoproterenol and theophylline. Pick (1977) and others (Koopman *et al.*, 1973; Block *et al.*, 1978; Oropeza-Rendon *et al.*, 1979) then examined the effect of migration inhibitory factor (MIF) for its effect on cAMP but found that this lymphokine (or lymphokine mixtures containing MIF activity) did not increase guinea pig peritoneal macrophage levels of cAMP. In fact, Pick (1977) found that MIF reduced cAMP and inhibited its increase by other agents. Moreover, the action of MIF to inhibit migration of macrophages was itself prevented by simultaneous addition of cAMP, β-adrenergic agents, or PGE_1 or PGE_2.

Chemotaxis, the directed migration of cells toward increasing concentrations of chemotactic substances such as activated complement components or bacterial products, is similarly inhibited by cAMP (Gallin *et al.*, 1978). It is significant that the administration of ethanol, a stimulant of cAMP in monocytes and lymphocytes (Atkinson *et al.*, 1977), results in reduced mobilization of pulmonary alveolar macrophages after bacterial challenge (Guarneri and Laurenzi, 1968). In contrast to cAMP, several agents such as serotonin, carbamylcholine, levamisole, and ascorbic acid were shown to raise cGMP levels and to enhance chemotaxis in human monocytes (Sandler *et al.*, 1975a,b; Wright *et al.*, 1977; Gallin *et al.*, 1978). Agents that increased cAMP inhibited the cGMP increases and locomotion (Gallin *et al.*, 1978).

The assay of chemotaxis requires considerable time, making it difficult to assess the critical early effects of agents on cyclic nucleotides. Stephens and Snyderman (1982) found that the initial morphological response, polarization (changing from a round to a triangular motile configuration), occurs in monocytes within 45 sec after exposure to chemoattractants such as forml methionyl leucyl phenylalanine (FMLP). Using this assay they found consistent augmentation by all the agents shown above to stimulate cGMP, as well as by α–adre-

TABLE 1. EFFECTS ON MACROPHAGE CYCLIC NUCLEOTIDES[a,b]

Agent	cGMP Increase	cGMP No change	cAMP Increase	cAMP No change	cAMP Decrease
A23187	Ge6; Re32	Ge4,27; Ba27; Hb10[c]	Ge5; Hb10; Re13,32	Ge6; Ba27; Re32[e]	Ge15[e]
Acetylcholine		Ge4			
Adenosine	Ge6		Hb22		
Alcohol			Ba2		
Arachidonate		Ge4	Ge5		
Ascorbic acid	Ge4,6; Hb10			Ge6	
Azide, sodium	Ge4,6	Ge27		Ge6	
Bradykinin	Hb30				
Calcitonin			Me23		
Calcium	Ge4		Ge5	Re32	
Carbamylcholine	Ge28; Hb29				
Cholera toxin		Ba27; Ge4	Ge15[d],18; Me23; Mr23; Re11		
Colchicine			Ge5	Ge15[d],18[d]; Re11[d],12[d]	
Con A			Ge5[d]	Ge40[d]; Re11[d]	
Con A–Sepharose				Ge16	
Epinephrine			Ge25		
5,8,11,14-Eicosatetraynoic acid			e: Ge18,25; Me23; Mr9,23; Re32		
Fluoride, sodium				Ge5[d]	

FMLP				Ge18[c]	
Glucagon				Ge25; Re32	
GTP				Ge18[d,e]	
HETE					
Histamine	Hb14	Hb29			
Hydrocortisone	Hb30		Hb22	Ge25	
Hydroxylamine			Hb22[d]		
IgE (agg)	Ge4			Rr7	
IgG (agg)	Rr7			Ge6	
Indomethacin	Ge6			Ge6;26[c,e]; Re32[c]	
Infection (Toxoplasma)	Ge6				Mr9[e]
Interferon	C34,35		C34,35; Mr40		
Isoproterenol			Ge3,15,16,18,19,25,28; Hb21; Me37,38; Re11,32		
Leukocyte dialysate	Hb31				
Levamisole	Hb39				
Listeria activator	Ge6			Ge6	
Lymphokines					
Unfractionated	Ge6,28		Ge26[e]	Ge28	
MIF-enriched			Ga20	Ga20,Ge3	Ge24[c]
MIF-poor	Ge6			Ge6	
MGF-enriched	Ge6		Ge36	Ge6	
MDP	Ge6,17			Ge6	
Melatonin	Hb30			Hb30	
Methylxanthines	Ge4		Ge5,19[d]; Ba2; Me37		
MNNG	Ba27; Ge6,27				
Nitrite, sodium	Ge4		Me23	Re32	
Parathyroid hormone			Re11		Mr23
PGA$_1$, A$_2$					

(continued)

TABLE 1. (Continued)

Agent	cGMP Increase	cGMP No change	cAMP Increase	cAMP No change	cAMP Decrease
PGE$_1$, E$_2$		Hb10[c]	Ba2; Ge15,16,18,25; Hb10,21; Mr8; Re11,12,32		
PHA	Ge6			Ge6,16[d]; Re11	
PMA	Ge6		Ge5	Ge6	
Polystyrene beads		Ge4	Hb10,30		
Prostacyclin		Hb10[c],30	Re1		
Serotonin	Hb10,29,30	Ge4,27			
Serum		Ge4	Ge25[e]	Hb30	
Superoxide					
Transfer factor	Hb31				
Tuftsin	Me33				Me33
Tumor presence			Ge5		
WGA					
Zymosan	Re32	Ge27	Ge5; Re32	Re32[e]	Mr8[e]

[a] B, rabbit; C, cell line; G, guinea pig; H, human; M, mouse; R, rat; a, alveolar; b, blood; e, peritoneal, elicited; r, peritoneal, resident.

[b] References: 1, Adolfs and Bonta (1982); 2, Atkinson et al. (1977); 3, Block et al. (1978); 4, Bromberg and Pick (1980); 5, Bromberg and Pick (1981); 6, Coffey, Hadden, Hadden, Ito, England, Sadlik, and Schindler (unpublished observations); 7, Dessaint et al. (1980); 8, Diamantstein and Ulmer (1976); 9, Droller and Remington (1975); 10, Gallin et al. (1978); 11, Gemsa et al. (1975); 12, Gemsa et al. (1977); 13, Gemsa et al. (1979); 14, Goetzl et al. (1980); 15, Grunspan-Swirsky and Pick (1978); 16, Grunspan-Swirsky and Pick (1979); 17 Hadden and Englard (1977); 18, Hagmann and Fishman (1980); 19, Higgins and David (1976); 20, Higgins et al. (1976); 21, Kalisker et al. (1977); 22, Marone et al. (1980); 23, Minkin et al. (1977); 24, Pick (1977); 25, Remold-O'Donnell (1974); 26, Remold-O'Donnell and Remold (1974); 27, Rohrer and Atkinson (1980); 28, Rouveix et al. (1981); 29, Sandler et al. (1975a); 30, Sandler et al. (1975b); 31, Sandler et al. (1980); 32, Smith et al. (1980); 33, Stabinsky et al. (1980); 34, Tovey and Rochette-Egly (1980); 35, Tovey et al. (1979); 36, Wahl et al. (1979); 37, Welscher and Cruchaud (1976); 38, Welscher and Cruchaud (1978); 39, Wright et al. (1977); 40, Degré and Rollag (1982).

[c] Diminishes the increase caused by other agents.

[d] Augments the increases caused by other agents.

[e] Studies involved isolated cyclase assay.

nergic agents (phenylephrine, clonidine). Each of these agents alone stimulated chemokinesis but not chemotaxis, and caused a transient polarization that was absolutely dependent on external Ca^{2+}. Like chemotaxis, the polarization to chemoattractants was inhibited by several agents that increase cAMP levels (theophylline, histamine, and isoproterenol).

It would be expected from the above findings that chemotactic agents might reduce cAMP and increase cGMP levels in the responding cells. Interestingly, in human neutrophils, both FMLP and C5a caused transient increases in cAMP (Simchowitz et al., 1980). Such increases have not been observed in macrophages, however. The effects of the chemotactic peptide FMLP were described by Hagmann and Fishman (1980) with reference to cAMP in guinea pig peritoneal macrophages. While causing a small decrease in cAMP, FMLP treatment greatly reduced the sensitivity of the cells to cAMP stimulants such as isoproterenol and PGE_1. This effect is probably secondary to the cell spreading caused by FMLP and can be mimicked by allowing the cells to spread on a plastic surface for 1–4 hr. Colchicine prevented these responses to FMLP and caused the cells to respond dramatically to cAMP stimulants in association with a change to a round morphology.

We are not aware of any reports of FMLP causing an increase in macrophage cGMP levels, but would expect that this and other chemotactic substances might do so from the following rationale: The hydroxyeicosatetraenoic acids (HETEs) are fatty acid derivatives that have been shown to stimulate increases in cGMP in association with both chemotaxis and chemokinesis in human monocytes and neutrophils (Goetzl et al., 1980). These compounds, especially the 5-HETE and 5,12-diHETE (leukotriene B_4), are also thought to be increased intracellularly and to play important roles in response to other chemotactic substances (Goetzl et al., 1980). The HETEs are derived through a series of reactions described below.

Phospholipid transmethylation may be an important membrane trigger signal for chemotaxis of human monocytes, neutrophils, and guinea pig macrophages (Pike and Snyderman, 1981). As described in other cells (Hirata and Axelrod, 1980), phosphatidylethanolamine is converted by the sequential action of two transmethylation enzymes to form phosphatidylcholine (see Fig. 1). Translocation of the phospholipids, increased membrane fluidity, increased Ca^{2+} uptake, and activation of a Ca^{2+}-dependent phospholipase then occur rapidly. Macrophages contain Ca^{2+}-dependent phospholipase A_2 and C, which, when activated, lyse membrane phospholipids to produce arachidonic acid (Wightman et al., 1981a,b; Hsueh et al., 1981; Homma et al., 1982; Humes et al., 1980). Arachidonic acid is further metabolized via the cyclooxygenase pathway to form the prostaglandins, or via lipoxygenases to form various hydroperoxyeicosatetraenoic acids (HPETEs), HETEs, and leukotrienes. All of these arachidonic acid metabolites have been demonstrated in macrophages activated by a variety of chemotactic and other stimuli (Bonney et al., 1980b,c; Gemsa et al., 1979; Goetzl et al., 1980; Hamilton, 1980; Kurland et al., 1977; Rigaud et al., 1979; Valone et al., 1980).

It is thus of interest that transmethylation reactions were found to regulate

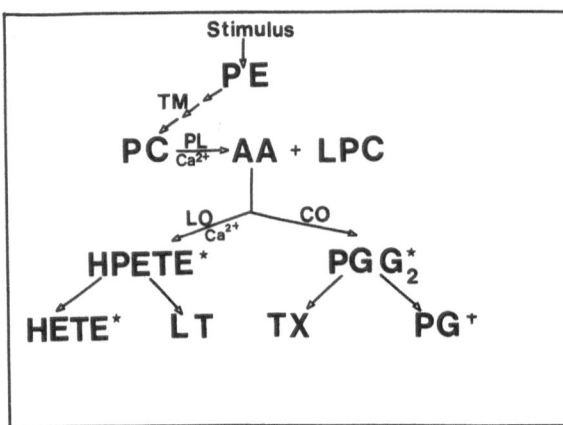

FIGURE 1. AA, arachidonic acid; CO, cyclooxygenase; HETE, hydroxyeicosatetraenoic acids; HPETE, hydroperoxyeicosatetraenoic acids; LO, lipoxygenase; LPC, lysophosphatidylcholine; LT, leukotrienes; PC, phosphatidylcholine; PE, phosphatidylethanolamine; PG, prostaglandins; PGG_2, prostaglandin endoperoxide; PL, phospholipase; TX, thromboxanes; TM, transmethylases. *, guanylate cyclase stimulant; †, adenylate cyclase stimulant.

the affinity of chemotactic factor receptors on macrophages (Pike and Snyderman, 1982). Inhibitors of methyltransferase reactions blocked chemotaxis of macrophages (Pike *et al.*, 1978) as well as neutrophils (Hirata *et al.*, 1979). Inhibition of the phospholipase A_2 activity also blocked chemotaxis. An apparent paradox remains to be explained: chemoattractants inhibit rather than stimulate the methylation of phospholipids in mononuclear phagocytes (Snyderman and Goetzl, 1981).

Of the many arachidonic acid metabolites, only the prostaglandins of the E and A series [and prostacyclin (PGI_2)] have been shown to stimulate cAMP in macrophages (see Table 1). Interestingly, PGE_2 prevents PGI_2-induced elevations of cAMP in rat macrophages (Adolfs and Bonta, 1982). This may explain, in part, why resident peritoneal macrophages, which produce higher levels of prostaglandins than elicited cells, are less responsive to PGE_2 and PGI_2 (Bonney *et al.*, 1980a). The endoperoxides PGG_2 and PGH_2, the thromboxanes, the HPETEs, and certain HETEs have been shown to stimulate guanylate cyclase and cGMP levels in intact and broken preparations of several types of hemopoietic cells (Coffey and Hadden, 1981; Goldberg *et al.*, 1978; Goetzl *et al.*, 1980). The scheme outlined in Fig. 1 may account for mitogen-induced increases in cGMP in lymphocytes (Coffey and Hadden, 1981; Coffey *et al.*, 1981) and cGMP increases induced by other Ca^{2+} uptake-stimulating substances in other cells (Craven and DeRubertis, 1982). This scheme may prove to be descriptive of the mechanism of cGMP changes occurring in macrophages in response to chemotactic factors and agents stimulating other functions in these phagocytes.

3. MACROPHAGE ACTIVATION AND PROLIFERATION

An important consequence of the immune response is the activation of macrophages for enhanced phagocytosis and killing of pathogens and tumor cells (Nathan and Cohn, 1980; North, 1981). The activated macrophage differs from the unactivated one in several morphological and metabolic characteristics including greater size and spreading, increased motility and microbicidal capacity, decreased alkaline phosphodiesterase and 5'-nucleotidase activity, elevated activities and secretion of acid hydrolases and neutral proteases, increased activity of the hexose monophosphate shunt, and enhanced production of superoxide and hydrogen peroxide (North, 1981; Soberman and Karnovsky, 1981; Edelson, 1981; Klebanoff, 1982) and of prostaglandins (Friedman *et al.*, 1979).

Another consequence of immune reactions is the enhanced proliferation of macrophages (Hadden and England, 1977; Hadden *et al.*, 1978; North, 1981). Both activation and proliferation are mediated *in vivo* by T-lymphocyte-produced lymphokines, termed macrophage-activating factor (MAF) and macrophage growth factor (MGF), respectively (Hadden and Englard, 1977; Hadden *et al.*, 1979a). Activation but not proliferation is induced by IFN (Schultz, 1980). IFN induces a rapid stimulation of cGMP and, several hours later, an increase in cAMP (Tovey *et al.*, 1979; Tovey and Rochette-Egly, 1980). It is suspected that activation properties of IFN may be linked to cGMP and that the capacity to inhibit cell replication is mediated by cAMP. In some instances, data suggest that a proliferation-dependent differentiation step of the macrophage may precede activation (Hadden and Englard, 1977). Alternatively, different subsets of macrophages may be involved in the activation and proliferation responses.*

In recent *in vitro* studies of cyclic nucleotide roles in these processes, investigators have used a variety of triggering and modulating substances in addition to the lymphokines. Sandler *et al.* (1975c) attributed the adjuvant effect of dialyzable transfer factor to increased cGMP in human monocytes. Tuftsin, a tetrapeptide derived from IgG and discovered to bind to and to activate macrophages, was shown to increase cGMP and decrease cAMP levels in macrophages as well as neutrophils (Stabinsky *et al.*, 1980). Tuftsin also increased guanylate cyclase directly in supernatants of neuroblastoma cells (Deguchi and Yoshioka, 1982). Dessaint *et al.* (1980) reported that the activation of uninduced rat peritoneal macrophages by aggregated IgE resulted in a six-fold increase in cGMP within 10 min. Like many biological activations of cGMP, Ca^{2+} was essential. M. Ito and J. W. Hadden (unpublished observations) have noted similar changes after adding aggregated IgG to guinea pig peritoneal exudate macrophages. In addition, we found that an MAF derived from *Lysteria monocytogenes* increased cGMP in guinea pig peritoneal macrophages.

Muramyl dipeptide (MDP), an adjuvant derived from the cell wall of BCG, is one of the most potent of naturally occurring substances for macrophage activation (Chedid *et al.*, 1978; Hadden *et al.*, 1979b; Wahl *et al.*, 1979; Leclerc and Chedid, 1982). Preliminary work (Hadden and England, 1979; J. W. Hadden, T. E. Schindler, and R. G. Coffey, unpublished observations) indicates that addition of MDP to mineral oil-induced guinea pig peritoneal macrophages elicits increases in cGMP within 10–20 min. Wahl *et al.* (1979) found that in addition to the early increase in cGMP, MDP also elicits an elevation in cAMP levels after 18 hrs of incubation, and suggested that this was dependent on prostaglandin synthesis. Similarly, incubation for 24 hr with a crude mixture of lymphokines stimulated adenylate cyclase activity in guinea pig peritoneal casein-induced

---

*The identity of gamma IFN with MAF has now been established beyond doubt. See, for example, Nathan *et al.* (1984).

macrophages (Remold-O'Donnell and Remold, 1974). This stimulation was blocked by indomethacin, again suggesting an indirect effect mediated by prostaglandins. The effect of MDP to induce macrophage activation to kill *L. monocytogenes* is unaffected by indomethacin, which prevents prostaglandin synthesis, and appears to be related to the increases of cGMP levels (Hadden and Englard, 1979). It is notable that the effects of MDP to act *in vivo* as an immunoadjuvant and to protect animals from bacterial challenge are unaffected by treatment with indomethacin. Only the effects of MDP to induce fever (pyrogen synthesis) are blocked by this treatment. It appears then that MDP's main action as a macrophage activator is mediated by cGMP. Its side effects to induce fever and collagenase production, and to inhibit macrophage proliferation as a result of cAMP production, derive from prostaglandin synthesis.

Other agents capable of inducing macrophage activation include poly(A:U), the Ca^{2+} ionophore A23187, and lipopolysaccharide (LPS) (Alexander and Evans, 1971). The latter substance increases cGMP in B lymphocytes (Watson, 1977), but confirmation of this observation in macrophages awaits further studies. The action of LPS may be complex, as it induces the release of IFN, which activates as discussed above.

Proliferation of macrophages can be induced by mitogens such as phytohemagglutinin (PHA) and phorbol myristate acetate (PMA) as well as by the specific T-cell-derived lymphokine MGF (Hadden *et al.*, 1982). Both alveolar and peritoneal guinea pig macrophages respond to these substances with a brisk increase in cGMP, followed several days later by DNA synthesis and cell division (Hadden *et al.*, 1982). These results are thus consistent with mitogen-induced increases in cGMP levels of lymphocytes (Coffey *et al.*, 1977; Hadden *et al.*, 1972, 1975; Watson, 1977). Recent data suggest that highly purified MGF is identical to CSF (Sadlik *et al.*, 1983). Since Ziboh *et al.* (1982) have shown that CSF induces the release of arachidonic acid from phospholipids of peritoneal macrophages, it is possible that MGF acts through this mechanism to produce stimulants of cGMP (Fig. 1).

The participation of Ca^{2+} influx in macrophage proliferation has not been studied, but is suspected to be important by analogy to lymphocytes (Hadden *et al.*, 1975; Coffey *et al.*, 1977). Ca^{2+} influx is essential for mitogen stimulation of lymphocyte cGMP levels as well as DNA synthesis. Two key steps in the proposed pathway for guanylate cyclase activation (Fig. 1) require Ca^{2+}: phospholipase and lipoxygenase. It will be of great interest to analyze these enzymes in relationship to Ca^{2+} requirements for macrophage proliferation.

As in lymphocytes, glucocorticoids modulate the proliferation of macrophages (Duncan *et al.*, 1982). Production of MGF by lymphocytes is much more sensitive to steroid inhibition than the action of MGF on macrophages. cGMP-raising agents such as acetylcholine, imidazole, and 8-bromo-cGMP itself augment the basal proliferation of macrophages (Hadden and Englard, 1977, 1979). The observations (Grunspan-Swirsky and Pick, 1979) that lectin mitogens enhance the responsiveness of guinea pig peritoneal machrophage adenylate cyclase to stimulation by PGE_1 and isoproterenol may relate to effects of these substances to alter the morphology of the cells, as discussed above. Such effects are probably not related to early events in the triggering of macrophage proliferation since cAMP is antiproliferative in macrophages (Hadden *et al.*, 1978) as in most other systems. Moreover, the macrophage mitogen PMA is known to cause an uncoupling of adenylate cyclase from both β - and prostaglandin receptors in other cells (Marks, 1980; Rochette-Egly and Castagna, 1979).

Cyclic nucleotides also influence the development of macrophages. Elevations of cAMP by prostaglandin and isoproterenol have been linked to inhibition of proliferation of macrophage progenitors (CFU-c) induced by CSF (Kurland *et al.*, 1977; Taetle and Koessler, 1980; Oshita *et al.*, 1977). cGMP and agents that increase its levels (carbamylcholine, imidazole, $PGF_{2\alpha}$) increased the number of progenitor colonies (Kurland *et al.*, 1977; Oshita *et al.*, 1977; Taetle and Koessler, 1980).

4. MACROPHAGE PHAGOCYTOSIS

Macrophages have receptors for the Fc portion of IgG and for C3, and these function in recognition of certain opsonized microorganisms or other particles to be ingested (Hocking and Golde, 1979). Fc receptor expression is reduced by cAMP (Rhodes, 1975).

Several distinct steps subsequent to recognition have been described in the ingestion phase of phagocytosis: transmission of the message to initiate phagocytosis from receptor to effector, adhesion of the plasma membrane to the particle, assembly of pseudopodia, movement of pseudopodia to engulf the particle, and fusion of the pseudopodia (Stossel, 1976). Microfilaments and microtubules occur in areas of pseudopod formation, and polymerization and cross-linking of actin into microfilaments is activated by contact with particles to be ingested (Stossel and Hartwig, 1976). Myosin binds to actin and a cofactor in the complex and causes contraction of the gel, providing the force for pseudopod formation and engulfment of the particle (Stossel, 1976). Such a complex series of events offers many points for possible regulation.

A predictable effect of cAMP, based on observations with isolated enzyme systems (Kerrick and Hoar, 1981), would be the inactivation of myosin light-chain kinase through phosphorylation mediated by cAMP-dependent protein kinase. Myosin light-chain kinase requires Ca^{2+} and calmodulin to phosphorylate and activate myosin ATPase and contraction in macrophages (Trotter and Adelstein, 1979). The net effect of cAMP would thus be an inhibition of myosin function and consequently the prevention of phagocytosis.

Unequivocal inhibition of neutrophil phagocytosis by cAMP has been observed by several workers (for review see Ignarro, 1977). Several observations of a similar nature have also been made with mouse peritoneal macrophages (Lima *et al.*, 1974; Weissmann *et al.*, 1971; Welscher and Cruchaud, 1976; Stabinsky *et al.*, 1980). Not only does cAMP reduce phagocytosis of *Trypanosoma cruzi* by peritoneal macrophages, it also reduces the percentage of cells capable of incorporating the parasites (Wirth and Kierzenbaum, 1982). However, some lack of specificity of the nucleotide (Weissmann *et al.*, 1971) and reports of accumulation of cAMP in alveolar macrophages (Seyberth *et al.*, 1973) and human monocytes (Sandler *et al.*, 1975a) during phagocytosis of latex particles have raised doubts about the generality of the inhibition of cAMP. Since contact between lympho-cytes and latex particles results in cAMP increases (Manganiello *et al.*, 1971), definitive experiments with blood and alveolar macrophages must be performed with well-purified populations. Different inhibitory effects might be related to the different sources of energy required for particle ingestion: oxidative phos-phorylation provides the energy for alveolar macrophages, whereas glycolysis serves for peritoneal macrophages of the guinea pig (Hocking and Golde, 1979). Also uncertain at present is the question of transmethylation reactions in the phagocytosis signal: inhibitors of transmethylation were able to block phagocy-tosis by guinea pig and mouse peritoneal macrophages, but they were stimu-lated in human monocytes (Pike and Snyderman, 1981).

Phagocytic stimuli and a variety of inflammatory stimuli have been reported to induce the release of arachidonic acid and production of prostaglandins by macrophages (Brune *et al.*, 1979; Humes *et al.*, 1980). Indeed, an Fcγ receptor isolated from a macrophagelike cell line has an intrinsic phospholipase A_2 ac-tivity (Suzuki *et al.*, 1982). Reports of accompanying increases in cAMP induced by phagocytic stimuli have been sparse; Smith *et al.* (1980) have shown that one phagocytic stimulus, zymosan, induced an increase in cAMP that, if blocked by indomethacin, does not impair phagocytosis or the production of chemilumines-cence. A similar effect was observed with the calcium ionophore A23187. Degré and Rollag (1982) found that stimulation of enhanced phagocytosis by IFN was accompanied by increases in cAMP in mouse peritoneal macrophages. Howev-er, these effects were dissociated by *N*-ethylmaleimide, which prevented the increase in cAMP but not phagocytosis. These data indicate that the increases in macrophage prostaglandin levels and cAMP levels are not part of the initiation processes and may instead be involved in feedback inhibitory mechanisms. Interestingly, basal levels of cAMP in mouse peritoneal macrophages remained unaltered during phagocytosis of SRBC, zymosan, and aggregated IgG (Welscher and Cruchaud, 1976). On the other hand, phagocytosis of *S. aureus* by human monocytes is accompanied by a fall in cAMP (Merdrignac *et al.*, 1982). This is due to reduced adenylate cyclase within 10 min of exposure and, later, to increased phosphodiesterase activity.

In contrast to the inhibitory effects of cAMP, cGMP is positively linked to the induction of phagocytosis. Smith *et al.* (1980) observed that macrophage levels of cGMP are increased by both A23187 and zymosan. These increases were further shown to be dependent on Ca^{2+} and were not inhibited by indo-methacin. Pick *et al.* (1979) observed that lymphokine-rich fractions induce Ca^{2+} influx and it seems likely that both the ionophore and phagocytic stimuli will be shown to be associated with Ca^{2+} influx and/or mobilization in the mac-rophage, as they are in the granulocyte. Further support for a role of cGMP is found in the work of Stabinsky *et al.* (1980), who reported that stimulation of phagocytosis by tuftsin in mouse peritoneal macrophages was associated with increases in cGMP. Moreover, 8-bromo-cGMP itself stimulated phagocytosis. In addition, Lima *et al.* (1974) found that imidazole and levamisole, agents that raise cGMP in lymphocytes (Hadden *et al.*, 1975) and macrophages (Wright *et al.*, 1977), also augment phagocytosis of SRBC by mouse peritoneal macrophages.

Finally, elevated cGMP levels were detected in a mouse macrophage cell line when phagocytosis was occurring (Goodell *et al.*, 1978).

5. RESPIRATORY BURST AND RELEASE OF PROSTAGLANDINS AND PROTEINS BY MACROPHAGES

Macrophage activation and phagocytosis are difficult to separate pharmacologically because many phagocytic stimuli cause activation. Similarly, activation and release of biologically important molecules are difficult to separate because activation results in enhanced release (Soberman and Karnovsky, 1981).

It is generally believed that an early response to phagocytic stimuli is the "respiratory burst," which begins with an increase in NADPH and NADH oxidases, and results in high levels of O_2^- (superoxide), H_2O_2, and OH^- and chemiluminescence (Hocking and Golde, 1979; Soberman and Karnovsky, 1981; Klebanoff, 1982). The activation of NAD(P)H oxidase may be dependent on Ca^{2+} and calmodulin, as demonstrated in neutrophils (Jones *et al.*, 1982). Among the three forms of reduced oxygen, H_2O_2 is thought to be the agent responsible for microbicidal and perhaps tumoricidal activity (Nathan *et al.*, 1979a,b; Nathan and Cohn, 1980). Mouse resident or thioglycollate-induced peritoneal macrophages apparently do not undergo a significant respiratory burst during phagocytosis (Soberman and Karnovsky, 1981) and may therefore be useful in dissecting regulatory points for this versus other metabolic changes accompanying phagocytosis.

A variety of phagocytic as well as nonphagocytic stimuli are associated with stimulation of the phospholipid deacylation and arachidonic acid oxidation reactions discussed in Section 1, as well as the initiation of lysosomal enzyme synthesis and discharge and secretion of neutral protease (plasminogen activator) and of monokines such as LAF (North, 1981). For example, MDP, PMA, A23187, and zymosan all activate peritoneal macrophages for enhanced secretion of oxygen metabolites, lysosomal enzymes, neutral protease and PGE_2 production (Chang *et al.*, 1980; Pick and Keisari, 1981). The interdependence of these events is demonstrated by the mutual inhibition of PMA- or zymosan-induced protease and PGE_2 release by several protease inhibitors (Chang *et al.*, 1980) and by dexamethasone (Hamilton, 1980; Bonney *et al.*, 1980c).

Foster (1980) reviewed the inhibition of protease secretion by cAMP and several agents generating cAMP intracellularly and speculated that cGMP, formed by fatty acid peroxide stimulation of guanylate cyclase, promotes the secretion. The complexity of the reaction is indicated by studies of several other inhibitors including vinblastine, colchicine, vitamin A, and protein synthesis blockers(Vassalli *et al.*,1976a,b). Rosen *et al.*(1978) confirmed in a macrophagelike cell line that the cAMP inhibition of plasminogen activator secretion is mediated by cAMP-dependent protein kinase. Zymosan-induced lysosomal enzyme secretion was only partially inhibited by cAMP in resident mouse peritoneal macrophages (McMillan *et al.*, 1980), but immune complex- or opsonized SRBC-induced release was significantly inhibited by cAMP (Welscher and Cruchaud, 1976).

As mentioned above, aggregated IgE-provoked release of β-glucuronidase was associated with rapid and marked increases in cGMP (Dessaint *et al.*, 1980). Increased levels of cGMP were also observed within minutes of zymosan or A23187 addition to rat peritoneal macrophages (Smith *et al.*, 1980). These workers associated chemiluminescence induced by these agents with the lipoxygenase pathway of arachidonic acid metabolism (Smith and Weidemann, 1980). They showed that the simultaneous stimulation of the cyclooxygenase pathway and cAMP could be inhibited by indomethacin without affecting chemiluminescence or cGMP production. Others (Gemsa *et al.*, 1979; Bromberg and Pick, 1981) also reported that indomethacin inhibits the increase in cAMP by A23187, PMA, and other inducers of the oxidative burst in both rat and guinea pig peritoneal exudate macrophages. We interpret these findings to reflect activation of phospholipase and thus of both oxygenation pathways of arachidonic acid metabolism; only the lipoxygenase pathway gives rise to metabolites stimulating cGMP and chemiluminescence. In contrast, the cyclooxygenase pathway produces prostaglandins that stimulate cAMP, which may act as a negative feedback signal through inhibition of phospholipase (Lapetina and Cuatrecasas, 1979).

Bromberg and Pick (1980) have reported that lymphokine fractions containing MIF (and other lymphokines such as the mitogenic and chemotactic factor) and A23187 do not increase macrophage levels of cGMP. On the other hand, we have observed that similar lymphokine fractions increase cGMP in macrophages and have noted that a number of macrophage activators including MAF, MDP, *Listeria* factor, A23187, and PMA also increase macrophage levels of cGMP (Hadden and England, 1979; Hadden *et al.*, 1979b; Hadden, Schindler, and Coffey, Table 1 and unpublished observations). While the discrepancies between Bromberg and Pick's data and the data of ourselves and of Smith *et al.* (1980) are not easily resolvable, they most likely rest on technical problems involved in the measurement of cGMP levels in macrophages.

Another report involving monokines deserves mentioning in this section. Several years ago Diamantstein and Ulmer (1976) observed that the production and release of LAF from mouse peritoneal macrophages were stimulated by exogenous cGMP. Implicit in their discussion of the data was the suggestion that the production of LAF was cGMP dependent.

6. MACROPHAGE CYTOTOXICITY

The mechanisms responsible for the destruction of microbial pathogens and tumor cells are not known. Nathan *et al.* (1979a,b) and Nathan and Cohn (1980) have provided convincing evidence that mouse peritoneal macrophages, when activated by bacteria *in vivo*, release sufficient H_2O_2 to destroy neoplastic as well as bacterial cells *in vitro*. Most workers now concur that H_2O_2 mediates most of the cytotoxic activities of macrophages (North, 1981; Soberman and Karnovsky, 1981; Klebanoff, 1982). However, others (Weinberg *et al.*, 1978; Sorrell *et al.*,

1978) have presented evidence that reduced oxygen species were not involved in tumor cytoxicity. Proteases (Adams *et al.*, 1980) and/or phospholipases (Vadas *et al.*, 1981) secreted by macrophages may also participate in these reactions.

We are not aware of any reports on effects of cyclic nucleotides on H_2O_2 production, although H_2O_2 itself increase cGMP in some cells and might therefore act as a positive feedback regulator of activation. The effects of cAMP to inhibit phospholipase A_2 are believed to be indirect (Lapetina and Cuatrecasas, 1979) and thus may not be relevant to the control of the enzyme under circumstances in which it is secreted.

The roles of cyclic nucleotides in activation of macrophages for tumor cytotoxicity appear to be consistent with those in activation for phagocytosis. Schultz *et al.* (1978, 1979) have reported that IFN-mediated activation for tumor cytotoxicity was not inhibited by indomethacin, and is therefore independent of prostaglandins. Following activation, tumor cytotoxicity *per se* is also not inhibited by indomethacin and, in fact, may be enhanced (Shaw *et al.*, 1979; Taffet and Russell, 1981). Indeed, Schultz *et al.* (1978, 1979) and Schultz (1980) showed unequivocal inhibition of preactivated mouse peritoneal macrophage killing of tumor cells by PGE_1, PGE_2, cholera toxin, and hydrocortisone—all agents that increase cAMP levels. Dibutyryl cGMP and $PGF_{2\alpha}$ enhanced the cytotoxicity.

The influence of infections or tumor processes on host macrophage cyclic nucleotide metabolism is a separate but related issue. Droller and Remington (1975) found that infection of mice with *Toxoplasma*, a protozoan, resulted in reduced adenylate cyclase activity of the host's peritoneal macrophages in association with activation of these cells for tumor eradication. This finding supports the often-expressed view (North, 1981) that *in vivo* activation studies must be conducted in parallel with *in vitro* experiements in order to gain a complete understanding of relevant control mechanisms.

7. SUMMARY

In this survey of interrelated macrophage functions we have found that cAMP and agents that increase its levels are associated with inhibition of random and directed locomotion, Fc receptor expression, and responsiveness to lymphokines and other substances that signal the cells to become activated for enhanced phagocytosis, release of enzymes, bactericidal and tumoricidal activities, or to undergo proliferation. In contrast, cGMP and agents that raise its level are linked to enhancement of each of these functions. Many of these cGMP-raising agents act indirectly, possible through a Ca^{2+}-dependent pathway involving arachidonic acid release and metabolism by the lipoxygenase pathway. Other aspects of macrophage responses to lymphokines not discussed above that are apparently inhibited by cAMP and promoted by cGMP are aggregation (Rouveix *et al.*, 1980) and fusion (Papadimitrious and Sforcina, 1975). Mounting evidence suggests that cGMP, together with Ca^{2+}, may serve as second messengers to mediate some of these functions, particularly locomotion and proliferation.

The only positive aspects of cAMP action uncovered in macrophages so far appear to be the promotion of pyrogen and collagenase production in response to bacterial substances. These effects are linked to prostaglandin synthesis and secretion, and may serve an important role in attenuating at the proper time one or more responses involving membrane phospholipase activation and arachidonic acid release. This type of control mechanism might account for the fact that macrophages do not replicate as a result of phagocytosis. PGE and PGA are considered negative regulators of proliferation of a variety of hemopoietic cells (Moore, 1981).

None of the suggested mechanisms for cyclic nucleotide regulation of macrophage function will be proven until appropriate cyclic nucleotide-dependent kinases and their substrates are identified. Establishment of meaningful relationships between such molecules and biological effects will constitute the ambitious but necessary goal for the next decade.

ACKNOWLEDGMENTS. Portions of this work were supported by Grants CA-20178 and CA-08748 from the National Institutes of Health. We would like to acknowledge the participation of Drs. Arthur Englard, Matthew R. Duncan, Mashihiko Ito, Thomas E. Schindler, Elba M. Hadden, and John R. Sadlik in unpublished experiments cited in Table 1.

REFERENCES

Adams, D. O., Kao, K. -J., Farb, R., and Pizzo, S., 1980, Effector mechanisms of cytolytically activated macrophages. II. Secretion of a cytolytic factor of activated macrophages and its relationship to secreted neutral proteases, *J. Immunol.* **124**:293–300.

Adolfs, M. J. P., and Bonta, I. I., 1982, Low concentration of prostaglandin E_2 inhibit the prostacyclin-induced elevations of cyclic AMP in elicited populations of rat peritoneal macrophages, *Br. J. Pharmacol.* **75**:373–376.

Alexander, P., and Evans, R., 1971, Endotoxin and double stranded RNA render macrophages cytotoxic, *Nature New Biol.* **232**:76–78.

Atkinson, J. P., Sullivan, T. J., Kelly, J. P., and Parker, C. W., 1977, Stimulation by alcohols of cyclic nucleotide metabolism in human leukocytes, *J. Clin. Invest.* **60**:284–294.

Block, L. H., Aloni, B., Biemesderfer, D., Kashgarian, M., and Bitensky, M. W., 1978, Macrophage migration inhibition factor: Interactions with calcium, magnesium, and cyclic AMP, *J. Immunol.* **121**:1416–1421.

Bonney, R. J., Burger, S., Davies, P., Kuehl, F. A., Jr., and Humes, J. L., 1980a, Prostaglandin E_2 and prostacyclin elevate cyclic AMP levels in elicited populations of mouse peritoneal macrophages, *Adv. Prostaglandin Thromboxane Res.* **8**:1961–1963.

Bonney, R. J., Davies, P., Kuehl, F. A., Jr., and Humes, J. L., 1980b, Arachidonic acid oxygenation products produced by mouse peritioneal macrophages responding to inflammatory stimuli, *J. Reticuloendothel. Soc.* **28**:113S–115S.

Bonney, R. J., Wightman, P. D., Dahlgren, M. E., Davies, P., Kuehl, F. A., Jr., and Humes, J. L., 1980c, Effect of RNA and protein synthesis inhibitors on release of inflammatory mediators by macrophages responding to phorbol myristate acetate, *Biochim. Biophys. Acta* **633**:410–421.

Bourne, H. R., Lichtenstein, L. M., Melmon, K. L., Henney, C. S., Weinstein, Y., and Shearer, G. M., 1974, Modulation of inflammation and immunity by cyclic AMP, *Science* **184**:19–28.

Bromberg, Y., and Pick, E., 1980, Cyclic GMP metabolism in macrophages. I. Regulation of cyclic GMP levels by calcium and stimulation of cyclic GMP synthesis by NO-generation agents, *Cell. Immunol.* **52**:73–83.

Bromberg, Y., and Pick, E., 1981, Activation of macrophage adenylate cyclase by stimulants of the oxidative burst and by arachidonic acid—two distinct mechanisms, *Cell. Immunol.* **61**:90–103.

Brune, K., Kalin, H., Schmidt, R., and Hecker, E., 1979, Regulation of prostaglandin release from macrophages, *Adv. Inflammation Res.* **1**:467–476.

Chang, J., Wigley, F., and Newcombe, D., 1980, Neutral protease activation of peritoneal macrophage prostaglandin synthesis, *Proc. Natl. Acad. Sci. USA* **77**:4736–4740.

Chedid, L., Audibert, F., and Johnson, A. G., 1978, Biological activities of muramyl depeptide, a synthetic glycopeptide analogous to bacterial immunoregulating agents, *Prog. Allergy* **25**:63–105.

Coffey, R. G., and Hadden, J. W., 1981, Arachidonate and metabolites in mitogen activation of lymphocyte guanylate cyclase, in: *Advances in Immunopharmacology* (J. Hadden, L. Chedid, P. Mullen, and F. Spreafico, eds.), pp. 365–373, Pergamon Press, Elmsford, N.Y.

Coffey, R. G., Hadden, E. M., and Hadden, J. W., 1977, Evidence for cyclic GMP and calcium mediation of lymphocyte activation by mitogens, *J. Immunol.* **119**:1387–1394.

Coffey, R. G., Hadden, E. M., and Hadden, J. W., 1981, Phytohemagglutinin stimulation of guanylate cyclase in human lymphocytes, *J. Biol. Chem.* **256**:4418–4424.

Craven, P. A., and DeRubertis, F. R., 1982, Relationship of calcium stimulation of cyclic GMP and lipid peroxidation in the rat kidney: Evidence for involvement of calmodulin and separate pathways of peroxidation in cortex versus inner medulla, *Metab. Clin. Exp.* **31**:103–116.

Degré, M., and Rollag, H., 1982, Effect of murine beta-interferon preparation on phagocytosis and cyclic AMP levels in mouse peritoneal macrophages, *J Interferon Res.* **2**:151–158.

Deguchi, T., and Yoshioka, M., 1982, L-Arginine identified as an endogenous activator for soluble guanylate cyclase from neuroblastoma cells, *J. Biol. Chem.* **257**:10147–10151.

Dessaint, J., Waksman, B. H., Metzger, H., and Capron, A., 1980, Cytophilic binding of IgE to the macrophage. III. Involvement of cyclic GMP and calicum in macrophage activation by dimeric or aggregated rat myeloma IgE, *Cell. Immunol.* **51**:280–292.

Diamantstein, T., and Ulmer, A. 1976. Two distinct lymphocyte-stimulating soluble factors (LAF) released from murine peritoneal cells. I. The cellular source and the effect of cyclic GMP on their release, *Immunology* **30**:741–748.

Droller, M. J., and Remington, J. S., 1975, Lymphocyte and macrophage adenylcyclase activity in animals with enhanced cell-mediated resistance to infection and tumors, *Cell. Immunol.* **19**:349–355.

Duncan, M. R., Sadlik, J. R., and Hadden, J. W., 1982, Glucocorticoid modulation of lymphokine-induced macrophage proliferation, *Cell. Immunol.* **67**:23–26.

Edelson, P. J., 1981, Macrophage plasma membrane enzymes as differentiation markers of macrophage activation, *Lymphokines* **3**:57–84.

Foster, S., 1980, Cyclic nucleotides, possible intracellular mediators of macrophage activation and secretory processes, *Agents Actions* **10**:556–560.

Friedman, S. A., Remold-O'Donnell, E., and Piessens, W. F., 1979, Enhanced PGE production by MAF-treated peritoneal exudate macrophages, *Cell. Immunol.* **42**:213–218.

Gallin, J., Sandler, J. A., Clyman, R. I., Manganiello, V. C., and Vaughan, M., 1978, Agents that increase cyclic AMP inhibit accumulation of cGMP and depress human monocyte locomotion, *J. Immunol.* **120**:492–496.

Gemsa, D., Steggemann, L., Menzel, J., and Till, G., 1975, Release of cyclic AMP from macrophages by stimulation with prostaglandins, *J. Immunol.* **114**:1422–1423.

Gemsa, D., Steggemann, L., Till, G., and Resch, K., 1977, Enhancement of the PGE_1 response of macrophages by concanavalin A and colchicine, *J. Immunol.* **119**:524–529.

Gemsa, D., Seitz, M., Kramer, W., Grimm, W., Till, G., and Resch, K., 1979, Ionophore A23187 raises cyclic AMP levels in macrophages by stimulating prostaglandin E formation, *Exp. Cell Res.* **118**:55–62.

Goetzl, E. J., Derian, C., and Valone, F. H., 1980, The extracellular and intracellular roles of hydroxyeicosatetraenoic acids in the modulation of polymorphonuclear leukocyte and macrophage function, *J. Reticuloendothel. Soc.* **28**(Suppl.):105–111.

Goldberg, N. D., Graff, G., Haddox, M. K., Stephenson, J. H., Glass, D. B., and Moser, M. E., 1978, Redox modulation of splenic cell soluble guanylate cyclase activity: Activation by hydrophilic and hydrophobic oxidants represented by ascorbic and dehydroascorbic acids, fatty acid hydroperoxides, and prostaglandin endoperoxides, *Adv. Cyclic Nucleotide Res.* **9**:101–130.

Goodell, E. M., Bilgen, S., and Carchman, R. A., 1978, Biochemical characteristics of phagocytosis in the P388 D_1 cell, *Exp. Cell Res.* **114**:57–62.

Grunspan-Swirsky, A., and Pick, E., 1978, Enhancement of macrophage adenylate cyclase by microtubule disrupting drugs, *Immunopharmacology* **1**:71–82.

Grunspan-Swirsky, A., and Pick, E., 1979, Facilitation of adenylate cyclase stimulation in macrophages by lectins, *Cell. Immunol.* **45**:415–427.

Guarneri, J. J., and Laurenzi, G. A., 1968, Effect of alcohol on the mobilization of alveolar macrophages, *J. Lab. Clin. Med.* **72**:40–51.

Hadden, E. M., Sadlik, J. R., Coffey, R. G., and Hadden, J. W., 1982, Effects of phorbol myristate acetate and a lymphokine on cyclic 3′, 5′-guanosine monophosphate levels and proliferation of macrophages, *Cancer Res.* **42**:3064–3069.

Hadden, J. W., and Englard, A., 1977, Molecular aspects of macrophage activation and proliferation, in: *Immunopharmacology*, Volume 3 (J. W. Hadden, R. G. Coffey, and F. Spreafico, eds.), pp. 87–100, Plenum Press, New York.

Hadden, J. W., and Englard, A., 1979, Molecular aspects of macrophage activation and proliferation, in: *10th International Course on Transplanation and Clinical Immunology*, pp. 279–296, Excerpta Medica, Amsterdam.

Hadden, J. W., Hadden, E. M., Haddox, M. K., and Goldberg, N. D., 1972, Guanosine cyclic 3′,5′-monophosphate: A possible intracellular mediator of mitogenic influences in lymphocytes, *Proc. Natl. Acad. Sci. USA* **69**:3024–3027.

Hadden, J. W., Johnson, E. M., Hadden, E. M., Coffey, R. G., and Johnson, L. D., 1975, Cyclic GMP and lymphocyte activation, in: *Immune Recognition* (A. S. Rosenthal, ed.), pp. 359–390, Academic Press, New York.

Hadden, J. W., Coffey, R. G., and Spreafico, F. (eds.), 1977, *Immunopharmacology*, Plenum Press, New York.

Hadden, J. W., Sadlik, J. R., and Hadden, E. M., 1978, The induction of macrophage proliferation in vitro by a lymphocyte produced factor, *J. Immunol.* **121**:231–238.

Hadden, J. W., Sadlik, J. R., Englard, A., Warfel, A., and Hadden, E., 1979a, Lymphokine-induced macrophage proliferation, activation, and fusion, in: *Biochemical Characterization of the Lymphokines* (A. deWeck, ed.), pp. 235–242, Academic Press, New York.

Hadden, J. W., Englard, A., Sadlik, J. R., and Hadden, E., 1979b, The comparative effects of isoprinosine, levamisole, muramyl dipeptide and SM1213 on lymphocyte and macrophage proliferation and activation in vitro, *Int. J. Immunopharmacol.* **1**:17–27.

Hagmann, J., and Fishman, P. H., 1980, Modulation of adenylate cyclase in intact macrophages by microtubules: Opposing actions of colchicine and chemotactic factor, *J. Biol. Chem.* **255**:2659–2662.

Hamilton, J. A., 1980, Stimulation of macrophage prostaglandin and neutrophil protease production by phorbol esters as a model for the induction of vascular changes associated with tumor promotion, *Cancer Res.* **40**:2273–2280.

Higgins, T. J., and David, J. R., 1976, Effect of isoproterenol and aminophylline on cyclic AMP levels of guinea pig macrophages, *Cell. Immunol.* **27**:1–10.

Higgins, T. J., Winston, C. T., and David, J. R., 1976. Effect of migration inhibitory factor (MIF) on cyclic AMP levels of guinea pig macrophages, *Cell. Immunol.* **27**:11–16.

Hirata, F., and Axelrod, J., 1980, Phospholipid methylation and biological signal transmission, *Science* **209**:1082–1090.

Hirata, F., Corcoran, B. A., Venkatasubramanian, K., Schiffmann, E., and Axlerod, J., 1979, Chemoattractants stimulate degradation of methylated phospholipids and release of arachidonic acid in rabbit leukocytes, *Proc. Natl. Acad. Sci. USA* **76**:2640–2645.

Hocking, W. G., and Golde, D. W., 1979, The pulmonary-alveolar macrophage, *N. Engl. J. Med.* **301**:580–587, 639–645.

Homma, Y., Onozaki, K., Hashimoto, T., Nagai, Y., and Takenawa, T., 1982, Differential activation of phospholipids metabolism by formylated peptide and ionophore A23187 in guinea pig peritoneal macrophages, *J. Immunol.* **129**:1619–1626.

Hsueh, W., Desai, U., Gonzalez-Crussi, F., Lamb, R., and Chu, A., 1981, Two phospholipase pools for prostaglandin synthesis in macrophages, *Nature (London)* **290**:710–713.

Humes, J. L., Burger, S., Galavage, M., Kuehl, F. A., Jr., Wightman, P. D., Dahlgren, M. E., Davies, P., and Bonney, R. J., 1980, The diminished production of arachidonic acid oxygenation products by elicited mouse peritoneal macrophages: Possible mechanisms, *J. Immunol.* **124:**2110–2116.

Ignarro, L. J., 1977, Regulation of polymorphonuclear leukocyte, macrophage, and platelet function, in: *Immunopharmacology* (J. W. Hadden, R. G. Coffey, and F. Spreafico, eds.), pp. 61–86, Plenum Press, New York.

Jones, H. P., Ghai, G., Petrone, W. F., and McCord, J. M., 1982, Calmodulin-dependent stimulation of the NADPH oxidase of human neutrophils, *Biochim. Biophys. Acta* **714:**152–156.

Kalisker, A., Nelson, H. E., and Middleton, E., 1977, Drug-induced changes of adenylate cyclase activity in cells from asthmatic and nonasthmatic subjects, *J. Allergy Clin. Immunol.* **60:**259–265.

Kerrick, W. G. L., and Hoar, P. E., 1981, Inhibition of smooth muscle tension by cyclic AMP-dependent protein kinase, *Nature (London)* **292:**253–255.

Klebanoff, S. J., 1982, Oxygen-dependent cytotoxic mechanisms of phagocytes, in: *Phagocytic Cells.* (J. I. Gallin and A. S. Fauci, eds.), pp. 111-162, Raven Press, New York.

Koopman, W. J., Gillis, M. H., and David, J. R., 1973, Prevention of MIF activity by agents known to increase cellular cyclic AMP, *J. Immunol.* **110:**1609–1614.

Kurland, J. I., Hadden, J. W., and Moore, M. A. S., 1977, Role of cyclic nucleotides in the preparation of committed granulocyte-macrophage progenitor cells, *Cancer Res.* **37:**4535–4538.

Lapetina, E. G., and Cuatrecasas, P., 1979, Rapid inactivation of cyclooxygenase activity after stimulation of intact platelets, *Proc. Natl. Acad. Sci. USA* **76:**121–125.

Leclerc, C., and Chedid, L., 1982, Macrophage activation by synthetic muramyl peptides, *Lymphokines* **7:**1–22.

Lima, A. O., Javierre, M. Q., Dias da Silva, W., and Camara, D. S., 1974, Immunological phagocytosis: Effect of drugs on phosphodiesterase activity, *Experientia* **30:**945–946.

Manganiello, V., Evans, W. H., Stossel, T. P., Mason, R. J., and Vaughan, M., 1971, The effect of polystyrene beads on cyclic 3′,5SFT-adenosine monophosphate concentration in leukocytes, *J. Clin. Invest.* **50:**2741–2744.

Marks, F., 1980, Prevention of phorbol ester-induced catecholamine refractoriness by inhibitors of protein and RNA biosynthesis in mouse epidermis in vivo, *FEBS Lett.* **114:**261–264.

Marone, G., Lichtenstein, L. M., and Plaut, M., 1980, Hydrocortisone and human lymphocytes—Increases in cyclic AMP and potentiation of adenylate cyclase-activating agents, *J. Pharmacol. Exp. Ther.* **215:**469–478.

McMillan, R. M., MacIntrye, D. E., Beesley, J. E., and Gordon, J. L., 1980. Regulation of macrophage lysosomal enzyme secretion: Role of arachidonate metabolites, divalent cations and cyclic AMP, *J. Cell Sci.* **44:**299–316.

Merdrignac, G., Duval, J., Gouranton, J., and Genetet, B., 1982, Changes in cyclic AMP metabolism during phagocytosis of S. aureus by human monocytes, *J. Reticuloendothel. Soc.* **32:**209–218.

Minkin, C., Blackman, L., Newbrey, J., Pokress, S., Posek, R., and Walling, M., 1977, Effects of parathyroid hormone and calcitonin on adenylate cyclase in murine mononuclear phagocytes, *Biochem. Biophys. Res. Commun.* **76:**875–881.

Moore, M. A. S., 1981, Macrophage regulatory networks, in: *The Lymphokines: Biochemistry and Biological Activity* (J. W. Hadden and W. E. Steward, II, eds.), pp. 305–326, Humana Press, Clifton, N.J.

Nathan, C. F., and Cohn, Z. A., 1980, Role of oxygen-dependent mechanisms in antibody-induced lysis of tumor cells by activated macrophages, *J. Exp. Med.* **152:**198–208.

Nathan, C. F., Bruckner, L. H., Silverstein, S. C., and Cohn, Z. A., 1979a, Extracellular cytolysis by activated macrophages and granulocytes. I. Pharmacologic triggering of effector cells and the release of hydrogen peroxide, *J. Exp. Med.* **149:**84–99.

Nathan, C. F., Silverstein, S.C., Bruckner, L. H., and Cohn, Z. A., 1979b, Extracellular cytolysis by activated macrophages and granulocytes. II. Hydrogen peroxide as a mediator of cytotoxicity, *J. Exp. Med.* **149:**100–113.

North, R. J., 1981, An introduction to macrophage activation, *Lymphokines* **3:**1–10.

Oropeza-Rendon, R. L., Speth, V., Hiller, G., Weber, K., and Fischer, H., 1979, Prostaglandin E_1

  reversibly induces morphological changes in macrophages and inhibits phagocytosis, *Exp. Cell Res.* **119:**365–371.

Oshita, A. K., Rothstein, G., and Lonngi, G., 1977, cGMP stimulation of stem cell proliferation, *Blood* **49:**585–592.

Papadimitrious, J. M., and Sforcina, D., 1975, The effects of drugs on monocytic fusion in vivo, *Exp. Cell Res.* **91:**233–236.

Pick, E., 1972, Cyclic AMP affects macrophage migration, *Nature New Biol.* **238:**176–177.

Pick, E., 1977, The mechanism of action of soluble lymphocyte mediators. IV. Effect of migration inhibitory factor (MIF) on macrophage cyclic AMP and on responsiveness to adenylate cyclase stimulators, *Cell. Immunol.* **32:**329–340.

Pick, E., and Keisari, Y., 1981, Superoxide anion and hydrogen peroxide production by chemically elicited peritoneal macrophages, *Cell. Immunol.* **59:**301–318.

Pick, E., Seger, M., Honig, S., and Griffel, B., 1979, Intracellular mediation of lymphokine action: Mimicry of migration inhibitory factor (MIF) action by phorbol myristate acetate (PMA) and the ionophore A23187, *Ann. N.Y. Acad. Sci.* **332:**378–394.

Pike, M. C., and Synderman, R., 1981, Requirement of transmethylation reactions for immune effector functions, *Lymphokines* **3:**424–444.

Pike, M. C., and Snyderman, R., 1982, Transmethylation reactions regulate affinity and functional activity of chemotactic factor receptors on macrophages, *Cell* **28:**107–114.

Pike, M. C., Kredich, N. M., and Snyderman, R., 1978, Requirement of S-adenosyl-L-methionine-mediated methylation for human monocyte chemotaxis, *Proc. Natl. Acad. Sci. USA* **75:**3928–3932.

Remold-O'Donnell, E., 1974, Stimulation and desensitization of macrophage adenylate cyclase by prostaglandins and catecholamines, *J. Biol. Chem.* **249:**3615–3621.

Remold-O'Donnel, E., and Remold, H. G., 1974, The enhancement of macrophage adenylate cyclase by products of activated lymphocytes, *J. Biol. Chem.* **249:**3622–3627.

Rhodes, J., 1975, Modulation of macrophage Fc receptor expression in vitro by insulin and cyclic nucleotides, *Nature (London)* **257:**597–599.

Rigaud, M., Durand, J., and Breton, J. C., 1979, Transformation of arachidonic acid into 12-hydroxy-5,8,10,14-eicosatetraenoic acid by mouse peritoneal macrophages, *Biochim. Biophys. Acta* **573:**408–412.

Rochette-Egly, C., and Castagna, M., 1979, A tumor-promoting phorbol ester inhibits the cyclic AMP response of rat embryo fibroblasts to catecholamines and prostaglandin E_1, *FEBS Lett.* **103:**38–42.

Rohrer, S. D., and Atkinson, J. P., 1980, The effect of potential agonists and phagocytic stimuli on the cyclic GMP concentrations in several macrophage populations, *J. Reticuloendothel. Soc.* **28:**343–356.

Rosen, N., Schneck, J., Bloom, B. R., and Rosen, O. M., 1978, Inhibition of plasminogen activator secretion by cyclic AMP in a macrophage-like cell line, *J. Cyclic Nucleotide Res.* **4:**345–358.

Rouveix, B., Badenoch-Jones, P., Larno, S., and Turk, J. L., 1980, Lymphokine-induced macrophage aggregation: The possible role of cyclic nucleotides, *Immunopharmacology* **2:**319–326.

Sadlik, J. R., Hadden, E. M., and Hadden, J. W., 1983, Lymphokine-induced macrophage proliferation: Purification and characterization of antigen induced MGF/CSF, in: *Advances in Immunopharmacology*, Volume 2 (J. W. Hadden, L. Chedid, P. Dukor, F. Spreafico, and, D. Willoughby, eds.) pp. 221–227, Pergamon Press, Elmsford, New York.

Sandler, J. A., Gallin, J. I., and Vaughan, M., 1975a, Effects of serotonin, carbamylcholine, and ascorbic acid on leukocyte cyclic GMP and chemotaxis, *J. Cell Biol.* **67:**480–483.

Sandler, J. A., Clyman, R. I., Manganiello, V. C., and Vaughan, M., 1975b, Effect of serotonin and derivatives on guanosine 3′,5′-monophosphate in human monocytes, *J. Clin. Invest.* **55:**431–435.

Sandler, J. A., Smith, T. K., Manganiello, V. C., and Kirkpatrick, C. H., 1975c, Stimulation of monocyte cGMP by leukocyte dialysates—Antigen-independent property of dialyzable transfer factor, *J. Clin. Invest.* **56:**1271–1279.

Schultz, R. M., 1980, Macrophage activation by interferons, *Lymphokine Rep.* **1:**463–98.

Schultz, R. M., Pavlidis, N. A., Stylos, W. A., and Chirigos, M. A., 1978, Regulation of macrophage tumoricidal function: A role for prostaglandins of the E series, *Science* **202:**320–321.

Schultz, R. M., Pavlidis, N. A., Stoychkov, J. N., and Chirigos, M. A., 1979, Prevention of macrophage tumoricidal activity by agents known to increase cellular cyclic AMP, *Cell. Immunol.* **42**:71–78.

Seyberth, H. W., Schmidt-Gayk, H., Jakobs, K. H., and Hackenthal, E., 1973, Cyclic adenosine monophosphate in phagocytizing granulocytes and alveolar macrophages, *J. Cell Biol.* **57**:567–571.

Shaw, J. O., Russell, S. W., Printz, M. P., and Skidgel, R. A., 1979, Macrophage-mediated tumor cell killing: Lack of dependence on the cyclooxygenase pathway of prostaglandin synthesis, *J. Immunol.* **123**:50–54.

Simchowitz, L., Fischbein, L. C. , Spilberg, I., and Atkinson, J. P., 1980, Induction of a transient elevation in intracellular levels of adenosine 3′,5′-cyclic monophosphate by chemotactic factors: An early event in human neutrophil activation, *J. Immunol.* **124**:1482–1491.

Smith, R. L., and Weidemann, M. J., 1980, Reactive oxygen production associated with arachidonic acid metabolism by peritoneal macrophages, *Biochem. Biophys. Res. Commun.* **96**:973–980.

Smith, R. L., Hunt, N. H., Merritt, J. E., Evans, T., and Weidemann, M. J., 1980, Cyclic nucleotide metabolism and reactive oxygen production by macrophages, *Biochem. Biophys. Res. Commun.* **96**:1079–1087.

Snyderman, R., and Goetzl, E. J., 1981, Molecular and cellular mechanisms of leukocyte chemotaxis, *Science* **213**:830–837.

Soberman, R. J., and Karnovsky, M. L., 1981, Biochemical properties of activated macrophages, *Lymphokines* **3**:11–31.

Sorrell, T. C., Lehrer, R. I., and Cline, M. J., 1978, Mechanism of nonspecific macrophage-mediated cytotoxicity: Evidence for lack of dependence upon oxygen, *J. Immunol.* **120**:347–352.

Stabinsky, Y., Bar-Shavit, A., Fridkin, M., and Goldman, R., 1980, On the mechanism of action of the phagocytosis-stimulating peptide tuftsin, *Mol. Cell. Biochem.* **30**:71–77.

Stephens, C. G., and Snyderman, R., 1982, Cyclic nucleotides regulate the morphologic alterations required for chemotaxis in monocytes, *J. Immunol.* **128**:1192–1197.

Stossel, T. P., 1976, The mechanism of phagocytosis, *J. Reticuloendothel. Soc.* **19**:237–245.

Stossel, T. P., and Hartwig, J. H., 1976, Interactions of actin, myosin, and a new actin-binding protein of rabbit pulmonary macrophages. II. Role in cytoplasmic movement and phagocytosis, *J. Cell Biol.* **68**:602–619.

Suzuki, T., Saito-Takai, T., Sadasivan, R., and Nitta, T., 1982, Biochemical signal transmitted by Fcγ receptors: Phospholipase A_2 activity of Fcγ2b receptors of murine macrophage cell line P388D$_1$. *Proc. Natl. Acad. Sci. USA* **79**:591–595.

Taetle, R., and Koessler, A., 1980, Effects of cyclic nucleotides and prostaglandins on normal and abnormal human myeloid progenitor proliferation, *Cancer Res.* **40**:1223–1229.

Taffet, S. M., and Russell, S. W., 1981, Macrophage-mediated tumor cell killing: Regulation of expression of cytolytic activity by prostaglandin E, *J. Immunol.* **126**:424–430.

Thompson, W. J., Ross, C. P., Strada, S. J., Hersh, E. M., and Lavis, V. R., 1980, Comparative analyses of cyclic adenosine 3′,5′-monophosphate phosphodiesterases of human peripheral blood monocytes and cultured P388D$_1$ cells, *Cancer Res.* **40**:1955–1960.

Tovey, M. G., and Rochette-Egly, C., 1980, The effect of interferon on cyclic nucleotides, *Ann. N.Y. Acad. Sci.* **350**:266–278.

Tovey, M. G., Rochette-Egly, C., and Castagna, M., 1979, Effect of interferon on concentrations of cyclic nucleotides in cultured cells, *Proc. Natl. Acad. Sci. USA* **76**:3890–3893.

Trotter, J. A., and Adelstein, R. S., 1979, Macrophage myosin: Regulation of actin-activated ATPase activity by phosphorylation of the 20,000-dalton light chain, *J. Biol. Chem.* **254**:8781–8785.

Vadas, P., Wasi, S., Movat, H. Z., and Hay, J. B., 1981, Extracellular phospholipase A_2 mediates inflammatory hyperaemia, *Nature (London)* **293**:583–585.

Valone, F. H., Franklin, M., Sun, F. F., and Goetzl, E. J., 1980, Alveolar macrophage lipoxygenase products of arachidonic acid: Isolation and recognition as the predominant constituents of the neutrophil chemotactic activity elaborated by alveolar macrophages, *Cell. Immunol.* **54**:390–401.

Vassalli, J. D., Hamilton, J., and Reich, E., 1976a, Macrophage plasminogen activator: Modulation of enzyme production by anti-inflammatory steroids, mitotic inhibitors, and cyclic nucleotides, *Cell* **8**:271–281.

Vassalli, J. D., Hamilton, J., and Reich, E., 1976b, Macrophage plasminogen activator: Induction by concanavalin A and phorbol myristate acetate, *Cell* **11**:695–705.

Wahl, S., Wahl, L., McCarthy, J., Chedid, L., and Mergenhagen, S., 1979, Macrophage activation by mycobacterial water soluble compounds and synthetic muramyl dipeptide, *J. Immunol.* **122**:2226–2231.

Watson, J., 1977, Involvement of cyclic nucleotides as intracellular mediators in the induction of antibody synthesis, in: *Immunopharmacology* (J. W. Hadden, R. G. Coffey, and F. Spreafico, eds.), pp. 29–45, Plenum Press, New York.

Wedner, H. J., Chan, B. Y., Parker C. S., and Parker, C. W., 1979, Cyclic nucleotide phosphodiesterase activity in human peripheral blood lymphocytes and monocytes, *J. Immunol.* **123**:725–732.

Weinberg, J. B., Chapman, H. A., Jr., and Hibbs, J. B., Jr., 1978, Characterization of the effects of endotoxin on macrophage tumor cell killing, *J. Immunol.* **121**:72–80.

Weissmann, G., Dukor, P., and Zurier, R. B., 1971, Effects of cyclic AMP on release of lysosomal enzymes from phagocytes, *Nature New Biol.* **231**:131–133.

Welscher, H. D., and Cruchaud, A., 1976, The influence of various particles and 3′,5′ cyclic adenosine monophosphate on release of lysosomal enzymes by mouse macrophages, *J. Reticuloendothel. Soc.* **20**:405–420.

Welscher, H. D., and Cruchaud, A., 1978, Conditions for maximal synthesis of cyclic AMP by mouse macrophages in response to adrenergic stimulation, *Eur. J. Immunol.* **8**:180–184.

Wightman, P. D., Humes, J. L., Davies, P., and Bonney, R. J., 1981a, Identification and characterization of two phospholipase A_2 activities in resident mouse peritoneal macrophages, *Biochem. J.* **195**:427–433.

Wightman, P. D., Dahlgren, M. E., Hall, J. C., Davies, P., and Bonney, R. J., 1981b, Identification and characterization of a phospholipase C activity in resident mouse peritoneal macrophages: Inhibition of the enzyme by phenothiazines, *Biochem. J.* **197**:523–526.

Wirth, J. J., and Kierzenbaum, F., 1982, Inhibitory action of elevated levels of cyclic AMP on phagocytosis: Effects on macrophage–*Trypanosoma cruzi* interaction, *J. Immunol.* **129**:2759–2762.

Wright, D. G., Kirkpatrick, I. C. H., and Gallin, J. I., 1977, Effects of levamisole on neutrophils and mononuclear cells from normal individuals and from patients with abnormal leukocyte chemotaxis, in: *Progress in Cancer Research and Therapy II* (M. A. Chirigos, ed.), pp. 227–234, Raven Press, New York.

Zendegui, J. G., and Klein, T. W., 1982, Reduction in cyclic 3′,5′-adenosine monophosphate phosphodiesterase activity in exudate and cultured mouse peritoneal macrophages, *J. Reticuloendothel. Soc.* **31**:455–468.

Ziboh, V. A., Miller, A. M., Wu, M.-C., Yunis, A. A., Jimenez, J., and Wong, G., 1982, Induced release and metabolism of arachidonic acid from myeloid cells by purified colony-stimulating factor, *J. Cell. Physiol.* **113**:67–72.

3

The Biology of Mast Cell Secretion and Its Pharmacologic Modulation

ROBERT F. LEMANSKE, JR., and MICHAEL A. KALINER

1. INTRODUCTION

Exocytosis is the process by which cells transfer intracellularly manufactured products into the extracellular milieu. Many cells utilize this process and its presence is, for the most part, essential to homeostasis and the ultimate survival of the organism. In some cases, however, the release of intracellular chemical contents, albeit under specific control mechanisms, may have untoward consequences to the surrounding tissues. Such is the case for mast cell or basophil secretion, which is the initial cellular event in evoking immediate hypersensitivity reactions.

The human mast cell and basophil are secretory cells that are capable of releasing both preformed as well as newly synthesized molecules termed mediators, which actually cause the allergic reaction. These mediators play diverse roles in the pathogenesis of various immunologic and inflammatory processes, including immediate and late-phase allergic reactions, host defence against parasitic infestations, and numerous skin conditions. In addition to their role in inflammatory reactions, the mast cell and basophil have provided useful insights into general mechanisms of secretion. This chapter will, therefore, focus on the mast cell and basophil as a model to provide an overview of the biologic phenomenon of secretion and its modulation. Before exploring this subject in detail, however, it may be helpful to provide a general description of the origin, distribution, morphology, and immunologic function of these cells.

ROBERT F. LEMANSKE, JR. • Departments of Pediatrics and Medicine, University of Wisconsin Medical School, Madison, Wisconsin 53792.   MICHAEL A. KALINER • Allergic Diseases Section, Laboratory of Clinical Investigation, National Institute of Allergy and Infectious Diseases, National Institutes of Health, Bethesda, Maryland 20205.

1.1. ORIGIN, DISTRIBUTION, AND MORPHOLOGY

Both the mast cell and the basophil were first described by Paul Ehrlich while he was a medical student approximately 100 years ago. He noted the mast cell to be a deeply staining metachromatic cell and, because of its "overfed" appearance, derived its name from the German "mastüng," which means to masticate or to chew.

Although it has been suggested that the mast cell may be derived from various precursor cells such as histiocytes, fibroblasts, undifferentiated mes-enchymal cells, endothelial cells, eosinophils, plasmatocytes, lymphocytes, plasma cells, thymocytes, and reticular cells (Selye, 1965), its precise derivation is unknown. Experiments involving both irradiated beige mice (Kitamura *et al.*, 1977) and congenitally mast cell-deficient mice of the w^v genotype (Kitamura and Hatanaka, 1978) suggest that murine mast cells may be derived from bone mar-row precursors. In the mouse, thymus cells appear to differentiate into mast cells under a variety of conditions (Ginsburg and Sachs, 1962; Ishizaka *et al.*, 1976). Further, lymphocyte derived-growth factors promote mast cell prolifera-tion in cultures of mouse lymphoid tissue, suggesting that, regardless of the nature of the mast cell precursor, mast cell number may be regulated by lympho-cyte-derived factors (Ginsburg *et al.*, 1978).

The mammalian mast cell is generally ovoid or irregularly elongate in tissue and varies in size from 10 to 30 μm. The characteristic feature of the mast cell is the presence of dense cytoplasmic granules. Each granule averages 0.2–0.4 μm in diameter and stains intensely with a variety of metachromatic dyes such as toluidine blue. In the rat, the granule is amorphous in character; in man, the granule contains lattice or scroll-like structures (Caulfield *et al.*, 1980), which become amorphous during degranulation. The nucleus of the mast cell in hema-toxylin and eosin-stained sections is similar to that of the plasma cell. The normal complement of subcellular organelles is present including mitochondria, rough endoplasmic reticulum, a sparse Golgi complex, and abundant sub-membranous filaments (Benditt and Lagunoff, 1964).

In human tissues, mast cells are relatively abundant in the skin, lymphoid tissue, uterus, urinary bladder, tongue, synovia, mesentery, subserosal and submucosal layers of the digestive tract, and around large and small blood vessels. In the lungs, mast cells are found both in bronchial airway connective tissues and in peripheral intraalveolar spaces. Human skin contains approx-imately 10,000 mast cells/mm^3, which are found in greatest numbers near blood vessels, hair follicles, and sebaceous and sweat glands.

Recent observations have emphasized that mast cells may exhibit intra-species as well as interspecies heterogeneity (Barrett and Pearce, 1982; Leman-ske *et al.*, 1983a,b; Pearce *et al.*, 1982; Lichtenstein *et al.*, 1979). In the rat gastroin-testinal tract, for example, at least three types of granulated cells can be differentially stained with metachromatic dyes. The granulated cells that reside in the submucosal areas have been termed "typical" mast cells; those in the mucosa have been termed "atypical" or mucosal mast cells; and a third cell type that contains large granules resides in the intraepithelial regions and has been termed a globule leukocyte (Lemanske *el al.*, 1983a,b). Interestingly, in addition to the morphologic differences ascribed to typical and atypical mast cells, functional differences in response to mast cell secretagogues and various pharmacologic agents have also been reported (Pearce *et al.*, 1982). Recent technologic advances have allowed the separation of relatively pure preparations of human pulmonary mast cells (Schulman *et al.*, 1982), and preliminary data have suggested that some of the biochemical events involved in mediator release may differ from those previously observed in the rat peritoneal mast cell (Schulman *et al.*, 1982). These observations emphasize that, while a conceptual framework for the biochemical events involved in mast cell secretion can be formulated in one system (i.e., rat peritoneal mast cells), extrapolations of these findings to other mast cell (or basophil) populations may not always be possible.

In contrast to some lower vertebrates in which it appears that a single type of metachromatic-staining cell both circulates in the blood and populates the connective tissues, the human basophil and mast cell are clearly distinct. Human basophils are first detected in the third month of embryonic life and appear to originate from azurophilic granulocytes in the bone marrow as do other blood leukocytes (Parwaresch, 1976). During maturation, there is a gradual accumulation of characteristic metachromatic granules and segmented nuclei. Basophils are circulating blood cells that rarely occur in extravascular sites other than bone marrow (Dvorak, 1978). Their absolute numbers in peripheral blood vary between 20 and 45 cells/mm^3. In contrast to mast cells, basophils have nuclei that are polymorphous, and the cytosol contains fewer (Dvorak *et al.*, 1980) but larger granules that take up metachromatic stains less intensely than do mast cells.

1.2. THE MAST CELL IN IMMUNOLOGIC REACTIONS

The appreciation of the role of the mast cell in immunologic reactions evolved through studies carried out concurrently with the biologic and biochemical studies of the mast cell and led eventually to the discovery of IgE antibody. In 1902, Portier and Richet first described the phenomenon of anaphylaxis. They observed that not all dogs injected with sea anemone toxin died. Animals that survived exhibited a dramatic reaction if subsequently injected with much smaller quantities of toxin. The manifestations included shortness of breath, diarrhea, bloody vomitus, and death—all occurring within several minutes. Subsequently, it was shown that serum obtained from animals after an initial immunization contained a circulatory factor capable of transferring this hypersensitivity to normal animals.

The initial report which indicated that anaphylactic sensitivity could be passively transferred in humans involved a physician who was transfused with the serum from a subject who was allergic to horses. The recipient subsequently developed asthma upon grooming his own horse (Ramirez, 1919). Prausnitz and Küstner (1921) demonstrated that serum transferred into the skin of a normal recipient induced an allergic reaction upon contacting antigen to which the original donor was sensitive. The Prausnitz–Küstner test demonstrated two principles fundamental to allergy. (1) Allergic serum contains a sensitizing factor that can be transferred to normal recipients; and (2) sensitization persists for a long time after transfer. The search for this factor, known as reagin, continued for an additional 45 years before final identification of the IgE molecule (Ishizaka *et al.*, 1966; Johansson and Bennich, 1967). In the late 1960s, reagin was isolated from normal serum (Ishizaka *et al.*, 1966) and found to be a unique class of immunoglobulin, designated IgE, that bound principally to mast cells and basophils.

1.3. IMMEDIATE HYPERSENSITIVITY

Immediate hypersensitivity reactions are those in which an antigen interacts with corresponding antigen-specific IgE on the surface of either tissue mast cells or circulating basophils and results in the discharge of their granular contents. Preformed mediators contained in the granules are capable of producing immediate tissue effects including the generation of additional, newly synthesized molecules that participate in the genesis of the immediate reaction; in addition, mast cell and basophil activation leads to the gradual release of molecules from the granule matrix that are capable of producing additional effects lasting for hours (Table 1). In some instances, IgE-mediated release of granular contents can further result in late-phase reactions both in the skin and in the lung, which occur approximately 6–8 hr after the initial antigen exposure (Atkins *et al.*, 1973;

TABLE 1. MAST CELL-DERIVED MEDIATORS

Preformed, rapidly eluted under physiologic conditions
  Histamine
  Eosinophil chemotactic factors
  Neutrophil chemotactic factors
  Superoxide
  Arylsulfatase A
  Exoglycosidases
  Serotonin[a]
Preformed, firmly associated with the granule under physiologic conditions
  Heparin
  Chymotrypsin/trypsin
  Inflammatory factor[a]
  Peroxidase[a]
  Superoxide dismutase[a]
  Arylsulfatase B
Mediators generated as a consequence of mast cell activation/secretion
  Slow-reacting substance (leukotrienes C, D, and E)
  Prostaglandins
  Thromboxanes
  Platelet-activating factor
  Prostaglandin-generating factor

[a]Demonstrated in the mast cells of species other than human.

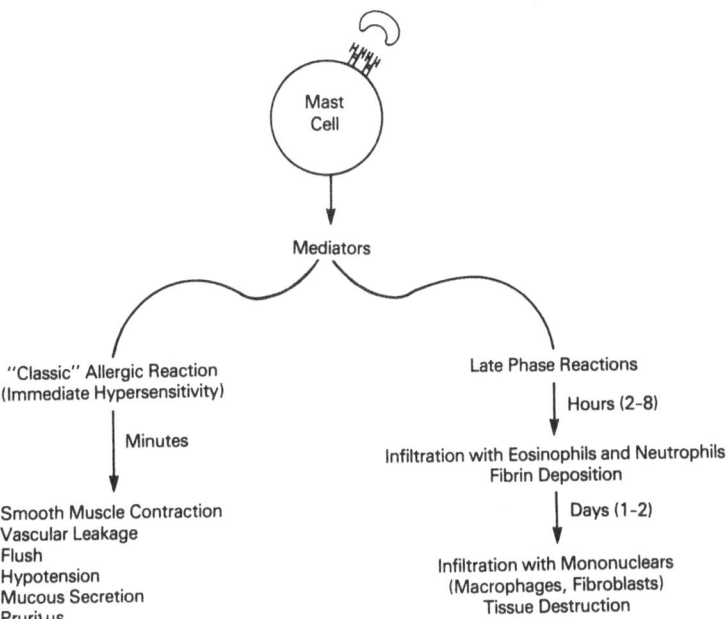

FIGURE 1.   Consequences of mediator release. Degranulation of mast cells produces immediate tissue changes as a result of the release of preformed as well as newly generated mediators. Factors released from the granule may also lead to the development of delayed inflammatory changes, termed "late-phase allergic reactions." (Reprinted with permission from Oertel and Kaliner, 1981, *J. Immunol.* **127:**1398.)

Dolovich *et al.*, 1973; Lemanske and Kaliner, 1983) (Fig. 1). Histologically, these late-phase reactions in the skin are characterized by a prominent neutrophil, eosinophil, basophil, and mononuclear cell infiltrate (Solley *et al.*, 1976; De Shazo *et al.*, 1979).

The fundamental immunologic component of immediate hypersensitivity is the production of an immunoglobulin of the ϵ class. IgE is a typical monomeric immunoglobulin consisting of two heavy and two light chains. IgE has a higher molecular mass than the other monomeric immunoglobulins (180,000 daltons), a relatively high carbohydrate content (about 12.3%), and a faster sedimentation coefficient (7.92 S) (Bennich and Johansson, 1971). The polypeptide mass is about 11,000 daltons greater than that of IgG or IgA, and it has been suggested that the additional portion of the IgE heavy chain is the region that fixes to the surface of the mast cell or basophil (Ishizaka *et al.*, 1970). IgE molecules bind to the surface of mast cells and basophils by the attachment of their Fc region to specific membrane receptors.

The physicochemical characteristics of the IgE receptor on rat mast cells and rat leukemic basophils have been critically analyzed and recently reviewed (Metzger *et al.*, 1982). The receptor *in situ* is unclustered, mobile, and univalent, and its aggregation into dimers and higher oligomers triggers degranulation.

The receptor is a glycoprotein composed of two subunits, an α chain with a molecular mass of approximately 50,000 daltons and a β chain with a molecular mass of 30,000 daltons. Both α and β chains are composed of at least two domains labeled α_1 and α_2, and β_1 and β_2, respectively. Receptors with IgE-binding capability have also been described in human B (Gonzales-Molina and Spiegelberg, 1977) and T lymphocytes (Yodoi and Ishizaka, 1979), human monocytes (Spiegelberg and Melewicz, 1980), and human and rat eosinophils (Capron *et al.*, 1981). However, the binding site of these nonmast cell or basophil receptors is of relatively low affinity and less specific; in addition, such receptors appear to be structurally distinct.

Aggregation of IgE receptors on mast cell and basophil membranes is sufficient to initiate degranulation (Ishizaka, 1982). Thus, although the IgE molecule functions as the recognition unit of the IgE–receptor complex, it is the aggregation of the receptors that induces the biochemical events leading to the degranulation process. The number of IgE receptors on nonatopic human basophils has been estimated to be approximately 20,000 to 50,000, of which 10% are occupied *in vivo*. In contrast, atopic basophils contain between 100,000 and 500,000 receptors on their cell surface, of which 95% are occupied *in vivo*. This suggests either that the number of IgE receptors is genetically determined along with the propensity for the production of IgE or that the serum level of IgE may have an enhancing capacity for the generation of IgE receptors on basophils (Malveaux *et al.*, 1978).

2. BIOCHEMICAL EVENTS IN MAST CELL AND BASOPHIL SECRETION

Secretion literally means a process to separate, elaborate, or release a product. The potential for the process of cellular secretion is present in eukaryotic cells in that they possess both an endoplasmic reticulum and a Golgi complex, which are necessary for the synthesis, segregation, transport, concentration, and storage of various molecules (Palade, 1975). Synthesized macromolecules may be stored intracellularly by surrounding them with a lipid bilayer membrane. Such molecular packages in mast cells and basophils are termed granules. The movement of macromolecular constituents from the intracellular to the extracellular environment is termed exocytosis and occurs in a wide variety of cell types in man including the adrenal medullary cell, pancreatic exocrine cell, hepatocyte, nerve endings, and cells from both the anterior and the posterior pituitary gland.

The process of secretion may be triggered by a number of signals that differ depending on the cell in question. For example, secretion by the anterior pituitary gland is regulated through signals traveling down nerves originating in the hypothalamus, whereas mast cells and basophils may be stimulated by antigen–IgE interactions; several proteins derived from activation of the complement cascade (Frank, 1979); and by various nonimmunologic activators including polyanions, such as compound 48/80, and antibiotics, such as polymyxin B and amphotericin B (Selye, 1965). Once the cell-specific signal is received, however, the actual process of secretion involves a number of events that are shared by most secretory cells (Palade, 1975). Secretion requires metabolic energy which may be generated through anaerobic or aerobic glycolysis or through oxidative phosphorylation. The absolute need for calcium in the secretion process has been demonstrated in a number of systems and has led to the hypothesis termed "stimulus–secretion coupling" first proposed by Douglas and Rubin in 1961.

Another common feature in the secretory process is the important role played by cyclic nucleotides, such as cAMP. Intracellular cAMP may function to activate various protein kinases that in turn phosphorylate and thereby activate proteins that regulate numerous metabolic processes. Although increased levels of cAMP appear to facilitate secretion in a number of systems (Becker and Henson, 1973), agents capable of increasing cellular cAMP have been shown to exert an inhibitory influence on most effector cells involved in immunologic or inflammatory events (Becker and Henson, 1973; Kaliner and Austen, 1974a; Bourne et al., 1974).

The phosphorylation of specific intracellular proteins by various protein kinases is an important means by which regulatory substances such as cyclic nucleotides, steroid hormones, and calcium initiate biochemical changes that affect intracellular processes (Greengard, 1978). cAMP-dependent protein kinases may be involved in the regulation of neurotransmitter biosynthesis (Lovenberg et al., 1975), microtubular function (Sloboda et al., 1975), and mast cell histamine release (Holgate et al., 1980). These findings suggest that this mechanism is important in the normal expression of cellular exocytosis. In addition, phosphorylation of membrane phospholipids accompanies mast cell secretion (Kennerly et al., 1979a,b; Marquardt et al., 1981), indicating that phosphorylation reactions are not restricted to events occurring within the cell.

Membrane phospholipids also undergo successive methylation reaction following the induction of exocytosis (Hirata and Axelrod, 1980). In the mast cell, such changes are associated with increased membrane fluidity, calcium movement, and the *de novo* synthesis of prostaglandins (Hirata and Axelrod, 1980; Ishizaka, 1982).

The molecular aspects of perigranule membrane fusion with the cell membrane have been studied in mast cells (Chandler and Heuser, 1980), pancreatic β cells (Orci et al., 1977), plasmalemmal vesicles (Palade and Bruns, 1968), and Limulus sperm (Tilney et al., 1979) using a number of microscopic techniques. The interpretations of the ultrastructure of these membrane-related events differ depending on the techniques utilized. Electron microscopic analysis has suggested that the granule membranes often contact the plasma membrane at sites where the intervening cytoplasm has been expressed, forming "pentalaminar figures" (Palade and Bruns, 1968). Freeze-fracture as well as other techniques (Lawson et al., 1977) have suggested the presence of intramembranous protein particles that are displaced laterally away from the fusing granular and plasma membranes during the fusion process. Recent work by Chandler and co-workers (Chandler and Heuser, 1980), however, demonstrated the presence of single, narrow-necked pores joining single granules with the plasma membrane. Intramembranous particle displacement and extensive contact between fusing membranes were not detected.

Overall, the secretory process is a complex sequence of events. Much has been learned regarding these processes through the study of isolated mast cells and basophils obtained from a number of mammalian species. In the remaining portion of this chapter, the previous discussion will be enlarged by dissecting the secretory process into individual stages and detailing specific biochemical events as well as their pharmacologic modulation. The compartmentalization resulting from such a discussion should not in any way detract from the process as a whole; indeed, the biology of secretion is a meshwork of interrelated events that are difficult, if not impossible, to separate.

The analyses of mast cell secretion have involved biochemical and morphologic techniques, which have led to the appreciation of a number of events in the secretory process (Table 2). Each of the events will be discussed in some detail in order to define the processes involved as well as their pharmacologic and physiologic modulation.

2.1. SERINE ESTERASE

A membrane-associated serine esterase is present in both mast cells (Becker and Henson, 1973) and basophils (Pruzansky and Patterson, 1973) and its early activation may be important in the secretory process (Kaliner and Austen, 1973; Becker and Henson, 1973) following cell stimulation by a number of secretagogues including antigen, Con A, dextran, lysosomal granule proteins, and polymyxin B. Analysis of the sequence of events during either rat mast cell secretion or human lung mediator release indicates that activation of the esterase

TABLE 2. EVENTS IN MAST CELL SECRETION

Biochemical
    Activation of serine esterase
    Calcium movement
    Cyclic nucleotide formation
    cAMP utilization
    cAMP-dependent protein kinase activation
    Phospholipid turnover
    Arachidonic acid metabolism
    Energy utilization
    Microtubule assembly
    Actomyosin activation
Morphologic
    Pore formation
    Granule swelling
    Microfilament organization
    Cistern formation
    Granule dissolution

occurs prior to energy utilization and an initial calcium-requiring EDTA-inhibita-ble step (Becker and Henson, 1973; Kaliner and Austen, 1973; Ranadive and Cochrane, 1971). The evidence indicating that activation of the serine esterase plays a role in the secretory process is indirect, however, since it comes from inhibition studies employing agents, such as diisopropyl fluorophosphate, that are capable of phosphorylating serine residues in proteins, thereby inactivating enzymes that contain serine in their active site. Moreover, data suggest that these inhibitors may affect the release reaction by inhibiting metabolic energy production (Taurog et al., 1979).

2.2. CALCIUM

The concept of "stimulus–secretion" coupling, proposed by Douglas and Rubin in 1961, focuses on the importance of calcium in the secretion process. In the case of the mast cell, abundant evidence has accumulated in the past decade suggesting that the movement of calcium across the plasma membrane is a link between cell stimulation and subsequent secretion. The supporting evidence includes (1) the ability of calcium chelators to completely inhibit the release reaction (Foreman and Mongar, 1975), (2) the ability of the calcium ionophore A23187 to stimulate release through its ability to transport calcium intracellularly (Foreman et al., 1973), (3) the capacity of direct intracellular injection of calcium but not magnesium using microinjection techniques to produce mast cell de-granulation (Kanno et al., 1973), and (4) the demonstration that purified mast cells secrete histamine when fused to phospholipid vesicles containing calcium but not potassium or magnesium (Theoharides and Douglas, 1978).

The level of intracellular calcium is not only influenced by agents that per-mit influx into the cell but also by processes occurring within the cell. It has been shown that calcium exists in at least two cellular compartments (Donlon et al., 1979): (1) a rapidly exchangeable EGTA-chelatable pool that is unrelated to the quantity of histamine released, and (2) a slow-exchange compartment (EGTA-nonchelatable) that is correlated with histamine release. With the exception of compound 48/80, most mast cell secretagogues require extracellular calcium for histamine release. If mast cells are depleted of intracellular calcium by prolonged incubation in calcium-free buffers and subsequently challenged with compound 48/80, an internal calcium requirement can be demonstrated (Atkinson et al., 1979). Therefore, compound 48/80-induced exocytosis requires existing pools of intracellular calcium. It has been proposed that this calcium is bound to the inner aspect of the cell membrane.

The mechanism by which changes in intracellular levels of calcium affect mediator release is unknown. The presence of this divalent cation, however, has been shown to be necessary for a number of steps involved in the secretory process including the action of cyclic nucleotides on protein phosphorylation, the action of phospholipase A_2 on its substrate arachidonic acid, the activation of serine esterase, and microtubular function.

2.3. CYCLIC NUCLEOTIDES

Since their discovery in the early 1960s, a large body of evidence has accumulated suggesting that intracellular levels of cAMP and cGMP modulate or mediate a variety of secretory processes (Sutherland *et al.*, 1968; Hardman, 1971; Goldberg *et al.*, 1975). Following hormonal stimulation, cAMP and ccGMP levels may change in opposite directions with opposing effects on the cell in question (Goldberg *et al.*, 1975). The observation of this relationship led Goldberg and co-workers to propose the so-called "yin yang" hypothesis, named for the two natural forces of Chinese cosmology that are frequently in opposition to each other but may, under certain circumstances, act in concert (Steer, 1977; Goldberg *et al.*, 1975).

cAMP and cGMP are formed by the action of the enzymes adenylate cyclase or guanylate cyclase on the substrates ATP and GTP, respectively. Although both cyclases have been well studied, the mechanism(s) by which various agents may interact with them has been characterized best for adenylate cyclase. This enzyme is apparently bound to the cytoplasmic side of the plasma membrane and various drugs, such as β-adrenergic agents, bind to cell surface receptors and initiate a sequence of events culminating in the activation of adenylate cyclase (Rodbell, 1980).

Cell surface receptors are capable of lateral mobility along the plasma membrane. There is evidence to suggest that the proper positioning of receptors with adenylate cyclase is important to its activation. This process may involve sequential methylations of phospholipids, resulting in decreased membrane viscosity (Hirata and Axelrod, 1980). The incorporation of a radiolabeled methyl group from S-adenosylmethionine into reticulocyte ghost membranes is increased in a dose-dependent manner upon stimulation with isoproterenol (Hirata and Axelrod, 1980). Thus β-adrenergic agents may interact with their appropriate receptor, stimulate phospholipid methylation, and increase membrane fluidity, facilitating receptor coupling to adenylate cyclase activation. Once hormone, receptor, and enzyme are coupled, however, full activation of cyclase is also dependent on the presence of guanyl nucleotides and divalent cations such as magnesium and calcium (Steer, 1977). Pharmacologic agents capable of activating adenylate cyclase generate increased levels of intracellular cAMP. β-Adrenergic agents, histamine, adenosine, cholera toxin, and prostaglandins of the E series have all been shown to produce these effects in mast cells.

In addition to *de novo* generation, levels of cAMP may also be affected by preventing or augmenting its metabolic breakdown by phosphodiesterase. Methylxanthines are capable of inhibiting phosphodiesterase, thereby raising intracellular levels of cAMP. Imidazole, perhaps through its buffering action, augments phosphodiesterase activity, decreasing AMP levels.

Guanylate cyclase is, for the most part, a soluble enzyme not located on the plasma membrane. A number of agents including α-adrenergic and cholinergic drugs increase cellular cGMP levels, and it is likely that they do so through stimulation of guanylate cyclase. In some cases, the cGMP rise is associated with a concomitant rise in cAMP and cellular response is determined by the relative levels of each and their respective action on various intracellular processes (Steer, 1977).

The relationship between mast cell and basophil secretory events and cyclic nucleotides has received much attention over the past decade. It appears that alterations in cyclic nucleotide levels may modulate (either enhance or inhibit) the release process, accompany the process as a concomitant event (either increasing, decreasing, or both), or be stimulated by secretory products (both histamine and prostaglandins alter cAMP and ccGMP levels). There is thus a complex interrelationship between mast cell secretion and the cyclic nucleotides. To complicate the relationships even more, studies have involved mast cell secretion in human tissues after isolation and exposure to multiple enzymes in order to partially purify these cells from human lung preparations. It is therefore not surprising that some observations are discordant.

The effects of alterations in cyclic nucleotide levels upon mast cell and basophil function have been studied in two ways. (1) The effects of pharmacologic agents known to increase cAMP or cGMP added to various tissues or cells prior to immunologic challenge may be determined; and (2) the levels of cyclic nucleotides in tissues or cells undergoing mediator release may be measured at various time points following challenge.

Experiments involving *in vitro* histamine release in antigen-challenged human lung and nasal mucosa have demonstrated inhibition of mediator release by agents known to increase levels of cAMP including epinephrine and isoproterenol (Orange et al., 1971a), prostaglandin E_1 and E_2 (Tauber et al., 1973), methylxanthines (Orange et al., 1971b), and cholera toxin (Kaliner et al., 1973). Further α-adrenergic agonists, such as phenylephrine and nonrepinephrine, enhance antigen-induced release of mediators in association with a reduction of total lung cAMP (Kaliner et al., 1972). Imidazole also increases mediator release in association with decreased cAMP levels (Kaliner and Austen, 1972). These data suggest an inverse relationship between mast cell cAMP levels and immunologically induced mediator release (Table 3). However, the levels of cyclic nucleotides measured in the lung reflect the total population of cells within the lung tissue while mediator release involves only a small population of mast cells.

Cholinergic stimulation of muscarinic receptor sites with physiologic concentrations of carbachol was found to increase total lung cGMP levels (Kaliner, 1977a) and to increase the immunologic release of mediators (Kaliner and Austen, 1972; Kaliner, 1977a). Exogenous cGMP also increases mediator release (Kaliner and Austen, 1972). Prostaglandin $F_{2\alpha}$ is also capable of increasing cGMP (Kaliner, 1977a) and enhancing mediator release (Tauber et al., 1973). These findings suggest that cGMP acts in a reciprocal manner to cAMP, enhancing the immunologically stimulated secretory reaction.

Histamine may stimulate H_1 or H_2 receptors in the human lung (Platshon and Kaliner, 1978). H_1 stimulation increases total lung cGMP whereas H_2 stimulation induces increases in cAMP. However, stimulation of either H_1 nor H_2 receptors fails to influence the immunologic release of mast cell-derived mediators (Kaliner, 1978). Thus, not all changes in lung cyclic nucleotide levels reflect

TABLE 3. AGENTS THAT MODULATE THE RELEASE OF MEDIATORS IN ASSOCIATION
WITH ALTERATIONS IN CYCLIC NUCLEOTIDE LEVELS

Agents that increase cAMP levels and inhibit release
   cAMP
   β-Adrenergic agonists
   Methylxanthines
   Cholera toxin
   PGE, PGD_2, PGI_2
   Histamine
   Adenosine
Agents that reduce cAMP levels and enhance release
   α-Adrenergic agonists
   Imidazole
Agents that increase cGMP levels and enhance release
   cGMP
   $PGF_{2\alpha}$
   Cholinergic agonists

mast cell-related phenomena or, alternately, the mast cell may lack functional histamine receptors.

Studies involving cyclic nucleotide changes in purified mast cells have focused primarily on the use of rat peritoneal mast cells and analysis of the effects of cAMP-active agents on both immunologically and nonimmunologically induced degranulation (Lewis *et al.*, 1979; Sullivan *et al.*, 1975; Sullivan and Parker, 1976). Rat mast cell cAMP may be increased in a dose-related fashion by methylxanthines or dibutyryl cAMP (Sullivan and Parker, 1976). The combination of methylxanthines and prostaglandin E_2 acts synergistically to both increase mast cell cAMP and inhibit the immunologically induced release of histamine (Kaliner and Austen, 1974b). These observations strongly suggest that increases in intracellular cAMP inhibit histamine release in isolated mast cell preparations.

Although mast cells have been demonstrated to have high-affinity β-adrenergic receptors on their cell surface (Donlon *et al.*, 1982; Marquardt and Wasserman, 1982), β-adrenergic stimulation either fails to increase mast cell cAMP (Kaliner and Austen, 1974b) or increases cAMP without inhibition of histamine release (Sullivan and Parker, 1976; Marquardt and Wasserman, 1982). These observations suggest that mast cells, once purified, have uncoupled their β-adrenergic/adenylate cyclase systems or that subcellular pools of cAMP stimulated by β-adrenergic agonists that do not affect secretion. The capacity of β-adrenergic agonist to inhibit rat peritoneal mast cell secretion *in vivo* (Koopman *et al.*, 1970) suggests that mast cell isolation procedures may alter agonist–receptor–enzyme interactions.

Histamine may inhibit human basophil mediator release through stimulation of H_2 receptors associated with increases in cAMP levels (Bourne *et al.*, 1971). The observation that human lung mast cells failed to respond to physiologic concentrations of histamine (Kaliner, 1978) stimulated the analysis of histamine's effects on rat mast cell degranulation (Wescott and Kaliner, 1980, 1981). Histamine at concentrations up to 1000 μM failed to inhibit mast cell degranulation and, indeed, appeared to increase mediator release unless phosphodiesterase activity was simultaneously inhibited (Wescott and Kaliner, 1981). Under conditions in which metabolism of cAMP was impaired, very large concentrations of histamine were able to inhibit mast cell degranulation in association with increases in cAMP. Of interest was the observation that the receptor involved in these actions was of the H_1 type. Thus, mast cells do have histamine receptors of the H_1 class functionally linked to adenylate cyclase (Wescott and Kaliner, 1981). However, due to the concentrations of agonist involved, it is unlikely that this action of histamine has any physiologic relevance.

Kinetic experiments involving mast cells undergoing immunologically induced degranulation indicate that there is an initial reduction in total cAMP associated with a depletion of cellular ATP (Kaliner and Austen, 1974b). Subsequent studies have demonstrated an earlier rise in cAMP followed by reductions (Sullivan *et al.*, 1975; Sullivan and Parker, 1976) or a biphasic elevation not accompanied by a reduction (Lewis *et al.*, 1979). Thus, at this time, it is not possible to definitively state what changes cAMP levels may undergo accompanying the secretory process.

The possible mechanisms by which alterations in cAMP levels may influence mast cell degranulation include modulation of membrane-associated phospholipid methylation (Hirata and Axelrod, 1980; Ishizaka, 1982), suppression of membrane phospholipid turnover (Kennerly *et al.*, 1979b), and alterations in microtubule function (Kaliner, 1977b). An additional mechanism includes phosphorylation of essential proteins through activation of cAMP-dependent protein kinases (Holgate *et al.*, 1980).

2.4. PHOSPHOLIPIDS

A detailed analysis of the lipid composition of rat mast cell plasma membranes indicates that the primary phospholipids include phosphatidylcholine, 29.6 ± 3.3%; sphingomyelin, 19.8 ± 2.2%; and phosphatidylserine plus phosphatidylinositol, 16.1 ± 2.0% (Strandberg and Westerberg, 1976). The composition of mast cell membrane phospholipids is similar to human red blood cells and many other cells.

Following mast cell activation, various phospholipids may undergo a number of chemical reactions; two that have been studied in detail include phosphorylation and methylation. Kennerly *et al.* (1979a), using incorporation of $^{32}PO_4$ into individual phospholipid classes, demonstrated that mast cells stimulated with either anti-IgE, Con A, A23187, or compound 48/80 showed striking increases in the labeling of phosphatidic acid, which was detected as early as 8 sec after stimulation. Increased labeling of phosphatidylcholine and phosphatidylinositol was apparent by 30 sec. Secretion-associated phosphorylation of these phospholipids was inhibited by theophylline and dibutyryl cAMP, suggesting that increases in cAMP act to inhibit the release reaction prior to the phosphorylating step (Kennerly *et al.*, 1979b). In addition, 5,8,11,14-eicosatetraenoic acid (ETYA), an acetylenic derivative of arachidonic acid that inhibits mast cell degranulation (Sullivan and Parker, 1979), was also found to inhibit phosphate incorporation into lipids, suggesting that an ETYA-inhibitable step also precedes the phosphorylation reaction (Sullivan and Parker, 1979).

Calcium-dependent protein phosphorylation accompanying histamine secretion has also been demonstrated (Sieghart *et al.*, 1978). Stimulation of rat peritoneal mast cells with either A23187 or compound 48/80 results in the rapid phosphorylation of proteins having molecular masses of 68,000, 59,000, and 42,000 daltons and within 30–60 sec phosphorylation of a fourth protein with a molecular mass of 78,000 daltons occurs. Moreover, these phosphorylated proteins display different rates of dephosphorylation following mast cell activation.

Disodium cromoglycate, a drug that inhibits *in vitro* mast cell histamine release in response to antigen challenge, compound 48/80 (Johnson *et al.*, 1978), or A23187 (Johnson and Bach, 1975) may affect mast cell secretion by regulating phosphorylation of a specific mast cell protein (Theoharides *et al.*, 1980). Incubation of rat peritoneal mast cells with cromoglycate induced the incorporation of radioactive phosphate into a single protein band with a molecular mass of 78,000 daltons and resulted in the inhibition of histamine release following stimulation with compound 48/80. It was suggested that the increased phosphorylation of this protein by cromoglycate may inhibit degranulation through its effects on calcium flux within the cell. Thus, phosphorylation of membrane or intracellular proteins may be important in both the generation and the modulation of the release reaction as it proceeds to completion.

Methylation of phospholipids has also been demonstrated to be an important event in the exocytotic process. Two distinct methyltransferases incorporate individual methyl groups on (1) the substrate phosphatidylcholine, and (2) the intermediate phosphatidyl-N-monomethylethanolamine, leading to the formation of phosphatidylethanolamine (Hirata and Axelrod, 1980; Ishizaka, 1982). The reaction sequence is known to proceed from the cytoplasmic to the external surface of the plasma membrane and occurs prior to the release of histamine (Hirata and Axelrod, 1980; Ishizaka, 1982). Methyltransferase inhibitors, such as adenosyl homocysteine, inhibit both phospholipid methylation and histamine release, indicating a coupled system (Hirata *et al.*, 1979; Ishizaka *et al.*, 1980). It is significant to note that degranulating agents, such as compound 48/80 and A23187, which do not involve the cross-linking of membrane-associated IgE receptors, show no stimulation of phospholipid methylation (Hirata *et al.*, 1979). Thus, the activation of methylation is closely related to Con A or anti-IgE bridging of IgE surface receptors followed by the activation of lipid methylation.

Membrane phospholipids also serve as precursor molecules for chemical mediators that are generated during the sequence of events surrounding exocytosis (Table 1). The release of arachidonic acid by the action of phospholipase A_2 on membrane phospholipids appears to be a pivotal point for two important pathways (Fig. 2). Derivatives of the cyclooxygenase pathway of arachidonate metabolism include endoperoxides, prostaglandins, and thromboxanes, whereas derivatives of the lipoxygenase pathway include various mono- and dihydrox-

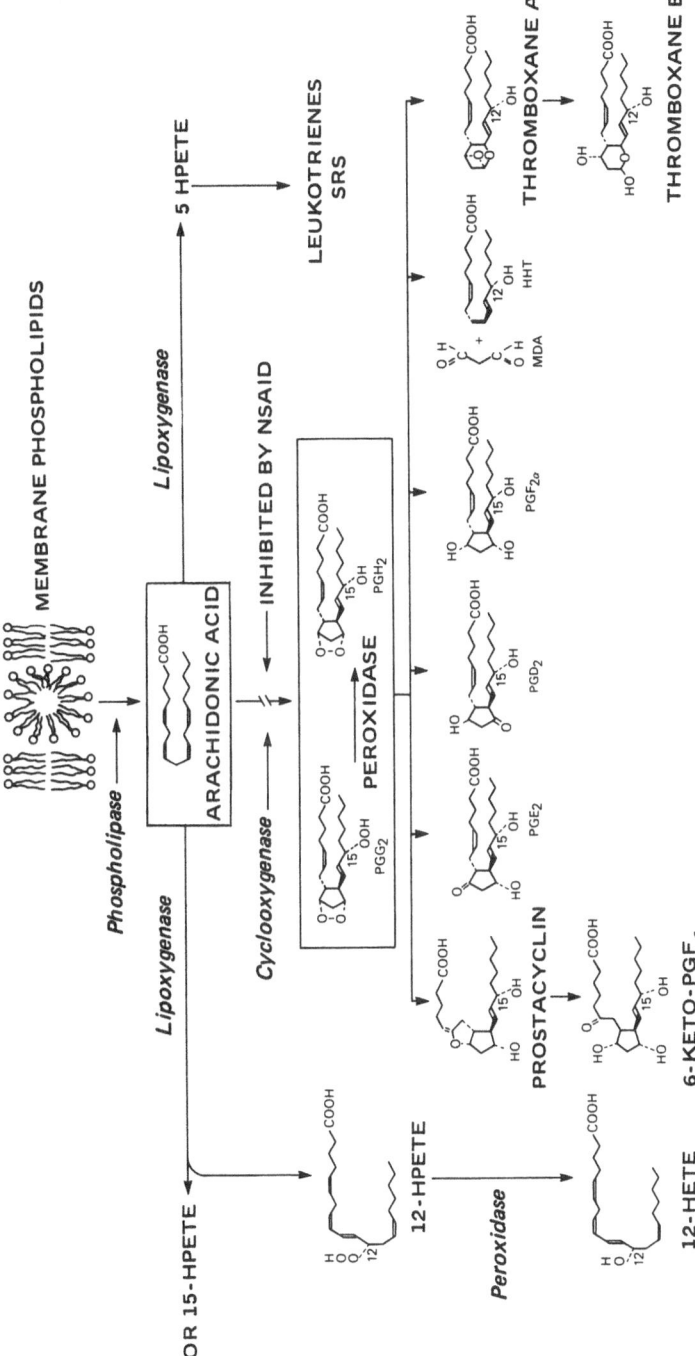

FIGURE 2. The arachidonic acid cascade. The release of arachidonic acid from membrane phospholipids is a pivotal point for two important biochemical pathways. Derivatives of the lipoxygenase pathway include various mono- and dihydroxyeicosatetraenoic acids (HETEs) and leukotrienes, whereas derivatives of the cyclooxygenase pathway include endoperoxides, prostaglandins, and thromboxanes.

yeicosatetraenoic acids (HETEs) and leukotrienes. The nature and amount of the various intermediates that are formed along either pathway may differ depending on the species and cell type. In addition to the formation of newly synthesized mediators, there is evidence to suggest that these pathways are also important in influencing the magnitude of the exocytotic process once initiated.

The influence of cyclooxygenase and lipoxygenase products upon the secretory process has been studied using pharmacologic agents that are capable of inhibiting these pathways. Nonsteroidal antiinflammatory drugs (NSAID), such as indomethacin, meclofenamic acid, and aspirin, are potent inhibitors of cyclooxygenase (Flower, 1974), whereas ETYA blocks both lipoxygenase and cyclooxygenase pathways of arachidonic acid metabolism (Flower, 1974; Hammarström, 1977). The effect of these agents on mediator release appears to depend on the cell used for study, the initiating stimulus, and the time of their introduction into the reaction sequence. In human basophils, antigen-induced histamine release is completely inhibited with ETYA, whereas NSAID enhance mediator release (Marone *et al.*, 1979). Arachidonic acid, but not other fatty acids including linoleic, linolenic, and stearic acids, was found to augment histamine release, an effect that was not influenced by preincubation with NSAID. Further, indomethacin counteracted the inhibition of mediator release produced by agents known to modulate basophil histamine release through increases in cAMP without attenuating the rises in cAMP (Marone *et al.*, 1979). These data suggest that the product(s) of arachidonic acid metabolism formed via the lipoxygenase pathway is involved in antigen-induced basophil mediator release and that these effects may be produced through the modulation of control mechanisms associated with cAMP.

Studies employing rat mast cells, however, have yielded conflicting results. In one study, mediator release was not found to be affected by aspirin or indomethacin. Further, arachidonic acid alone did not initiate mediator release but inhibited release induced by anti-IgE or Con A. This inhibition of release was blocked if aspirin or indomethacin was present, suggesting the involvement of cyclooxygenase products (Sullivan and Parker, 1979). Stenson *et al.* (1980), however, demonstrated that two lipoxygenase pathway products, 5-OH-6,8,11,14-eicosatetraenoic and 12-OH-5,8,10,14-eicosatetraenoic acids, were able to augment anti-IgE histamine release. Furthermore, ETYA inhibited mediator release induced by anti-IgE, Con A, A23187 (Stenson *et al.*, 1980), suggesting that products of the lipoxygenase pathway may also influence rat mast cell exocytosis. However, the ability of ETYA to inhibit mediator release by secretagogues dependent on extracellular calcium (antigen, Con A), but its failure to influence secretagogues capable of mobilizing intracellular calcium (compound 48/80) suggests that its effects may be produced by its action on early calcium movement (Nemeth and Douglas, 1980).

2.5. ENERGY

Noncytotoxic histamine release is an energy-dependent process (Chakravarty, 1962; Peterson, 1974a; Diamant, 1975). Under anoxic conditions and in the absence of glucose, anaphylactic histamine release is inhibited but is reconstituted by the addition of glucose (Chakravarty, 1962, 1965). Antimycin A, which blocks electron transfer between cytochromes b and c, inhibits histamine release in the absence but not in the presence of exogenous glucose (Peterson, 1974b). These data suggest that the energy requirement for histamine release may be derived from either oxidative (aerobic) metabolism or anaerobic glycolysis.

A close correlation exists between mast cell ATP content and the capacity of these cells to secrete histamine (Peterson, 1974a; Peterson and Diamant, 1974). Glucose has been demonstrated to be capable of maintaining ATP levels in mast cells through anaerobic glycolysis under anoxic conditions. 2-Deoxyglucose, an inhibitor of the glycolytic pathway, reduces the ATP content of mast cells with concomitant suppression of responsiveness to antigen or compound $^{48}/_{80}$ (Johansen and Chakravarty, 1975). Oligomycin inhibits oxidative ATP production and also inhibits histamine release (Peterson, 1974b). Not only does inhibition of the synthesis of ATP prevent histamine release, but there is also a direct correlation between ATP utilization by mast cells and histamine release. Stimulation of secretion is followed within seconds by a significant reduction in ATP levels occurring simultaneously with the release reaction (Kaliner and Austen, 1974b; Johansen, 1979). Finally, ATP itself, when added to a suspension of mast cells, may initiate degranulation (Keller, 1966), and this release process is temperature dependent, requires cellular energy utilization, and is dependent on the presence of calcium. The precise nature by which ATP exerts its effects on secretion is unknown but may involve the exchange of ions within cellular compartments, the assembly and function of microtubules, the phosphorylation of proteins and phospholipids either directly from ATP or via cAMP-dependent protein kinases, and the utilization of ATP as the source of intracellular cAMP.

The potential importance of this ATP-induced mast cell degranulation is the observation that ATP may be the secretory product released from nerve endings of the purinergic nervous system (Burnstock, 1972). ATP discharged from purinergic nerves in the vicinity of mast cells could thus potentially induce mast cell degranulation.

2.6. MICROTUBULES AND MICROFILAMENTS

Microtubules and microfilaments are subcellular organelles that are both ultrastructurally and chemically distinct and are found in all eukaryotic cells (Bryan, 1974). Microtubules appear to be involved in secretory processes in a variety of cell types (Goldstein *et al.*, 1973; Malaisse *et al.*, 1975; Wolff and Bhattacharyya, 1975; Poisner and Bernstein, 1971). They are long, tubelike organelles and in cross-sections of glutaraldehyde-fixed, osmium-stained preparations appear as an electron-dense annulus surrounding an electron-lucent core (Bryan, 1974). The basic unit of the microtubule is a protein complex (tubulin) of approximately 110,000 daltons, sedimentation velocity 6 S, and dimeric structure composed of two monomeric subunits (α and β) whose protein composition differs by only a few amino acid residues (Bryan, 1974). Pharmacologic agents known to affect microtubular structure or function have been used to study the relationship of microtubules to the secretory process.

Colchicine and vinblastine are agents that appear to exert their biologic effects by preventing reaggregation of depolymerized microtubules (Wilson *et al.*, 1974). Following 3 hr of pretreatment with colchicine, histamine release from rat mast cells in response to compound 48/80 or polymyxin B is inhibited 20–70%, suggesting that microtubule function may be involved in mast cell secretion (Lagunoff and Chi, 1976; Tolone *et al.*, 1974; Orr *et al.*, 1972). Antigen-induced stimulation of histamine release from human basophils or human lung fragments is inhibitable by colchicine only when incubation at 4°C is also included (Kaliner, 1977b; Levy and Carlton, 1969). The effect of incubation of cells at 4°C is to depolymerize microtubules (Wilson, 1975). In addition to effects on secretion, colchicine exhibits a profound effect on the morphology of rat peritoneal mast cells (Lagunoff and Chi, 1976; Padawer and Gordon, 1955) and is associated with a loss of ultrastructurally visible microtubules. The disruption of normal microtubular function by these agents, however, appears to be dependent on their ability to bind to depolymerized tubular proteins which are in equilibrium with their polymerized counterparts. Thus, cells possessing stable polymerized microtubules would be more resistant to these pharmacologic agents (Wilson, 1975).

All eukaryotic cells also possess microfilamentous structures that represent actomyosin-contractile elements. Electron microscopy has demonstrated these structures in the cortical cytoplasm of rat (Röhlich *et al.*, 1971) and human mast cells (Caulfield *et al.*, 1980). Using specific binding of heavy meromyosin in glycerinated rat mast cells, it was demonstrated that these filaments bind heavy meromyosin in the form of arrowhead complexes (Röhlich, 1975), indicating that they are actin filaments. There is roughly twice the concentration of filaments in the subplasmalemmal cytoplasm as compared with other cytoplasmic areas (Röhlich *et al.*, 1971). Many of the filaments are attached to the inner surface of the plasma membrane and in some instances to the membranes of cytoplasmic granules.

While the existence of microfilaments in mast cells is well documented, their functional role remains unclear. Cytochalasin A and B inhibit mast cell degranulation by compound 48/80 (Orr *et al.*, 1972), implicating microfilaments in the exocytosis process. However, cytochalasin B can inhibit exocytosis in isolated mast cells by interfering with glucose utilization (Doulgas and Ueda, 1973), probably by blocking glucose uptake. Cytochalasin A may inhibit mast cell secretion through a reaction with sulfhydryl groups located on the outer surface of the cell membrane. This hypothesis is supported by the capacity of glutathione, which does not readily enter normal mast cells, to prevent inhibition by cytochalasin A (Lagunoff and Wan, 1979). The location of large numbers of microfilaments in subcortical areas of mast cells and their integral association with both plasma and perigranular membranes suggest that microfilaments play some role in the secretion process. However, the exact nature of the participation of microfilaments in the mechanism(s) of granule exocytosis has not been precisely defined.

3. CONCLUSION

Since their initial description approximately 100 years ago, the mast cell and basophil have contributed a great deal to our understanding of the secretory process. Many of the biochemical events that occur following stimulation of these cells are now known and it is apparent that the process is complex with many interrelated pathways. Once activated, these cells are destined to secrete into the surrounding tissues molecules that are capable of producing numerous biologic effects. The pathologic effects of this process have been extensively studied in immediate hypersensitivity reactions. However, the abundance of mast cells in various human tissues suggests that they may also play a significant role in normal tissue homeostasis. The relationship of this role to the secretory process will be an important area for future investigation.

ACKNOWLEDGMENT. The authors express gratitude to Karen Leighty for editorial assistance in the preparation of the manuscript.

REFERENCES

Atkins, P. G., Green, G., and Zweiman, B., 1973. Histologic studies of human skin test responses to ragweed, compound 48/80, and histamine, *J. Allergy Clin. Immunol.* **51**:263.

Atkinson, G., Ennis, M., and Pearce, F., 1979, The effect of alkaline earth cations on the release of histamine from rat peritoneal mast cells treated with compound 48/80 and peptide 401, *Br. J. Pharmacol.* **65**:395.

Barrett, K. E., and Pearce, F. L., 1982, A comparative study of histamine release from rat peritoneal and pleural mast cells, *Agents Actions* **12**:186.

Becker, E. L., and Henson, P. M., 1973; *In vitro* studies of immunologically induced secretion of mediators from cells and related phenomena, *Adv. Immunol.* **17**:93.

Benditt, E. P., and Lagunoff, D., 1964, The mast cell: Its structure and function, *Prog. Allergy* **8**:195.

Bennich, H., and Johansson, S. G. O., 1971, Structure and function of immunoglobulin E, *Adv. Immunol.* **13**:1.

Bourne, H. R., Melmon, K. L., and Lichtenstein, L. M., 1971, Histamine augments leukocyte adenosine 3',5'-monophosphate and blocks antigenic histamine release, *Science* **173**:743.

Bourne, H. R., Lichtenstein, L. M., Melmon, K. L., Hennery, C. S., Weinstein, Y., and Shearer, G. M., 1974, Modulation of inflammation and immunity by cyclic AMP, *Science* **184**:19.

Bryan, J., 1974, Biochemical properties of microtubules, *Fed. Proc.* **33**:152.

Burnstock G., 1972, Purinergic nerves, *Pharmacol. Rev.* **24**:509.

Capron, M., Capron, A., Dessaint, J., Torpier, G., Gunnar, S., Johansson, O., and Prin, L., 1981, Fc receptors for IgE on human and rat eosinophils, *J. Immunol.* **126**:2087.

Caulfield, J. P., Lewis, R. A., Hein, A., and Austen, K. F., 1980, Secretion in dissociated pulmonary mast cells: Evidence for solubilization of granule contents before discharge, *J. Cell Biol.* **85**:299.

Chakravarty, N., 1962, Inhibition of anaphylactic histamine release by 2-deoxyglucose, *Nature (London)* **194**:1182.

Chakravarty, N., 1965, Glycolysis in rat peritoneal mast cells, *J. Cell Biol.* **25**:123.

Chandler, D. E., and Heuser, J. E., 1980, Arrest of membrane fusion events in mast cells by quick-freezing, *J. Cell Biol.* **86**:666.

De Shazo, R. D., Levinson, A. I., Dvorak, H. F., and Davis, R. W., 1979, The late-phase skin reaction: Evidence for activation of the coagulation system in an IgE-dependent reaction in man, *J. Immunol.* **122**:692.

Diamant, B., 1975, Energy production in rat mast cells and its role for histamine release, *Int. Arch. Allergy Appl. Immunol.* **49**:155.

Dolovich, J., Hargreave, F. E., Chalmers, R., Shier, K. G., Gauldie, J., and Bienenstock, J., 1973, Late cutaneous allergic responses in isolated IgE-dependent reactions, *J. Allergy Clin. Immunol.* **52**:38.

Donlon, M., Bland, C., Catravas, G. N., and Kaliner, M., 1979, Characterization of two cellular calcium compartments in the isolated rat peritoneal mast cell, *J. Cell Biol.* **83**:289.

Donlon, M., Hunt, W. A., Catravas, G. N., and Kaliner, M., 1982, Identification of beta-adrenergic receptors on perigranular membranes of rat peritoneal mast cells, *Life Sci.* **31**:411.

Douglas, W. W., and Rubin, R. P., 1961, The role of calcium in the secretory response of the adrenal medulla to acetylcholine, *J. Physiol (London)* **159**:40.

Douglas, W. W., and Ueda, Y., 1973, Mast cell secretion (histamine release) induced by 48/80: Calcium-dependent exocytosis inhibited strongly by cytochalasin only when glycolysis is rate limiting, *J. Physiol. (London)* **234**:97P.

Dvorak, A. M., 1978, Biology and morphology of basophilic leukocytes, in: *Immediate Hypersensitivty: Modern Concepts and Developments* (M. K. Bach, ed.), pp. 369–405, Dekker, New York.

Dvorak, A. M., Newball, H. H., Dvorak, H. F., and Lichtenstein, L. M., 1980, Antigen-induced IgE-mediated degranulation of human basophils, *Lab Invest.* **43**:126.

Flower, R. J., 1974, Drugs which inhibit prostaglandin biosynthesis, *Pharmacol. Rev.* **26**:33.

Foreman, J. C., and Mongar, J. L., 1975, Calcium and the control of histamine secretion from mast cells, in: *Calcium Transport in Contraction and Secretion* (E. Carafoli, ed.), p. 175, North-Holland, Amsterdam.

Foreman, J. C., Mongar, J. L., and Gomperts, B. D., 1973, Calcium ionophores and movement of calcium ions following the physiologic stimulus to a secretory process, *Nature (London)* **245**:249.

Frank, M., 1979, The complement system in host defense and inflammation, *Rev. Infect. Dis.* **1**:483.

Ginsburg, H., and Sachs, L., 1962, Formation of pure suspensions of mast cells in tissue culture by differentiation of lymphoid cells from the mouse, *J. Natl. Cancer Inst.* **31**:1.

Ginsburg, H., Hammel, N. I., Eren, R., Weissman, B. A., and Naot, Y., 1978, Differentiation and activity of mast cells following immunization in cultures of lymph node cells, *Immunology* **35**:485.

Goldberg, N. D., Haddox, M. K., Nicol, S. E., Glass, D. B., Sanford, C. H., Kuehl, F. A., Jr., and Estensen, R., 1975, Biological regulation through opposing influences of cyclic GMP and cyclic AMP: The yin-yang hypothesis, *Adv. Cyclic Nucleotide Res.* **5**:307.

Goldstein, I., Hoffstein, S., Gallin, J., and Weissman, G., 1973, Mechanisms of lysosomal enzyme release from human leukocytes: Microtubule assembly and membrane fusion induced by a component of complement, *Proc. Natl. Acad. Sci. U.S.A.* **70**:2916.

Gonzales-Molina, A., and Spiegelberg, H. L., 1977, A subpopulation of normal human peripheral B lymphocytes that bind IgE, *J. Clin, Invest.* **59**:616.

Greengard, P., 1978, Phosphorylated proteins as physiological effectors, *Science* **199**:146.

Hammarström, S., 1977, Selective inhibition of platelet lipoxygenase by 5,8,11-eicosatriynoic acid, *Biochim. Biophys, Acta* **487**:517.

Hardman, J. G., 1971, Other cyclic nucleotides, in: *Cyclic AMP* (G. A. Robison, R. W. Butcher, and E. W. Sutherland, eds), pp. 400–420, Academic Press, New York.

Hirata, F., and Axelrod, J., 1980, Phospholipid methylation and biological signal transmission, *Science* **209**:1082.

Hirata, F., Axelrod, J., and Crews, F. T., 1979, Concanavalin A stimulates phospholipid methylation and phosphatidylserine decarboxylation in rat mast cells, *Proc. Natl. Acad. Sci. U.S.A.* **76**:4813.

Holgate, S. T., Lewis, R. A., and Austen, K. F., 1980, 3′,5′-Cyclic adenosine monophosphate-dependent protein kinase of the rat serosal mast cell and its immunologic activation, *J. Immunol.* **124**:2093.

Ishizaka, K., Ishizaka, T., and Hornbrook, M. M., 1966, Physiochemical properties of reaginic antibody. V. Correlation of reaginic activity with γE-globulin antibody, *J. Immunol.* **97**:840.

Ishizaka, T., 1982, Biochemical analysis of triggering signals induced by bridging of IgE receptors, *Fed. Proc.* **14**:17.

Ishizaka, T., Ishizaka, K., and Lee, E. H., 1970, Biologic function of the Fc portion of IgE molecules, *J. Allergy* **95**:124.

Ishizaka, T., Okudaira, H., Mauser, L. E., and Ishizaka, K., 1976, Development of rat mast cells in vitro. I. Differentiation of mast cells from thymus cells, *J. Immunol.* **116**:747.

Ishizaka, T., Hirata, F., Ishizaka, K., and Axelrod, J., 1980, Stimulation of phospholipid methylation, Ca²⁺ influx, and histamine release by bridging of IgE receptors on rat mast cells, *Proc. Natl. Acad. Sci. U.S.A.* **77**:1903.

Johansen, T., 1979, Adenosine triphosphate levels during anaphylactic histamine release in rat mast cells in vitro: Effects of glycolytic and respiratory inhibitors, *Eur. J. Pharmacol.* **58**:107.

Johansen, T., and Chakravarty, N., 1975, The utilization of adenosine triphosphate in rat mast cells during histamine release induced by anaphylactic reaction and compound 48/80, *Naunyn-Schmiedebergs Arch. Pharmacol.* **288**:243.

Johansson, S. G. O., and Bennich, H., 1967, Immunological studies of an atypical myeloma immunoglobulin, *Immunology* **13**:381.

Johnson, H. G., and Bach, M. K., 1975, Prevention of calcium ionophore-induced release of histamine in rat mast cells by disodium cromoglycate, *J. Immunol.* **114**:514.

Johnson, H. G., Van Hout, J., and Wright, B., 1978, *Int. Arch. Allergy Appl Immunol.* **56**:416.

Kaliner, M., 1977a, Human lung tissue and anaphylaxis. I. The role of cyclic GMP as a modulator of the immunologically induced secretory process, *J. Allergy Clin. Immunol.* **60**:204.

Kaliner, M., 1977b, Human lung tissue and anaphylaxis: Evidence that cyclic nucleotides modulate the immunologic release of mediators through effects on microtubular assembly, *J. Clin. Invest.* **60**:951.

Kaliner, M., 1978, Human lung tissue and anaphylaxis: The effect of histamine upon the immunologic release of mediators, *Am. Rev. Respir. Dis.* **118**:1015.

Kaliner, M., and Austen, K. F., 1972, Hormonal control of the immunological release of histamine and slow-reacting substance of anaphylaxis from human lung, in: *Cyclic AMP, Cell Growth, and the Immune Response* (W. Braun, L. M. Lichtenstein, and C. W. Parker, eds), pp. 163–175, Springer-Verlag, Berlin.

Kaliner, M. A., and Austen, K. F., 1973, The sequence of biochemical events in the release of chemical mediators from sensitized human lung tissue, *J. Exp. Med.* **138**:1077.

Kaliner, M., and Austen, K. F., 1974a, Cyclic nucleotides and modulation of effector systems of inflammation, *Biochem. Pharmacol.* **23**:763.

Kaliner, M., and Austen, K. F., 1974b, Cyclic AMP, ATP, and reversed anaphylactic histamine release from rat mast cells, *J. Immunol.* **112**:664.

Kaliner, M., Orange, R. P., and Austen, K. F., 1972, Immunological release of histamine and slow-reacting substance from human lung. IV. Enhancement by cholinergic and alpha adrenergic stimulation, *J. Exp. Med.* **136**:556.

Kaliner, M., Wasserman, S. I., and Austen, K. F., 1973, Immunologic release of chemical mediators from human nasal polyps, *N. Engl. J. Med.* **289**:277.

Kanno, T., Cochrane, D. E., and Douglas, W. W., 1973, Exocytosis (secretory granule extrusion) induced by injection of calcium into mast cells, *Can. J. Physiol. Pharmacol.* **51**:1001.

Keller, R., 1966, Tissue mast cells in immune reactions, *Monogr. Allergy* **2**:1.

Kennerly, D. A., Sullivan, T. J., and Parker, C. W., 1979a, Activation of phospholipid metabolism during mediator release from stimulated mast cells, *J. Immunol.* **122**:152.

Kennerly, D. A., Secosan, C. J., Parker, C. W., and Sullivan, T. J., 1979b, Modulation of stimulated phospholipid metabolism in mast cells by pharmacologic agents that increase cyclic 3′,5′-adenosine monophosphate levels, *J. Immunol.* **123**:1519.

Kitamura, Y., and Hatanaka, K., 1978, Decrease in mast cells in wᵛ mice and their increase by bone marrow transplantation, *Blood* **52**:446.

Kitamura, Y., Shimada, M., Hatanaka, K., and Miyano, Y., 1977, Development of mast cells from grafted bone marrow cells in irradiated mice, *Nature (London)* **268**:442.

Koopman, W. J., Orange, R. P., and Austen, K. F., 1970, Immunochemical and biologic properties of rat IgE. III. Modulation of the IgE-mediated release of slow-reacting substance of anaphylaxis by agents influencing the level of cyclic 3′,5′-adenosine monophosphate, *J. Immunol.* **105**:1096.

Lagunoff, D., and Chi, E. Y., 1976, Effect of colchicine on rat mast cells, *J. Cell Biol.* **71**:182.

Lagunoff, D., and Wan, H., 1979, Inhibition of histamine release from rat mast cells by cytochalasin A and other sulfydryl reagents, *Biochem. Pharmacol.* **28**:1765.

Lawson, D., Roff, M. C., Gomperts, B. D., Fewtrell, C., and Gilula, N. B., 1977, Molecular events during membrane fusion: A study of exocytosis in rat peritoneal mast cells, *J. Cell Biol.* **72**:242.

Lemanske, R. F., and Kaliner, M. A., 1983, Late phase allergic reactions, *Int. J. Dermatol.* **22**:401.

Lemanske, R. F., Atkins, F. M., and Metcalfe, D. D., 1983a, Gastrointestinal mast cells in health and disease (Part I), *J. Pediatr.* **103**:177.

Lemanske, R. F., Atkins, F. M., and Metcalfe, D. D., 1983b, Gastrointestinal mast cells in health and disease (Part II), *J. Pediatr.* **103**:343.

Levy, D. A., and Carlton, J. A., 1969, Influence of temperature on the inhibition of colchicine of allergic histamine release, *Proc. Soc. Exp. Biol. Med.* **130**:1333.

Lewis, R. A., Holgate, S. T., Roberts, L. J., Maguire, J. F., Oates, J. A., and Austen, K. F., 1979, Effects of indomethacin on cyclic nucleotide levels and histamine release from rat serosal mast cells, *J. Immunol.* **123**:1663.

Lichtenstein, L. M., Foreman, J. C., Conroy, M. C., Marone, G., and Newball, H. H., 1979, Differences between histamine release from rat mast cells and human basophils and mast cells, *in: The Mast Cell: Its Role in Health and Disease* (J. Pepys and A. M. Edwards, eds), p. 83, Pitman Press, Kent, England.

Lovenberg, W., Bruckwick, E. A., and Hanbauer, I., 1975, ATP, cyclic AMP, and magnesium increase the affinity of rat striatal tyrosine hydroxylase for its cofactor, *Proc. Natl. Acad. Sci. U.S.A.* **72**:177.

Malaisse, W. J., Malaisse-Lange, F., Van Obbergiten, E., Somero, G., Devis, G., Ravazzolla, N., and Orci, L., 1975, Role of microtubules in the phasic pattern of insulin release, *Ann. N.Y. Acad. Sci.* **253**:630.

Malveaux, F. J., Conroy, M. C., Adkinson, N. F., and Lichtenstein, L. M., 1978, IgE receptors on human basophils, *J. Clin. Invest.* **61**:176.

Marone, G., Kagey-Sobotka, A., and Lichtenstein, L., 1979, Effects of arachidonic acid and its metabolites on antigen-induced histamine release from human basophils in vitro, *J. Immunol.* **123**:1669.

Marquardt, D. L., and Wasserman, S. I., 1982, Characterization of the rat mast cell beta-adrenergic receptor in resting and stimulated cells by radioligand binding, *J. Immunol.* **129**:2122.

Marquardt, D. L., Nicolotti, R. A., Kennerly, D. A., and Sullivan, T. J., 1981, Lipid metabolism during mediator release from mast cells: Studies of the role of arachidonic acid metabolism in the control of phospholipid metabolism, *J. Immunol.* **127**:845.

Metzger, H., Goetze, A., Kanellopoulos, J., Holowka, D., and Fewtrell, C., 1982, Structure of the high affinity mast cell receptor for IgE, *Fed. Proc.* **41**:8.

Nemeth, E. F., and Douglas, W. W., 1980, Differential inhibitory effects of the arachidonic acid analog ETYA on rat mast cell exocytosis evoked by secretagogues utilizing cellular or extracellular calcium, *Eur. J. Pharmacol.* **67**:439.

Oertel, H. L., and Kaliner, M., 1981, The biologic activity of mast cell granules. III. Purification of inflammatory factors of anaphylaxis (IF-A) responsible for causing late phase reactions, *J. Immunol.* **127**:1398.

Orange, R. P., Kaliner, M. A., LaRaia, P. J., and Austen, K. F., 1971a, Immunological release of histamine and slow-reacting substance of anaphylaxis from human lung. II. Influence of cellular levels of cyclic AMP, *Fed. Proc.* **30**:1725.

Orange, R. P., Austen, W. G., and Austen, K. F., 1971b, Immunological release of histamine and slow reacting substance of anaphylaxis from human lung. I. Modulation by agents influencing cellular levels of cyclic 3′,5′-adenosine monophosphate, *J. Exp. Med.* **134**(Suppl.):136.

Orci, L., Perrelet, A., and Friend, D. S., 1977, Freeze fracture of membrane fusions during exocytosis in pancreatic β cells, *J. Cell Biol.* **75**:23.

Orr, T. S. C., Hall, D. E., and Allison, A. C., 1972, Role of contractile microfilaments in the release of histamine from mast cells, *Nature (London)* **236**:350.

Padawer, J., and Gordon, A. S., 1955, Effects of cholchicine on mast cells of the rat, *Proc. Soc. Exp. Biol. Med.* **88**:522.

Palade, G., 1975, Intracellular aspects of the process of protein synthesis, *Science* **189**:347.

Palade, G. E., and Bruns, R. R., 1968, Structural modulation of plasmalemmal vesicles, *J. Cell Biol.* **37**:633.

Parwaresch, M. R., 1976, *The Human Basophil*, p. 1, Springer-Verlag, Berlin.

Pearce, F. L., Befus, A. D., Gauldie, J., and Beinenstock, J., 1982, Mucosal mast cells. II. Effects of anti-allergic compounds on histamine secretion by isolated intestinal mast cells, *J. Immunol.* **128**:2481.

Peterson, C., 1974a, Role of energy metabolism in histamine release: A study of isolated rat mast cells, *Acta Physiol. Scand.* **413**(Suppl.):1.

Peterson, C., 1974b, Inhibitory action of antimycin A on histamine release from isolated rat mast cells, *Acta Pharmacol. Toxicol.* **34**:347.

Peterson, C., 1974c, Histamine release induced by compound 48/80 from isolated rat mast cells: Dependence on endogenous ATP, *Acta Pharmacol. Toxicol.* **34**:356.

Peterson, C., and Diamant, B., 1974, Increased utilization of endogenous ATP in isolated rat mast cells during histamine release induced by compound 48/80, *Acta Pharmacol. Toxicol.* **34**:337.

Platshon, L., and Kaliner, M., 1978, The effect of the immunological release of histamine upon human lung cyclic nucleotide levels and prostaglandin generation, *J. Clin. Invest.* **62**:1113.

Poisner, A. M., and Bernstein, J., 1971, A possible role of microtubules in catecholamine release from the adrenal medulla: Effect of colchicine, vinca alkaloids and deuterium oxide, *J. Pharmacol. Exp. Ther.* **177**:102.

Portier, P., and Richet, C., 1902, De l'action anaphylactique de certaine venins, *C.R. Soc. Biol.* **54**:170.

Prausnitz, C., and Küstner, H., 1921, Studien über die ÜberempFindlichkeit, *Zentralbl. Bakteriol. Parasitenkd. Infektionskr. Hyg. Abt.* **86**:160.

Pruzansky, J. J., and Patterson, R., 1973, The diisopropylfluorophosphate inhibitable steps in antigen-induced histamine release from human leukocytes, *J. Immunol.* **17**:93.

Ramirez, M. A., 1919, Horse asthma following blood transfusion, *J. Am. Med. Assoc.*, **73**:984.

Ranadive, N. S., and Cochrane, C. G., 1971, Mechanisms of histamine release from mast cells by cationic protein (band 2) from neutrophil lysosomes, *J. Immunol.* **106**:506.

Rodbell, M., 1980, The role of hormone receptors and GTP-regulatory proteins in membrane transudation, *Nature (London)* **284**:17.

Röhlich, P., 1975, Membrane-associated actin filaments in the cortical cytoplasm of the rat mast cell, *Exp. Cell Res.* **93**:293.

Röhlich, P., Anderson, P., and Uvnäs, B., 1971, Electron microscope observations on compound 48/80 induced degranulation in rat mast cells: Evidence for sequential exocytosis of storage granules, *J. Cell Biol.* **51**:465.

Schulman, E. S., MacGlashan, D. W., Peters, S. P., Schleimer, R. P., Newball, H. H., and Lichtenstein, L. M., 1982, Human lung mast cells: Purification and characterization, *J. Immunol.* **129**:2662.

Selye, H., 1965, *The Mast Cell*, p. 1, Butterworths, London.

Sieghart, W., Theoharides, T., Alper, S., Douglas, W. W., and Greenhard, P., 1978, Calcium-dependent protein phosphorylation during secretion by exocytosis in the mast cell, *Nature (London)* **275**:329.

Sloboda, R. D., Rudolph, S. A., Rosenbaum, J. L., and Greengard, P., 1975, Cyclic AMP-dependent endogenous phosphorylation of a microtubule-associated protein, *Proc. Natl. Acad. Sci. U.S.A.* **72**:177.

Solley, G., Gleich, G., Jordan, R., and Shroeter, A., 1976, The late phase of the immediate wheal and flare skin reaction: Its dependence on IgE antibody, *J. Clin. Invest.* **58**:408.

Spiegelberg, H. L., and Melewicz, F. M., 1980, Fc receptors specific for IgE on subpopulations of human lymphocytes and monocytes, *Clin. Immunol. Immunopathol.* **15**:424.

Steer, M. L., 1977, Adrenergic receptors, in: *Clinics in Endocrinology and Metabolism* (L. Landsberg, ed.), pp. 577–598, Saunders, Philadelphia.

Stenson, W. F., Parker, C. W., and Sullivan, T. J., 1980, Augmentation of IgE-mediated release of histamine by 5-hydroxyeicosatetraenoic acid and 12-hydroxyeicosatetraenoic acid, *Biochem. Biophys. Res. Commun.* **96**:1045.

Strandberg, K., and Westerberg, S., 1976, Composition of phospholipids and phospholipid fatty acids in rat mast cells, *Mol. Cell. Biochem.* **11**:103.

Sullivan, T. J., and Parker, C. W., 1976, Pharmacologic modulation of inflammatory mediator release by rat mast cells, *Am. J. Pathol.* **85**:437.

Sullivan, T. J., and Parker, C. W., 1979, Possible role of arachidonic acid and its metabolites in mediator release from mast cells, *J. Immunol.* **122**:431.

Sullivan, T. J., Parker, K. L., Stenson, W., and Parker, C. W., 1975, Modulation of cyclic AMP in purified rat mast cells. I. Response to pharmacologic, metabolic, and physical stimuli, *J. Immunol.* **114**:1473.

Sutherland, E. W., Robison, G. A., and Butcher, R. W., 1968, Some aspects of the biological role of adenosine 3',5'-monophosphate (cyclic AMP), *Circulation* **37**:279.

Tauber, A. I., Kaliner, M., Stechschulte, D. J., and Austen, K. F., 1973, The immunologic release of histamine and slow reacting substance of anaphylaxis from human lung. V. Effect of prostaglandin on histamine release, *J. Immunol.* **111**:27.

Taurog, J. D., Fewtrell, C., and Becker, E. L., 1979, IgE-mediated triggering of rat basophil leukemia cells: Lack of evidence for serine esterase activation, *J. Immunol.* **122**:2150.

Theoharides, T. C., and Douglas, W. W., 1978, Secretion in mast cells induced by calcium entrapped within phospholipid vesicles, *Science* **201**:1143.

Theoharides, T. C., Sieghart, W., Greengard, P., and Douglas, W. W., 1980, Antiallergic drug cromolyn may inhibit histamine secretion by regulating phosphorylation of a mast cell protein, *Science* **207**:80.

Tilney, L. G., Clain, J. G., and Tilney, M. S., 1979, Membrane events in the acrosomal reaction of *Limulus* sperm: Membrane fusion, filament-membrane particle attachment and the source and formation of new membrane surface, *J. Cell Biol.* **81**:229.

Tolone, G., Bonasera, L., and Parrinello, N., 1974, Histamine release from mast cell: Role of microtubules, *Experientia* **30**:426.

Wescott, S., and Kaliner, M., 1980, The effect of histamine on mast cell cAMP *J. Allergy Clin. Immunol.* **65**:198.

Wescott, S., and Kaliner, M., 1981, The effects of histamine and PGD_2 on rat mast cell cyclic AMP and mediator release, *J. Allergy Clin. Immunol.* **68**:383.

Wilson, L., 1975, Action of drugs on microtubules, *Life Sci.* **17**:303.

Wilson, L., Bamberg, J. R., Mizel, S. B., Grisham, L. M., and Creswell, J1974, Interaction of drugs with microtubule proteins, *Fed. Proc.* **33**:158.

Wolff, J., and Bhattacharyya, B., 1975, Microtubules and thyroid hormone mobilization, *Ann. N.Y. Acad. Sci.* **253**:763.

Yodoi, J., and Ishizaka, K., 1979, Lymphocytes bearing Fc receptors for IgE. I. Presence of human and rat T lymphocytes with Fc epsilon receptors, *J. Immunol.* **122**:2577.

4

Release of Lipid Mediators from Macrophages and Its Pharmacological Modulation

RÉGINE ROUBIN and JACQUES BENVENISTE

1. INTRODUCTION

When macrophages encounter inflammatory stimuli, they respond by releasing a number of products that may account for the central role of this cell in chronic inflammatory diseases. These products include hydrolytic enzymes, components of both the classical and the alternate pathway of complement, and factors modulating responses of lymphocytes to antigens. Recently, macrophages have also been shown to release lipid mediators, both arachidonic acid metabolites and Paf-acether or platelet-activating factor. Quantitative and/or qualitative variations in the release of these compounds occur depending on the local environment from which the macrophages were obtained. Peritoneal macrophages obtained from untreated animals are defined as resident. Those obtained after the introduction of a sterile irritant such as thioglycollate broth, sodium caseinate, protease peptone, or mineral oil are defined as elicited, and macrophages obtained from animals immunologically sensitized to a specific antigen or following bacterial infection are defined as activated. These three macrophage populations have distinct biological properties.

Since the release of lipid mediators varies from one population to another, one might question whether it is related to some of the properties of the macrophage and what the effects of the lipid mediators on other cell types are. Since our knowledge of the biosynthetic pathways of these mediators and the availability of snythetic compounds are fairly recent, little is yet known on these aspects.

RÉGINE ROUBIN and JACQUES BENVENISTE • INSERM U-200, Université Paris-Sud, 92140 Clamart, France.

2. PROSTAGLANDINS

2.1. BIOSYNTHESIS

Since mammalian cells contain very little free arachidonic acid, the release of unesterified arachidonic acid from phospholipids is a prerequisite for the synthesis of prostaglandins (and also leukotrienes) from intact cells (Kuehl and Egan, 1980). It has been assumed for many years that a phospholipase A_2 produces arachidonic acid (Van den Bosch, 1980), but it is likely that a phospholipase C also participates (Bell et al., 1979). Wightman et al. (1981a) have shown that homogenates of mouse peritoneal macrophages contain two phospholipase A_2 activities. One is active at pH 4.5 and is independent of Ca^{2+} and the other is active at pH 8.5 and is Ca^{2+} dependent. They found that the pH 8.5 activity hydrolyzes purified phospholipids very efficiently whereas the pH 4.5 one hydrolyzes phosphatidylethanolamine (PE) and phosphatidylcholine (PC) better when they are mixed with other polar lipids. These authors suggested for the pH 4.5 activity a lysosomal origin. At the same time, Hsueh et al. (1981) showed that rabbit alveolar macrophages contain two phospholipase A_2 pools, one in the lysosome and the other elsewhere, presumably in the membrane. Depending on the type of stimulus, phagocytic or provoking Ca^{2+} influx, the lysosomal and/or the membranous pool is activated.

The release of arachidonic acid can also result from the activation of the phosphatidylinositol (PI) cycle. Indeed, years ago, Karnovsky and Wallach (1961) and Graham et al. (1967) showed that phagocytizing macrophages preferentially incorporated ^{32}P into PI. This rapid turnover of PI involves the action of a phospholipase C. The generated diacylglycerol is a substrate for a diacyl lipase that hydrolyzes fatty acids including arachidonic acid. Also, the diacylglycerol can be phosphorylated into phosphatidic acid, which on the one hand can reenter the PI cycle and on the other hand acts as a Ca^{2+} ionophore favoring Ca^{2+} mobilization. The latter activates the Ca^{2+}-dependent phospholipase A_2, which deacylates other phospholipids, including PC, generating arachidonic acid. This coupling was shown first to be operative in platelets (for a review see Lapetina, 1982). Macrophage homogenates contain a phospholipase C activity (Wightman et al., 1981b) that is inhibited by phenothiazines, a finding that fits well with the inhibition of prostaglandin release in intact cells by these compounds (Humes et al., 1979).

Of the phospholipids of macrophage membranes, 20–25% of their total fatty acid content is arachidonic acid (Mahoney et al., 1977; Scott et al., 1980), making this cell type a good model for studying arachidonic acid metabolism. Among the cells involved in the immune response, macrophages appear to be the largest producers of prostaglandins (Kurland and Bockman, 1978). In Fig. 1 is illustrated the biosynthesis of prostaglandins and thromboxane via the cyclooxygenase pathway. These end products are formed from two short-lived cyclic endoperoxides, prostaglandins (PG) G_2 and H_2 (Samuelsson et al., 1978). Prostacyclin (PGI_2) and thromboxane TxA_2 possess great biological activities although they

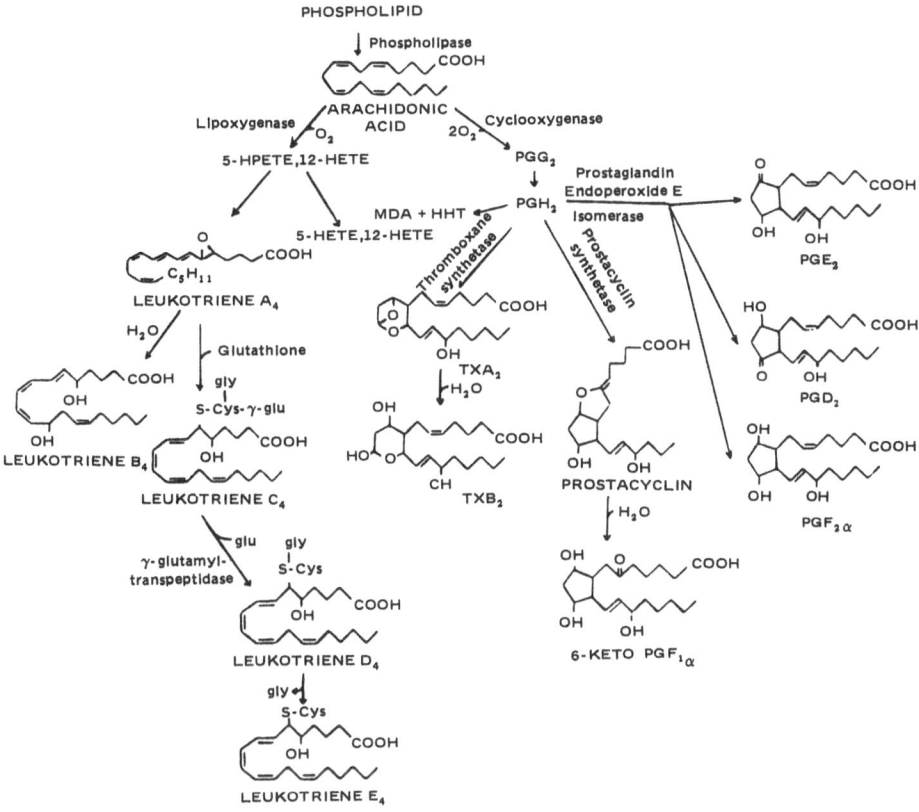

FIGURE 1.   Metabolism of arachidonic acid into prostaglandins, thromboxanes, and leukotrienes.

are very unstable and are quickly transformed into 6-keto-PGF$_{1\alpha}$ and TxB$_2$, respectively.

2.2. ASSAY

Before the chemical identification of the various prostaglandins and their synthesis, the detection of prostaglandins was performed by bioassay on a number of isolated tissues. Now two novel assays are available: radioimmunoassays, which provide highly sensitive measurements of the various products, and a variety of chromatographic systems, which allow prostaglandin identification by comparison of their mobility with known synthetic compounds. The latter assays are based on the preincorporation of radiolabeled arachidonic acid into cellular phospholipids. The advantage of the chromatographic systems is that they allow identification of the whole range of prostaglandins but without quantitation, whereas the radioimmunoassay does measure prostaglandins, but only the type one is looking for. Finally, definitive identification is assessed by mass spectrometry.

2.3. STIMULI

Prostaglandins are not storage products but are synthesized and immediately released in the extracellular medium upon various stimuli, the most physiologically relevant being lymphokines (Gordon *et al.*, 1976; Friedman *et al.*, 1979) and the phagocytic process. Phagocytosis of zymosan (Humes *et al.*, 1977), bacteria (Gemsa *et al.*, 1979a) and immunoglobulin-coated erythrocytes (Brune *et al.*, 1978) triggers PGE release, whereas phagocytosis of latex particles (a noninflammatory agent) does not. However, when latex is coated with IgG, even in the presence of an inhibitor of phagocytosis, prostaglandin release is obtained. This indicates that phagocytosis *per se* is not a prerequisite for prostaglandin synthesis; rather, an interaction between a ligand and the Fc receptor is the critical step in this process (Rouzer *et al.*, 1980a). Recently the release of PGE_2 after exposure of macrophages to particulate IgE immune complexes has been obtained (Rouzer *et al.*, 1982a).

The Ca^{2+} ionophore A23187 (Gemsa *et al.*, 1979b) and the well-known tumor promoter, phorbol myristate acetate (PMA) (Bonney *et al.*, 1980), are also very efficient in inducing prostaglandin release. Lipopolysaccharide (LPS) of gram-negative bacteria, in contrast to other stimuli, exhibits a slow action, the maximal PGE_2 release occurring after 10 hr of incubation (Gemsa *et al.*, 1980). In contrast to these inflammatory compounds, colchicine, an antiinflammatory one, is capable of inducing a high level of PGE release, indicating that components of the cytoskeleton may influence biosynthesis of prostaglandins (Gemsa *et al.*, 1980).

2.4. RELEASE FROM RESIDENT MACROPHAGES

Twenty-four-hour macrophage monolayers incubated with [^{3}H]arachidonic acid incorporated 40–60% of the label within 4 hr (Bonney *et al.*, 1978a). Analysis of phospholipids indicated that the bulk of the label was incorporated into PC and PE. Unstimulated cells produced low amounts of prostaglandins; however, upon adequate stimulation the basal rate could be greatly increased. Zymosan added to cultures of resident macrophages prelabeled with [^{3}H]arachidonic acid caused the release of large amounts of [^{3}H]arachidonic acid derivatives. Approximately 67% of the radiolabel was recovered as prostaglandins and the remaining as lipoxygenase products (Scott *et al.*, 1980). The release started 5–7 min after zymosan addition and continued for at least 24 hr (Humes *et al.*, 1977; Scott *et al.*, 1980). Chromatography of these [^{3}H]-labeled oxygenation compounds indicated that the major products were PGE_2 (51%) and 6-keto-$PGF_{1\alpha}$ (16%), the stable metabolite of PGI_2 (Bonney *et al.*, 1978a; Scott *et al.*, 1980). $PGF_{2\alpha}$ was not detected in significant amounts, and TxB_2 was present in very low amounts

(Brune *et al.*, 1978; Drapier *et al.*, 1983). Analysis of cell cultures exposed to zymosan showed that the majority of [^{3}H]arachidonic acid was released from PC (Bonney *et al.*, 1978a; Hsueh *et al.*, 1979; Drapier *et al.*, 1983). A diminished PGE$_2$ and a higher PGI$_2$ synthesis occurred in macrophages cultured for 2 hr and stimulated with zymosan as compared to 24 hr (Bonney *et al.*, 1981; Rouzer *et al.*, 1982a; Drapier *et al.*, 1983).

Resident macrophages also have the capacity to metabolize exogenous arachidonic acid in concentrations up to 1 μM without loss of viability and in the absence of a trigger (Scott *et al.*, 1982a). After a 20-min incubation, one-third of the fatty acid was found esterified in cell phospholipids and two-thirds was metabolized to oxygenated products that were recovered in the culture medium. In these conditions, HETE, PGI$_2$, and PGE$_2$ were found in a proportion of 67:24:9, i.e., quite different from that found in response to a phagocytic stimulus. These observations show that resident macrophages are capable of exhibiting high levels of cyclooxygenase and lipoxygenase activity.

2.5. RELEASE FROM INFLAMMATORY PERITONEAL MACROPHAGES

Humes *et al.* (1977) showed that, in contrast to resident macrophages, macrophages from mice stimulated with thioglycollate broth have a greatly diminished capacity for synthesizing and releasing prostaglandins in response to a zymosan challenge. They extended their study to the effect of various *in vivo*

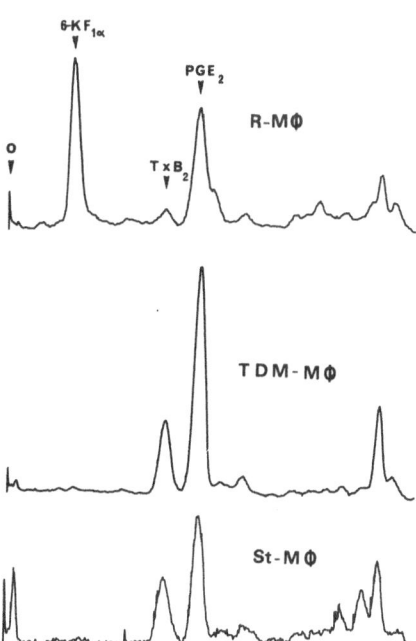

FIGURE 2. Autoradiogram scans showing the different patterns of cyclooxygenase derivatives released by resident (R-Mφ), trehalose dimycolate (TDM-Mφ); and *Streptococcus* (St-Mφ)-activated macrophages. (From Drapier *et al.*, 1983, with permission from Elsevier.)

inflammatory stimuli, including immunogenic stimuli such as BCG and *Corynebacterium parvum*. All stimuli induced macrophages with a lower capacity to synthesize prostaglandins (Humes *et al.*, 1980). They attributed this lower capacity to a diminished arachidonic acid deacylation rate in inflammatory macrophages. These results were later confirmed by Scott *et al.* (1982b) and Drapier *et al.* (1983), both of these groups finding, in addition, a channeling in the synthesized prostaglandins different from that found in resident macrophages. Indeed, a reduced PGI_2 synthesis and an increased TxA_2 synthesis were the distinct features of the macrophages obtained with *C. parvum* (Scott *et al.*, 1982b) or with a chemically defined extract of *Mycobacterium tuberculosis*, trehalose dimycolate (Drapier *et al.*, 1983) (Fig. 2). However, as opposed to Scott *et al.* (1982b), Drapier *et al.* (1983) did not conclude that a diminished arachidonic acid metabolism, but rather this different prostaglandin channeling, was a criterion of macrophage activation. These results are at variance with those reported by Bärlin *et al.* (1981), who found that unstimulated macrophages obtained from mice treated with *C. parvum* release larger amounts of PGE_2 than do resident cells. It is noteworthy that peritoneal macrophages from mice bearing a fibrosarcoma release large quantities of PGE_2 and PGI_2 (Pelus and Bockman, 1979).

2.6. RELEASE FROM ALVEOLAR MACROPHAGES

Rabbit alveolar macrophages produce PGD_2, E_2, $F_{2\alpha}$, and I_2 when stimulated by zymosan but not by latex (Hsueh *et al.*, 1979). When exogenous arachidonic acid is supplied, unstimulated rat alveolar macrophages release high amounts of TxB_2 and no PGI_2 (Arnoux *et al.*, 1981a), a result in keeping with activated peritoneal macrophages. Similar results were reported by Rouzer *et al.* (1982b) in mouse pulmonary macrophages.

3. LEUKOTRIENES

3.1. HISTORICAL BACKGROUND AND BIOSYNTHESIS

Slow-reacting substance (SRS) was first discovered by Feldberg and Kellaway (1938) in the perfusate of lung treated with cobra venom. This substance, which caused a characteristic contraction of selected smooth muscle preparations, was later found in the perfusates of sensitized lungs challenged with antigen (Orange *et al.*, 1971). For many years, progress on the study of SRS was hampered by the very low quantities available. The use of A23187-stimulated mouse mastocytoma cells (Murphy *et al.*, 1979) or rat basophilic leukemia cells (Morris *et al.*, 1980) has led to the generation of SRS in sufficient quantity to allow for its chemical characterization. SRS was identified as metabolites of arachidonic acid via the lipoxygenase pathway and were named leukotriene C and D (LTC, LTD) (Hammarström *et al.*, 1979; Örning *et al.*, 1980; Morris *et al.*, 1980). In Fig. 1 is illustrated the formation of the various leukotrienes. The unstable LTA_4 is either dihydroxylated into LTB_4 (a potent neutrophil chemotactic factor) or converted into LTC_4 by addition of glutathione at C_6 of the eicosatetraenoic acid. The cysteinyl-glycine derivative (LTD_4) is thought to be a degradation product of LTC_4 via a γ-glutamyl transpeptidase activity. The enzyme yielding the cysteine derivative (LTE_4) has not been identified.

3.2. ASSAY

SRS activity is bioassayed on an atropinized guinea pig ileum or isolated trachea in the presence of an antihistamine compound (Stechschulte *et al.*, 1967). The specificity of the slow and long-lasting contraction is assessed by its reversion in the presence of FPL 55712. Taking advantage of the specific absorption (280 nm) of the triene configuration of the molecules, the various leukotrienes can be detected after separation by high-pressure liquid chromatography. The retention time of the natural compound is compared with that of synthetic standards. Radioimmunoassays are not commercially available.

3.3. RELEASE FROM PERITONEAL MACROPHAGES

Resident rat and mouse peritoneal macrophages release SRS when stimulated with A23187 in the presence of large amount of cysteine (10 mM) (Bach and Brashler, 1974, 1978; Orange *et al.*, 1980). Bach *et al.* (1980) showed that the majority of the SRS activities belong to LTC and a few to LTD (Bach and Brashler, 1980). Macrophages stimulated by zymosan phagocytosis released LTC (Rouzer *et al.*, 1980b). The level of LTC increased for 60 min and remained constant thereafter. The release of LTC from 2-hr adherent macrophages appears lower than from 24-hr monolayers and in both cases the presence of cysteine in the incubation medium is not a prerequisite (Rouzer *et al.*, 1982a). Phagocytosis of IgG or IgE immune complexes (Rouzer *et al.*, 1980c, 1982a), or bacteria (Roubin and Benveniste, 1981a) induced LTC release but to a lesser extent than zymosan. Soluble membrane-mediated inflammatory stimuli (PMA, LPS) as opposed to phagocytized inflammatory material (zymosan) do not induce leukotriene release although they are good stimuli for prostaglandin synthesis (Humes *et al.*, 1982). These authors propose that two pools of arachidonic acid exist in macrophage membranes, one accessible to both the cyclooxygenase and the lipoxygenase pathway and the other only to the cyclooxygenase. Fusion of lysosomes with phagocytic vacuoles would make the arachidonic acid produced by the lysosomal phospholipase A_2 accessible to both the lipoxygenase—possibly a soluble enzyme (Jakschik and Lee, 1980)—and the cyclooxygenase, an endoplasmic reticulum-associated activity (Rollins and Smith, 1979). In the case of a soluble stimulus, interaction with the plasma membrane would activate membrane phospholipase A_2, making arachidonate only accessible to the cyclooxygenase. Such a concept has also been formulated by Hsueh *et al.* (1981).

As for prostaglandin release, the state of macrophage activation induces

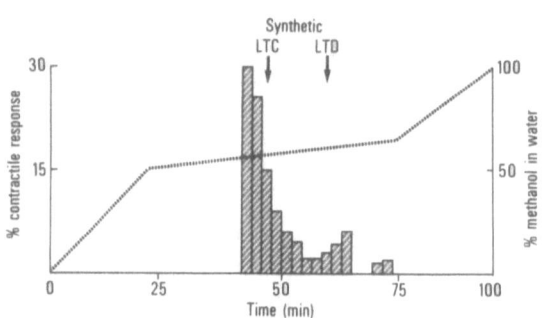

FIGURE 3. Reverse-phase HPLC elution profiles of slow-reacting substance derived from resident macrophages stimulated by zymosan phagocytosis. Contractile response (bar) was measured on a guinea pig ileum in the presence of atropine and an antihistamine compound. A gradient of methanol in water (.....) was used to elute the column. (From Roubin *et al.*, 1982a, with permission from Verlag Chemie.)

qualitative and/or quantitative variations in leukotriene formation. We have compared the ability of thioglycollate-elicited, BCG-activated or resident macrophages to release SRS (Roubin and Benveniste, 1981a,b; Roubin *et al.*, 1982a). When stimulated by ionophore or zymosan, thioglycollate macrophages were the only cells exhibiting markedly reduced SRS release, whereas resident macrophage and BCG macrophage SRS induced comparable contractile respones. The striking difference between resident macrophages and BCG macrophages resided in the leukotriene composition of the SRS released. SRS from these two populations was chromatographed by HPLC and LTC and LTD identified by retention time in comparison with the synthetic compounds synthesized as in Rokach *et al.* (1980) and kindly furnished by Dr. Rokach (Merck Frosst Laboratories, Pointe-Claire-Dorval, Canada). We found, as already described by Bach *et al.* (1980) and Bach and Braschler (1980) that most (80%) of the contractile response derived from resident macrophages migrated as LTC and a small amount as LTD (20%) (Fig. 3), whereas in BCG macrophages LTC and LTD activities were of equal proportion (Fig. 4). Since LTD is 10 times more potent than LTC in contracting guinea pig ileum (Piper *et al.*, 1981; Roubin *et al.*, 1982a) we concluded that BCG-activated macrophages release, on a molar basis, lower amounts of LTC than resident macrophages. We extended the study to two other types of activated macrophages obtained after injection of streptococci or trehalose dimycolate and found that a lower release of LTC was a common feature of inflammatory macrophages (Drapier *et al.*, 1983). Similar results were recently reported by Scott *et al.* (1982b) using *C. parvum*-activated macrophages.

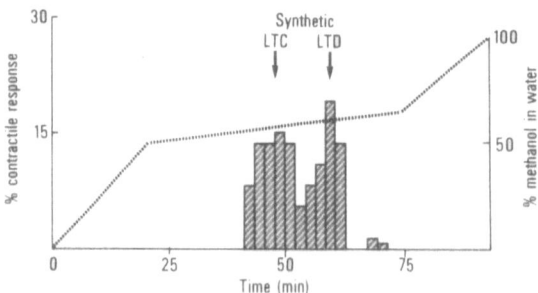

FIGURE 4. Reverse-phase HPLC elution profiles of slow-reacting substance derived from BCG-activated macrophages stimulated by zymosan phagocytosis. (From Roubin *et al.*, 1982a, with permission from Verlag Chemie.)

Of interest is the greater amount of LTD in activated macrophages than in resident cells. This could be due to a higher γ-glutamyl transpeptidase activity (the enzyme thought to convert LTC to LTD) in activated cells than in resident cells. Indeed, Rouzer et al. (1982c) reported this to be the case. However, these authors have not correlated this greater enzyme activity with an increased release of LTD from the C. parvum-activated macrophages.

3.4. RELEASE FROM LUNG MACROPHAGES

Considerable work in the past has shown that IgE-sensitized lung tissue produces SRS when challenged with a specific antigen. Studies of purified pulmonary mast cells have indicated that they are not capable of releasing large quantities of leukotrienes (Orange et al., 1971; Lewis and Austen, 1981), suggesting that macrophages could be the source of SRS in this reaction. However, Orange et al. (1980) did not find increased amounts of SRS activity in alveolar macrophages harvested by intratracheal lavage of rat lung and stimulated by ionophore even in the presence of cysteine. In contrast, Rankin et al. (1982) reported the release of LTC from rat alveolar macrophages upon ionophore stimulation or upon challenge with IgE antibody and specific antigen. Arnoux et al. (1981a) investigated whether exogenous arachidonic acid could enhance SRS production by alveolar macrophages. Identification and quantitation of arachidonate metabolites were performed using high-efficiency glass capillary column gas chromatography coupled with mass spectrometry. Only 12-HETE was detected and again not the 5,8,9,11,15-HETE isomer [the precursor(s) of SRS]. Rouzer et al. (1982b) compared the arachidonate metabolism of mouse pulmonary alveolar macrophages, obtained by intratracheal lavage, and pulmonary tissue macrophages, obtained by enzymatic digestion of the lung. They found that the tissue macrophages—surely a mixture of interstitial and alveolar macrophages—released greater amounts of arachidonate metabolites than the exclusively alveolar ones. It is probable that constantly stimulated alveolar macrophages lose their ability to release arachidonate metabolites as do inflammatory peritoneal macrophages. These authors found that interstitial pulmonary macrophages stimulated by zymosan phagocytosis release as much LTC and HETEs as do resident peritoneal macrophages.

4. PAF-ACETHER

4.1. HISTORICAL BACKGROUND, DEFINITION, AND ASSAY

A leukocyte-dependent histamine-releasing mechanism was described by Barbaro and Zvaifler (1966) and a soluble intermediate subsequently detected (Siraganian and Osler, 1971). It was considered "lytic" for platelets but remained uncharacterized. The methodology for its routine preparation was described by Benveniste et al. (1972) who started its characterization, named it platelet-activating factor (PAF), and demonstrated its release from IgE-sensitized rabbit basophils. Its presence in man (Benveniste, 1974), its effect on human platelets (Benveniste *et al.*, 1975), and most of its known physicochemical characteristics including its phospholipid nature (Benveniste *et al.*, 1977) were revealed later. The proposed structure was that of a glycerophospholipid with a choline polar head group, an ester-linked acyl chain at C_2, and no ester link at C_1 (Benveniste *et al.*, 1977), thereby creating a new class of phospholipid mediator. Finally, the procedure for its purification was described (Tencé *et al.*, 1980), its structure was elucidated as being a 1-O-alkyl-2-acetyl-sn-glyceryl-3-phosphorylcholine (Benveniste *et al.*, 1979; Demopoulos *et al.*, 1979), and its total synthesis was achieved (Godfroid *et al.*, 1980). Given the numerous substances present in biological fluids and cell supernatants that can activate platelets, it was necessary to strictly define Paf-acether. For several years, even before the knowledge of its molecular structure, the following criteria were used to precisely distinguish it from, for example, arachidonic acid, thrombin, ADP, and prostaglandins: (1) platelet aggregation (or release of labeled serotonin) in the presence of aspirin or indomethacin and of ADP scavengers, (2) elution pattern identical to that of hog leukocyte (and now synthetic) Paf-acether on silicic acid thin-layer or high-pressure liquid chromatography, and (3) inactivation by phospholipases A_2, C, and D and resistance to lipase from *Rhizopus arrhizus*.

4.2. RELEASE FROM PERITONEAL MACROPHAGES

Paf-acether was first demonstrated as originating from IgE-sensitized basophils challenged with antigen, thus suggesting its origin from mast cells. Rat peritoneal cells release Paf-acether and histamine when stimulated by A23187. However, when mast cells and macrophages are purified on a Ficoll gradient, Paf-acether and histamine are found to be released from two different populations. Paf-acether-producing cells are also capable of secreting acid phosphatase (Fig. 5), indicating that macrophages and not mast cells are responsible for Paf-acether production (Mencia-Huerta and Benveniste, 1979).

Paf-acether production by macrophages can be observed in response to a variety of stimuli, either unspecific such as A23187 or specific such as phagocytosis of zymosan, bacteria, erythrocytes coated with IgG, or immune complexes (Mencia-Huerta and Benveniste, 1981) (Fig. 6). It is noteworthy that latex particles neither cause inflammation *in vivo* nor stimulate greatly Paf-acether production in contrast to both bacteria and zymosan, which cause inflammation *in vivo* and markedly stimulate Paf-acether production *in vitro*. Since latex particles are ingested avidly by macrophages in culture but do not stimulate Paf-acether production, it appears that phagocytosis *per se* is not a sufficient stimulus for Paf-acether production (nor for the release of arachidonic acid derivatives; see above). Indeed, blockade of phagocytosis by cytochalasin B did not inhibit Paf-acether production (Mencia-Huerta and Benveniste, 1981). The release started 5 min after ionophore stimulation and was maximal at 60 min (Roubin *et al.*, 1982b).

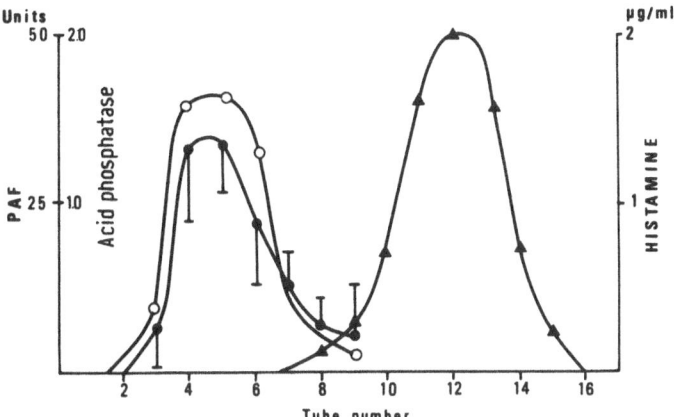

FIGURE 5.   Ability of Ficoll gradient-fractionated rat peritoneal cells to release Paf-acether (●), acid phosphatase (○), and histamine (▲). Paf-acether activity was found in cells containing acid phosphatase (i.e., macrophages) and not in cells containing histamine (i.e., mastocytes). (From Mencia-Huerta and Benveniste, 1979, with permission from Verlag Chemie.)

Contrary to what is observed for prostaglandin or leukotriene production, 24-hr adherent macrophages lose their ability to form Paf-acether.

Macrophages obtained from inflammatory sites produce less Paf-acether than do resident macrophages. We have studied the release of Paf-acether from mouse peritoneal macrophages elicited with thioglycollate broth or sodium caseinate, or activated with viable BCG. We found that elicited macrophages released lower amounts of mediator than do resident ones (Roubin and Benveniste, 1981b; Roubin et al., 1982a) although they released a large amount of the deacetylated Paf-acether derivative 2-lyso-Paf-acether (Roubin et al., 1982b). This

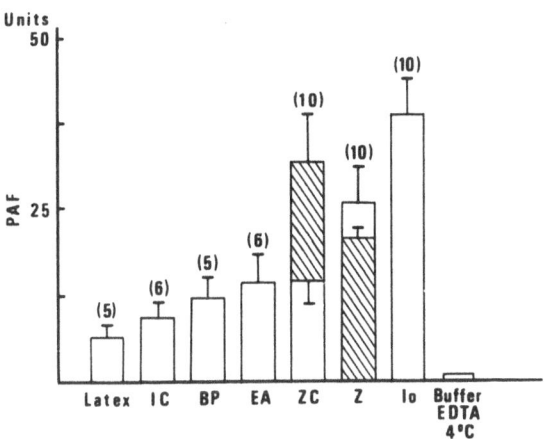

FIGURE 6.   Release of Paf-acether from peritoneal macrophages stimulated for 1 hr at 37°C with latex particles, immune complexes (IC), *Bordetella pertussis* (BP), erythrocytes coated with IgE (EA), zymosan (Z) coated with complement (ZC), or ionophore A23187 (Io), with (hatched bars)or without (clear bars) agitation. Number of experiments shown in parentheses. (From Mencia-Huerta and Benveniste, 1981, with permission from Academic Press.)

impairment has been attributed to a lower acetyltransferase activity exhibited by thioglycollate-induced macrophages (see Section 4.4.2). In contrast to the impaired release of Paf-acether from elicited macrophages, the BCG-activated ones released in the extracellular medium a larger amount of mediator than resident macrophages (Roubin *et al.*, 1982a) (Fig. 7). Whether or not this production can influence lymphocyte response in delayed hypersensitivity reactions is under investigation.

Recently we observed that Paf-acether synthesized by macrophages was not entirely released in the extracellular medium. The total amount of mediator was obtained after ethanol extraction of cell lipids. Resident macrophages released only 4% of that synthesized (Benveniste *et al.*, 1982a). However, it is still not known whether the mediator is on the membrane or inside the cells and this point needs clarification. Reconsidering our data on BCG macrophages, we found that although Paf-acether was released in the extracellular medium with a higher efficiency than from resident macrophages, the total amount of mediator formed was lower (unpublished observation). We have extended this study to macrophages obtained after injection of killed streptococci or chemically defined extract of *M. tuberculosis*, trehalose dimycolate, and found that a lower formation of Paf-acether from these activated macrophages was indeed a general feature of inflammatory macrophages (Drapier *et al.*, 1983). However, as found for BCG macrophages, trehalose dimycolate-induced macrophages released a larger amount of Paf-acether in the extracellular medium than do resident cells (Table 1). An interesting question concerns the finding that some types of macrophages exhibit a ratio of release to formation of Paf-acether that is higher than others. Are regulatory molecules involved in such a phenomenon or are the kinetics of the release different in activated macrophages as compared to resident ones?

These data indicate that local environment alters Paf-acether generation by

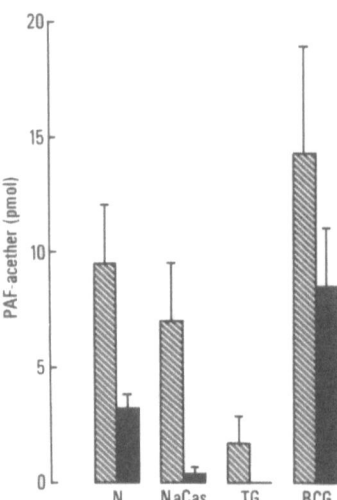

FIGURE 7.   Release of Paf-acether from resident (normal = N), sodium caseinate (NaCas)-, thioglycollate (TG)-, and BCG-induced macrophages stimulated with ionophore A23187 (hatched bars) or zymosan (clear bars) phagocytosis. (From Roubin *et al.*, 1982a, with permission from Verlag Chemie.)

TABLE 1. FORMATION OF 2-LYSO-PAF-ACETHER AND PAF-ACETHER UPON ZYMOSAN CHALLENGE BY VARIOUS MACROPHAGE POPULATIONS[a]

Macrophages	2-lyso-Paf-acether	Paf-acether	
		Released	Membrane-bound
Resident	526.3 ± 73.7	9.3 ± 1.2	148.6 ± 4.5
Trehalose dimycolate-activated	363.1 ± 97.4	13.3 ± 1.9	15.1 ± 0.3
Streptococcus-activated	302.6 ± 7.10	0	5.8 ± 0.8

[a]Paf-acether released in the extracellular medium or recovered after ethanolic extraction (membrane-bound) of macrophage monolayers was measured by aggregation of washed rabbit platelets. 2-Lyso-Paf-acether was measured after chemical acetylation as Paf-acether. Membrane-bound and released 2-lyso-Paf-acether have been summed. Results are expressed in pg/μg protein and are the mean ± S.D. of four to six experiments.

macrophages. Whether or not such changes are relevant to vascular changes (permeability, blood pressure) at various stages of the inflammatory process has still to be determined.

4.3. RELEASE FROM ALVEOLAR MACROPHAGES

Paf-acether is released from rat, rabbit, monkey, and human alveolar macrophages upon stimulation with A23187. In contrast, the release of Paf-acether by zymosan or opsonized zymosan varies from species to species. Rat and rabbit alveolar macrophages release Paf-acether in the presence of zymosan, opsonized or not, whereas alveolar macrophages from monkey or human cannot, although they readily phagocytized zymosan or opsonized zymosan. This is probably due to a failure of the triggering mechanism since human alveolar macrophages release Paf-acether upon ionophore challenge. This release is dependent on the dose of ionophore used for stimulation (Arnoux et al., 1980). The lack of Paf-acether release from human and monkey alveolar macrophages stimulated by zymosan or opsonized zymosan as opposed to rat and rabbit alveolar macrophages might be explained by species difference but also by raising and environmental conditions.

The release of Paf-acether from alveolar macrophages in humans with various pathologies and presenting with or without smoker's habit was studied (Arnoux et al., 1981b). Ionophore-stimulated alveolar macrophages from nonsmoker healthy subjects were compared to macrophages from either smoker or nonsmoker sarcoidosis patients, smoker idiopathic pulmonary fibrosis patients, and nonsmoker asthmatic patients. Alveolar macrophages from smokers with any pathology released higher amounts of Paf-acether than nonsmokers. Another interesting finding was the greater release of Paf-acether from alveolar macrophages in the different pathologies—except from asthmatic patients— than from healthy donors. Indeed, the release of Paf-acether from alveolar macrophages of asthmatic patients was not dependent on the dose of ionophore.

However, they released Paf-acether (Arnoux *et al.*, 1982) and lysosomal enzymes (Joseph *et al.*, 1983) when stimulated with the specific allergen. The allergens used were those inducing a positive Prick test or *in vitro* basophil degranulation test. Such allergens could not induce the release of Paf-acether and lysosomal enzymes from alveolar macrophages of normal donors.

The specific release of Paf-acether by alveolar macrophages of asthmatic patients obtained with sensitizing allergens may represent a new pathway in the physiopathology of human asthma disease. Indeed, Paf-acether, TxA$_2$, and PGF$_{2\alpha}$ (see Section 3.4) are all potent bronchoconstrictors either directly or via platelet activation (Vargaftig *et al.*, 1980,1981; Denjean *et al.*, 1981). Thus, besides the well-recognized role of bronchial mast cells in the pathogenesis of asthma, the participation of alveolar macrophages must also be taken into account in the IgE-dependent mechanisms of allergic disease (Fig. 8).

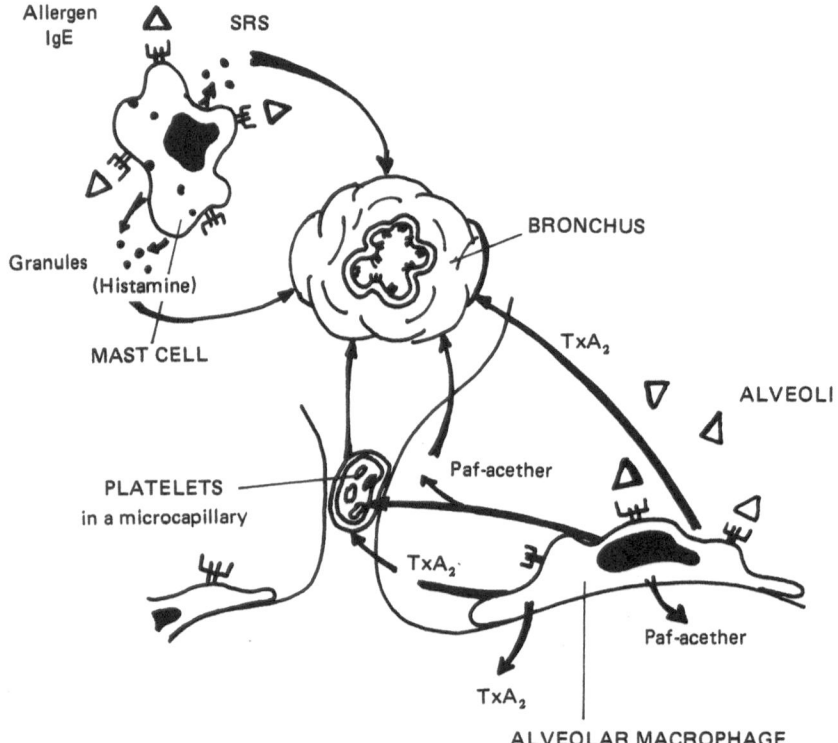

FIGURE 8.   The two pathways inducing bronchus contraction. On the one hand, the binding of allergen with IgE fixed on mast cells leads to the release of their granule contents (e.g., histamine) and slow-reacting substance. On the other hand, alveolar IgE-sensitized macrophages are capable of releasing Paf-acether (and thromboxane A$_2$), which, either directly or through platelet activation, induce bronchoconstriction. (From Arnoux *et al.*, unpublished schema.)

4.4. PAF-ACETHER METABOLISM

4.4.1. PHOSPHOLIPASE A$_2$-DEPENDENT RELEASE OF PAF-ACETHER

The release of Paf-acether from macrophages was abolished by EDTA, bromophenacyl bromide, mepacrine, and 874 CB (Clin-Midy) (Benveniste and Mencia-Huerta, 1978; Mencia-Huerta and Benveniste, 1979). These results suggested the intervention of a phospholipase A$_2$ in Paf-acether formation. More recently, Polonsky *et al.* (1980) have demonstrated the simultaneous release from hog leukocytes incubated overnight at pH 9.6, of Paf-acether and of its nonacetylated derivative 2-lyso-Paf-acether (1-*O*-alkyl-glyceryl-3-phosphorylcholine). This result suggested (1) the activation of a phospholipase A$_2$ yielding 2-lyso-Paf-

Ether phospholipids

(1-0-alkyl-2-0-acyl-<u>sn</u>-glyceryl-3-phosphorylcholine)

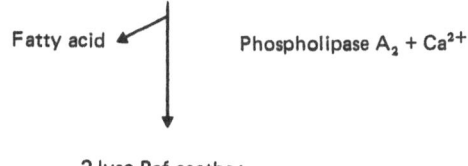

2-lyso Paf-acether

(1-0-alkyl-<u>sn</u>-glyceryl-3-phosphorylcholine)

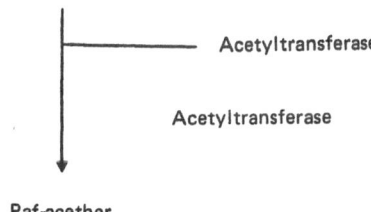

Paf-acether

(1-0-alkyl-2-0-acetyl-<u>sn</u>-glyceryl-3-phosphorylcholine)

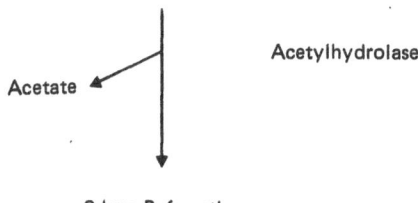

2-lyso Paf-acether

(1-0-alkyl-sn-glyceryl-3-phosphorylcholine)

FIGURE 9.   Model of Paf-acether metabolism.

acether from membrane ether phospholipids [indeed, in macrophages a significant amount of the choline phosphoglyceride is of the alkyl ether type (Sugiura et al., 1982)] and (2) the existence of an enzyme capable of acetylating 2-lyso-Paf-acether into Paf-acether or of hydrolyzing Paf-acether into 2-lyso-Paf-acether (Fig. 9).

Thereafter, the release of 2-lyso-Paf-acether was found to occur not only at pH 9.6 (Optimal pH for phospholipase A_2 activity), but also with physiological stimuli that induce Paf-acether release (Benveniste et al., 1982a,b; Roubin et al., 1982b). However, direct evidence for the role of a phospholipase A_2 at early stages of Paf-acether formation in macrophages is still lacking.

4.4.2 ACETYLTRANSFERASE

The demonstration of a large release of 2-lyso-Paf-acether from various cells associated with a poor release of Paf-acether questioned whether acetate donors could be a limiting factor in Paf-acether synthesis. Indeed, adding acetyl-CoA or sodium acetate to zymosan-stimulated macrophages enhanced the release of Paf-acether (Mencia-Huerta et al., 1981a, 1982), whereas palmitoyl-CoA, butyryl-CoA, or CoA itself was inefficient. Direct proof of the incorporation of the acetyl moiety of acetate donors into the Paf-acether molecule was obtained from experiments using radiolabeled substrates. Incubation of tritiated acetate or acetyl-CoA with macrophages (Mencia-Huerta et al., 1981a, 1982) yielded radiolabeled Paf-acether (Figs. 10A, B). That indeed 2-lyso-Paf-acether was a precursor for Paf-acether was demonstrated by experiments in which cold acetyl-CoA and tritiated 2-lyso-Paf-acether were added to macrophages. Again, radiolabeled Paf-acether was obtained (Mencia-Huerta et al., 1982) (Figs. 10A, C). The enzyme capable of linking the two precursors, acetate and 2-lyso-Paf-acether, was present in lysates and microsomal preparations from macrophages (Ninio et al., 1982a,b). An enzyme with identical properties has been described in various rat tissues (spleen, lung and lymph nodes) by Wykle et al. (1980). The acetyltransferase is stereospecific since it cannot acetylate the optical isomer of 2-lyso-Paf-acether (Wykle et al., 1980). By contrast, it can also use the 1-ester analog of 2-lyso-Paf-acether as substrate although it is well known that the reaction product, 1-O-acyl-2-O-acetyl-glyceryl-3-phosphorylcholine, possesses much lower biological activity than Paf-acether (Demopoulos et al., 1979; Tencé et al., 1981). Data reported by Snyder's group (Wykle et al., 1980) show that acetyltransferase is different from acyltransferase, the enzyme responsible for the transfer of palmitate to glycerolipids, although both are inhibited by the same products, p-bromophenacyl bromide and diisopropylfluorophosphate. The enzyme found in macrophages has its activity modulated by the state of cell activation. When macrophages are stimulated by the A23187 or zymosan, acetyltransferase activity increased more than threefold over control (Ninio et al., 1982b, 1983). In contrast, in thioglycollate-elicited macrophages, the basal enzymatic activity is much lower than in normal macrophages (Roubin et al., 1982b; Ninio et al., 1982b). Such a modulation of acetyltransferase activity may represent one of the regulatory mechanisms of Paf-acether production.

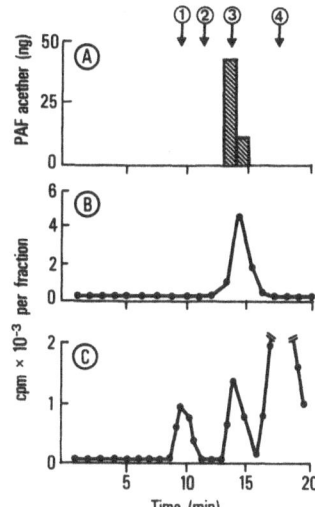

FIGURE 10.   Biosynthesis of Paf-acether by intact murine macrophages stimulated by zymosan phagocytosis in tbe presence of either [³H]acetylCoA (B) or [³H]-2-lyso-Paf-acether (C). Radioactivity coeluted with biological activity (A) after HPLC. (From Mencia-Huerta *et al.*, 1982, with permission from the American Association of Immunologists.)

4.4.3.   OTHER ENZYMES

A number of enzymes are capable of hydrolyzing and synthesizing 1-*O*-alkyl-2-acetyl-glyceryl-3-phosphorylcholine. However, their actual function in Paf-acether metabolism is still lacking since there is no evidence for their localization in Paf-acether-producing cells. These enzymes are acetylhydrolase (Blank *et al.*, 1981), choline phosphotransferase (Renooij and Snyder, 1981), and alkyl-monooxygenase (Lee *et al.*, 1981).

5.   PHARMACOLOGIC MODULATION OF LIPID MEDIATOR BIOSYNTHESIS

Modulation of macrophage lipid metabolism occurs at the level of phospholipase A_2, cyclooxygenase and lipoxygenase pathways, and probably acetyltransferase. Table 2 summarizes the effect of various drugs known to inhibit the synthesis of mediators in various cell types. However, not all of them have been tested on macrophages. Phospholipase A_2 is thought to be the common enzyme for the three major classes of mediators we have described although proof is still lacking that deacylation of ether phospholipids yields both 2-lyso-Paf-acether and arachidonic acid formation. Blockade of phospholipase A_2 is obtained (1) by more or less specific inhibitors of the enzyme such as bromophenacyl bromide, mepacrine, 874 CB (Clin-Midy); (2) by Ca^{2+}-chelating agents (e.g., EDTA); (3) by Ca^{2+} channel blockers (e.g., Verapamil, Nifedipine); (4) by agents known to increase cAMP level (e.g., dibutyryl-cAMP); and (5) by corticosteriods which induce the formation of macrocortin. In addition to the specific inhibitors of cyclooxygenase or lipoxygenase activities described in Table 1, various structural analogs are potent inhibitors of prostaglandin and/or leukotriene synthesis (Jak-

TABLE 2. PHARMACOLOGICAL MODULATION

Drug	Enzyme inhibited	Effects
Bromophenacyl bromide Mepacrine 874 CB EDTA Nifedipine Corticosteroid Dibutyryl cAMP	Phospholipase A$_2$	↓ Prostaglandins, thromboxane, HETE, leukotrienes, Paf-acether and, in platelets, 2-lyso-Paf- acether (Bach and Braschler, 1974; Bray and Gordon, 1976, 1978; Glatt *et al.*, 1977; Bonney *et al.*, 1978b; Mencia-Huerta *et al.*, 1980; Bromberg and Pick, 1981; Vadas, 1982; Benveniste *et al.*, 1982c; Jouvin-Marche *et al.*, 1983)
Aspirine Indomethacin Other NSAID	Cyclooxygenase	↓ Prostaglandins, thromboxane (Bonney *et al.*, 1978b; Bray and Gordon, 1978)
Imidazole derivatives	Thromboxane synthetase	↓ Thromboxane (Leung and Mihich, 1980)
BW755 Benoxaprofen	Cyclo- and lipoxygenase	↓ Prostaglandins, HETE, leuko- trienes (Radmark *et al.*, 1980; Walker and Dawson, 1979) ↓ Only prostaglandins in mac- rophages (Bonney *et al.*, 1978b)
Serine borate complex	γ-Glutamyl transpeptidase	↓ LTD (Örning and Hammarström, 1980)
Buthionine sulfoximine	Glutamyl cysteine synthetase	↓ LTC (Rouzer *et al.*, 1981)

schik *et al.*, 1981). No such structural analogs have yet been found for Paf-acether.

6. CONCLUSION

We have reviewed three classes of lipid mediators released from macrophages upon various stimuli including phagocytosis and the IgE-dependent mechanisms establishing a role for these mediators in allergic and inflammatory reactions. It is noteworthy that very often the same stimulus can induce the release of the three classes of mediators in a similar fashion, i.e., with rapid and identical kinetics. All these mediators are very potent in inducing various biological effects including enhanced vascular permeability, smooth muscle contraction, bronchospasm, cardiac arrhythmia, and/or blood pressure modifications. A few of them exert effects that can counteract the effects of mediators. TxA$_2$ and Paf-acether are very potent platelet-aggregating agents, whereas PGI$_2$ antagonizes their effects. Also, PGE$_2$ and PGF$_{2\alpha}$ have opposite effects (relaxation versus contraction) on bronchial tissue. On the contrary, LTC, LTD, TxA$_2$, and Paf-acether exhibit very powerful bronchospasm effects. If one must consider the stimulatory effect of the mediators by themselves in triggering the release of other ones and/or in amplifying the effect of others, one might propose the existence of regulatory mechanisms to avoid effects that are too noxious. For example, Paf-acether by itself can induce the release of lipo- and/or cyclooxygenase-dependent arachidonate metabolites from various cell types and organs (Mencia-Huerta *et al.*, 1981b; McManus *et al.*, 1980; Voelkel *et al*, 1982; Chilton *et al.*, 1982). Fortunately, these mediators increase cAMP levels of the target cells, which, as a feedback effect, decreases the ability of these cells to release other mediators; for example, PGE_1 is a good inhibitor of Paf-acether release in macrophages (Mencia-Huerta *et al.*, 1980). Future research will bring more light to the comprehension of the complex set of events that represents inflammation.

REFERENCES

Arnoux, B., Duval, D., and Benveniste, J., 1980, Release of platelet-activating factor (PAF-acether) from alveolar macrophages by the calcium ionophore A 23187 and phagocytosis, *Eur. J. Clin. Invest.* **10**:437.

Arnoux, B., Durand, J., Rigaud, M., Masse, R., and Benveniste, J., 1981a, Arachidonic acid metabolites in rat alveolar macrophages, *Am. Rev. Respir. Dis.* **123**:22a.

Arnoux, B., Cerrina, J., Jouvin, E., and Benveniste, J., 1981b, Release of platelet-activating factor (PAF-acether) from monocytes and alveolar macrophages in pulmonary diseases, *Eur. J. Clin. Invest.* **11**:2a.

Arnoux, B., Simoes-Caeiro, M. H., Landes, A., Mathieu, M., Duroux, P., and Benveniste, J., 1982, Alveolar macrophages from asthmatic patients release platelet-activating factor (PAF-acether) and lyso-PAF-acether when stimulated with the specific allergen, *Am. Rev. Respir. Dis.* **125**:70a.

Bach, M. K., and Brashler, J. R., 1974, In vivo and in vitro production of a slow-reacting substance in the rat upon treatment with calcium ionophore, *J. Immunol.* **113**:2040.

Bach, M. K., and Brashler, J. R., 1978, Ionophore A 23187-induced production of slow-reacting substance of anaphylaxis (SRS-A) by rat peritoneal cells in vitro: Evidence for production by mononuclear cells, *J. Immunol.* **120**:998.

Bach, M. K., and Brashler, J. R., 1980, Identification of a component of rat mononuclear cell SRS as leukotriene D, *Biochem. Biophys. Res. Commun.* **93**:1121.

Bach, M. K., Brashler, J. R., Hammarström, S., and Samuelsson, B., 1980, Identification of leukotriene C-1 as a major component of slow-reacting substance from rat mononuclear cells, *J. Immunol.* **125**:115.

Barbaro, J. F., and Zvaifler, N. J., 1966, Antigen-induced histamine release from platelets of rabbits producing homologous PCA antibody, *Proc. Soc. Exp. Biol. Med.* **122**:1245.

Bärlin, E., Leser, H. G., Deimann, W., Resch, K., and Gemsa, D., 1981, In vivo activation of macrophages by *Corynebacterium parvum*, pyran copolymer and glucan: Differential effects of prostaglandin E release, tumor cytotoxicity and lymphocyte stimulation, *Int. Arch. Allergy Appl. Immunol.* **66**(Suppl. 1):182.

Bell, R. L., Kennerly, D. A., Stanford, N., and Majerus, P. W., 1979, Diglyceride lipase: A pathway for archidonate release from human platelets, *Proc. Natl. Acad. Sci. USA* **76**:3238.

Benveniste, J., 1974, Platelet-activating factor, a new mediator of anaphylaxis and immune complex deposition from rabbit and human basophils, *Nature (London)* **249**:581.

Benveniste, J., and Mencia-Huerta, J. M., 1978, Release of platelet-activating factor (PAF) by macrophages during phagocytosis, *Fed. Proc.* **37**:1554a.

Benveniste, J., Henson, P. M., and Cochrane, C. G., 1972, Leukocyte-dependent histamine release from rabbit platelets: The role of IgE, basophils and a platelet-activating factor, *J. Exp. Med.* **136**:1356.

Benveniste, J., Le Couedic, J. P., and Kamoun, P., 1975, Aggregation of human platelets by purified platelet-activating factor, *Lancet* **1**:344.

Benveniste, J., Le Couedic, J. P., Polonsky, J., and Tencé, M., 1977, Structural analysis of purified platelet-activating factor, *Nature (London)* **269**:170.

Benveniste, J., Tencé, M., Varenne, P., Bidault, J., Boullet, C., and Polonsky, J., 1979, Semi-synthèse et structure proposée du facteur activant les plaquettes (PAF): PAF-acether, un alkyl-éther analogue de la lysophosphatidylcholine, *C.R. Acad. Sci. Ser. D* **289**:1037.

Benveniste, J., Roubin, R., Chignard, M., Jouvin-Marche, E., and Le Couedic, J. P., 1982a, Release of platelet-activating factor (PAF-acether) and 2-lyso PAF-acether from three cell types, *Agents Actions* **12**:711.

Benveniste, J., Roubin, R., Jouvin-Marche, E., Mencia-Huerta, J. M., and Le Couedic, J. P., 1982b, Phospholipase A_2 (PLA_2)-dependent release of lyso-platelet-activating factor (L-PAF-acether) from inflammatory cells, *Fed. Proc.* **41**:233a.

Benveniste, J., Chignard, M., Le Couedic, J. P., and Vargaftig, B. B., 1982c, Biosynthesis of platelet-activating factor (PAF-acether). II. Involvement of phospholipase A_2 in the formation of PAF-acether and lyso-PAF-acether from rabbit platelets, *Thromb. Res.* **25**:375.

Blank, M. E., Lee, T. C., Fitzgerald, V., and Snyder, F., 1981, A specific acetylhydrolase for 1-alkyl-2-acetyl-*sn*-glycero-3-phosphocholine (a hypotensive and platelet-activating lipid), *J. Biol. Chem.* **256**:175.

Bonney, R. J., Wightman, P. D., Davies, P., Sadowski, S. J., Kuehl, F. A., Jr., and Humes, J. L., 1978a, Regulation of prostaglandin synthesis and of the selective release of lysosomal hydrolases by mouse peritoneal macrophages, *Biochem. J.* **176**:433.

Bonney, R. J., Davies, P., Kuehl, F. A., and Humes, J. L., 1978b, A comparison of several anti-inflammatory drugs regarding their ability to inhibit prostaglandin synthesis and release from macrophages, *Eur. J. Rheum. Inflam.* **1**:308.

Bonney, R. J., Wightman, P. D., Dahlgren, M. E., Davies, P., Kuehl, F. A., and Humes, J. L., 1980, Release of inflammatory mediators by macrophages exposed to phorbol myristate acetate: Effect of RNA and protein synthesis inhibitors, *Biochim. Biophys. Acta* **633**:410.

Bonney, R. J., Wightman, P. D., Dahlgren, M. E., Humes, J. L., and Davies, P., 1981, The pathways of biosynthesis for prostaglandins by the stimulus-triggered macrophage, *Scand. J. Rheumatol.* **40**(Suppl.):53.

Bray, M. A., and Gordon, D., 1976, Effects of anti-inflammatory drugs on macrophage prostaglandin biosynthesis, *Br. J. Pharmacol.* **57**:466.

Bray, M. A., and Gordon, D., 1978, Prostaglandin production by macrophages and the effect of anti-inflammatory drugs, *Br. J. Pharmacol.* **63**:635.

Bromberg, Y., and Pick, E., 1981, Activation of macrophage adenylate cyclase by stimulants of the oxidative burst and by archidonic acid: Two distinct mechanisms, *Cell. Immunol.* **61**:90.

Brune, K., Glatt, M., Kalin, H., and Peskar, B. A., 1978, Pharmacological control of prostaglandin and thromboxane release from macrophages, *Nature (London)* **274**:261.

Chilton, F. H., O'Flaherty, J. T., Walsh, C. E., Thomas, M. H., Wykle, R. L., De Chatelet, L. R., and Waite, B. M., 1982, Platelet-activating factor: Stimulation of the lipoxygenase pathway in polymorphonuclear leukocytes by 1-O-alkyl-2-O-acetyl-*sn*-glycero-3-phosphocholine, *J. Biol. Chem.* **257**:5402.

Demopoulos, C. A., Pinckard, R. N., and Hanahan, D. J., 1979, Platelet-activating factor: Evidence for 1-O-alkyl-2-acetyl-*sn*-glyceryl-3-phosphorylcholine as the active component (a new class of lipid chemical mediators), *J. Biol. Chem.* **254**:9355.

Denjean, A., Arnoux, B., Benveniste, J., Lockhart, A., and Masse, R., 1981, Bronchoconstriction induced by intratracheal administration of platelet-activating factor (PAF-acether) in baboons, *Agents Actions* **11**:567.

Drapier, J. C., Roubin, R., Petit, J. F., and Benveniste, J., 1983, Lipid mediator synthesis in peritoneal macrophages from mice injected with immunostimulants, *Biochim. Biophys. Acts* **751**:90.

Feldberg, W., and Kellaway, C. H., 1938, Liberation of histamine and formation of lysolecithine-like substances by cobra venom, *J. Physiol. (London)* **94**:187.

Friedman, S. A., Remold-O'Donnell, E., and Piessens, W. F., 1979, Enhanced PGE production by MAF-treated peritoneal exudate macrophages, *Cell, Immunol.* **42**:213.

Gemsa, D., Seitz, M., Menzel, J., Grimm, W., Kramer, W., and Till, G., 1979a, Modulation of phagocytosis induced prostaglandin release from macrophages, *Adv. Exp. Med. Biol.* **114**:421.

Gemsa, D., Seitz, M., Kramer, W., Grimm, W., Till, G., and Resch, K., 1979b, Ionophore a 23187 raises cyclic AMP levels in macrophages by stimulating prostaglandin E formation, *Exp. Cell Res.* **118**:55.

Gemsa, D., Kramer, W., Brenner, M., Till, G., and Resch, K., 1980, Induction of prostaglandin E release from macrophages by colchicine, *J. Immunol.* **124**:376.

Glatt, M., Kälin, H., Wagner, K., and Brune, K., 1977, Prostaglandin release from macrophages: An assay system for anti-inflammatory drugs in vitro, *Agents Actions* **7**:321.

Godfroid, J. J., Heymans, F., Redeuilh, C., Steiner, E., and Benveniste, J., 1980, Platelet-activating factor (PAF-acether): Total synthesis of 1-O-octadecyl-2-O-acetyl-*sn*-glycero-3-phos-phorylcholine, *FEBS Lett.* **116**:161.

Gordon, D., Bray, M. A., and Morley, J., 1976, Control of lymphokine secretion by prostaglandins, *Nature (London)* **262**:401.

Graham, R. C., Karnovsky, M. J., Shofer, A. W., Glass, E. A., and Karnovsky, M. L., 1967, Metabolic and morphological observations on the effect of surface-active agents on leukocytes, *J. Cell Biol.* **32**:629.

Hammarström, S., Murphy, R. C., Samuelsson, B., Clark, D. A., Mioskowski, C., and Corey, E. J., 1979, Structure of leukotriene C: Identification of the amino acid part, *Biochem. Biophys. Res. Commun.* **91**:1266.

Hsueh, W., Kuh, C., and Needleman, P., 1979, Relationship of prostaglandin secretion by rabbit alveolar macrophages to phagocytosis and lysosomal enzyme release, *Biochem. J.* **184**:345.

Hsueh, W., Desai, U., Gonzalez-Crussi, F., Lamb, R., and Chu, A., 1981, Two phospholipase pools for prostaglandin synthesis in macrophages, *Nature (London)* **290**:710.

Humes, J. L., Bonney, R. J., Pelus, L., Dahlgren, M. E., Sadowski, S. J., Kuehl F. A., Jr., and Davies, P., 1977, Macrophages synthesize and release prostaglandins in response to inflammatory stimuli, *Nature (London)* **269**:149.

Humes, J. L., Ham, E. A., Egan, R. W., Bonney, R. J., Davies, P., and Kuehl, F. A., 1979, Pathways of arachidonic acid metabolism and modulation by drugs, *Agents Actions* **4**(Suppl):96.

Humes, J. L., Burger, S., Galavage, M., Kuehl, F. A., Jr., Wightman, P. D., Dahlgren, M. E., Davies, P., and Bonney, R. J., 1980, The diminished production of arachidonic acid oxygenation products by elicited mouse peritoneal macrophages: Possible mechanisms, *J. Immunol.* **124**:2110.

Humes, J. L., Sadowski, S., Galavage, M., Goldenberg, M., Subers, E., Bonney, R. J., and Kuehl, F. A., 1982, Evidence for two sources of arachidonic acid from oxidative metabolism by mouse peritoneal macrophages, *J. Biol. Chem.* **257**:1591.

Jakschik, B. A., and Lee, L. H., 1980, Enzymatic assembly of slow-reacting substance, *Nature (London)* **287**:51.

Jakschik, B. A., Sprecher, H., and Sams, A. R., 1981, Modulation of leukotriene formation, in: *SRS-A and Leukotrienes* (P.J. Piper, ed.), pp. 119–129, Wiley, New York.

Joseph, M., Tonnel, A. B., Torpier, G., Capron, A., Arnoux, B., and Benveniste, J., 1983, Involvement of immunoglobulin E in the secretory processes of alveolar macrophages from asthmatic patients, *J. Clin. Invest.* **71**:221.

Jouvin-Marche, E., Cerrina, J., Coëffier, E., Duroux, P., and Benveniste, J., 1983, Effect of the Ca^{2+}-antagonist nifedipine on the release of platelet-activating factor (Paf-acether), slow-reacting substance and β-glucuronidase from human neutrophils, *Eur. J. Pharmacol.* **89**:19.

Karnovsky, M. L., and Wallach, D. F. H., 1961, The biochemical basis of phagocytosis. III. Incorporation of inorganic phosphate into various classes of phosphatides during phagocytosis, *J. Biol. Chem.* **236**:1895.

Kuehl, F. A., and Egan, R. W., 1980, Prostaglandins, arachidonic acid and inflammation, *Science* **210**:978.

Kurland, J. I., and Bockman, R., 1978, Prostaglandin E production by human blood monocytes and mouse peritoneal macrophages, *J. Exp. Med.* **147**:952.

Lapetina, E. G., 1982, Regulation of arachidonic acid production: Role of phospholipases C and A_2, *Trends Pharmacol. Sci.* **3**:115.

Lee, T. C., Blank, M. L., Fitzgerald, V., and Snyder, F., 1981, Substrate specificity in the biocleavage of the O-alkyl bond: 1-Alkyl-2-acetyl-*sn*-glycero-3-phosphocholine (a hypotensive and platelet-activating lipid) and its metabolites, *Arch. Biochem. Biophys.* **208**:353.

Leung, K. H., and Mihich, E., 1980, Prostaglandin modulation of development of cell-mediated immunity in culture, *Nature (London)* **288**:597.

Lewis, R. A., and Austen, K. F., 1981, Mediation of local homeostasis and inflammation by leukotrienes and other mast cell-dependent compounds, *Nature (London)* **293**:103.

McManus, L. M., Hanahan, D. J., and Pinckard, R. N., 1980, Human platelet stimulation by acetyl glyceryl ether phosphorylcholine (AGEPC), *J. Clin. Invest.* **67**:903.

Mahoney, E. M., Hamill, A. L., Scott, W. A., and Cohn, Z. A., 1977, Response of endocytosis to altered fatty acyl composition of macrophage phospholipids, *Proc. Natl. Acad. Sci. USA* **74**:4895.

Mencia-Huerta, J. M., and Benveniste, J., 1979, Platelet-activating factor and macrophages. I. Evidence for the release from rat and mouse peritoneal macrophages and not from mastocytes, *Eur. J. Immunol.* **9**:409.

Mencia-Huerta, J. M., and Benveniste, J., 1981, Platelet-activating factor (PAF-acether) and macrophages. II. Phagocytosis-associated release of PAF-acether from rat peritoneal macrophages, *Cell, Immunol.* **57**:281.

Mencia-Huerta, J. M., Akerman, C., and Benveniste, J., 1980, Phospholipase A$_2$ (PLA$_2$), lipo (LO), cyclo (CO) oxygenases, and release of platelet-activating factor (PAF) and slow-reacting substance (SRS) from rat macrophages, *Fed. Proc.* **39**:691a.

Mencia-Huerta, J. M., Roubin, R., and Benveniste, J., 1981a, Acetyl-coenzyme A (Ac-CoA) and sodium acetate enhance the release of platelet-activating factor (PAF-acether) from murine peritoneal cells, *Int. Arch. Allergy Appl. Immunol.* **66**(Suppl. 1):178.

Mencia-Huerta, J. M., Hadji, L., and Benveniste, J., 1981b, Release of a slow-reacting substance from rabbit platelets, *J. Clin. Invest.* **68**:1586.

Mencia-Huerta, J. M., Roubin, R., Morgat, J., and Benveniste, J., 1982, Biosynthesis of platelet-activating factor (PAF-acether). III. Formation of PAF-acether from synthetic substrates by stimulated murine macrophages, *J. Immunol.* **129**:804.

Morris, H. R., Taylor, G. W., Piper, P. J., Samhoun, M. N., and Tippins, J. R., 1980, Slow-reacting substances (SRSs): The structure identification of SRSs from rat basophilic leukemia cells, *Prostaglandins* **19**:185.

Murphy, R. C., Hammarström, S., and Samuelsson, B., 1979, Leukotriene C: A slow-reacting substance from murine mastocytoma cells, *Proc. Natl. Acad. Sci. USA* **76**:4275.

Ninio, E., Mencia-Huerta, J. M., Heymans, F., and Benveniste, J., 1982a, Biosynthesis of platelet-activating factor. I. Evidence for an acetyltransferase activity in murine macrophages, *Biochim. Biophys. Acta* **710**:23.

Ninio, E., Roubin, R., Mencia-Huerta, J. M., and Benveniste, J., 1982b, Modulation of acetyltransferase activity (ATA) in murine macrophages (Mϕ) producing platelet-activating factor (PAF-acether), *Fed. Proc.* **41**:731a.

Ninio, E., Mencia-Huerta, J. M., and Benveniste, J., 1983, Biosynthesis of platelet-activating factor (Paf-acether). V. Enhancement of acetyltransferase activity in murine peritoneal cells by the calcium ionophore A23187, *Biochim. Biophys. Acta* **751**:298.

Orange, R. P., Austen, W. G., and Austen, K. F., 1971, Immunological release of histamine and slow-reacting substance from human lung. I. Modulation by agents influencing cellular level of cyclic 3'5'-adenosine monophosphate, *J. Exp. Med.* **134**:1368.

Orange, R. P., Moore, E. G., and Gelfand, E. W., 1980, The formation and release of slow-reacting substance of anaphylaxis (SRS-A) by rat and mouse peritoneal mononuclear cells induced by ionophore A 23187, *J. Immunol.* **124**:2264.

Örning, L., and Hammarström, S., 1980, Inhibition of leukotriene C and leukotriene D biosynthesis, *J. Biol. Chem.* **255**:8023.

Örning, L., Hammarström, S., and Samuelsson, B., 1980, Leukotriene D: A slow-reacting substance from rat basophilic leukemia cells, *Proc. Natl. Acad. Sci. USA* **77**:2014.

Pelus, L. M., and Bockman, R. S., 1979, Increased prostaglandin synthesis by macrophages from tumor-bearing mice, *J. Immunol.* **123**:2118.

Piper, P. J., Samhoun, M. N., Tippins, J. R., Williams, T. J., Palmer, M. A., and Peck, M. J., 1981, Pharmacological studies on pure SRS-A and synthetic leukotrienes C$_4$ and D$_4$, in: *SRS-A and Leukotrienes* (P. J. Piper, ed.), pp. 81–99, Wiley, New York.

Polonsky, J., Tencé, M., Varenne, P., Das, B. C., Lunel, J., and Benveniste, J., 1980, Release of 1-O-alkyl-glyceryl-3-phosphorylcholine, O-deacetyl platelet-activating factor from leukocytes: Chemical ionization mass spectrometry of phospholipids, *Proc. Natl. Acad. Sci. USA* **77**:7019.

Radmark, O., Malmsten, C., and Samuelsson, B., 1980, The inhibitory effects of BW755C on arachidonic acid metabolism in human polymorphonuclear leukocytes, *FEBS Lett.* **110**:213.

Rankin, J. A., Hitchcock, M., Merrill, W., Bach, M. K., Brashler, J. R., and Askenase, P. W., 1982, IgE-dependent release of leukotriene C₄ from alveolar macrophages, *Nature (London)* 297:329.

Renooij, W., and Snyder, F., 1981, Biosynthesis of 1-alkyl-2-acetyl-sn-glycero-3-phosphocholine (platelet-activating factor and a hypotensive lipid) by cholinephosphotransferase in various rat tissues, *Biochim. Biophys. Acta* 663:545.

Rokach, J., Girard, Y., Guindon, Y., Atkinson, J. G., Larue, M., Young, R. N., Masson, P., and Holme, G., 1980, The synthesis of a leukotriene with SRS-like activity, *Tetrahedron Lett.* 21:1485.

Rollins, T. E., and Smith, W. L., 1979, Subcellular localization of prostaglandin-forming cyclooxygenase in Swiss mouse 3T3 fibroblasts by electron microscopic immunocytochemistry, *J. Biol. Chem.* 255:4872.

Roubin, R., and Benveniste, J., 1981a, Release of leukotrienes C and D from inflammatory macrophages upon phagocytosis of zymosan and bacteris, *Agents Actions* 11:578.

Roubin, R., and Benveniste, J., 1981b, Release of platelet-activating factor (PAF-acether) and slow-reacting substance (SRS) from inflammatory mice macrophages (Mφ), *Fed. Proc.* 40:1068a.

Roubin, R., Mencia-Huerta, J. M., and Benveniste, J., 1982a, Release of platelet-activating factor (PAF-acether) and leukotrienes C and D from inflammatory macrophages, *Agents Actions* 12:141.

Roubin, R., Mencia-Huerta, J. M., Landes, A., and Benveniste, J., 1982b, Biosynthesis of platelet-activating factor (PAF-acether). IV. Impairment of acetyl-transferase activity in thioglycollate-elicited mouse macrophages, *J. Immunol.* 129:809.

Rouzer, C. A., Scott, W. A., Kemp, J., and Cohn, Z. A., 1980a, Prostaglandin synthesis by macrophages requires a specific receptor–ligand interaction, *Proc. Natl. Acad. Sci. USA* 77:4279.

Rouzer, C. A., Scott, W. A., Cohn, Z. A., Blackburn, P., and Manning, J. M., 1980b, Mouse peritoneal macrophages release leukotriene C in response to a phagocytic stimulus, *Proc. Natl. Acad. Sci. USA* 77:4928.

Rouzer, C. A., Scott, W. A., Hamill, A. L., and Cohn, Z. A., 1980c, Dynamics of leukotriene C production by macrophages, *J. Exp. Med.* 152:1236.

Rouzer, C.A., Scott, W. A., Griffith, O. W., Hamill, A. L., and Cohn, Z. A., 1981, Depletion of glutathione selectively inhibits synthesis of leukotriene C by macrophages, *Proc. Natl. Acad. Sci. USA* 78:2532.

Rouzer, C. A., Scott, W. A., Hamill, A. L., Liu, F. T., Katx, D. H., and Cohn, Z. A., 1982a, Secretion of leukotriene C and other arachidonic acid metabolites by macrophages challenged with immunoglobulin E immune complexes, *J. Exp. Med.* 156:1077.

Rouzer, C. A., Scott, W. A., Hamill, A. L., and Cohn, Z. A., 1982b, Synthesis of leukotriene C and other arachidonic acid metabolites by mouse pulmonary macrophages, *J. Exp. Med.* 155:720.

Rouzer, C. A., Scott, W. A., Griffith, O. W., Hamill, A. L., and Cohn, Z. A., 1982c, Glutathione metabolism in resting and phagocytozing peritoneal macrophages, *J. Biol. Chem.* 257:2002.

Samuelsson, B., Goldyne, M., Granström, E., Hamberg, M., Hammarström, S., and Malmsten, C., 1978, Prostaglandins and thromboxanes, *Annu. Rev. Biochem.* 47:997.

Scott, W. A., Zrike, J. M., Hamill, A. L., Kempe, J., and Cohn, Z. A., 1980, Regulation of arachidonic acid metabolites in macrophages, *J. Exp. Med.* 152:324.

Scott, W. A., Pawlowski, N. A., Andreach, M., and Cohn, Z. A., 1982a, Resting macrophages produce distinct metabolites from exogenous arachidonic acid, *J. Exp. Med.* 155:535.

Scott, W. A., Pawlowski, N. A., Murray, H. W., Andreach, M., Zrike, J., and Cohn, Z. A., 1982b, Regulation of arachidonic acid metabolism by macrophage activation, *J. Exp. Med.* 155:1148.

Siraganian, R. P., and Osler, A. G., 1971, Destruction of rabbit platelets in the allergic response of sensitized leukocytes. I. Demonstration of a fluid phase intermediate, *J. Immunol.* 106:1244.

Stechschulte, D. J., Austen, K. F., and Bloch, K. J., 1967, Antibodies involved in antigen-induced release of slow-reacting substance of anaphylaxis (SRS-A) in the guinea-pig and rat, *J. Exp. Med.* 125:127.

Sugiura, T., Onuma, Y., Sekiguchi, N., and Waku, K., 1982, Ether phospholipids in guinea-pig polymorphonuclear leukocytes and macrophages: Occurrence of high levels of 1-O-alkyl-2-acyl-sn-glycero-3-phosphocholine, *Biochim. Biophys. Acta* 712:515.

Tencé, M., Polonsky, J., Le Couedic, J. P., and Benveniste, J., 1980, Release, purification and characterization of platelet-activating factor (PAF), *Biochimie* 62:251.

Tencé, M., Coëffier, E., Heymans, F., Polonsky, J., Godfroid, J. J., and Benveniste, J., 1981, Structural analogs of platelet-activating factor (PAF-acether), *Biochimie* **63**:723.

Vadas, P., 1982, The efficacy of anti-inflammatory agents with respect to extracellular phospholipase A_2 activity, *Life Sci.* **30**:155.

Van den Bosch, H., 1980, Intracellular phospholipase A, *Biochim. Biophys. Acta* **614**:191.

Vargaftig, B. B., Lefort, J., Chignard, M., and Benveniste, J., 1980, Platelet-activating factor induces a platelet-dependent bronchoconstriction unrelated to the formation of prostaglandin derivatives, *Eur. J. Pharmacol.* **65**:185.

Vargaftig, B. B., Chignard, M., Mencia-Huerta, J. M., Arnoux, B., and Benveniste, J., 1981, Pharmocology of arachidonate metabolites and of platelet-activating factor (PAF-acether), in: *Platelets in Biology and Pathology* (J. L. Gordon, ed.), Volume 2, pp. 373–406, Elsevier, Amsterdam.

Voelkel, N. F., Worthen, S., Reeves, J. T., Henson, P. M., and Murphy, R. C., 1982, Nonimmunological production of leukotrienes induced by platelet-activating factor, *Science* **218**:286.

Walker, J. R., and Dawson, W., 1979, Inhibition of rabbit PMN lipoxygenase activity by benoxaprophen, *J. Pharm. Pharmacol.* **31**:778.

Wightman, P. D., Humes, J. L., Davies, P., and Bonney, J., 1981a, Identification and characterization of two phospholipase A_2 activities in resident mouse peritoneal macrophages, *Biochem. J.* **195**:427.

Wightman, P. D., Dahlgren, M. E., Hall, J. C., Davies, P., and Bonney, R. J., 1981b, Identification and characterization of a phospholipase C activity in resident mouse peritoneal macrophages, *Biochem. J.* **197**:523.

Wykle, R. L., Malone, B., and Snyder, F., 1980, Enzymatic synthesis of 1-alkyl-2-acetyl-*sn*-glycero-3-phosphocholine, a hypotensive and platelet-aggregating lipid, *J. Biol. Chem.* **225**:10256.

5

Lymphokines
Pharmacologic Modulation of Their Production and Action

TAKESHI YOSHIDA and KAZUO KOBAYASHI

1. INTRODUCTION

Lymphocytes stimulated with specific antigens or polyclonal activators (mitogens) are able to produce a variety of soluble factors affecting a broad scope of target cells and thus influencing almost every aspect of immune response. Since the first description of macrophage migration inhibition factor (MIF) in 1966 (David, 1966; Bloom and Bennet, 1966), numerous biological activities have been detected in the culture supernatants of lymphocytes. They are now collectively called lymphokines, as proposed by Dumonde *et al.* (1969). Most of these *in vitro* activities are, however, only defined functionally and their biochemical entities are not yet completely clarified. Although lymphokines can be classified into functionally defined groups by a variety of criteria, there is no consensus on any single classification. Nevertheless, it may be useful for later discussion to introduce some examples of such attempts. As mentioned above, lymphokines can target on a variety of cells. These are illustrated in Table 1. Although not yet proven, it will not be surprising to find that currently unlisted types of cells, for example, hepatocytes or pneumocytes (type I and II) or even the cells in the neuroendocrine system, are affected by certain lymphokines directly or indirectly. Almost all functions of these cells may be influenced by lymphokines as exemplified in Table 2. From this information, several useful classifications of lymphokines become possible. For example, they can be divided into two groups, inflammatory and regulatory lymphokines. The former applies to those that influence mainly the functions of macrophages and polymorphonuclear cells and thus affect the inflammatory outcome of immune reactions. The latter

TAKESHI YOSHIDA and KAZUO KOBAYASHI • Department of Pathology, University of Connecticut Health Center, Farmington, Connecticut 06032.

TABLE 1. TARGET CELLS OF LYMPHOKINES

Macrophages (monocytes)
Polymorphonuclear cells
   Neutrophils
   Eosinophils
   Basophils
Lymphocytes
Fibroblasts
Endothelial cells
Platelets

refers to those affecting the function of lymphocytes, therefore directly responsible for modulation of immune responses. According to another concept, lymphokines can also be divided into "afferent" and "efferent" lymphokines, indicating their effects on the afferent and efferent limbs of immune response, respectively. For instance, growth factors for lymphocytes or macrophage differentiation factors belong to the former, and lymphocyte chemotactic factor and macrophage activation factor belong to the latter.

In addition to the cataloging of these various lymphokine activities, discussion of the mechanisms of production of lymphokines has also been the subject of many review articles by us and others (Yoshida and Cohen, 1974b; Ewan and Yoshida, 1979; Cohen and Yoshida, 1979; Yoshida and Suko, 1983; Rocklin *et al.*, 1980; David and David, 1972). Thus, we now know fairly well the kinetics of *in vitro* lymphokine production, the cell types that produce them, specific and nonspecific stimuli that trigger production, and evidence to support *in vivo* production of these molecules. On the other hand, our knowledge of regulatory mechanisms acting on production and activity of lymphokines, particularly *in vivo*, is still rather limited. However, this area of study is now rapidly progressing mostly due to the availability of well-characterized lymphokines. In this chapter, therefore, we will focus discussions on the modulatory mechanisms or regulation of lymphokine activities *in vitro* and *in vivo* as well as those of lymphokine production *in vitro* and *in vivo*.

TABLE 2. CELLULAR FUNCTIONS AFFECTED BY LYMPHOKINES

Function	Examples of lymphokines
Proliferation	Mitogenic (or growth) factors
	Cytotoxic factors
Differentiation	Activation factors
	Differentiation factors
Mobility	Migration inhibition or enhancing factors
	Chemotactic factors
Phagocytosis	Activation factors
Secretion	Activation factors

2. PHARMACOLOGIC MODULATION OF LYMPHOKINE ACTIVITIES

2.1. *IN VITRO* MODULATION

In vitro activities of a given lymphokine can be modulated theoretically at three different phases: (1) the lymphokine molecule itself, (2) its interaction with target cells, and (3) target cell responses. Since the second and third phases are difficult to distinguish from each other in the studies of lymphokines at the present time, we will discuss the modulation of lymphokine activities only at two phases, namely the modulation of molecules, and either of molecule–cell interaction or of target cells. The modulation of activities could be either enhancing or suppressing. Whenever such information is available, both types of modulation will be discussed.

2.1.1. Modulation of Lymphokine Molecules

Several endogenous and exogenous materials that inactivate lymphokines have been described. Since most lymphokine molecules are known to be proteins or glycoproteins, enzymes such as proteinases and neuraminidases can destroy their activities (reviewed in Yoshida, 1979). Therefore, it is likely that endogenous enzymes such as esterases and proteases could suppress lymphokine activities. In fact, it was shown that macrophage MIF could be inactivated by several kinds of esterases on the macrophage surface (Remold, 1974). It has been shown that myeloperoxidase and hydrogen peroxide induced by chemotactic stimuli may destroy chemotactic factors by oxidation of their methionine residue (Clark and Szot, 1982; Clark, 1982). On the other hand, a lymphokine itself sometimes represents enzymatic activity. Thus, human leukocyte migration inhibition factor (LIF) has been shown to be a serine esterase and/or protease that is modulated by cGMP (Bendtzen, 1976; Rocklin, 1975; Rocklin and Rosenthal, 1977; Bendtzen and Rocklin, 1980). Various serine esterase inhibitors such as diisopropylfluorophosphate and phenylmethylsulfonylfluoride have been shown to irreversibly inhibit LIF.

Another way to inhibit or neutralize lymphokine activities is the use of antibodies raised against these molecules. The available antibodies against various lymphokines have been produced either as heterologous antiserum by conventional immunization procedures (reviewed in Yoshida, 1979; Rocklin *et al.*, 1980; Onozaki *et al.*, 1980) or as monoclonal antibodies by using hybridoma techniques (Luben and Mahler, 1980; Stadler *et al.*, 1982; Gillis *et al.*, 1981). All of these antibodies were able to specifically bind and neutralize the corresponding lymphokine in a reversible manner, suppressing the lymphokine's activity *in vitro*. It has been shown that those antibodies are useful not only for neutralization of the activities, but also for purification of lymphokines by the use of affinity column chromatography. Recently, it was reported that a monoclonal antibody was raised against the putative receptor of interleukin-2 (IL-2) (Osawa and Diamantstein, 1983). Obviously, this type of antibody would be interesting for modulating lymphokine–cell interactions.

In contrast to the above-mentioned suppression of lymphokine activities, very few reports are available concerning enhancement of the activity by directly modifying any lymphokine molecules. It is anticipated, however, that such enhancing agents may become available as soon as the more exact nature of active principles of each lymphokine is revealed by studies such as those on the use of monoclonal antibodies. As one of such rare reports, Aune and Pierce (1983) have described that soluble immune response suppressor (SIRS), which nonspecifically suppresses immune response *in vitro*, can be oxidized by hydrogen peroxide to become an active suppressor factor. Strictly speaking, therefore, this is an example of the conversion of a precursor lymphokine to an active form by chemical modification of the molecule, rather than the enhancement of the existing activity.

2.1.2. Modulation of Lymphokine–Target Cell Interactions

It was initially shown by Remold (1973) that among many monosaccharides, α-L-fucose specifically blocks the biologic activity of guinea pig MIF. Since then, various monosaccharides have been shown to inhibit the *in vitro* activities of many lymphokines including human MIF and LIF, and guinea pig chemotactic factors (Rocklin, 1976a; Amsden *et al.*, 1978). This inhibition is supposedly effected by monosaccharides competing with the terminal sugars of cellular receptors to which lymphokines bind. It is also possible to inhibit lymphokine activity by treating target cells with enzymes that destroy surface receptors. For example, trypsin or fucosidase treatment of macrophages could destroy their receptors for MIF in a reversible fashion; the treated macrophages become responsive to MIF after 24 hr incubation (Leu *et al.*, 1972; Remold, 1973).

Other categories of substances that may suppress the interaction between lymphokines and target cells include corticosteroids and prostaglandins (PGE_1 and PGE_2). Corticosteroids were first shown to interfere with the interaction between MIF and guinea pig macrophages (Weston *et al.*, 1973; Balow and Rosenthal, 1973). Furthermore, it was shown that glucocorticosteroids can inhibit human monocyte chemotactic responses and monocyte activation for bactericidal activity as well as lymphokine-induced macrophage proliferation (Masur *et al.*, 1982; Rinehart *et al.*, 1974; Duncan *et al.*, 1982). Although the exact nature of the suppression by corticosteroid is unknown, it is most likely that the general cellular functions such as motility and enzyme activities of target cells may be affected through this hormone's effect on microtubules and microfilaments as well as other intracellular biochemical pathways including changes in cyclic nucleotides (see Coffey and Hadden, this volume).

PGE_1 and E_2 were shown to suppress the activity of MIF when they were directly added to the *in vitro* assay system (Koopman *et al.*, 1973; Yoshida *et al.*, 1982). It was also shown that macrophage mitogenic factor activity could be inhibited by PGEs (Hadden *et al.*, 1980). It is as yet unresolved if these prostaglandins inhibit the cell-surface interaction of macrophage with MIF or if instead they modify the intracellular responsiveness to the stimulus from such interaction. Similarly, fatty acids such as sodium linoleate were effective to suppressing macrophage migration inhibition probably through its metabolism to prostaglandins by macrophages (Utermohlen *et al.*, 1980).

As mentioned above, lymphokines may be destroyed by serine sterase and/or proteases present on the target cell surface. Thus, it was shown that the addition of exogenous esterase inhibitors could enhance the activity of lymphokines. For example, physiologic concentrations of the plasma esterase and protease inhibitors α_2-macroglobulin, α_1-antitrypsin, C1-inhibitor, and antithrombin-heparin cofactor enhance the *in vitro* response of macrophages to MIF (Remold and Rosenberg, 1975). Similarly, human monocytes pretreated with the esterase inhibitors antithrombin III and soybean trypsin inhibitor showed increased responsiveness to macrophage activation factor (MAF) by their enhanced cytotoxicity for tumor cells (Cameron and Churchill, 1980).

Two more ways to modulate the cellular receptor for lymphokines have been reported. It was shown that fucose-binding protein (fucolectin from *Lotus tetragonolobus*) could trigger the putative MIF "receptor" on macrophages, of which migration was inhibited and enzymatic activities were enhanced (Leu *et al.*, 1980). Recently, modulation of the immune response was attempted using monoclonal antibody possibly directed against lymphokine receptors. The monoclonal antibody raised against the IL-2 "receptor" could inhibit the proliferative responses of lymphocytes (Osawa and Diamantstein, 1983). However, in view of previous studies on interaction between antireceptor ligands and cell-surface receptors, it may also be possible that monoclonal antibodies against any lymphokine receptor will be stimulatory, instead of inhibitory, to cellular functions depending on the conditions in which such antibodies are reacted with target cells.

There are a group of substances that can nonspecifically modulate target cell behavior, thus causing either enhancement or suppression of the responsiveness to lymphokines. It has been known that colchicine and vinblastine at certain concentrations significantly inhibit microtubule assembly and impair monocyte mobility, causing the suppression of their responsiveness to MIF as well as to chemotactic factors (Zakhireh and Malech, 1980; Pick and Abrahamer, 1973). Blocking of protein synthesis of target cells by puromycin and cycloheximide can either inhibit or enhance the cellular responsiveness to lymphokines; MIF (Pick and Manheimer, 1973) and LIF (Bendtzen, 1975) activities can be suppressed, whereas lymphotoxin can exert enhanced activity (Williams and Granger, 1969). By examining the oxygen metabolism of macrophages treated with MIF, Keisari and Pick (1980) have proposed a novel hypothesis; unstable products of oxygen reduction, such as O_2^-, OH^-, and $O_2^{\frac{1}{2}}$ or the more stable H_2O_2, may be responsible for most of the effects of MIF. This is an intriguing concept and most of the predictions from such a hypothesis can be tested experimentally. In general, the elevation of cAMP levels in target cells by treatment with cAMP itself, β-adrenergic stimulators, or phosphodiesterase inhibitors causes a reduction of lymphokine activity (Bendtzen and Palit, 1977; Koopman *et al.*, 1973; Kotkes and Pick, 1975; Lomnitzer *et al.*, 1976; Pick and Manheimer, 1974; Prieur and Granger, 1975). Although agents that elevate cellular cGMP levels also seem to modulate lymphokine activities, the results have been less conclusive, compared with those on cAMP (Bendtzen and Palit, 1977; Kotkes and Pick, 1975; Pick and Manheimer, 1974; see Coffey and Hadden, this volume). Interestingly, a well-known immune adjuvant, muramyl dipeptide (MDP), has been shown to increase tumoricidal activity of rat alveolar macrophages treated with a noneffective dose of MAF, thus indicating the presence of synergism between a lymphokine and MDP to activate macrophage function (Sone and Fidler, 1980). Similarly, the activity of macrophage mitogenic factor was decreased in the presence of MDP (Hadden et al, 1979). Other immunomodulating compounds may also increase lymphokine activities (see Schindler et al., this volume).

2.2. *IN VIVO* MODULATION

Although most lymphokines have been defined as mediators of *in vitro* correlates of cell-mediated immune responses, a variety of evidence indicates that lymphokines participate in immunologic reactions *in vivo* as summarized in Table 3 (reviewed in Yoshida and Cohen, 1974b). These include either the recovery of lymphokinelike activities in tissue extracts and fluid from DTH reaction sites or, conversely, the induction of DTH reactions in normal recipients by injecting lymphokine preparations produced *in vitro*. Using these systems, only a very few reported studies have examined the *in vivo* modulation of lymphokine activities.

α-L-Fucose and L-rhamnose, inhibitors of guinea pig MIF and chemotactic factors *in vitro* as discussed above, were injected intravenously into immune guinea pigs. The DTH skin reaction was found to be suppressed (Baba et al., 1979). Similarly, inhibition was achieved in the macrophage disappearance reaction (MDR) when such monosaccharides were injected intraperitoneally (Ochiai et al., 1982); the MDR has been shown to be an *in vivo* correlate as indicated in Table 3. Furthermore, it was recently shown that intravenous injection of α-L-fucose could partially abrogate the lymphokine-dependent phase of desensitiza-

TABLE 3. *IN VIVO* ROLES OF LYMPHOKINES[a,b]

In vivo reactions	Lymphokines recovered	Reactions reproduced by
DTH skin reaction	SRF, MCF	Lk (SRF)
Macrophage disappearance reaction (MDR)	MIF, MCF	Lk (MIF)
Monocyte disappearance phenomenon	MIF, IFN, Des.F	Lk (MIF)
Hypersensitivity Granulomas	MIF, ESP, MCF FSF, FCF, MFF	Lk (GFF)

[a]Note: Several lymphokines were reported in other tissues such as joint fluid and lymph.
[b]Abbreviations: SRF, skin reactive factor; MCF, macrophage chemotactic factor; MIF, migration inhibition factor; IFN, interferon; Des.F, desensitization factor; ESP, eosinophil stimulation promoter; FSF, fibroblast stimulation factor; FCF, fibroblast chemotactic factor; MFF, macrophage fusion factor; GFF, granuloma formation factor.

tion of delayed hypersensitivity (Baba *et al.*, 1983). It was previously shown that the anergy state of DTH was induced by intravenous injection of a large amount of specific antigen in immune gunea pigs, and that this anergy state was paradoxically due to a large amount of circulating lymphokines (Yoshida and Cohen, 1974a). In this system, α-L-fucose but not arabinose injected simultaneously with antigen could inhibit the expression of the anergy state. This is probably due to the inhibition by L-fucose of the interaction between a circulating lymphokine (e.g., MIF) and target monocytes, thus preventing the production of suppressor substances (e.g., PGE_1 and PGE_2) from the latter (Baba *et al.*, 1983).

As discussed previously, various polyclonal as well as monoclonal antibodies against some of the lymphokines are currently available. The use of such antibodies to neutralize the *in vivo* effects of lymphokines, however, has rarely been reported. It was initially found that systemic injection of antilymphokine antibodies could suppress an active, induced DTH skin reaction (Yoshida *et al.*, 1975), as well as MDR (Yoshida, unpublished). The activity of skin reactive factor (SRF) has also been shown to be suppressed by these antibodies. Unfortunately, these antibodies were not monospecific to a particular lymphokine (Kuratsuji *et al.*, 1976; Geczy *et al.*, 1975), and therefore, the observed effects could have been induced by their influence on multiple lymphokines *in vivo*. The definitive experiments should be performed using monoclonal antibodies now available to some of the lymphokines.

Many hormones and metabolic inhibitors such as corticosteroids and cycloheximide have been known to suppress DTH reactions *in vivo* (reviewed in Turk, 1980). In view of their known activities on lymphokines *in vitro* as discussed above, the *in vivo* suppression by these drugs is considered due to their inhibitory effects on lymphokine action.

3. PHARMACOLOGIC MODULATION OF LYMPHOKINE PRODUCTION

3.1. *IN VITRO* MODULATION

There are a variety of factors and agents reported to influence positively or negatively the production of lymphokines *in vitro*. These substances may be classified tentatively into two major groups, one with direct effects on lymphokine production, and the other with indirect effects probably through natural (or endogenous) feedback mechanisms. Naturally, this may represent a somewhat arbitrary categorization, but may conveniently permit us to speculate on their cause–effect relationship as much as possible from the limited information available on this complex issue.

3.1.1. Agents and Factors Directly Affecting Lymphokine Production

As in the case of inhibitors of lymphokine activities, there are a series of substances known to affect intracellular metabolism. These materials, therefore, could affect nonspecifically the production of lymphokines by effector lymphocytes. For example, cycloheximide, puromycin, and actinomycin D were all shown to inhibit MIF, MAF, as well as LIF production (Varesio *et al.*, 1981a; Bendtzen *et al.*, 1981; Bendtzen, 1975; Gorski *et al.*, 1976; Mizoguchi *et al.*, 1973; Pekarek *et al.*, 1976). Furthermore, the production of MIF and LIF has also been shown to be suppressed by elevation of cAMP levels with cAMP itself, agonists, and phosphodiesterase inhibitors (Pick, 1974; Bendtzen *et al.*, 1981). These agents could also inhibit the production of lymphotoxin (Lies and Peter, 1973; Williams and Granger, 1969; Prieur and Granger, 1975). Interestingly, *in vitro* production of most of the inflammatory lymphokines does not require either DNA synthesis or cell proliferation. For example, it was shown that mitomycin C, X-irradiation, and 5-bromo-2-deoxyuridine with light treatments had no effect on either MIF or LIF production (Mizoguchi *et al.*, 1973; Rocklin, 1973; Rocklin *et al.*, 1980; Salvin and Nishio, 1972).

On the other hand, some substances are known to enhance the production of lymphokines. Thus, phorbol myristate acetate (PMA) or other phorbol ester analogs were shown to enhance interferon (IFN)-γ as well as IL-2 production (Farrar *et al.*, 1981; Yip *et al.*, 1981). This could represent rather indirect effects of these materials than direct ones; for example, through IL-1 produced by the stimulated macrophages with PMA. As discussed below, IL-1 may trigger the production of IL-2. A similar enhancement of MIF production was observed when cimetidine (H-2 receptor antagonist) was used *in vitro* (Lipsmeyer, 1980). This enhancement may have been caused by suppression of histamine-receptor-bearing lymphocytes, which has been shown to inhibit the effector cell for cell-mediated immunity (Rocklin, 1976b, 1977).

Besides the above-mentioned substances, endogenously a variety of regulatory cells have been described to modulate the production of lymphokines *in vitro*. Recent reports indicate that these modulatory cells are T cells suppressing the production of various lymphokines including MIF, IL-2, and IFN-γ (Gullberg and Larrson, 1982; Gullberg *et al.*, 1981; Northoff *et al.*, 1980; Palacios and Moller, 1981; Torres *et al.*, 1982a; Chensue, 1980; Chensue *et al.*, 1983). Most of these studies in mice show that such suppressor T cells belong to the Ly-1$^-$,23$^+$ subpopulation. Histamine-receptor-bearing cells in man also seem to belong to a suppressor T-cell population showing surface markers such as IgGFc and OKT8 (Rocklin, 1976b, 1977). Soluble mediators, if any, from these suppressor cells are yet to be characterized. Although we have included all of these regulatory cells in the category of those directly acting on the production of lymphokines, this is probably due to our current lack of knowledge on their relationship to the known regulatory circuit in lymphokine production as discussed below. Then, it would not be surprising if well-defined soluble products from these regulatory cells become available to modulate the production of lymphokines *in vivo*.

3.1.2. Feedback Regulation of Lymphokine Production

Our own studies on an *in vivo* phenomenon called "desensitization" of DTH have been extremely revealing on the nature of the feedback regulation of lymphokine production (Yoshida *et al.*, 1982; Yoshida and Cohen, 1982). Although this system is discussed below in Section 3.2 on *in vivo* modulation, the essential findings also relate to the regulation of *in vitro* lymphokine production. In essence, lymphokine (e.g., MIF)-treated macrophages release suppressor substances including PGE_1 and E_2 that can abrogate the production of various lymphokines by lymphocytes stimulated with antigen. Similar results have been reported by others on MIF and MAF (Taramelli *et al.*, 1981; Varesio and Holden, 1980; Varesio *et al.*, 1981b) and on IL-2 (Chouaib and Fradelizi, 1982; Rappaport and Dodge, 1982; Tilden and Balch, 1982), partially confirming the earlier studies on direct inhibitory effects of PGE_1 and E_2 on lymphokine production *in vitro* (Gordon *et al.*, 1975). The presence of this type of regulation preventing excessive mediator production may explain the previous observation that more lymphokines are produced when the culture medium is changed at 24 or 48 hr after the initial incubation. In this context, it may also be relevant to mention another regulatory mechanism in which B cells capable of making MIF under certain conditions (e.g., polyclonal activation) may be inhibited to do so by a mediator called MIF-inhibitory factor (MIFIF) generated by antigen-stimulated T cells (Cohen and Yoshida, 1977). Although the biologic significance of B-cell lymphokines is not known, it is speculated that the deregulation of B-cell lymphokine production may cause some abnormality in autoimmune status as discussed later.

    Another possible pathway of negative feedback regulation on lymphokine production may be through the effect of lymphokines on the action of corticosteroid hormones. As discussed in the previous section, corticosteroids are suppressive of lymphokine activities, probably through their effects on target cells of lymphokines. However, it is well known that corticosteroids could affect lymphocytes and, more specifically, T-cell functions, thus inhibiting lymphokine production (Gillis *et al.*, 1979a,b; Wahl *et al.*, 1975; Duncan *et al.*, 1982). In this context, it is very interesting that some investigators, although in an *in vivo* situation, could detect the increased level of serum corticosteroids after intravenous injection of Con A-stimulated lymphocyte culture supernatants (Besedovsky *et al.*, 1981). This means that there may be a feedback regulatory loop between lymphokines and corticosteroids. Since there has been no *in vitro* system available to examine the phenomenon, the exact cellular interactions involved, particularly the target cell of such lymphokine action, are still unknown.

    There are at least a few positive feedback regulatory pathways of lymphokine production. For the last few years, numerous reports are available concerning lymphocyte growth-promoting factors or mitogenic lymphokines including IL-2, IL-3, and B-cell growth factor (BCGF) (Torres *et al.*, 1982; Schrader and Clark-Lewis, 1982; Frank *et al.*, 1981; Mier and Gallo, 1982; Ihle *et al.*, 1981; Falkoff *et al.*, 1982; Muraguchi *et al.*, 1982; Howard *et al.*, 1982). It is not hard to understand that such lymphocyte growth factors would facilitate the production of more lymphokines, recruiting resting lymphocytes for activation and proliferation, although no direct evidence has been obtained indicating the amplified production of lymphokines by brief stimulation of normal lymphocytes with these factors. In fact, however, a variety of T-cell lines and clones established by the use of IL-2 would speak for such an augmentation mechanism (to cite a few: Swain and Dutton, 1982; Palacios, 1982; Prystowsky *et al.*, 1982; Kelso *et al.*, 1982; Mckimm-Breschkin *et al.*, 1982; Matsuyama *et al.*, 1982; Conta *et al.*, 1983). Further enhancing this amplifying mechanism of lymphokine production, IL-1 can promote the production of IL-2 (Smith *et al.*, 1980; Mizel and Mizel, 1981). Since the production of IL-1 by macrophages can be enhanced by a lymphokine, MAF, another loop of positive feedback is likely to occur, namely MAF → IL-1 → IL-2 → MAF. Yet another positive feedback regulation is probable through the long-studied but still elusive factor, transfer factor (TF) or leukocyte dialysates. Several reports indicate that TF preparations could recruit normal lymphocytes to produce LIF and MIF (Borkowsky *et al.*, 1981; Wilson *et al.*, 1980; Philp *et al.*, 1981).

Although the exact biologic significance should be clarified by further studies, some endogenous factors such as PMN-derived factor to increase DNA synthesis by T cells (Yoshinaga *et al.*, 1980) or lymphokines that affect the development of Ia antigens (Steinman *et al.*, 1980; Scher *et al.*, 1980; Steeg *et al.*, 1980) may be operating as the positive regulatory mechanisms of lymphokine production. The former factor may play a role in the enhanced production of lymphokines at inflammatory sites if such a factor is generated by stimulation of PMNs with lymphokines. Since the production of various lymphokines, particularly the regulatory lymphokines, is Ia-dependent (Lattime *et al.*, 1982). the Ia-inducing factor may facilitate the generation of lymphokines in general. Another interesting lymphokine that directly or indirectly regulates the production of various lymphokine molecules is IFN-γ. Functionally, this type of IFN does not differ significantly from other types of IFNs. Thus, this immune IFN as a lymphocyte product can either enhance or suppress lymphokine production through its effect on different phases of cell-mediated immune responses (Kadish *et al.*, 1980; Steeg *et al.*, 1982; Fitzpatrick and Stringfellow, 1980; Friedman *et al.*, 1980; Itoh *et al.*, 1980).

3.2. *IN VIVO* MODULATION

3.2.1. Desensitization Model of Delayed Hypersensitivity

To illustrate the *in vivo* modulation of lymphokine production, the results of our studies on an *in vivo* model system, called "desensitization," will be discussed briefly. Desensitization of DTH can be achieved by systemic administration of antigen into a previously immunized animal showing DTH (Uhr and Pappenheimer, 1958). The unresponsive state is initially antigen-nonspecific and transient, being similar to the anergy state found in various clinical conditions, and then followed by an antigen-specific unresponsive phase. Initially, Kantor (1975) suggested that the maintenance of the desensitized state might involve the presence of a suppressive factor in the anergic animal. Our study showed that desensitization led to the transient appearance of MIF in the circulation, and that the intravenous injection of MIF-containing supernatants into immune animals led to a period of unresponsiveness indistinguishable from anergy (Yoshida and Cohen, 1974a). In this context it is also interesting that MIF could inhibit the action of macrophage mitogenic factor (MMF) (Hadden *et al.*, personal communication). These findings suggested that circulating lymphokines in the desensitized animals may be responsible for the inhibition of lymphokine-dependent reactions such as cutaneous DTH reactions and MDR. In fact, the later studies have shown that anergy can be passively transferred with serum from desensitized animals into immune animals (Papermaster *et al.*, 1978). It was also shown that the serum of a desensitized animal could be suppressive of lymphokine production *in vitro* (Yoshida *et al.*, 1982). The responsible suppressive factor in the serum has been considered to be monokines including prostaglandins or their complexes with carrier proteins. Our most recent studies have revealed that antigen-specific unresponsiveness of DTH reactions at the later phase of desensitization is mediated by antigen-specific suppressor T cells, which can be identified within lymph nodes of the desensitized animals (Kobayashi *et al.*, 1984). These *in vivo* studies clearly indicate that there are at least two major down-regulation mechanisms: lymphokine-induced, macrophage-dependent, antigen-nonspecific inhibition, and suppressor T-cell-dependent, antigen-specific inhibition.

3.2.2. Modulation of Lymphokine Production

Including our own studies, numerous reports are available of lymphokinelike activities detected in various disease states (reviewed in Yoshida and Cohen, 1974b, and Rocklin *et al.*, 1980; Bertotto *et al.*, 1981; Petrini *et al.*, 1982; Rea and Yoshida, 1982). From the studies on the desensitization model mentioned above, it is most likely that such circulating lymphokines are playing an important role in regulatory circuits of cell-mediated immunity in man. In this context, it is extremely interesting that, as alluded to before, the immunodeficiency state in the aged or autoimmune rodents may be due to a deficiency of IL-2 production (Dauphinee *et al.*, 1981; Ortiz-Ortiz and Weigle, 1982; Gilman *et al.*, 1982). Recent findings indicate that such immunodeficient mice usually contain MIF-like activity in their circulation (Yoshida *et al.*, unpublished). This indicates that the deficiency of IL-2 production in such animals may be regulated by the feedback mechanisms through circulating lymphokines. It is our contention, however, that we should be extremely cautious in the interpretation of these findings, since the *in vivo* environment naturally involves multifactorial modulations interacting each other. Nevertheless, the recent attempts to determine the effects of IL-2 *in vivo* by direct administration of the purified material have been encouraging, since such studies should eventually reveal complex cause–effect relationships among various lymphokines and pharmacologic agents *in vivo* (Hefeneider *et al.*, 1983; Cheever *et al.*, 1982). Similarly, the *in vivo* effect of IL-1 was also examined (Staruch and Wood, 1983). As discussed in Section 3.1 on *in vitro* modulation of lymphokine production, it is conceivable that such treatment by a regulatory monokine triggers a chain of events involving various lymphokine activities.

As far as suppressor cells that regulate *in vivo* lymphokine production are concerned, the presence of these cells has been observed in many clinical states including tuberculosis patients (Joffe and Rabson, 1981; Ellner, 1978; Tsuyuguchi *et al.*, 1980), or experimental animal models such as schistosome-induced granulomatous inflammation (Chensue *et al.*, 1980; Chensue *et al.*, 1983). At the present time, however, our knowledge in this area is rather deficient on how these cells modulate the production of lymphokines *in vivo*. In this context, the recent report indicating the presence of IL-2 inhibitor in serum and its control by a suppressor cell population is quite intriguing (Hardt *et al.*, 1981).

Finally, although its biologic significance is still uncertain, there is an interesting report that serum from guinea pigs injected with niridazole contained a suppressor factor to block the production of MIF *in vitro* (Daniels *et al.*, 1975). The cellular interaction involved in the generation of such a suppressor "metabolite" of niridazole should be informative in the elucidation of *in vivo* pharmacologic modulation of lymphokines.

4. CONCLUSION

In this chapter we have attempted to review the pharmacologic regulation of lymphokines. Rapidly accumulating data have been indicative of the ubiquitous nature of lymphokine activities in a variety of biologic responses. Although this group of substances is produced by lymphocytes as a result of an immune response, their effects are far-reaching and complex. In view of their profound influence on physiologic as well as pathologic states of the host, it is crucial for us to know how to manipulate these effects to the host's advantage.

In spite of the recent advances in this field, however, it is painfully clear to us that the deficiency of our current knowledge on regulatory mechanisms of lymphokines is great. Most of the materials known to modulate lymphokine action and production are only available in vague biologic terms. As discussed in this chapter, we know of only a very few examples of chemically well-defined substances that can modulate action and production of lymphokines. With a rapid increase in our knowledge in this line, our strategies to manipulate this important group of biologic substances should certainly improve.

REFERENCES

Amsden, A., Ewan, V., Yoshida, T., and Cohen, S., 1978, Studies on cellular receptors for lymphokines. I. Interaction of chemotactic factors with monosaccharides, *J. Immunol.* **120**:542.

Aune, T. M., and Pierce, C. W., 1983, Characterization and mechanisms of action of soluble immune response suppressor (SIRS), in: *Advances in Immunopharmacology* (J. W. Hadden, L. Chedid, P. Dukor, F. Spreafico, and D. Willoghby, eds.)., pp. 597–602, Pergamon Press, Elmsford, N.Y.

Baba, T., Yoshida, T., and Cohen, S., 1979, Suppression of cell-mediated immune reactions by alpha-L-fucose, *J. Immunol.* **122**:838.

Baba, T., Yoshida, T., and Cohen, S., 1983, Desensitization III: The role of lymphokines in the maintenance of the anergic state during desensitization, *J. Exp. Pathol.* **1**:39.

Balow, J. E., and Rosenthal, A. S., 1973, Glucocorticoid suppression of macrophage migration inhibitory factor, *J. Exp. Med.* **137**:1031.

Bendtzen, K., 1975. Drug effects on human leukocyte migration and migration inhibitory activity from lymphocytes stimulated with concanavalin A, *Acta Pathol. Microbiol. Scand.* **83**:447.

Bendtzen, K., 1976, Some physicochemical properties of human leukocyte migration inhibitory factor (LIF), *Acta Pathol. Microbiol. Scand.* **84**:471.

Bendtzen, K., and Palit, J., 1977, Modulation of human leukocyte migration inhibitory factor (LIF) by 3'5'-cyclic AMP, 3'5'-cyclic GMP and agents known to influence intracellular cyclic nucleotide metabolism, *Acta Pathol. Microbiol. Scand.* **85**:317.

Bendtzen, K., and Rocklin, R. E., 1980, Use of benzoyl-L-phenylalanyl-L-valyl-arginine (^{3}H) methyl ester as a sensitive and selective substrate for the human lymphokine, leukocyte migration inhibitory factor (LIF), *J. Immunol.* **125**:1775.

Bendtzen, K., Mahoney, R., and Rocklin, R. E., 1981, Production of human leukocyte migration inhibitory factor (LIF) by lymphocytes stimulated with phytohemagglutinin. 1. Effect of various metabolic inhibitors, *Clin. Immunol. Immunopathol.* **18**:212.

Bertotto, A., Caprino, D., Vaccaro, R., and Sonaglia, F., 1981, Serum migration-inhibitory activity in children with acute infectious mononucleosis, *Clin. Immunol. Immunopathol.* **19**:314.

Besedovsky, H. O., del Rey, A., and Sorkin, E., 1981, Lymphokine-containing supernatants from Con A-stimulated cells increase corticosterone blood levels, *J. Immunol.* **126**:385.

Bloom, B. R., and Bennet, B., 1966, Mechanism of a reaction in vitro associated with delayed-type hypersensitivity, *Science* **153**:80.

Borkowsky, W., Suleski, P., Bhardwaj, N., and Lawrence, H. S., 1981, Antigen-specific activity of murine leukocyte dialysate containing transfer factor on human leukocytes in the leukocyte migration inhibition assay, *J. Immunol.* **126**:80.

Cameron, D. J., and Churchill, W. H., 1980, Chemical modification of macrophages enhances their response to human macrophage activation factor, *Cell. Immunol.* **55**:201.

Cheever, M. A., Greenberg, P. D., Fefer, A., and Gillis, S., 1982, Augmentation of the anti-tumor therapeutic efficacy of long-term cultured T lymphocytes by in vivo administration of purified interleukin 2, *J. Exp. Med.* **155**:968.

Chensue, S. W., Boros, D. L., and David, C. S., 1980, Regulation of granulomatous inflammation in murine schistosomiasis: In vitro characterization of T lymphocyte subsets involved in the production and suppression of migration inhibition factor, *J. Exp. Med.* **151**:1398.

Chensue, S. W., Boros, D. L., and David, C. S., 1983, Regulation of granulomatous inflammation in murine schistosomiasis. II. Suppressor cell-derived, I-C subregion-encoded soluble suppressor factor mediates regulation of lymphokine production, *J. Exp. Med.* **157**:219.

Chouaib, S., and Fradelizi, D., 1982, The mechanism of inhibition of human IL-2 production. *J. Immunol.* **129**:2463.

Clark, R. A., 1982, Chemotactic factors trigger their own oxidative inactivation by human neutrophils, *J. Immunol.* **129**:2725.

Clark, R. A., and Szot, S., 1982, Chemotactic factor inactivation by stimulated human neutrophils mediated by myeloperoxidase-catalyzed methionine oxidation, *J. Immunol.* **128**:1507.

Cohen, S., and Yoshida, T., 1977, Suppression of B cell MIF production by T cells and soluble T cell-derived factors, *J. Immunol.* **119**:719.

Cohen, S., and Yoshida, T., 1979, Lymphokine-mediated reactions, in: *Immunopathology* (S. Cohen, P. A. Ward, and R. T. McCluskey, eds.), pp. 49–68, Wiley, New York.

Conta, B. S., Powell, M. B., and Ruddle, N. H., 1983, Production of lymphotoxin, gamma-, alpha-, and beta-IFN by murine T cell lines and clones, *J. Immunol.* **130**:2231.

Daniels, J. C., 1975, Two stages in lymphocyte mediator production by differential susceptibility to blockade using niridazole, *Proc. Natl. Acad. Sci. USA* **72**:4569.

Daniels, J. C., Fajardo, I., and David, J. R., 1975, Two stages in lymphocyte, *Proc. Natl. Acad. Sci. USA.*

Dauphinee, M. J., Kipper, S. B., Wofsy, D., and Talal, N., 1981, Interleukin 2 deficiency is a common feature of autoimmune mice, *J. Immunol.* **127**:2483.

David, J. R., 1966, Delayed hypersensitivity in vitro: Its mediation by cell-free substances formed by lymphoid cell–antigen interaction, *Proc. Natl. Acad. Sci. USA* **56**:72.

David, J. R., and David, R. A., 1972, Cellular hypersensitivity and immunity: Inhibition of macrophage migration and the lymphocyte mediators, *Prog. Allergy* **16**:300.

Dumonde, D. C., Wolstencroft, R. A., Panayi, G. S., Matthew, M., Morley, J., and Howson, W. T., 1969, "Lymphokine": Non-antibody mediators of cellular immunity generated by lymphocyte activation, *Nature (London)* **224**:38.

Duncan, M. R., Sadlik, J. R., and Hadden, J. W., 1982, Glucocorticoid modulation of lymphokine-induced macrophage proliferation, *Cell Immunol.* **67**:23.

Ellner, J. J., 1978, Suppressor adherent cells in human tuberculosis, *J. Immunol.* **121**:2573.

Ewan, V., and Yoshida, T., 1979, Lymphokines and cytokines, in: *Chemical Messengers of the Inflammatory Process* (J. Houck, ed.), pp. 197–227, Elsevier/North-Holland, Amsterdam.

Falkoff, R. J. M., Zhu, L. and Fauci, A. S., 1982, Separate signals for human B cell proliferation and differentiation in response to *Staphylococcus aureus*: Evidence for a two-signal model of B cell activation, *J. Immunol.* **129**:97.

Farrar, J. F., Hilfiker, M. L., Farrar, W. L., and Farrar, J. J., 1981, Phorbol myristic acetate enhances the production of interleukin 2, *Cell Immunol.* **58**:156.

Fitzpatrick, F. A., and Stringfellow, D. A., 1980, Virus and interferon effects on cellular prostaglandin synthesis, *J. Immunol.* **125**:431.

Frank, M. B., Watson, J., Mochizuki, D., and Gillis, S., 1981, Biochemical and biological characterization of lymphocyte regulatory molecules. VIII. Purification of interleukin 2 from a human T cell leukemia, *J. Immunol.* **127**:2361.

Fridman, W. H., Gressor, I., Bandu, M. T., Aguet, M., and Neauport-Santes, C., 1980, Interferon enhances the expression of Fc-gamma receptors, *J. Immunol.* **124**:2436.

Geczy, C. L., Friedrich, W., and de Weck, A. L., 1975, Production and in vivo effect of antibodies against guinea pigs lymphokines, *Cell Immunol.* **19**:65.

Gillis, S., Crabtree, G. R., and Smith, K. A., 1979a, Glucocorticoid-induced inhibition of T cell growth factor production I. The effect on mitogen-induced lymphocyte proliferation, *J. Immunol.* **123**:1624.

Gillis, S., Crabtree, G. R., and Smith, K. A., 1979b, Glucocorticoid-induced inhibition of T cell growth factor production. II. The effect on the in vitro generation of cytolytic T cells, *J. Immunol.* **123**:1632.

Gillis, S., Gillis, A. E., and Henney, C. S., 1981, Monoclonal antibody directed against interleukin 2. I. Inhibition of T lymphocyte mitogenesis and the in vitro differentiation of alloreactive cytolytic T cells, *J. Exp. Med.* **154**:983.

Gilman, S. C., Rosenberg, J. S., and Feldman, J. D., 1982, T lymphocytes of young and aged rats. II. Functional defects and the role of interleukin 2, *J. Immunol.* **128**:644.

Gordon, D., Bray, M. A., and Morley, J., 1975, Control of lymphokine secretion by prostaglandins, *Nature (London)* **262**:401.

Gorski, A. J., Dupont, B., Hansen, J. A., and Good, R. A., 1976, leukocyte migration inhibitory factor (LMIF) production in unidirectional mixed lymphocyte cultures, *J. Immunol.* **117**:865.

Gullberg, M., and Larrson, E.-L., 1982, Studies on induction and effector functions of concanavalin A-induced suppressor cells that limit TCGF production, *J. Immunol.* **128**:746.

Gullberg, M., Ivars, F., Coutinho, A., and Larrson, E.-L., 1981, Regulation of T cell growth factor production: Arrest of TCGF production after 18 hours in normal lectin-stimulated mouse spleen cell cultures, *J. Immunol.* **127**:407.

Hadden, J. W., Englard, A., Sadlik, J. R., and Hadden, E. M., 1979, The comparative effects of isoprinosine, levamisole, muramyl dipeptide and SM1213 on lymphocyte and macrophage proliferation and activation in vitro, *Int. J. Immunopharmacol.* **1**:17.

Hadden, J. W., Sadlik, J. R., Englard, A., Warfel, A. H., and Hadden, E. M., 1980, Lymphokine-induced macrophage proliferation, activation and fusion, in: *Biochemical Characterization of Lymphokines* (A. L. de Weck, F. Kristensen, and M. Landy, eds.), pp. 235–242, Academic Press, New York.

Hardt, C., Rollinghoff, M., Pfizenmaier, K., Mosmann, H., and Wagner, H., 1981, Lyt-23⁺ cyclophosphamide-sensitive T cells regulate the activity of an interleukin 2 inhibitor in vivo, *J. Exp. Med.* **154**:262.

Hefeneider, S. H., Conlon, P. J., Henney, C. S., and Gillis, S., 1983, In vivo interleukin 2 administration augment the generation of alloreactive cytolytic T lymphocytes and resident natural killer cells, *J. Immunol.* **130**:222.

Howard, M., Farrar, J., Hilfiker, M., Johnson, B., Takatsu, K., Hamaoka, T., and Paul, W. E., 1982, Identification of a T cell-derived B cell growth factor distinct from interleukin 2, *J. Exp. Med.* **155**:914.

Ihle, J. N., Pepersack, L., and Rebar, L., 1981, Regulation of T cell differentiation: In vitro induction of 20 alpha-hydroxysteroid dehydrogenase in splenic lymphocytes is mediated by a unique lymphokine, *J. Immunol.* **126**:2184.

Itoh, K., Inoue, M., Kataoka, S., and Kumagai, K., 1980, Differential effect of interferon expression of IgG- and IgM-Fc receptors on human lymphocytes, *J. Immunol.* **124**:2589.

Joffe, M. I., and Rabson, A. R., 1981, Suppression of LIF production but not blastogenesis in patients with tuberculous meningitis, *Clin. Immunol. Immunopathol.* **18**:245.

Kadish, A. A., Tansey, F. A., Yu, G. S. M., Doyle, A. T., and Bloom, B. R., 1980, Interferon as a mediator of human lymphocyte suppression, *J. Exp. Med.* **151**:637.

Kantor, F. S., 1975, Infection, anergy and cell-mediated immunity, *N. Engl. J. Med.* **292**:629.

Keisari, Y., and Pick, E., 1980, Lymphokine mimicry by phorbol myristate acetate (PMA) and the ionophore A23187—A new hypothesis for explaining the action mechanism of migration inhibitory factor (MIF), in: *Biochemical Characterization of Lymphokines* (A. L. de Weck, F. Kristensen, and M. Landy, eds.), pp. 113–121, Academic Press, New York.

Kelso, A., Glasebrook, A. L., Kanagawa, O., and Brunner, K. T., 1982, Production of macrophage-activating factor by T lymphocyte clones and correlation with other lymphokine activities, *J. Immunol.* **129**:550.

Kobayashi, K., Yoshida, T., and Cohen, S., 1984, (submitted for publication).

Koopman, W. J., Gillis, H. H., and David, J. R., 1973, Prevention of MIF activity by agents known to increase cellular cyclic AMP, *J. Immunol.* **110**:1609.

Kotkes, P., and Pick, E., 1975, in: *The Immunological Basis of Connective Tissue Disorders* (L. G. Silvestri, ed.), pp. 141–153, North-Holland, Amsterdam.

Kuratsuji, T., Yoshida, T., and Cohen, S., 1976, Anti-lymphokine antibody. II. Specificity of biological activity, *J. Immunol.* **117**:1985.

Lattime, E. C., Gillis, S., Pecoraro, G., and Stutman, O., 1982, Ia-dependent interleukin 2 production in syngeneic cellular interactions, *J. Immunol.* **128**:480.

Leu, R. W., Eddleston, A. L. W. F., Hadden, J. W., and Good, R. A., 1972, Mechanism of action of migration inhibitory factor (MIF). I. Evidence for a receptor for MIF present on the peritoneal macrophage but not on the alveolar macrophage, *J. Exp. Med.* **136**:589.

Leu, R. W., Brewer, M. A., and Huddleston, D. J., 1980, Similarities in enhanced glucosamine incorporation by macrophages stimulated with migration inhibitor factor and the fucolectin from *Lotus tetragonolobus*, *Cell. Immunol.* **55**:227.

Lies, R. B., and Peter, J. B., 1973, Cyclic AMP inhibition of cytotoxin ("lymphotoxin") elaboration by stimulated lymphocytes, *Cell. Immunol.* **8**:332.

Lipsmeyer, E. A., 1980, Effect of cimetidine on delayed hypersensitivity, *Clin. Immunol. Immunopathol.* **16**:166.

Lomnitzer, R., Rabson, A. R., and Koornhof, H. J., 1976, The effects of cyclic AMP on leukocyte inhibitory factor (LIF) production and on the inhibition of leukocyte migration, *Clin. Exp. Immunol.* **24**:42.

Luben, R. A., and Mahler, M. A., 1980, Use of in vitro immunization in production of monoclonal antibodies against osteoclast activating factor: A method with general applicability to lymphokines, *Biochemical Characterization of Lymphokines* (A. L. de Weck, F. Kristensen, and M. Landy, eds.), pp. 55–65, Academic Press, New York.

Mckimm-Breschkin, J. L., Mottram, P. L., Thomas, W. R., and Miller, J. F. A. P., 1982, Antigen-specific production of immune interferon by T cell lines, *J. Exp. Med.* **155**:1204.

Masur, H., Murray, H. W., and Jones, T. C., 1982, Effect of hydrocortisone on macrophage response to lymphokine, *Infect. Immun.* **35**:709.

Matsuyama, M., Sugamura, K., Kawade, Y., and Hinuma, Y., 1982, Production of immune interferon by human cytotoxic T cell clones, *J. Immunol.* **129**:450.

Mier, J. W., and Gallo, R. C., 1982, The purification and properties of human T cell growth factor, *J. Immunol.* **128**:1122.

Mizel, S. B., and Mizel, D., 1981, Purification to apparent homogeneity of murine interleukin 1, *J. Immunol.* **126**:834.

Mizoguchi, Y., Yamamoto, S., and Morisawa, S., 1973, Studies on the biosynthesis of macrophage migration inhibitory factor in delayed hypersensitivity. I. Effects of inhibitors of nucleic acid and protein synthesis on the production of macrophage migration inhibitory factor, *J. Biochem. (Tokyo)* **73**:467.

Muraguchi, A., Kasahara, T., Oppenheim, J. J., and Fauci, A. S., 1982, B cell growth factor and T cell growth factor produced by mitogen-stimulated normal human peripheral blood T lymphocytes are distinct molecules, *J. Immunol.* **129**:2486.

Northoff, H., Carter, C., and Oppenheim, J. J., 1980, Inhibition of concanavalin A-induced human lymphocyte mitogenic factor (interleukin-2) production by suppressor T lymphocytes, *J. Immunol.* **125**:1823.

Ochiai, T., Baba, T., Mizushima, A., Onozaki, K., and Yaoita, H., 1982, Induction of macrophage disappearance reaction by immunoadsorbed MIF, *Cell. Immunol.* **71**:346.

Onozaki, K., Haga, S., Miura, K., Homma, Y., and Hashimoto, T., 1980, Production of an antibody against guinea pig MIF. II. Analysis of the antibody-reacting material using radiolabelled lymphokines, *Cell. Immunol.* **55**:465.

Ortiz-Ortiz, L., and Weigle, W. O., 1982, Activation of effector cells in experimental allergic encephalomyelitis by interleukin 2 (IL2), *J. Immunol.* **128**:1545.

Osawa, H., and Diamantstein, T., 1983, The characteristics of a monoclonal antibody that binds specifically to rat T lymphoblasts and inhibits IL 2 receptor functions, *J. Immunol.* **130**:51.

Palacios, R., 1982, Cloned lines of interleukin 2 producer human T lymphocytes, *J. Immunol.* **129**:2586.

Palacios, R., and Moller, G., 1981, T cell growth factor abrogates concanavalin A-induced suppressor cell function, *J. Exp. Med.* **153**:1360.

Papermaster, V., Yoshida, T., and Cohen, S., 1978, Desensitization. II. Passive transfer to the desensitized state by serum from desensitized animals, *Cell. Immunol.* **35**:378.

Pekarek, J., Svejcar, J., Nonza, K., and Johnovsky, J., 1976, Effect of immunosuppressive drugs on an in vitro correlate of cell-mediated immunity, *Immunology* **31**:773.

Petrini, M., Azzara, A., Polidori, R., Vatteroni, M. L., Caracciolo, F., Carulli, G., and Ambrogi, F., 1982, Serum factors inhibiting some leukocytic functions in Hodgkin's disease, *Clin. Immunol. Immunopathol.* **23**:124.

Philp, J. R., McCormack, J. G., Moore, A. L., and Johnson, J. E., III, 1981, A lymphokine resembling transfer factor that stimulates MIF production by nonsensitive lymphocytes, *J. Immunol.* **126**:1469.

Pick, E., 1974, Soluble lymphocyte mediators. I. Inhibition of macrophage migration inhibitory factor production by drugs, *Immunology* **26**:649.

Pick, E., and Abrahamer, H., 1973, Blocking of macrophage migration inhibitory factor by microtubular disruptive drugs, *Int. Arch. Allergy Appl. Immunol.* **44**:215.

Pick, E., and Manheimer, S., 1973, The mechanism of action of macrophage migration inhibitory factor, *Int. Arch. Allergy Appl. Immunol.* **45**:295.

Pick, E., and Manheimer, S., 1974, The mechanism of action of soluble lymphocyte mediators. II. Modification of macrophage migration and migration inhibitory action by drugs, enzymes and cationic environment, *Cell. Immunol.* **11**:30.

Prieur, A., and Granger, G. A., 1975, The effect of agents which modulate levels of the cyclic nucleotides on human lymphotoxin secretion and activity in vitro, *Transplantation* **20**:331.

Prystowsky, M. B., Ely, J. M., Beller, D. I., Eisenberg, L., Goldman, J., Goldman, M., Goldwasser, E., Ihle, J., Quintans, J., Remold, H., Vogel, S. N., and Fitch, F. W., 1982, Alloreactive cloned T cell lines. VI. Multiple lymphokine activities secreted by helper and cytolytic cloned T lymphocytes, *J. Immunol.* **129**:2337.

Rappaport, R. S., and Dodge, G. R., 1982, Prostaglandin E inhibits the production of human interleukin 2, *J. Exp. Med.* **155**:943.

Rea, T., and Yoshida, T., 1982, Migration inhibitory activity detected in leprosy patients, *J. Invest. Dermatol.* **79**:336.

Remold, H. G., 1973, Requirement for alpha-L-fucose on the macrophage membrane receptor for MIF, *J. Exp. Med.* **138**:1065.

Remold, H. G., 1974, The enhancement of MIF activity by inhibition of macrophage associated esterases, *J. Immunol.* **112**:1571.

Remold, H. G., and Rosenberg, R. D., 1975, Enhancement of migration inhibitory factor activity by plasma esterase inhibitors, *J. Biol. Chem.* **250**:6608.

Rinehart, J. J., Balcerzak, S. P., Sagone, A. L., and LoBuglio, A. F., 1974, Effect of corticosteroids on human monocyte function, *J. Clin. Invest.* **54**:1337.

Rocklin, R. E., 1973, Production of migration inhibitory factor by non-dividing lymphocytes, *J. Immunol.* **110**:674.

Rocklin, R. E., 1975, Partial characterization of leukocyte inhibitory factor by concanavalin A-stimulated human lymphocytes (LIFConA), *J. Immunol.* **114**:1161.

Rocklin, R. E., 1976a, Role of monosaccharides in the interaction of two lymphocyte mediators with their target cells, *J. Immunol.* **116**:816.

Rocklin, R. E., 1976b, Modulation of cellular immune responses in vivo and vitro by histamine receptor-bearing lymphocytes, *J. Clin. Invest.* **57**:1051.

Rocklin, R. E., 1977, Histamine-induced suppressor factor (HSF): Effect on migration inhibitory factor (MIF) production and proliferation, *J. Immunol.* **118**:1734.

Rocklin, R. E., and Rosenthal, A. S., 1977, Evidence that human leukocyte inhibitory factor (LIF) is an esterase, *J. Immunol.* **119**:249.

Rocklin, R. E., Bendtzen, K., and Greineder, D., 1980, Mediators of immunity: Lymphokines and monokines, *Adv. Immunol.* **29**:55.

Salvin, S. B., and Nishio, J., 1972, Lymphoid cells in delayed hypersensitivity. III. The influence of X-irradiation on passive transfer and on in vitro production of soluble mediators, *J. Exp. Med.* **135**:985.

Scher, M. G., Beller, D. I., and Unanue, E. R., 1980, Demonstration of a soluble mediator that induces exudates rich in Ia-positive macrophages, *J. Exp. Med.* **152**:1684.

Schrader, J. W., and Clark-Lewis, I., 1982, A T cell-derived factor stimulating multipotential hematopoietic stem cells: Molecular weight and distinction from T cell growth factor and T cell-derived granulocyte-macrophage colony-stimulating factor, *J. Immunol.* **129**:30.

Smith, K. A., Lackman, L. B., Oppenheim, J. J., and Favata, M. F. 1980, The functional relationship of the interleukins, *J. Exp. Med.* **151**:1551.

Sone, S., and Fidler, I. J., 1980, Synergistic activation by lymphokines and muramyl dipeptide of tumoricidal properties in rat alveolar macrophages, *J. Immunol.* **125**:2454.

Stadler, B. M., Berenstein, E. H., Siraganian, R. P., and Oppenheim, J. J., 1982, Monoclonal antibody against human interleukin 2 (IL2). I. Purification of IL 2 for the production of monoclonal antibodies, *J. Immunol.* **128**:1620.

Staruch, M. J., and Wood, D. D., 1983, The adjuvanticity of interleukin 1 in vivo, *J. Immunol.* **130**:2191.

Steeg, P. S., Moore, R. N., and Oppenheim, J. J., 1980, Regulation of murine macrophage Ia-antigen by products of activated spleen cells, *J. Exp. Med.* **152**:1734.

Steeg, P. S., Moore, R. N., Johnson, H. M., and Oppenheim, J. J., 1982, Regulation of murine macrophage Ia antigen expression by a lymphokine with immune interferon activity, *J. Exp. Med.* **156**:1780.

Steinman, R. M., Nogueira, N., Witmer, M. D., Tydings, J. D., and Mellman, I. S., 1980, Lymphokine enhances the expression and synthesis of Ia antigens on cultured mouse peritoneal macrophages, *J. Exp. Med.* **152**:1248.

Swain, S. L., and Dutton, R. W., 1982, Production of a B cell growth-promoting activity from a cloned T cell line and its assay on the BLL, B cell tumor, *J. Exp. Med.* **156**:1821.

Taramelli, D., Holden, H. T., and Varesio, L., 1981, In vitro induction of tumoricidal and suppressor macrophages by lymphokines: Possible feedback regulation, *J. Immunol.* **126**:2123.

Tilden, A. B., and Balch, C. M., 1982, A comparison of PGE_2 effects on human suppressor cell function and on interleukin 2 function, *J. Immunol.* **129**:2469.

Torres, B. A., Yamamoto, J. K., and Johnson, H. M., 1982a, Cellular regulation of gamma interferon production: Lyt phenotype of the suppressor cell, *Infect. Immun.* **35**:770.

Torres, B. A., Farrar, W. L., and Johnson, H. M., 1982b, Interleukin 2 regulates immune interferon production by normal and suppressor cell cultures, *J. Immunol.* **128**:2217.

Tsuyuguchi, I., Shiratsuchi, H., Teraoka, O., and Hirano, T. 1980, Increase in T cell-bearing IgG-Fc receptors in peripheral blood of patients with tuberculosis by in vitro stimulation with purified protein derivative, *Am. Rev. Respir. Dis.* **121**:951.

Turk, J. L., 1980, *Delayed Hypersensitivity*, Elsevier/North-Holland, Amsterdam.

Uhr, J. W., and Pappenheimer, A. M., Jr., 1958, Delayed hypersensitivity. III. Specific desensitization of guinea pigs sensitized to protein antigens, *J. Exp. Med.* **108**:891.

Utermohlen, V., Besner, G., and Berkowitz, M. G., 1980, The effect of fatty acid addition in vitro on direct migration inhibition with paramyxoviral antigen, *Clin. Immunol. Immunopathol.* **16**:324.

Varesio, L., and Holden, H. T., 1980, Suppression of lymphokine production. I. Macrophage-mediated inhibition of MIF production, *Cell Immunol.* **56**:16.

Varesio, L., Holden, H. T., and Taramelli, D., 1981a, Mechanism of lymphocyte activation. II. Requirements for macromolecular synthesis in the production of lymphokines, *J. Immunol.* **125**:2810.

Varesio, L., Holden, H. T., and Taramelli, D., 1981b, Suppression of lymphokine production. II. Macrophage-dependent inhibition of production of macrophage activating factor, *Cell. Immunol.* **63**:279.

Wahl, S. W., Altman, L. C., and Rosenstreich, D. L., 1975, Inhibition of in vitro lymphokine synthesis by glucocorticosteroids, *J. Immunol.* **115**:476.

Weston, W. L., Krueger, G. G., and Claman, H. N., 1973, Site of action of cortisol in cellular immunity, *J. Immunol.* **110**:880.

Williams, T. W., and Granger, G. A., 1969, Lymphocyte in vitro cytotoxicity: Correlation of depression with release of lymphotoxin from human lymphocytes, *J. Immunol.* **103**:170.

Wilson, G. B., Fudenberg, H. H., Johnson, H. T., Jr., and Smith, C. L., 1980, Effects of dialyzable leukocytes extracts (DLE) with transfer factor activity on leukocyte migration in vitro. IV. Two distinct effects of DLE on leukocyte migration can be produced by prostaglandins, *Clin. Immunol. Immunopathol.* **16**:90.

Yip, Y. K., Pang, R. H. L., Oppenheim, J. J., Nachbar, M. S., Henriksen, D., Zerebekyj-Eckhardt, I., and Vilcek, J., 1981, Stimulation of human gamma interferon production by diterpene esters, *Infect. Immun.* **34**:131.

Yoshida, T., 1979, Purification and characterization of lymphokines, in: *Biology of Lymphokines* (S. Cohen, E. Pick, and J. J. Oppenheim, eds.), pp. 259–290, Academic Press, New York.

Yoshida, T., and Cohen, S., 1974a, Lymphokine activity in vivo in relation to circulating monocyte levels and delayed skin reactivity, *J. Immunol.* **112**:1540.

Yoshida, T., and Cohen, S., 1974b, In vivo manifestations of lymphokine or lymphokine-like activity, in: *Mechanisms of Cell-Mediated Immunity* (R. T. McCluskey and S. Cohen, eds.), pp. 43–60, Wiley, New York.

Yoshida, T., and Cohen, S., 1982, Biologic control of lymphokine function, *Fed. Proc.* **41**:2480.

Yoshida, T., and Suko, M., 1983, Immunopathology of delayed hypersensitivity, in: *Immunopathology*, Volume III (N. Rose and B. V. Siegel, eds.), pp. 397–428, Plenum Press, New York.

Yoshida, T., Biazzi, P. E., and Cohen, S., 1975, The production of anti-guinea pig lymphokine antibody, *J. Immunol.* **114**:688.

Yoshida, T., Suko, M., Baba, T., and Cohen, S., 1982, Feedback regulation of delayed-type hypersensitivity by lymphokine-activated macrophages, in: *Self-Defense Mechanisms: Role of Macrophages* (D. Mizuno and N. Ishida, eds.), pp. 159–165, Elsevier, Amsterdam.

Yoshinaga, M., Nishime, K., Nakamura, S., and Goto, F., 1980, A PMN-derived factor that enhances DNA-synthesis in PHA or antigen-stimulated lymphocytes, *J. Immunol.* **124**:94.

Zakhireh, B., and Malech, H. L., 1980, The effect of colchicine and vinblastine on the chemotactic response of human monocytes, *J. Immunol.* **125**:2143.

6

Effects of Nonspecific Inflammation on the Reticuloendothelial System

ROBERT M. FAUVE

1. INTRODUCTION

The first review concerning the influence of inflammation on host resistance was written by Metchnikoff (1892). He had already pointed out the significance and the importance of the mobilization of amoebocytes in primitive metazoans facing an aggression, and later on, showed that phagocytosis was a cornerstone of host resistance. As reviewed again by Metchnikoff (1901) in *Immunity in Infectious Diseases*, he made it clear that inflammation is one of the oldest phylogenetic mechanisms of resistance. In the same book, it was also reported that an increased resistance against bacteria can be induced at the site of an inflammatory reaction. Indeed, it had been observed during the last two decades of the 19th century that animals injected in the peritoneal cavity with different nonantigenic phlogogens are able to survive a lethal inoculum of pathogens. The explanation given for such an increased resistance was the increased influx of phagocytic cells into the site of infection. He also regarded these inflammatory phagocytes as being stimulated. Today, it is known that these phagocytic cells are not the only effectors responsible for such stimulation; nevertheless, the importance of inflammation as a nonspecific resistance mechanism is now well established. Moreover, it is also widely accepted by immunologists interested in *in vivo* immunity that specific immune effectors (antibodies and lymphocytes) are responsible for the induction of inflammatory reactions in the vicinity of specific targets. Since macrophages are among the most potent actors in host–invader relationships, one may wonder what elements of the tangled web of inflammation can modulate macrophage functions. In order to answer this question, we

ROBERT M. FAUVE • Unit of Cellular Immunophysiology, Pasteur Institute, 75724 Paris Cedex 15, France.

will consider, in the inflammatory focus, the different modulators of macrophages.

Today, it is known that the different facets of an inflammatory process do reflect the interactions of different systems not only locally but also at a distance from the inflammatory focus. The increased synthesis of acute-phase proteins, fever, and modifications of blood counts are, among many others, examples of such remote actions on the functions of distant tissues. These obvious interactions led us to postulate (Fauve and Hevin, 1975) that the granulomas induced in laboratory animals with many immunostimulants are responsible, at least in part, for the increased resistance against invaders. As will be shown, a nonspecific inflammatory reaction is able, indeed, to increase strikingly the resistance of laboratory animals against bacteria, parasites, and malignant cells when the inflammatory reaction is induced with nondiffusible, nonantigenic, nonbiodegradable phlogogens injected at a distance from the site of introduction, persistence, or multiplication of the pathogens. Known and hypothetical modulators of macrophages will be considered.

2. DEFINITION AND INDUCTION OF NONSPECIFIC INFLAMMATION

An inflammation is nonspecific when its induction does not result from the interactions of an antigen with the specific effectors of the immune response. This definition implies that the phlogogen used and its split products are not antigenic.

Among the many techniques used to induce inflammatory reactions, one can distinguish those using physical means from those using the injection of phlogogens.

Physical Stresses

Physical stresses used to induce inflammatory reactions are X-rays, heat, and trauma. These inflammations result from local reaction to tissue injury and are nonspecific except when this tissue injury is induced on skin or in tissues in which are introduced bacterial contaminants against which the host is already sensitized.

Introduction of Phlogogens

Phlogogens introduced into the tissues constitute two groups: biodegradable or nonbiodegradable irritants.

Biodegradable Irritants.   The most often used are glycogen, dextran, carrageenan, and agar. The possible presence of antigens of animal or bacterial origin must be determined, for as shown by Nelson and Boyden (1963), minute amounts of endotoxin may influence peritoneal cells. The same antigenic contamination has to be taken into consideration with a well-known irritant used to elicit macrophages from the peritoneal cavity: the thioglycollate medium. Hirsch and Fedorko (1969) and Robineaux *et al.* (1971) have demonstrated that the agar present in this broth is found in the phagosomes of peritoneal macrophages.

Nonbiodegradable Irritants.   These include nondigestible mineral oils, different substances such as silica, bentonite, talc, berylium, glass, silver nitrate, and copper. Plastics are of some interest, such as polyvinylchloride. Recently, it was found that polyacrylamide beads used for exclusion chromatography can be used to induce inflammatory reactions, and interesting differences were observed with regard to the pore size of the beads (Fontan and Fauve, 1983; Fauve *et al.*, 1984). Usually, these nonbiodegradable phlogogens are good inducers of foreign body granulomas in which epithelioid and Langhans giant multinucleated cells may develop (Boros, 1978).

3. LOCAL EFFECTS OF NONSPECIFIC INFLAMMATION BY-PRODUCTS ON MACROPHAGES

The inflammatory process has recently been reviewed in several excellent books (Vane and Ferreira, 1978; Movat, 1979; Houck, 1979; Weissman, 1980). Here, while summarizing the different cascades of events and the different systems involved in the inflammatory process, we shall consider the by-products that are known to act directly on macrophages.

When a tissue injury is induced and direct damage to vascular walls of capillaries, arterioles, or venules occurs, the result is a leakage of blood or plasma and, later, edema, fibrin formation, platelet aggregation, and leukocyte accumulation. Most of the time, in carefully induced inflammation, mast cell degranulation is one of the first steps. Following degranulation, mediators are released. Many of these are known to trigger the inflammatory process. These mediators will induce a cascade of events starting with vasodilation followed rapidly by increased vascular permeability, adherence of blood cells to the vascular endothelium, and leukocyte diapedesis. This increased vascular permeability allows the exudation of plasma with all the "actors" of the coagulation, fibrinolytic, complement, and kinin systems, and an increased concentration of different serum factors, among them the acute-phase proteins. Following leukocyte diapedesis, their movements are controlled by chemotactic factors. Within the extravascular space, leukocytes release metabolic products. Among them, free radicals and enzymes contribute to a great extent in changing the environment. Thus, it is clear that, in the inflammatory focus, macrophage functions can be modified by different factors. We will now consider the effect on macrophages of substances released by mast cells, the by-products of the activation of the coagulation, fibrinolytic, complement, and kinin systems, and the metabolic products of leukocytes. As summarized by Metcalf and Kaliner (1981), some of these preformed mediators are released rapidly under physiologic conditions, others are released more slowly, and some are generated as a consequence of mast cell activation or secretion.

3.1. SUBSTANCES RELEASED BY MAST CELLS

3.1.1. Histamine

As reviewed by Busse (1979), histamine is released immediately and its known actions are mediated through H_1 or H_2 receptors. Among them, some, such as increased vascular permeability and irritant-receptor stimulation (H_1 receptor mediated), explain in part how mast cell degranulation can start an inflammatory reaction. Other mediators are released at the same time: eosinophil and neutrophil chemotactic factors, arylsulfatase A, exoglycosidases, and serotonin. Although there have been no reported effects of these substances on macrophages, these mast cell products are obviously of importance in the induction of the inflammatory reaction. Among other mediators, released more slowly, chymotrypsin, trypsin, and arylsulfatase B have an adjuvant effect on the inflammatory process.

3.1.2. Heparin

This glycosaminoglycan acts indirectly on macrophages either by its well-known anticomplement activity, or, following its anticoagulant effect, by decreasing the encapsulation of macrophages in a fibrin clot.

Besides heparin, other substances able to act on macrophages are prostaglandins and platelet-activating factor (PAF). Others, such as peroxidase, superoxide dismutase, and superoxide, will be considered later.

3.1.3. Prostaglandins

Like other arachidonic acid metabolites, prostaglandins are released by almost every cell following adequate stimulation. For instance, they are generated by monocytes and macrophages, and it has been claimed that macrophage-derived PGE is involved in part in the suppression of T-cell response. As reviewed by Higgs (1982), despite the many reports concerning macrophages and prostaglandins, it is difficult today to draw a clear picture. Furthermore, since prostaglandins are produced by phagocytic mononuclear cells and since this synthesis is increased followed membrane receptor activation (Passwell et al., 1979), macrophage–prostaglandin interactions are very complex.

PGE_2 was shown to enhance the monocyte chemotactic response (McClatchey and Snyderman, 1973). PGE_1 induces reversible morphologic changes in macrophages and inhibits phagocytosis (Oropeza-Rendon et al., 1979). Of great interest is the finding that PGEs regulate the macrophage's tumoricidal function (Schultz et al., 1978).

3.1.4. PAF

This compound, an acetylated glycerylether phosphorylcholine, has been synthesized and its properties reviewed (Vargaftig et al., 1981). Although both the mast cell and the basophil are implicated, the principal cellular origin of PAF seems to be polymorphonuclear cells and mononuclear phagocytes. Concerning its activity on macrophages, PAF has been demonstrated to be chemotactic. More recently, it was found that monocyte aggregation is dependent on glycolysis and divalent cations (Yasaka *et al.*, 1982).

3.2. BY-PRODUCTS OF THE COAGULATION AND FIBRINOLYTIC SYSTEMS

Thrombin, following its action on fibrinogen, generates fibrinopeptide B, a chemoattractant.

Fibrin has been known for a long time to act as a framework for the migration of inflammatory cells and to help phagocytosis.

Fibrin degradation products have been found to be chemotactic for macrophages.

Plasminogen activator, besides its key role during the formation of plasmin, is also chemotactic and increases the adhesion of macrophages. It is also worthy of note that upon reaction of plasminogen activator with guinea pig serum, a macrophage migration inhibitory factor is generated (Roblin *et al.*, 1977).

Plasmin has been shown to increase the spreading of macrophages.

3.3. BY-PRODUCTS OF THE COMPLEMENT SYSTEM

For a long time, antigen–antibody complexes were considered to be a prerequisite for the activation of complement. Today, as reported in reviews of the subject (Hügli and Müller-Eberhard, 1978; Minta and Movat, 1979; Müller-Eberhard and Schreiber, 1980; Götze and Sundsmo, 1982), it is evident that the activation of C3 can be initiated following the activation of either the classical or the alternate pathway. Moreover, it has been shown that C-reactive protein (CRP) is able to activate the classical pathway. This finding is important since CRP is one of the acute-phase reactants whose serum level is strikingly increased during inflammation. Thus, it is evident that even in the absence of antibody, complement can be activated in an inflammatory focus. Using purified complement fractions, it was demonstrated that C5a, Ba, and the complex C567 are chemotactic for phagocytic cells. It was also found that C3b can induce the release of lysosomal hydrolases from mouse or guinea pig peritoneal macrophages (Götze *et al.*, 1980).

3.4. BY-PRODUCTS OF THE KININ SYSTEM

Following the action of Hageman factor and of plasmin, prekallikrein is transformed to kallikrein, which cleaves kininogens to produce kinins. There are two types of kininogens: low and high molecular weight. Following the action of kallikrein, a nonapeptide (bradykinin) is removed from kininogen. At the same time, from the high-molecular-weight kininogen, two fragments are formed and these have transient vascular permeability-enhancing activity. Another effect of these fragments is to inhibit the contact activation of Hageman factor. Besides the vasodilation induced by the by-products of the kinin system, other activities have been reported. Kallikrein is chemotactic for monocytes (Garcia Leme, 1978). Bradykinin, which increases the spreading of macrophages *in vitro* (Fauve and Hevin, 1977b; Stahl *et al.*, 1978), is quickly broken down by kininases. The resulting split products are claimed to be inactive. This is certainly true of their vasoactive function but, as will be reported below, these products may have other functions.

3.5. METABOLIC PRODUCTS OF LEUKOCYTES

It is well known that inflammatory macrophages display a striking stimulation of their metabolism (Cohn, 1978), which explains in part their increased ability to spread and the increased pinocytosis and phagocytosis. Besides prostaglandins, PAF, and some complement factors that are produced by macrophages and whose activity was mentioned above, some products synthesized by these cells are important not only because they help to keep the inflammatory process going, but also because they act as modulators of macrophage functions. Among the many factors synthesized by macrophages, we shall consider in this review only those acting on these cells.

As we have seen, plasminogen activator is chemotactic and increases the adhesion of macrophages. We shall consider:

3.5.1. Free Radicals

A recent excellent review on oxygen-derived free radicals and metabolites in leukocyte-dependent inflammatory reactions (Fantone and Ward, 1982) emphasizes the importance of these compounds in inflammatory reactions. In response to different stimuli such as phagocytosis or various substances, leukocytes undergo a respiratory burst. In conjunction, these cells release superoxide anion and hydrogen peroxide. Other highly reactive oxygen-derived metabolites are found such as hydroxyl radicals and singlet oxygen. These free radicals have a very short life. For instance, delta singlet oxygen has a half-life in water of approximately 2 μsec. Besides the importance of these free radicals in the bactericidal activity of phagocytes, they are toxic to a variety of eukaryotic cells. Furthermore, these radicals react with other molecules, generating compounds with interesting properties. For example, if human plasma is incubated in a system that generates superoxide and hydrogen peroxide, a chemotactic lipid is generated from arachidonic acid and is active at a concentration of 3 ng/ml. It seems that these free radicals are involved in the lysis of polymorphonuclear leukocytes. But, besides scavengers such as coeruloplasmin, α-tocopherol, and transferrin, macrophages are protected against these toxic effects by two enzymes: catalase and glutathione oxidase.

3.5.2. Colony-Stimulating Factor

CSF is secreted by activated macrophages. When added to bone marrow cells *in vitro*, CSF stimulates the growth of macrophage colonies. The biologic activity of CSF concerns not only hemopoiesis but also the natural resistance of the host. Handman and Burgess (1979) demonstrated that pure CSF is able to stimulate *in vitro* the killing of *Leishmania tropica* by macrophages, in contrast to normal macrophages in which *L. tropica* survive unharmed and multiply. It remains to be shown whether the concentration of CSF is great enough to allow such an activation of macrophages in an inflammatory focus.

3.5.3. α_2-Macroglobulin (α_2M)

α_2M is produced mainly by mononuclear phagocytes (Hovi *et al.*, 1977). This high-molecular-weight protein has polyvalent affinities and binds to many proteases. Besides its effect on lymphocytes, it has been shown (Vischer and Berger, 1980) that following the endocytosis of α_2M–trypsin complexes, the production of proteases by these cells is strikingly increased. Thus, despite the neutralizing effect of α_2M on the many proteases in an inflammatory focus, the increased synthesis of hydrolases may explain in part the self-perpetuation of some forms of inflammation.

3.5.4. Split Products of Serum Proteins

Split products of serum proteins are present in an inflammatory focus. Many are cleaved in biologically active fragments. Among them, fragments of both fibronectin and immunoglobulins modulate macrophage activity.

3.5.4a. Fragments of Fibronectin. As reviewed by Pearlstein *et al.* (1980), fibronectin, a cold-insoluble protein of high molecular weight, is a major cell-associated substance interacting with cytoskeletal elements and is involved in cell attachment and spreading, wound healing, and clearance by the RES. It has long been known that the effective clearing ability of the RES is dependent on a plasma factor, known today as fibronectin. Moreover, the phagocytic activity of liver and spleen macrophages has been directly correlated with plasma levels of fibronectin. More recently, some doubts have been raised concerning the possibility that the entire fibronectin molecule is involved in opsonization. Czop *et al.* (1981) have found that intact plasma fibronectin fails to augment SRBC phagocytosis by human monocytes. Following cleavage of the molecule with trypsin, a proteolytically derived form of fibronectin was found to be active. Since multiple forms of fibronectin can be generated from the intact molecule *in vitro* by plasmin or trypsin (Chen *et al.*, 1977; Ruoslahti *et al.*, 1979), the existence of a fibronectin fragment in an inflammatory focus is thus possible.

3.5.4b. Fragments of Immunoglobulins (IgG). Among these, Fc fragments and tuftsin have been found to modulate macrophage functions. Following the addition of Fc fragments to macrophages, their synthesis of collagenase and PGE_2 is increased (Passwell *et al.*, 1980). Tuftsin, a basic tetrapeptide occupying amino acid residues 289–292 in all the IgG subclasses, is liberated.

As reviewed by Najjar (1982), tuftsin (Thr-Lys-Pro-Arg) is cleaved from residues 289–292 of IgG following the action of two enzymes: tuftsin endocarboxypeptidase and a surface leukokininase. This product modulates motility, phagocytosis, bactericidal activity, and cytotoxicity against malignant cells. Goldman and Bar-Shavit (1982) found that tuftsin binds rapidly to cells of the granulocyte–macrophage series and that the number of binding sites is 7.2×10^4/cell. Binding is always followed by an increased phagocytic response. Tuftsin induces a dose-dependent increase in intracellular cGMP level and decreased cAMP content, which are good biochemical correlates of the phagocytic capacity of macrophages (Cox and Karnovsky, 1973; Ignarro and Cech, 1976).

4. REMOTE EFFECTS OF NONSPECIFIC INFLAMMATION ON MACROPHAGES

One obvious condition to study the remote effects of inflammation on macrophage is to induce a local inflammatory reaction with phlogogens that are nondiffusible, nonbiodegradable, and nonantigenic. Needless to say, the site of inflammation has to be distant from the site where the macrophages are studied. For these reasons, we have used different sterilized irritants such as silicone rubber, stainless steel, polyacrylamide beads, talc, and calcium phosphate gels. For most experiments, mice were injected in the dorsal area with talc particles embedded in a gel of calcium phosphate, care being taken to avoid contamination with bacteria and endotoxin. Under these conditions, a granuloma develops containing polymorphonuclear leukocytes, mainly macrophages and giant cells. As with the above-mentioned irritants, 3 days following the induction of the inflammatory reaction, the resistance of the mice against *Listeria monocytogenes* is increased to a point that in contrast with control animals, which die 4 days after infection, all treated animals survive (Fauve and Hevin, 1975; Zerial *et al.*, 1980). These results led us to study in more detail this inflammation-mediated immunostimulation. It became obvious that this stimulation of resistance was also manifested against *Salmonella typhimurium* (Fauve and Hevin, 1975), *Candida albicans* (Hurtrel *et al.*, 1978), *Schistosoma mansoni* (Fauve and Dodin, 1976), *Plasmodium berghei* (Michel *et al.*, 1982), and even against one of the more maligant murine tumors, the Lewis carcinoma (Fauve and Hevin, 1977a). These results encouraged us to study and to elucidate the complex mechanisms of such increased host resistance against invaders. The methodology used and the results obtained have been reviewed recently (Fauve *et al.*, 1982). We shall consider here only the remote effects of inflammation on macrophages.

4.1. INCREASED PHAGOCYTOSIS AND BACTERIAL KILLING BY MACROPHAGES

Since treated mice are more resistant to bacterial infections following an intravenous challenge, one may wonder if such animals are able to clear bacteria more rapidly from their blood. When mice are injected intravenously with 3 × 10^7 virulent salmonellae, 2 hr later, in contrast to control animals in which 8 × 10^6 bacteria are found per milliliter of blood, 1000-fold fewer salmonellae are found in the blood of treated mice. Such increased clearance was not found to reflect increased opsonic or bactericidal activities of the serum. Thus, such increased clearance is the consequence of an activation of spleen and liver macrophages.

Since the pioneering work of Mackaness (1962), it has been known that the fate of *L. monocytogenes* is dependent on the ability of macrophages to kill them. When control and treated animals are infected intravenously with 3 × 10^5 *Listeria* organisms, 2 hr later, the numbers of bacteria in the spleens of controls are more than 10-fold greater than in the spleens of treated mice. Forty-eight and seventy-two hours later, between 100- and 10,000-fold fewer bacteria are found in the spleens and livers of treated animals. Such stimulation is also found in germfree nude C3H mice.

4.2. INCREASED PHAGOCYTOSIS AND BACTERIAL KILLING OF MACROPHAGES FOLLOWING THE TREATMENT OF MICE WITH A CELL-FREE EXTRACT OF GRANULOMA

Since the inflammatory reaction is focused in the dorsal area of the animals, these results suggested to us that some mediators, in the broadest sense of the term, were involved in such stimulation of the RES. Among these compounds, one has to consider (1) the "classic" mediators of inflammation (kinins, archidonic acid metabolites, serotonin, histamine, etc.), (2) the acute-phase reactants, and (3) other substances present in the granuloma. In preliminary experiments, an increased listericidal activity was found in the spleens of mice injected with the cell-free extract of a 5-day-old granuloma. Following ammonium sulfate precipitation, preparative electrophoresis on Pevikon C870, gel chromatography, isoelectrophoresis, and SDS–polyacrylamide gels, it was found (Fontan and Fauve, 1980, 1983; Fontan *et al.*, 1983) that the active substance is a protein with an isoelectric point of 4.9 and a molecular weight of 58,000. Its activity is such that 0.5 μg of this fraction injected intravenously 12 hr before challenge increases significantly the resistance of mice against a lethal inoculum of *Listeria*.

4.3. INCREASED *IN VITRO* CYTOTOXIC ACTIVITY OF NORMAL RESIDENT MACROPHAGES INCUBATED *IN VITRO* AGAINST LEWIS CARCINOMA CELLS IN THE PRESENCE OF SERUM OR AN EXTRACT OF A GRANULOMA FROM TREATED MICE

When an inflammatory reaction is induced in C57BL/6 mice, 1 day following the subcutaneous injection of 5 × 10^5 Lewis carcinoma cells in the rear footpad, the growth of the tumor is delayed and the number of lung metastases is decreased. This same increased resistance is found in athymic nude mice. Following sequential tissue sections of tumors, Dauge *et al.* (1982) observed that in comparison with control animals, vascularization was even more evident in the tumors from the treated animals, in association with fewer mitotic figures in the tumors. One may wonder if such a decreased multiplication of Lewis carcinoma cells does not reflect a general effect of the inflammatory process on cell multiplication in the treated host. Following a pulse of $[^{125}I]$-UdR in control and treated mice, it was found that for 12 days, the incorporation was not modified in the testis, whereas from days 3 to 12, the incorporation of the isotope was significantly increased in bone marrow, spleen, thymus, and even the popliteal lymph nodes of treated mice. Again, such results can be explained only by a remote control of the effectors of host resistance against maligant cells. Usually, when resident macrophages are added to Lewis carcinoma cells *in vitro*, no decrease of $[^{125}I]$-UdR incorporation is observed in maglignant cells. In contrast, when the serum from treated animals or 0.5 µg/ml of the granuloma inflammatory protein is added to macrophages and malignant cells the incorporation of $[^{125}I]$-UdR is 100-fold smaller than with normal mouse serum or an extract from noninflammatory murine tissues. Thus, it is evident that some compound in the serum from treated mice is able to activate macrophages against the Lewis carcinoma. Further work is needed in order to characterize the active substance(s) responsible for such activation of macrophages against Lewis carcinoma cells.

4.4.   INCREASED *IN VIVO* ACTIVITIES OF MACROPHAGES FOLLOWING THE TREATMENT OF MICE WITH KININS

As mentioned above, it was relevant to consider the possible activity of the "classic" mediators of inflammation. In preliminary experiments, we had found that following the intravenous injection of different doses of histamine, serotonin, various prostaglandins, and bradykinin, only the latter was able to activate spleen and liver macrophages against *Listeria*. Since bradykinin is quickly split off in the blood circulation, we tested three synthetic peptides, Arg-Pro-Pro-Gly-Phe, Ser-Pro, and Phe-Arg. Only the pentapeptide was found to increase the ability of spleen and liver macrophages to ingest *Salmonella* and to kill *Listeria*. The same pentapeptide and some of its analogs were found to increase significantly the resistance of mice against the Lewis carcinoma. How the pentapeptide increases bacterial killing by macrophages is unknown, but preliminary experiments suggest that its action on macrophages is indirect.

5.   CONCLUSIONS

It is evident from the aforementioned results that an inflammatory reaction can modulate macrophage functions either *locally* or *at a distance*. Among the "actors" in a local modulation, others than those reported are certainly of great importance. Clearly, one can expect to find in inflammatory foci other compounds of interest. Furthermore, some split products of serum proteins or of tissue compounds are good candidates for the modulation of macrophage functions. Tuftsin is a good example of such a compound. Another field worthy of interest is the interplay between giant cells and macrophages. It is evident from our preliminary experimental work that the greater the number of giant cells in a granuloma, the greater is the local and remote influence of the granuloma on host resistance.

Concerning the remote effects on macrophages, among the possible mediators able to stimulate the resistance against invaders, one has to consider the acute-phase reactants (Koj, 1974). Among them, the activity of complement fractions C3 and C5 are well known. Of interest also is C3e, a low-molecular-weight acidic fragment of C3 which induces the release of leukocytes from bone marrow (Rother, 1972; Ghebrehiwet and Müller-Eberhard, 1978). Other acute-phase reactants such as haptoglobin and $\alpha_2 M$ are known to modulate the immune system by different mechanisms. CRP was recently found to have opsonic properties *in vivo* (Nakayama *et al.*, 1982). This protein has also been shown to induce an increased in splenic sequestration and a decrease in hepatic sequestration. The fraction we isolated from the granuloma, which has been found to have a very high specific activity, will be a possible mediator if its presence can be demonstrated in the serum of mice. As we have seen, fibronectin fragments are also possible mediators of greater interest since it has been shown, as reviewed by Pearlstein *et al.* (1980), that levels of fibronectin correlate with the innate resistance of man against various aggressors. Kallikrein was reported, following its injection into rats, to increase the mitosis of marrow cells (Rixon and Whitfield, 1973). These findings may be related to the known effect of inflammatory exudates and inflammatory serum on the multiplication of bone marrow cells. Our findings with bradykinin and its 1–5 pentapeptide fragment, despite the latter's significant but low activity, are interesting since the fragment and some of its active analogs are devoid of apparent toxicity. More interesting is the fact that a fragment devoid of kininlike activity is involved in a different sphere of activity.

Despite the complex interactions of all these factors in inflammation, it is obvious that the inflammatory process is one of the cornerstones of direct or remote macrophage modulation.

ACKNOWLEDGMENTS. The author's work discussed in this review was supported by grants from DGRST (80.7.0223), DRET (82.212), and CNAMTS.

REFERENCES

Boros, D. L., 1978, Granulomatous inflammations, *Prog. Allergy* **24**:183.

Busse, W. W., 1979, Histamine: Mediator and modulator in inflammation, In: *Chemical Messengers of the Inflammatory Process* (J. C. Houck, ed.), pp. 1–45, Elsevier/North-Holland, Amsterdam.

Chen, A. B., Amrani, D. L., and Mosesson, M. W., 1977, Heterogeneity of the cold-insoluble globulin of human plasma (CIg), a circulating cell surface protein, *Biochim. Biophys. Acta* **493**:310.

Cohn, Z. A., 1978, The maturation and activation of mononuclear phagocytes: Fact, fancy and future, *J. Immunol.* **121**:813.

Cox, J. D., and Karnovsky, M. D., 1973, The depression of phagocytosis by exogeneous cyclic nucleotides, prostaglandins and theophylline, *J. Cell Biol.* **59**:480.

Czop, J. K., Kadish, J. L., and Austen, K. F., 1981, Augmentation of human monocyte opsonin independent phagocytosis by fragments of human plasma fibronectin, *Proc. Natl. Acad. Sci. USA* **78**:3649.

Dauge, M. C., Hevin, M. B., and Fauve, R. M., 1982, Inflammation et résistance antitumorale. III. Effects précoces d'une réaction inflammatoire sur l'évolution de la tumeur de Lewis, *Ann. Immunol. (Inst. Pasteur)* **133C**:133.

Fantone, J. C., and Ward, P. A., 1982, Role of oxygen-derived free radicals and metabolites in leukocyte dependent inflammatory reactions, *Am. J. Pathol.* **107**:397.

Fauve, R. M., and Dodin, A., 1976, Influence d'une réaction inflammatoire provoquée par le BCG ou par un irritant non biodégradable sur la résistance des souris à la bilharziose, *C.R. Acad. Sci.* **282**:131.

Fauve, R. M., and Hevin, M. B., 1975, Influence d'une réaction inflammatoire sur la résistance des souris à l'infection par *Listeria monocytogenes* et *Salmonella typhimurium*, *C.R. Acad. Sci.* **281**:2037.

Fauve, R. M., and Hevin, M. B., 1977a, Inflammation et résistance antitumorale. I. Retard de croissance et inhibition du développement des métastases de la tumeur de Lewis chez des souris porteuses d'une réaction inflammatoire distante du site d'inoculation des cellules malignes, *Ann. Immunol. (Inst. Pasteur)* **128C**:923.

Fauve, R. M., and Hevin, M. B., 1977b, Inflammation et résistance antitumorale. II. Effets antagonistes de la bradykinine et d'une fraction isolée d'un surnageant de culture de cellules malignes sur l'étalement des macrophages, *Ann. Immunol. (Inst. Pasteur)* **128C**:1079.

Fauve, R. M., Fontan, E., and Hevin, M. B., 1982, Remote control of macrophage activation: Influence of a nonspecific inflammation, In: *Phagocytosis—Past and Future* (M. L. Karnovsky and L. Bolis, eds.), pp. 295–322, Academic Press, New York.

Fauve, R. M., Jusforgues, H., and Hevin, M. B., 1983, Maintenance of granuloma macrophages in serum free medium, *J. Immunol. Meth.* **64**:345.

Fontan, E., and Fauve, R. M., 1980, Inflammation et résistance antibactérienne. II. Isolement, par une nouvelle technique d'isoélectrofocalisation d'une fraction immunostimulante provenant d'un granulome inflammatoire de souris, *Ann. Immunol. (Inst. Pasteur)* **131D**:97.

Fontan, E., and Fauve, R. M., 1983, Inflammation et résistance antibactérienne. III. Influence d'une réaction inflammatoire induite par l'injection de gels de polyacrylamide sur la résistance des souris à l'infection par *Listeria monocytogenes*, *Ann. Immunol. (Inst. Pasteur)* **134C**:255.

Fontan, E., Fauve, R. M., Hevin, B., and Jusforgues, H., 1983, Immunostimulatory mouse granuloma protein, *Proc. Natl. Acad. Sci. USA* **80**:6395.

Garcia Leme, J., 1978, Bradykinin-system, in: Inflammation (J. R. Vane and S. H. Ferreira, eds.), pp. 464–522, Springer-Verlag, Berlin.

Ghebrehiwet, B., and Müller-Eberhard, H. J., 1978, Description of an acidic fragment (C3e) of human C3 having leukocytosis-producing activity, *J. Immunol.* **120**:1774.

Goldman, R., and Bar-Shavit, Z., 1982, Phagocytosis—Modes of particle recognition and stimulation by natural peptides, in: Phagocytosis—Past and Future (M. L. Karnovsky and L. Bolis, eds.), pp. 259–285, Academic Press, New York.

Götze, O., and Sundsmo, J. S., 1982, A role of complement proteins in the stimulation of human mononuclear phagocytes, in: Phagocytosis—Past and Future (M. L. Karnovsky and L. Bolis, eds.), pp. 357–373, Academic Press, New York.

Götze, O., Bianco, C., Sundsmo, J. S., and Cohn, Z. A., 1980, The stimulation of mononuclear phagocytes by components of the classical and the alternative pathways of complement activation, in: Mononuclear Phagocytes, Part II (R. van Furth, ed.), pp. 1421–1442, Nijhoff, The Hague.

Handman, E., and Burgess, A. W., 1979, Stimulation by granulocyte-macrophage-colony-stimulating factor of *Leishmania tropica* killing by macrophages, *J. Immunol.* **122**:1134.

Higgs, G. A., 1982, Arachidonic acid metabolism in leukocytes, in: *Phagocytosis—Past and Future* (M. L. Karnovsky and L. Bolis, eds.), pp. 105–129, Academic Press, New York.

Hirsch, J. G., and Fedorko, M. E., 1969, Morphology of mouse mononuclear phagocytes, in: *Mononuclear Phagocytes* (R. van Furth, ed.), pp. 7–42, Blackwell, Oxford.

Houck, J. C. (ed.), 1979, *Chemical Messengers of the Inflammatory Process*, Volume 1, Elsevier/North-Holland, Amsterdam.

Hovi, T., Mosher, D., and Vaheri, A., 1977, Cultured human monocytes synthesize and secrete α_2-macroglobulin, *J. Exp. Med.* **145**:1580.

Hügli, T. E., and Müller-Eberhard, H. J., 1978, Anaphylatoxins: C3a and C5a, *Adv. Immunol.* **26**:1.

Hurtrel, B., Lagrange, P. H., and Michel, J. C., 1978, Influence d'une réaction inflammatoire sur la résistance de souris à l'infection par *Candida albicans*, *Ann. Immunol. (Inst. Pasteur)* **129C**:843.

Ignarro, L. J., and Cech, S. Y., 1976, Bidirectional regulation of lysosomal enzyme secretion and phagocytosis in human neutrophils by guanosine 3',5'-monophosphate and adenosine 3',5'-monophosphate, *Proc. Soc. Exp. Biol. Med.* **151**:448.

Koj, A., 1974, Acute phase reactants, in: *Structure and Function of Plasma Proteins*, Volume 1 (A. C. Allison, ed.), pp. 73–131, Plenum Press, New York.

McClatchey, W., and Snyderman, R., 1973, Prostaglandins and inflammation: Enhancement of monocyte chemotactic responsiveness by prostaglandin E_2, *Prostaglandins* **12**:415.

Mackaness, G. B., 1962, Cellular resistance to infection, *J. Exp. Med.* **116**:381.

Metcalf, D. D., and Kaliner, M., 1981, Mast cells and basophils, in: *Cellular Functions in Immunity and Inflammation* (J. J. Oppenheim, D. L. Rosenstreich, and M. Potter, eds.), pp. 301–322, Elsevier/North-Holland, Amsterdam.

Metchnikoff, E., 1892, *Leçons sur la pathologie comparé de l'inflammation*, Masson, Paris.

Metchnikoff, E., 1901, *L'immunité dans les maladies infectieuses*, Masson, Paris.

Michel, J. C., Hurtrel, B., and Lagrange, P. H., 1982, Influence d'une réaction inflammatoire sur la résistance des souris au paludisme expérimental provoqué par *Plasmodium berghei*, *Ann. Immunol. (Inst. Pasteur)* **133C**:97.

Minta, J. O., and Movat, H. Z., 1979, The complement system and inflammation, *Curr. Top. Pathol.* **68**:136.

Movat, H. Z. (ed.), 1979, *Curr. Top. Pathol.* **68**.

Müller-Eberhard, H. J., and Schreiber, R. D., 1980, Molecular biology and chemistry of the alternative pathway of complement, *Adv. Immunol.* **29**:1.

Najjar, V. A., 1982, Biochemistry and physiology of tuftsin: Thr-Lys-Pro-Arg, in: *The Reticuloendothelial System: A Comprehensive Treatise*, Volume 2 (A. J. Sbarra and R. R. Strauss, eds.), pp. 45–71, Plenum Press, New York.

Nakayama, S., Mold, C., Gewurz, H., and Duclos, T. W., 1982, Opsonic properties of C-reactive protein *in vivo*, *J. Immunol.* **128**:2435.

Nelson, D. S., and Boyden, S. W., 1963, The loss of macrophages from peritoneal exudates following the injection of antigen into guinea pigs with delayed-type hypersentivity, *Immunology* **6**:264.

Oropeza-Rendon, R. L., Speth, V., Hillier, G., Weber, K., and Fischer, H., 1979, Prostaglandin E_1 reversibly induces morphological changes in macrophages and inhibits phagocytosis, *Exp. Cell Res.* **199**:365.

Passwell, J. H., Dayer, J. M., and Merler, E., 1979, Increased prostaglandin production by human monocytes after membrane receptor activation, *J. Immunol.* **123**:115.

Passwell, J. H., Dayer, J. M., Gass, K., and Edelson, P. J., 1980, Regulation by Fc fragments of the secretion of collagenase, PGE_2 and lysozyme by mouse peritoneal macrophages, *J. Immunol.* **125**:910.

Pearlstein, E., Gold, L. I., and Garcia-Pardo, A., 1980, Fibronectin: A review of its structure and biological activity, *Mol. Cell. Biochem.* **29**:103.

Rixon, R. H., and Whitfield, J. F., 1973, Kalliknein, Kinin, and cell proliferation, in: *Kininogenases* (G. L. Haberland and J. W. Roten, eds.), p. 131, Schattauer, Stuttgart.

Robineaux, R., Anteunis, A., and Bona, C., 1971, Ultrastructure des macrophages de cobaye, *Ann. Inst. Pasteur (Paris)* **120**:329.

Roblin, R. O., Hammond, E., Bensky, N. D., Dvorak, A. M., Dvorak, H. F., and Black, P. H., 1977, Generation of macrophage migration inhibitory activity by plasminogen activators, *Proc. Natl. Acad. Sci. USA* **74**:1570.

Rother, K., 1972, Leukocyte immobilizing factor: A new biologic activity derived from the third component of complement, *Eur. J. Immunol.* **2**:550.

Ruoslahti, E., Hayman, E. G., Kuusela, P., Shively, J. E., and Engvall, E., 1979, Isolation of a tryptic fragment containing the collagen-binding site of plasma fibronectin, *J. Biol. Chem.* **254**:6054.

Schultz, R. M., Parlidis, N. A., Stylos, W. A., and Chirigos, M. A., 1978, Regulation of macrophage tumoricidal function: A role for prostaglandins of the E series, *Science* **202**:320.

Stahl, K. W., Lambert, D., Rosenfeld, C., Muller, O., and Mathé, G., 1978, Characterization of a phagotoxic tumour peptide from rat, *Eur. J. Rheumatol. Inflam.* **1**:330.

Vane, J. R., and Ferreira, S. H. (eds.), 1978, *Inflammation*, Springer-Verlag, Berlin.

Vargaftig, B. B., Chignard, M., Benveniste, J., Lefort, J., and Wal, F., 1981, Background and present status of research on platelet-activating factor "PAF-acether," *Proc. N.Y. Acad. Sci.* **370**:119.

Vischer, T. L., and Berger, D., 1980, Activation of macrophages to produce neutral proteinases by endocytosis of α_2M–trypsin complexes, *J. Reticuloendothel. Soc.* **28**:427.

Weissman, G. (ed.), 1980, *The Cell Biology of Inflammation*, Elsevier/North-Holland, Amsterdam.

Yasaka, T., Boxer, L. A., and Baehner, R. L., 1982, Monocyte-aggregation and superoxide anion release in response to formyl-methionyl-leucyl-phenylalanine (FMLP) and platelet-activating factor (PAF), *J. Immunol.* **128**:1939.

Zerial, A., Floc'h, F., and Werner, G. H., 1980, Comparative effects of an inflammatory reaction on the resistance of mice to bacterial and viral infections, *Ann. Immunol. (Inst. Pasteur)* **131C**:177.

7

The Role of Macrophage-Derived Arachidonic Acid Oxygenation Products in the Modulation of Macrophage and Lymphocyte Function

RICHARD M. SCHULTZ

1. INTRODUCTION

Among the many functional activities of mononuclear phagocytes, the production and release of metabolites derived from arachidonic acid has recently attracted particular attention. Approximately 25% of the total fatty acid content of mouse resident peritoneal macrophages (Scott *et al.*, 1980), rabbit alveolar macrophages (Mason *et al.*, 1972), and human blood monocytes (Stossel *et al.*, 1974) is esterified arachidonic acid. There are now abundant studies showing that mononuclear phagocytes secrete certain arachidonic acid oxygenation products after treatment with a variety of phagocytizable particulates and soluble agents *in vitro*. Prostaglandin (PG) E_2 and 6-keto-PGF$_{1\alpha}$, the stable metabolite of prostacyclin (PGI$_2$), appear to be major products of most macrophage/monocyte populations studied, although some populations also synthesize PGF$_{2\alpha}$, PGI$_2$, thromboxane (Tx) A$_2$, and products of the lipoxygenase pathway (Davies *et al.*, 1980; Doig and Ford-Hutchinson, 1980; Rigaud *et al.*, 1979; Scott *et al.*, 1980; Valone *et al.*, 1979). Data will be reviewed in Section 2 on the synthesis of arachidonic acid oxygenation products by various mononuclear phagocyte populations.

The liberation of free arachidonic acid from cellular phospholipids initiates the formation of various arachidonic acid oxygenation products. The release of

RICHARD M. SCHULTZ • Department of Immunology, Lilly Research Laboratories, Indianapolis, Indiana 46285.

arachidonic acid is catalyzed by phospholipase A_2 (Flower and Blackwell, 1976) or, alternatively, by phospholipase C (Kennedy et al., 1979), which forms diacylglycerol, part of which is subsequently degraded by diacylglycerol lipase to yield free arachidonic acid. Macrophages appear to contain a phospholipase C and two phospholipase A_2 activities, one of lysosomal origin (Hsueh et al., 1981a,b). The free arachidonic acid is oxygenated in two distinct pathways (Fig. 1). The cyclooxygenase pathway of the cascade results in the formation of the stable primary prostaglandins of the E, F, and D series as well as the two newly discovered products, TxA_2 and PGI_2. The synthesis of these products proceeds through two labile endoperoxide intermediates (PGG_2 and PGH_2). The lipoxygenase pathway of the arachidonic acid cascade results in the synthesis of various hydroperoxy and hydroxy fatty acids.

Macrophages appear to be the major, although not the sole source of prostaglandins at sites of inflammation. The release of prostaglandins by macrophages was first described by Bray et al. (1974), who demonstrated the release of PGE-like material from guinea pig exudate cells. Subsequent studies have demonstrated that human macrophages release PGE_2 and $PGF_{2\alpha}$ using cells obtained either from human synovia (Sturge et al., 1978) or from implanted intrauterine devices (Myatt et al., 1975). Prostaglandins, depending on their structure, are considered to play a variety of important roles in the initiation and control of the inflammatory process (Bonta et al., 1977; Ferreira, 1979).

E-type prostaglandins have been proposed to have a regulatory role in controlling changes in macrophage metabolism and function induced by activation stimuli. Since the activated macrophage releases high concentrations of PGE_2 (Bray et al., 1974; Kurland and Bockman, 1978; Meltzer and Wahl, 1979), several authors have suggested that PGE_2 may have an important role in negative feeback inhibition to limit overzealous macrophage activity (Kennedy and Stobo, 1980; Schultz et al., 1978; Taffet and Russell, 1981). The regulatory effects of PGEs appear to be extremely complex, being dependent on the nature of the activation stimulus, the concentration of PGEs, and the time of exposure of PGEs relative to exposure to the activation stimulus (Schultz, 1980b). While PGE

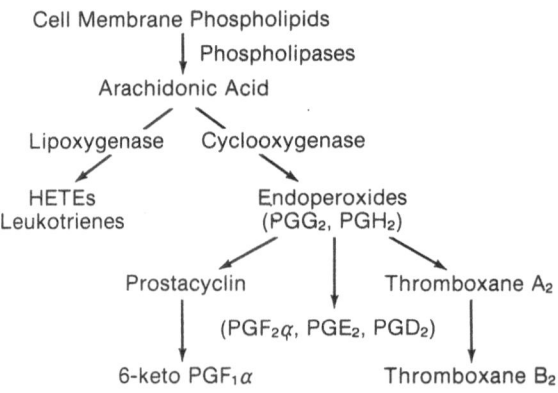

FIGURE 1.   The arachidonic acid cascade.

synthesis is required for collagenase production by LPS-stimulated macrophages (Wahl *et al.*, 1977), several other activities of macrophages including production of colony-stimulating factor (Moore *et al.*, 1979), interferon (IFN) (Moore *et al.*, 1980), plasminogen activator (Vassalli *et al.*, 1976), and oxygen intermediates (Metzger *et al.*, 1981) are potently inhibited by PGEs.

Exogenous PGEs also suppress the cytotoxic activity of activated macrophages (Schultz *et al.*, 1978; Taffet and Russell, 1981) and natural killer (NK) cells (Brunda and Holden, 1980). These latter findings raise the possibility that host resistance to neoplasia may be compromised by elevated levels of PGEs in the microenvironment of the tumor, since a large number of experimental animal tumors and spontaneous human neoplasms have been shown to contain and/or produce high concentrations of PGEs (Droller *et al.*, 1979; Goodwin, 1981; Sykes and Maddox, 1972). The ability of exogenous and endogenous PGEs to modulate macrophage functional activity is reviewed in Section 3.

There is also evidence (summarized in Section 4) that prostaglandins produced by macrophages may have an important role in the regulation of lymphocyte function. Exogenous PGEs have been demonstrated to potently suppress several lymphocyte functions including antigen-induced blastogenesis, tumor cytolysis, and lymphokine production (reviewed in Goldyne and Stobo, 1981). Since mononuclear phagocytes appear to be the major source of PGEs produced at sites of immune reactions (Ferraris *et al.*, 1974), it is reasonable to suppose that these mononuclear phagocyte-derived PGEs may act as physiologic regulators of lymphocyte function.

2. PRODUCTION OF ARACHIDONIC ACID METABOLITES BY MACROPHAGES

PGE_2 appears to be a major arachidonic acid oxygenation product of most macrophage/monocyte populations studied. A large variety of soluble and particulate stimuli have been shown to induce PGE_2 production by macrophages (Table 1). Since prostaglandins are not stored in cells and since mammalian cells contain very little free arachidonic acid, these diverse stimuli presumably act by stimulating arachidonic acid release from macrophage phospholipids. In addition to classical inflammation-inducing agents, a variety of immunologic stimuli including antibody-coated erythrocytes (Glatt *et al.*, 1977; Brune *et al.*, 1978b), antigen–antibody complexes (Bonney *et al.*, 1979; Gartner *et al.*, 1981), endotoxin (Kurland and Bockman, 1978), *Corynebacterium parvum* (Grimm *et al.*, 1978; Stringfellow *et al.*, 1978), and poly(I:C) (Kurland *et al.*, 1979) induce PGE synthesis by murine splenic and peritoneal adherent cells and by human peripheral blood monocytes. In addition, the lymphokine macrophage-activating factor (MAF) has been reported to stimulate the synthesis of PGEs in guinea pig peritoneal exudate macrophages (Friedman *et al.*, 1979), although other factors contaminating the MAF preparations could have been responsible for PGE induction.

Several studies have concentrated on defining the conditions for PGE release

TABLE 1. SOME EXAMPLES OF CONDITIONS AND/OR STIMULI THAT INDUCE THE RELEASE OF PGE$_2$ FROM MONONUCLEAR PHAGOCYTES

Source of mononuclear phagocytes	In vivo stimulus	In vitro stimulus	References
Human intrauterine contraceptive devices	None	None	Myatt et al. (1975)
Human peripheral blood	None	Con A	Passwell et al. (1979), Pelus and Bockman (1979)
	None	Endotoxin	Kurland and Bockman (1978)
	None	Fc fragments of human IgG	Passwell et al. (1979), Bockman (1981)
	None	Zymosan	
Mouse peritoneum	None	Antibody-coated erythrocytes	Brune et al. (1978)
	None	Antigen–antibody complexes	Bonney et al. (1979), Gartner et al. (1981)
	None	Endotoxin	Kurland and Bockman (1978)
	None	Fc fragments of human IgG	Passwell et al. (1980)
	None	HEPES-buffered media	Brune (1980)
	None	Monosodium urate crystals	McMillan et al. (1981)
	None	Neutral protease	Chang et al. (1980)
	None	Particle binding to Fc receptor	Rouzer et al. (1980a)
	None	Phorbol myristate acetate	Brune et al. (1978a), Humes et al. (1978), Schultz et al. (1980)
	None	Zymosan	Bockman (1981)
Mouse spleen	Neoplastic growth	None	Pelus and Bockman (1979)
Mouse cell lines (WEHI-3, J774, RAW264)	None	Endotoxin	Kurland and Bockman (1978), Tracey et al. (1982)
Rat peritoneum	Freund's incomplete adjuvant	Leukotriene C	Feuerstein et al. (1981)
	Sodium caseinate	Colchicine	Gemsa et al. (1980)
	Sodium Caseinate, thioglycollate	A23187	Gemsa et al. (1979a), Lim et al. (1981)

by macrophages. To examine whether phagocytosis *per se* or the surface characteristics of the phagocytized particles play a role in the induction of prostaglandin release, Gemsa *et al.* (1979b) examined different particles and various opsonization procedures. They noted that latex particles, although interiorized avidly by macrophages, failed to induce PGE release. Moreover, PGE formation was higher after phagocytosis of *E. coli* coated with IgG and complement than with bacteria opsonized with either one alone, although phagocytosis by macrophages occurred to a comparable extent. Similarly, Rouzer *et al.* (1980a) examined the requirements of PGE synthesis for particle attachment, membrane interiorization, and phagosome–lysosome fusion. Macrophages that were preloaded with dextran sulfate and that exhibited a greater than 99% inhibition of phagosome–lysosome fusion produced normal amounts of PGEs after treatment with zymosan. Inhibition of membrane interiorization with cytochalasin D was similarly ineffective in abrogating PGE synthesis. The addition of large numbers of unmodified polystyrene latex beads, which were readily ingested by macrophages, failed to induce PGE synthesis. However, when macrophages were challenged with latex beads coated with immune complexes, an increased production of PGEs resulted. No response occurred if the complex was prepared with the $F(ab')_2$ fragment of IgG. Rouzer *et al.* (1980a) concluded that particle binding to the Fc receptor of the macrophage plasma membrane is a sufficient stimulus for PGE synthesis.

Humes *et al.* (1982) showed that the products of arachidonic acid oxygenations by resident mouse peritoneal macrophages depend on the nature of the stimulus. For example, soluble membrane-mediated inflammatory stimuli such as phorbol myristate acetate (PMA) and LPS stimulated the formation of PGE_2 via the cyclooxygenase pathway. In contrast, zymosan, a particulate, phagocytizable inflammatory mediator, stimulated leukotriene (LT) C_4 and B_4 synthesis via the lipoxygenase pathway in addition to stimulating PGE_2 synthesis. Their data suggested that the prostaglandin synthetase system can obtain substrate arachidonic acid from a source different from that for leukotriene synthesis. Similarly, studies by Hsueh *et al.* (1981a) of rabbit alveolar macrophages showing that the action of PMA is additive to maximal stimulatory doses of zymosan in affecting the release of prostaglandins, favor the concept that there are two phospholipases in the macrophage, one in the membrane and one in the lysosome. The ability of LPS and PMA to selectively stimulate PGE_2, but not LTC_4, synthesis and secretion (Humes *et al.*, 1982) suggests that these stimulants interact with the plasma membrane to activate a phospholipase resulting in the release of arachidonic acid for the selective oxygenation by the cyclooxygenase residing in the endoplasmic reticulum. In contrast, zymosan particles are internalized into lysosomal phagocytic vesicles within the cell, and a phopholipase A_2 with a pH optimum of 4.5 has been suggested to be lysosomal (Wightman *et al.*, 1980; Hsueh *et al.*, 1981b). Thus, a lysosomal phospholipase may release arachidonic acid in close proximity to both cyclooxygenase and 5-lipoxygenase.

Hsueh *et al.* (1979, 1981a) demonstrated that the time course of PGE and arachidonic acid secretion by zymosan-treated macrophages does not parallel that of particle engulfment *per se*, but of the release of lysosomal enzymes.

Although their initial results (Hsueh *et al.*, 1979) raised the possibility of a direct relationship between lysosomal enzyme release and secretion of prostaglandins, they observed that inhibition of PGE synthesis by indomethacin did not alter lysosomal enzyme release. Bonney *et al.* (1978) also reported the lack of effect of indomethacin on the release of lysosomal acid hydrolases in mouse peritoneal macrophages. The converse, that lysosomal enzymes influence prostaglandin synthesis and release, is more difficult to exclude. Chang *et al.* (1980) observed that the treatment of murine macrophages with specific bacterial and mammalian proteases can provoke the synthesis and release of PGE_2 and other radiolabeled metabolites. Protease-activated PGE_2 synthesis was inhibited by a variety of protease inhibitors and synthetic substrates for neutral proteases. Moreover, they showed that PMA-activated PGE_2 synthesis by macrophages was blocked by a variety of protease inhibitors, suggesting that an endogenous protease is responsible for the initiation of PGE_2 synthesis in macrophages.

Bockman (1981) demonstrated that the pattern and sequence of prostaglandins synthesized by human blood monocytes are in part a function of the *in vitro* culture conditions and time in culture. Thromboxane and PGE were the major products released by human blood monocytes and mouse peritoneal macrophages on day 1 of culture following cell adherence. If these cells were studied after 24 hr of adherence, thromboxane synthesis was markedly reduced and PGEs were the major secretory product. A day 1 type of pattern could be obtained from day 2 cultured cells if adherence was delayed until day 2 of culture. Bockman suggested that activation of the thromboxane synthetase pathway in monocytes and macrophages is primarily a consequence of cell adherence. PGEs and PGI_2 appeared to be the major products in response to inflammatory stimuli. Brune (1980) presented data that inclusion of HEPES buffer in the culture medium can induce PGE release from macrophages in cell culture.

Because of evidence supporting functional heterogeneity among human monocytes, Goldyne and Stobo (1979) examined whether or not heterogeneity exists in these cells to synthesize PGEs. Subjecting monocytes to discontinuous density gradient franctionation produced significant differences in PGE_1 and PGE_2 synthesis among the resulting monocyte subpopulations. In contrast, Bonney *et al.* (1981a) could not demonstrate a difference in PGE_2 secretion by populations of macrophages that vary in their expression of Ia determinants.

Several studies have shown that elicited and activated populations of macrophages have a much diminished capacity to synthesize prostaglandins as compared with resident populations (Humes *et al.*, 1977, 1980; Bonney *et al.*, 1978, 1981b; Debatin *et al.*, 1982; Scott *et al.*, 1982). The decreased production of prostaglandins in response to zymosan was observed in populations of macrophages elicited by thioglycollate broth (Humes *et al.*, 1977, 1980; Bonney *et al.*, 1978), carrageenan (Humes *et al.*, 1980), BCG, and *C. parvum* (Humes *et al.*, 1980; Bonney *et al.*, 1981b; Scott *et al.*, 1982). These alterations paralleled changes characteristic of elicited macrophages such as decreased 5'-nucleotidase and elevated leucine aminopeptidase activities (Humes *et al.*, 1980). The reduced capacity of elicited cells to synthesize prostaglandins when challenged in culture with zymosan may be accounted for by one or more of the following: (1) differences in the amount of zymosan phagocytized, (2) diminished activity of cyclooxygenase, (3) altered rates of phospholipid deacylation for the production of arachidonic acid, and (4) defective secretion of newly synthesized prostaglandins. Humes *et al.* (1980) showed that there was no difference in the amount of zymosan particles ingested per cell between resident and elicited populations of macrophages. Similarly, no defect in the extracellular release of prostaglandins was observed in elicited macrophages. However, these investigators observed a decreased release of [^{3}H]arachidonic acid by elicited macrophages in response to zymosan. Since the availability of arachidonic acid has been shown to be rate-limiting for prostaglandin synthesis in certain systems (Gryglewski *et al.*, 1975), this may account for the marked difference in the amount of prostaglandins produced by these two populations of cells. Other factors such as decreased cyclooxygenase activity are alternative explanations that remain to be conclusively investigated.

Although PGE$_2$ is the arachidonate metabolite whose production has been measured most frequently in macrophage cultures, there are two independent reports that TxB$_2$ is quantitatively the most prominent cyclooxygenase product in elicited macrophages (Murota *et al.*, 1978; Morley *et al.*, 1979). Cook *et al.* (1981) examined the ability of rat peritoneal macrophages to synthesize TxA$_2$ and PGI$_2$ in response to endotoxin by radioimmunoassay of their stable metabolites, TxB$_2$ and 6-keto-PGF$_{1\alpha}$. *In vitro* exposure to *Salmonella enteritidis* endotoxin induced a concentration-dependent increase in the rate of formation of TxB$_2$ and 6-keto-PGF$_{1\alpha}$. Their results suggested that macrophages may be a significant source of TxA$_2$ and PGI$_2$ in endotoxin shock. A study by Feuerstein and Ramwell (1981) demonstrates that OKY-1581 (sodium (E)-3-[4(-3-pyridylmethyl)phenyl]-2-methylacrylate) is a selective thromboxane synthetase inhibitor in LPS-stimulated macrophages. Brune *et al.* (1978b) suggested that the formation of vacuoles may be a crucial event for the formation and release of PGE$_2$ and TxB$_2$ from macrophages. They speculated that during phagocytosis, cell membranes become internalized and membrane phospholipids come in contact with the phospholipase–cyclooxygenase system in the cell interior, thus becoming the substrate for the synthesis of prostaglandins and thromboxanes.

Several recent reports have demonstrated that macrophages can synthesize PGI$_2$ (Humes *et al.*, 1977; Stringfellow *et al.*, 1978; Ahnfelt-Ronne *et al.*, 1980; Cook *et al.*, 1981). Stringfellow *et al.* (1978) attempted to determine if cellular conversion of arachidonic acid to PGI$_2$ could be correlated with the biologic activity of normal resting, stimulated, or activated peritoneal macrophages. They observed a statistically significant inverse correlation between the level of macrophage functional activity and the ability of cellular homogenates to produce PGI$_2$. Ahnfelt-Ronne *et al.* (1980) showed that peritoneal macrophages from adjuvant arthritic rats preferentially synthesize PGI$_2$ *in vitro* and have a diminished capacity to produce PGE$_2$.

LTC and its metabolites LTD and LTE collectively comprise the biologic activity referred to as slow-reacting substance (SRS) of anaphylaxis. Several recent studies show that murine peritoneal and alveolar macrophages release LTC in response to a phagocytic challenge with unopsonized zymosan (Baggiolini *et al.*, 1982; Rouzer *et al.*, 1980b, 1982a; Scott *et al.*, 1983) and to IgE immune complexes (Rouzer *et al.*, 1982b; Scott *et al.*, 1983). These results suggest that macrophages may be a major source of leukotrienes in acute inflammation and also in immediate-type hypersensitivity reactions. Studies by Scott *et al.* (1983) indicate that zymosan-stimulated peritoneal cells of a single animal produce a 100-fold excess of the 3–6 pmoles of LTC necessary to produce complete contraction of a guinea pig ileum, the standard biologic assay for SRS. Rouzer *et al.* (1981) showed that treatment of macrophages with buthionine sulfoximine, a specific inhibitor of glutathione synthesis, results in a time-dependent depletion of intracellular glutathione and a concomitant inhibition of LTC synthesis. The data suggest that glutathione is a direct precursor of LTC. Roubin *et al.* (1982) demonstrated that different *in vivo* environmental factors can influence the release of platelet-activating factor, an ether phospholipid mediator, and LTC–LTD from macrophages.

Studies by Feuerstein *et al.* (1981) suggest that endogenous LTC is involved in the stimulation of macrophages by LPS. They showed that rat peritoneal macrophages incubated with LTC exhibit a dose-dependent increase in the release of PGE_2 and 6-keto-$PGF_{1\alpha}$. Moreover, nordihydroguaiaretic acid, an inhibitor of lipoxygenase, prevented the stimulation of PGE release by LPS, but did not affect the release of prostaglandins from nonstimulated cells.

In addition to leukotrienes, macrophages also form and release monohydroxy derivatives (mono-HETES) of arachidonic acid. Doig and Ford-Hutchinson (1980) showed that rat peritoneal macrophages exposed to the ionophore A23187 release 5-, 12-, and 15-HETE. Rabinovitch *et al.* (1981) demonstrated that resident mouse peritoneal macrophages synthesize 5-, 8-, 9-, 11-, 12-, and 15-HETE when incubated with exogenous arachidonic acid. Chang *et al.* (1982) demonstrated that treatment of human pulmonary macrophage monolayers with A23187 or zymosan particles led to increased formation and release of 5- and 12-HETE.

3. MODULATION OF MACROPHAGE METABOLISM AND FUNCTION BY ARACHIDONIC ACID METABOLITES

3.1. EFFECTS OF EXOGENOUS ARACHIDONIC ACID METABOLITES ON VARIOUS MACROPHAGE ACTIVITIES

Prostaglandins of the E series, but not $PGF_{2\alpha}$, modulate a number of inducible macrophage activities *in vitro* (Table 2). Although the mechanism by which PGEs exert their inhibitory effects on macrophage function is unknown, these alterations appear to be mediated by cAMP. The reports that PGEs activate membrane-bound adenylate cyclase and increase intracellular levels of cAMP in macrophages (Remold-O'Donnell, 1974; Schmidt-Gayk *et al.*, 1975; Gemsa *et al.*, 1978; Bonta *et al.*, 1981) and that other agents known to increase intracellular levels of cAMP similarly possess inhibitory effects on macrophage function (Koopman *et al.*, 1973; Vassalli *et al.*, 1976; Gallin *et al.*, 1978; Schultz *et al.*, 1979b;

TABLE 2. SUMMARY OF EFFECTS OF PGE ON MACROPHAGE ACTIVITIES *IN VITRO*

Cell source	Cellular response	References
Human monocytes	Decreased randon locomotion	Gallin *et al.* (1978)
Guinea pig peritoneal macrophages	Prevention of lymphokine-induced inhibition of macrophage migration	Koopman *et al.* (1973)
Guinea pig peritoneal macrophages	Stimulation of collagenase production	Wahl *et al.* (1977)
Mouse bone marrow	Inhibition of proliferation of committed granulocyte–macrophage progenitor cells	Kurland *et al.* (1978a), Razin *et al.* (1981)
Mouse bone marrow	Inhibition of pinocytic activity	Oropeza-Rendon *et al.* (1980)
Mouse bone marrow	Inhibition of zymosan-induced chemiluminescence	Weidemann *et al.* (1978)
Mouse peritoneal macrophages	Inhibition of release of lysosomal hydrolases	Zurier *et al.* (1971)
Mouse peritoneal macrophages	Inhibition of plasminogen activator production	Vassalli *et al.* (1976), Foster (1980)
Mouse peritoneal macrophages	Inhibition of interferon-induced tumoricidal activity	Schultz *et al.* (1978, 1979a)
Mouse peritoneal macrophages	Inhibition of cell spreading and adhesion	Cantarow *et al.* (1978)
Mouse peritoneal macrophages	Inhibition of Ia expression	Snyder *et al.* (1982)
Mouse peritoneal macrophages	Inhibition of production of oxygen intermediates	Metzger *et al.* (1981)
Mouse peritoneal macrophages	Inhibition of colony-stimulating factor production	Moore *et al.* (1979)
Mouse peritoneal macrophages	Inhibition of interferon production	Moore *et al.* (1980)

Foster, 1980; Metzger *et al.*, 1981) point to a role for cAMP in the negative regulation of macrophage function.

The range of concentrations of PGEs found in inflammatory fluids [approximately 10^{-7} to 10^{-9} M (Higgs *et al.*, 1974; Robinson and Levine, 1974)] is generally the same as the concentration range of PGE_1 and PGE_2 found inhibitory for macrophage function *in vitro*. Moreover, Gemsa *et al.* (1978) reported that the process of phagocytosis enhances the sensitivity of macrophages to PGE_1 along with a subsequent release of PGE_1, providing a sensitive control mechanism that may regulate macrophage function under physiologic conditions. In addition, Bonney *et al.* (1980) showed that the cAMP production by elicited macrophages is far more sensitive to exogenous PGE_2 than by resident populations of cells.

Other arachidonate metabolites have been shown to modulate macrophage metabolism and function. Studies by McCarthy *et al.* (1981) suggested a role for LTB_4 in the induction of macrophage acid hydrolases. Feuerstein *et al.* (1981) showed that LTC stimulates PGE_2 release from rat peritoneal macrophages. Moreover, nordihydroguaiaretic acid, an inhibitor of lipoxygenase, prevented the stimulation of prostaglandin release by LPS-treated macrophages. Spagnuolo *et al.* (1980) demonstrated a role for thromboxanes in the surface activation of human monocytes. They demonstrated that the specific thromboxane synthetase inhibitor, imidazole, at 400 μg/ml, abrogated LPS- and lymphokine-induced monocyte adherence, and that rabbit anti-TxB_2 antibody inhibited LPS-stimulated monocyte adherence. Clearly, further studies are warranted to clarify the roles of the various arachidonate metabolites in the diverse functions of macrophages.

3.2. AUTOREGULATION OF MACROPHAGE FUNCTION BY PROSTAGLANDINS

The ability of various macrophage-activating agents to induce the synthesis and release of PGEs from macrophages (Kurland and Bockman, 1978; Meltzer and Wahl, 1979; Schultz *et al.*, 1979a) and the ability of physiologic concentrations of exogenous PGEs to modulate several macrophage activities *in vitro* suggest that PGEs may also serve as feedback inhibitors by which macrophages modulate their own metabolism and function. In this regard, Kennedy and Stobo (1980) provided evidence that macrophages are capable of responding to self-synthesized prostaglandins by elevating cAMP levels and also by down-regulating their receptors for these prostaglandins. Similarly, Gemsa *et al.* (1979a) showed that PGE_2 synthesis by macrophages after treatment with A23187 stimulates cAMP accumulation in the same cells. Studies by Picker *et al.* (1980) suggested that macrophage synthesis of prostaglandins is responsible for culture-dependent changes occurring in various macrophage enzymes. These authors showed that addition of indomethacin to macrophages blunted culture-dependent increases in the ectoenzyme, 5'-nucleotidase, but enhanced culture-dependent increases in the lysosomal enzyme, acid phosphatase. These alterations could be restored to normal by the simultaneous addition of exogenous PGE_2 (10^{-7} M) along with indomethacin. Similarly, Schnyder *et al.* (1981) found that indomethacin and diclofenac markedly increased plasminogen activator secretion in resting cells and even more so in the zymosan-activated cells. This enhancing effect was paralleled by spreading and an increase in the cellular levels of β-glucuronidase and alkaline phosphodiesterase I. In all instances, PGE_2 lowered or blocked, depending on the concentration used, the effects of indomethacin and diclofenac.

Most of the experiments supporting a role for PGEs in the autoregulation of macrophage function utilize agents such as indomethacin or aspirin, which block prostaglandin synthesis. However, care must be taken in interpreting the results since these agents increase the synthesis of several hydroperoxy- and hydroxy-fatty acids by allowing the precursors, which normally are converted to prostaglandins, to be utilized by other enzyme systems not sensitive to these agents. For example, macrophages produce and release leukotrienes in response to phagocytosis, and indomethacin enhances leukotriene production (Bretz *et al.*, 1980). Since prostaglandins form only one part of a larger, more complex, interrelated metabolic cascade, one must demonstrate that the observed effect is truly the result of blocking prostaglandin synthesis and not increasing substrate availability for other pathways. In addition, another important consideration is the possibility that other arachidonate metabolites can act as antagonists of the effects of PGEs. For example, Snyder *et al.* (1982) showed that PGEs are potent inhibitors of the expression of Ia antigens on macrophages and that TxB_2, another macrophage product, antagonizes the effect of PGEs. Similarly, Kennedy and Stobo (1981) demonstrated that PGE_2 and TxA_2 act as dual feedback regulators of macrophages. Their experiments demonstrated that PGE_2 can increase cAMP levels six-fold in human monocytes, but this stimulation is not augmented in the presence of a specific inhibitor of thromboxane synthesis (9,11-dizao,prosta-5,13-dienoic acid).

Several studies have suggested that the endogenous production of PGEs by macrophages may act to limit inflammatory tissue damage due to phlogistic products. Metzger *et al.* (1981) reported that the production of oxygen radicals by LPS-activated macrophages was inhibited when PGE_2 (10^{-5} to 10^{-9} M) was present during the incubation with LPS. In their studies, PGE_2 apparently interfered with an early event in the activation process. Similarly, Kunkel *et al.* (1982) showed that elicited or resident mouse macrophages, in suspension cultures, produced up to 40-fold greater PGE_2 levels as compared to cells that were adhered for 16 hr. Moreover, only macrophages that adhered for at least 4 hr could respond to PMA or zymosan with increased O_2^- generation. Bonta *et al.* (1981) examined the effect of PGE_2 on intracellular levels of cAMP in macrophages isolated from carrageen an-induced granulomas at various stages of inflammation. They observed that during infiltration of the macrophages into the inflammatory tissue, the sensitivity of adenylate cyclase to activation by PGE_2 increases. Perhaps the fall in endogenous PGE_2 production by granuloma macrophages (Humes *et al.*, 1980) may partially help to explain the increasing sensitivity of these cells to exogenous PGE_2.

Several studies suggest that granulocyte–macrophage progenitor cell (GM-CFC) proliferation is under the dual control of macrophage-derived colony-stimulating factors (CSF) and PGEs (Kurland and Moore, 1977; Kurland *et al.*, 1978a,b). Using *in vitro* culture systems, Kurland and his colleagues have shown that PGEs directly inhibit CSF-stimulated GM-CFC proliferation. Moreover, the ability of CSF preparations to directly induce macrophage release of PGEs suggests that inhibition by PGEs provides a self-regulatory feedback mechanism for myelopoiesis. However, Verma *et al.* (1981) warned that the *in vitro* experimental systems utilized by these authors (Kurland and Moore, 1977; Kurland *et al.*, 1978a,b) may not necessarily reflect the *in vivo* hemopoietic environment, since there is no convincing evidence that PGE production by macrophages is a constitutive process. They claimed that no *in vitro* experimental conditions are free of some inadvertent activation of macrophages. In addition, Verma *et al.* (1981)

showed that PGE_1 treatment of human marrow cells prior to their *in vitro* culture, augmented human granulocyte–macrophage progenitor cell growth *in vitro*. This augmentation appeared to result from the recruitment by PGE_1 of the noncycling (G_0 and long G_1) GM-CFC. Pelus *et al.* (1979) demonstrated that bone marrow-derived macrophages cultured at high density inhibited their own differentiation. This inhibition could be prevented by addition of indomethacin (10^{-6} M) to the culture medium. Similarly, Razin *et al.* (1980, 1981) examined the effect of indomethacin on the appearance and phagocytic activity of bone marrow-derived macrophages. Indomethacin treatment resulted in the accumulation of a macrophage population characterized by a relatively higher number and lower phagocytic activity.

Macrophages play a central, pivotal role in the initiation and subsequent regulation of both cell-mediated and humoral immunity. The ability of PGEs to directly modulate expression of macrophage Ia antigens (Pelus *et al.*, 1982; Snyder *et al.*, 1982; Steeg *et al.*, 1982) may, in part, explain the immunosuppressive effects of PGEs or their inducers. The expression of these glycoprotein antigens is essential for macrophages to function as antigen-presenting cells during the induction of immune responses (for review see Unanue, 1981). Steeg *et al.* (1982) presented evidence that bacterial LPS inhibits IFN-γ regulation of macrophage Ia antigen expression by stimulating macrophage PGE_2 production. They demonstrated that LPS inhibited both IFN-γ induction of macrophage Ia antigen expression and IFN maintenance of the Ia$^+$ state in a dose-dependent manner. In the absence of IFN-γ, LPS had no significant effect on macrophage Ia antigen expression. The inhibitory effects of LPS were abrogated by the addition of indomethacin into the culture medium. Furthermore, 10^{-10} to 10^{-6} M exogenous PGE_2 or 10^{-6} to 10^{-4} M exogenous dibutyryl cAMP also inhibited IFN-γ regulation of macrophage Ia antigen expression. Snyder *et al.* (1982) presented preliminary evidence that the loss of Ia by macrophages after exposure to PGEs is associated with reduced antigen presentation to immune T cells.

Work in this laboratory (Schultz *et al.*, 1978, 1979a) demonstrated that exogenous PGE_1 and PGE_2 suppress the cytotoxicity of IFN-activated macrophages, even when applied after the macrophages reached full morphologic activation. However, PGEs exerted their strongest inhibitory effect when presented simultaneously with IFN. PGEs required concentrations greater than 10^{-8} M to suppress tumor killing by IFN-treated macrophages *in vitro*. Other agents known to increase intracellular levels of cAMP, including cholera toxin and dibutyryl cAMP, produced similar inhibitory activity (Schultz *et al.*, 1979b), suggesting a role for cAMP in modulating macrophage cytotoxicity. Using a different cytotoxicity assay, Taffet and Russell (1981) demonstrated that PGE (2×10^{-9} M) inhibited tumor cytolysis by LPS-activated macrophages. In contrast, McCarthy and Zwilling (1981) reported that PGEs did not affect the tumoricidal activity of BCG-activated macrophages *in vitro*, but reduced their cytostatic effect on tumor cells.

Macrophage functions of tumor cytotoxicity and PGE_2 release completely dissociate, since certain potent activation stimuli including antigen-induced lymphokine and fibroblast-derived IFN do not cause macrophages to release more

PGE_2 than buffer-treated controls (Meltzer and Wahl, 1979; Schultz et al., 1979a). Moreover, macrophage-mediated tumor cell killing appears to be completely independent of the cyclooxygenase pathway of prostaglandin synthesis (Meltzer and Wahl, 1979; Shaw et al., 1979; Schultz and Jackson, 1981). However, Meltzer and Wahl (1979) showed that antigen-induced lymphokine and LPS acted synergistically in increasing both PGE_2 secretion and in vitro tumor cytotoxicity. Although virus-induced IFN, a potent inducer of macrophage cytotoxicity (for review see Schultz, 1980a), does not induce PGE_2 release from macrophages (Schultz et al., 1979a), Yaron et al. (1977) showed that fibroblasts treated with IFN or IFN inducers produce PGEs, indicating that local fibroblasts could serve a function in limiting IFN-induced macrophage function. Stringfellow (1978) demonstrated that PGEs restored the IFN response in hyporeactive animals, further showing complex interrelationships between production of these two mediators.

The contribution of macrophage-borne PGE_2 to the self-regulation of macrophage cytotoxic function remains to be fully elucidated. Since certain activating stimuli such as LPS induce macrophages to release PGE_2 (Kurland and Bockman, 1978; Schultz et al., 1979a), it has been proposed that PGEs may act as local feedback inhibitors of the activated tumoricidal state (Schultz, 1980b). In this regard, Taffet and Russell (1981) demonstrated that treatment of LPS-stimulated macrophages with 10^{-6} M indomethacin (or other cyclooxygenase inhibitors) prevented PGE synthesis and prolonged cytolytic activity. The latter effect could be reversed by adding PGE_2 to the cultures at a concentration of 10^{-8} M. Similarly, Prosser et al. (1979) demonstrated that indomethacin (10^{-6} M) inhibited PGE_2 production and enhanced the tumor cytotoxicity of macrophages activated by BCG cell wall material. Resident peritoneal macrophages from tumor-bearing mice have been reported to release significantly more PGE_2 spontaneously in culture (Pelus and Bockman, 1979). In this regard, it is interesting that Farram and Nelson (1980) demonstrated that indomethacin was capable of enhancing the tumoricidal activity of macrophages harvested from the peritoneal cavities of mice bearing the C-4 tumor. Recent observations by Cameron and O'Brien (1982) show that when indomethacin was added to peripheral blood monocytes obtained from breast cancer patients, the patients' monocytes became capable of killing tumor cells. These monocyte preparations obtained from breast cancer patients showed a 64% increase in the secretion of PGE_2, as compared to macrophages obtained from normal donors.

The potency of tumor promoters in experimental carcinogenesis has been reported to correlate with PGE secretion by macrophages exposed to promoter in vitro (Brune et al., 1978a). Several studies (Keller, 1979; Schultz and Jackson, 1981; Keller et al al., 1982) show that the strongest known promoter in mouse skin carcinogenesis, 12-O-tetradecanoylphorbol-13-acetate (TPA), inhibits macrophage and NK cell tumoridical function. In a recent study (Schultz and Jackson, 1981), indomethacin enhanced the cytotoxic activity of macrophages simultaneously exposed to TPA and either IFN or LPS, suggesting that endogenously produced PGEs had autoregulatory activity.

Taffet et al. (1981) reported that lymphokine preparations decrease the sensitivity of activated macrophages to the negative regulatory effects of PGEs and are responsible for maintenance of the tumoricidal state. Although the mechanism responsible for this lymphokine effect is not known, these authors showed that generalized inhibition of macrophage responsiveness to PGEs did not appear to be involved because lymphokine did not reduce the cAMP response of macrophages after they were exposed to PGEs. A rabbit polyclonal antibody against IFN-γ neutralized antiviral activity as well as the lymphokine activity that interfered with PGE$_2$-mediated negative regulation of macrophage activation, suggesting that the latter activity was attributable to IFN-γ (Russell and Pace, 1982).

4. ROLE OF MACROPHAGE-DERIVED PROSTAGLANDINS IN IMMUNOSUPPRESSION

An increasing body of *in vitro* and *in vivo* experimental evidence shows that macrophages have major positive and negative regulatory effects on lymphocyte function by the synthesis and release of various soluble factors (reviewed in Oehler *et al.*, 1978; Unanue, 1978). Included among these soluble factors is PGE$_2$, which can suppress such T-lymphocyte responses such as antigen- and mitogen-induced blastogenesis (Goodwin *et al.*, 1977a; Ellner and Spagnuolo, 1979; Muscoplat *et al.*, 1979; Novogrodsky *et al.*, 1979; Dememkoff *et al.*, 1980; Metzger *et al.*, 1980; Mullink and Blomberg, 1980; Rosenstein and Strausser, 1980), lymphokine secretion (Gordon *et al.*, 1976), and cytotoxicity (Henney *et al.*, 1972; Lichtenstein *et al.*, 1972; Strom *et al.*, 1973; Plaut, 1979; Garrigues *et al.*, 1981). In addition, macrophages are also capable of suppressing plaque-forming cell responses to heterologous erythrocytes via prostaglandin production (Melmon *et al.*, 1974; Mattingly and Kemp, 1979). This section will attempt to briefly summarize the *in vivo* significance of the PGE$_2$-producing suppressor macrophage.

4.1. NATURE OF THE PGE$_2$-PRODUCING CELL

Despite the ubiquitous nature of prostaglandin production, existing studies suggest that the monocyte/macrophage is the main source of immunoregulatory prostaglandins. PGE$_2$ appears to be the major prostaglandin having immunoregulatory activity (Goldyne, 1977; Goldyne and Stobo, 1980, 1981). Although PGE$_1$ is as potent as PGE$_2$ in suppressing lymphocyte function, the levels of PGE$_1$ produced by human peripheral blood monocytes are more than 10-fold lower than those of PGE$_2$ (Goldyne and Stobo, 1979). Goldyne and Stobo (1979) reported that PGE$_2$ synthesis by peripheral blood monocytes reflects a heterogeneous contribution from various monocyte subpopulations. Several authors have noted that removal of macrophages from human peripheral blood or animal splenic cell cultures leads to a marked loss in the recovery of PGE$_2$ from the macrophage-depleted cells, whereas the partially purified macrophage populations readily synthesize PGE_2 (Ferraris *et al.*, 1974; Goodwin *et al.*, 1977b; Grimm *et al.*, 1978; Kurland and Bockman, 1978; Bray *et al.*, 1981). Depletion experiments for eliminating the majority of macrophages from mixed cell cultures often involve adherence to rayon or nylon fiber or Sephadex G-10 columns or to glass or plastic dishes. One problem with these depletion experiments is that some macrophage subpopulations are only loosely adherent and the usual procedures fail to adequately deplete them. A variety of immunologic stimuli including *C. parvum* (Grimm *et al.*, 1978; Hsueh and Kuhn, 1979), Fc fragments of IgG (Passwell *et al.*, 1980), antigen–antibody complexes (Bonney *et al.*, 1979; Gartner *et al.*, 1981), and lymphokine preparations (Gordon *et al.*, 1976; Meltzer and Wahl, 1979) induce the synthesis and release of PGE_2 from murine splenic and peritoneal adherent cells and rabbit alveolar macrophages.

In contrast to data on macrophage, the ability of lymphocytes themselves to generate extracellular quantities of prostaglandins sufficient to modify immune responses is controversial. Synthesis of PGEs has been demonstrated to occur in human peripheral blood lymphocytes (Goodwin *et al.*, 1977a; Rapoport *et al.*, 1977), glass wool-adherent murine splenic lymphocytes (Webb and Nowowiejski, 1978), and murine thymocytes (Bauminger, 1978; Fitzpatrick *et al.*, 1979). A major problem with these studies is that data were not provided on the purity of the lymphocyte populations, and contamination by small numbers of macrophages could account for the observed prostaglandin production. In studies using highly purified human lymphocyte subpopulations containing $\leq 1\%$ monocytes, both T cells and B cells failed to synthesize detectable levels of PGE_2 (Kurland and Bockman, 1978; Yamamoto *et al.*, 1979; Kennedy *et al.*, 1980; Bray *et al.*, 1981). The relative inability of lymphocytes to generate prostaglandins, when compared to macrophages, may be related to low phospholipase A_2 activity in lymphocytes (Ferber *et al.*, 1980).

4.2. EFFECTS OF PROSTAGLANDINS ON IMMUNOLOGIC RESPONSES

Numerous studies have demonstrated that exogenous PGE_2 inhibits mitogen- and antigen-induced blastogenesis (Smith *et al.*, 1971; Stockman and Mumford, 1974; Goodwin *et al.*, 1977a,b, 1978; Novogrodsky *et al.*, 1979; Demenkoff *et al.*, 1980; Metzger *et al.*, 1980; Deimann *et al.*, 1981; Gemsa *et al.*, 1981). One troublesome aspect of some of these studies (Smith *et al.*, 1971; Strom *et al.*, 1973) is the high concentration required to suppress lymphocyte responses when added to cultures ($> 10^{-7}$ M), compared to the amount produced ($\simeq 10^{-8}$ M) by human leukocytes with optimal PHA stimulation (Ferraris *et al.*, 1974). Goodwin *et al.* (1977a) studied the effect of lower, more physiologic concentrations of prostaglandins on mitogenic stimulation of human T lymphocytes. They found reproducible inhibition with PGE_1 and PGE_2 at concentrations of 1 ng/ml (3×10^{-9} M) and 10 ng/ml (3×10^{-8} M). Moreover, the concentration range of PGE_2 (1–100 ng/ml) that Goodwin *et al.* (1977a) found inhibitory to mitogen-stimulated cultures is also the range of concentrations found in inflammatory fluids (Robinson and Levine, 1974). However, both quantitation of the amount of PGEs elaborated *in vitro* into the culture fluid by leukocytes and determination of the amount of PGEs present in inflammatory fluids may grossly underestimate those concentrations achievable at the lymphocyte surface. Studies by Goodwin *et al.* (1979a) showed specific reversible binding of PGE_1 and PGE_2 to human T cells with a K_D of $\simeq 2 \times 10^{-9}$ M and indicated a mean of 200 PGE binding sites per lymphocyte. Similar data have been generated for rat thymocytes (Schaumburg, 1973).

Stobo *et al.* (1979) demonstrated that the modulatory effect of PGE_2 depends on the T-lymphocyte subpopulation involved. Subpopulations of human T lymphocytes derived from peripheral blood by density gradient fractionation showed diametrically opposite responses to PGE_2 following PHA-induced blastogenesis: The blastogenic response was enhanced in lymphocytes from the low-density region of the gradient, whereas the response was inhibited in the higher density region. Since PGEs alter a response already initiated by some other primary stimulus, Goldyne and Stobo (1980) emphasized that the modulatory effect of PGE_2 on T-cell reactivity can vary and must, therefore, be defined in the context of the primary stimulus (Novogrodsky *et al.*, 1979), the specific reactivity under study (Yoneda and Mundy, 1979), and the population or subpopulation of T lymphocytes being tested (Stobo *et al.*, 1979).

Two other functional activities of T lymphocytes, cell-mediated cytotoxicity (Henney *et al.*, 1972; Lichtenstein *et al.*, 1972; Strom *et al.*, 1973, Plaut, 1979) and lymphokine secretion (Gordon *et al.*, 1976), are also inhibited by PGE_2. Henney *et al.* (1972) demonstrated that PGE ($\geq 10^{-8}$ M) inhibits the ability of sensitized T cells to kill their specific tumor targets. In contrast, recent studies by Chism and Stobo (unpublished observations) show that concentrations of PGE_2 in the range of 10^{-9} to 10^{-7} M do not significantly alter T-dependent cytotoxicity among primed, murine splenic T cells. Tracey and Adkinson (1980) reported that the tumor cytotoxicity of normal splenic NK cells and BCG-induced peritoneal NK cells is inhibited by PGE_2 at concentrations between 10^{-9} and 10^{-5} M. Gordon *et al.* (1976) demonstrated that PGE at 0.1 µg/ml inhibits the production of the lymphokine migration inhibition factor (MIF).

Several studies further suggest that endogenous production of PGE_2 by macrophages is involved in the normal regulation of the immune response. Depletion of macrophages from leukocyte cultures or use of prostaglandin synthetase inhibitors such as indomethacin or aspirin without removing macrophages alters the lymphocyte response in the direction expected by the removal of PGE_2 (Goodwin *et al.*, 1977a,b; Mattingly and Kemp, 1979; Novogrodsky *et al.*, 1979; Demenkoff *et al.*, 1980; Metzger *et al.*, 1980; Garrigues *et al.*, 1981). Similarly, the ability of prostaglandin synthetase inhibitors to potentiate lymphocyte mitogenesis *in vitro* has suggested that anergy in some patients with Hodgkin's disease (Goodwin *et al.*, 1977b), rheumatoid arthritis (Panayi and Corrigal, 1979), and sarcoidosis (Goodwin *et al.*, 1976b) is due to the overproduction of PGE_2 by monocytes/macrophages. Further studies are necessary to better define the roles of PGE_2 and other macrophage-derived arachidonate metabolites as physiologic and pathophysiologic modulators of lymphocyte function.

5. CONCLUDING REMARKS

It is now clear that mononuclear phagocytes synthesize significant amounts of various cyclooxygenase and lipoxygenase products of the arachidonic acid cascade depending on the environment from which the cells were obtained, the particular subpopulation(s) of cells under study, and the nature of the stimuli that the cells encounter in their pericellular environment. The data summarized in this review clearly implicate PGE_2 in the regulation of macrophage and lymphocyte function. Future investigations are warranted since other arachidonate metabolites released by macrophages may have important roles in the regulation of the immune system and may participate in reactions previously considered to be mediated solely by PGEs.

Several studies demonstrate that PGE_2 is involved in the autoregulation of macrophage function. Apparently prostaglandins do not initiate, but rather modulate responses in macrophages initiated by some other stimulus. Moreover, this prostaglandin-mediated modulation is variable depending on the stage of differentiation of the macrophage and its state of functional activation. In view of the pivotal role of the macrophage in the induction and maintenance of the immune response and its significant role as an effector cell in host defenses to infection and neoplasia, further definition of the conditions under which macrophages produce arachidonic acid oxygenation products and the respective role of these products in regulation of cell function is necessary to elucidate the physiologic and pathologic significance of these products.

ACKNOWLEDGMENT.   I thank Mrs. Mary Bolton and Mrs. Patsy Swisher for skillful assistance in manuscript preparation.

REFERENCES

Ahnfelt-Ronne, I., Binderup, L., Bramm, E., and Arrigoni-Martelli, E., 1980, Macrophages from adjuvant arthritic rats preferentially synthesize prostacyclin, *Agents Actions* **10**:85.

Baggiolini, M., Schnyder, J., Dewald, B., Bretz, U., and Payne, T. G., 1982, Phagocytosis-stimulated macrophages: Production of prostaglandins and SRS-A, and prostaglandin effects on macrophage activation, *Immunobiology* **161**:369.

Bauminger, S., 1978, Differences in prostaglandin formation between thymocyte subpopulations, *Prostaglandins* **16**:351.

Bockman, R. S., 1981, Prostaglandin production by human blood monocytes and mouse peritoneal macrophages: Synthesis dependent on *in vitro* culture conditions, *Prostaglandins* **21**:9.

Bonney, R. J., Wightman, P. D., Davies, P., Sadowski, S., Kuehl, F. A., Jr., and Humes, J. L., 1978, Regulation of prostaglandin synthesis and of selective release of lysosomal hydrolases by mouse peritoneal macrophages, *Biochem. J.* **176**:433.

Bonney, R. J., Naruns, P., Davies, P., and Humes, J. L., 1979, Antigen–antibody complexes stimulate the synthesis and release of prostaglandins by mouse peritoneal macrophages, *Prostaglandins* **18**:605.

Bonney, R. J., Burger, S., Davies, P., Kuehl, F. A., and Humes, J. L., 1980, Prostaglandin E_2 and prostacyclin elevate cyclic AMP levels in elicited populations of mouse peritoneal macrophages, in: *Advances in Prostaglandin and Thromboxane Research*, Volume 8 (B. Samuelsson, P. W. Ramwell, and R. Paoletti, eds.), pp. 1691–1693, Raven Press, New York.

Bonney, R. J., Beddini, J., Cameron, P., Davies, P., Gordon, J., Sadowski, S., and Humes, J. L., 1981a, Variations in prostaglandin E_2 and I_2 secretion by populations of macrophages that vary in their expression of Ia determinants, *Fed. Proc.* **40**:1161.

Bonney, R. J., Davies, P., and Humes, J. L., 1981b, Variations in the capacity for prostaglandin production by resident and elicited macrophages, in: *Mediation of Cellular Immunity in Cancer by Immune Modifiers* (M. A. Chirigos, ed.) pp. 43–48, Raven Press, New York.

Bonta, I. L., Parnham, M. J., Adolfs, M. J. P., and Van Vliet, L., 1977, Dual function of E-type prostaglandins in models of chronic inflammation, in: *Perspectives in Inflammation: Future Trends and Developments* (D. A. Willoughby, J. P. Giroud, and G. P. Velo, eds.), University Park Press, Baltimore.

Bonta, I. L., Adolfs, M. J. P., and Parnham, M. J., 1981, Prostaglandin E_2 elevation of cyclic-AMP in granuloma macrophages at various stages of inflammation: Relevance to anti-inflammatory and immunomodulatory functions, *Prostaglandins* **22**:95.

Bray, M. A., Gordon, D., and Morley, J., 1974, Role of prostaglandins in reactions in cellular immunity, *Br. J. Pharm.* **52**:453P.

Bray, M. A., Powell, R. G., and Lydyard, P. M., 1981, Prostaglandin generation by separated human blood mononuclear cell fractions, *Int. J. Immunopharmacol.* **3**:377.

Bretz, U., Dewald, B., Payne, T., and Schnyder, J., 1980, Phagocytosis stimulates the release of a slow reacting substance in cultured macrophages, *Br. J. Pharmacol.* **71**:631.

Brunda, M. J., and Holden, H. T., 1980, Prostaglandin-mediated inhibition of murine natural killer cell activity, in: *Natural Cell-Mediated Immunity against Tumors* (R. B. Herberman, ed.), pp. 721–734, Academic Press, New York.

Brune, K., 1980, HEPES-buffered media may induce prostaglandin release from macrophages in tissue culture, *Agents Actions* **10**:491.

Brune, K., Kalin, H., Schmidt, R., and Hecker, E., 1978a, Inflammatory, tumor initiating, and promoting activities of polycyclic aromatic hydrocarbons and diterpene esters in mouse skin as compared with their prostaglandin releasing potency *in vitro*, Cancer Lett. **4**:333.

Brune, K., Glatt, M., Kalin, H., and Peskar, H., 1978b, Pharmacological control of prostaglandin and thromboxane release from macrophages, *Nature (London)* **274**:261.

Cameron, D. J., and O'Brien, P., 1982, Relationship of the suppression of macrophage mediated tumor cytotoxicity in conjunction with secretion of prostaglandin from the macrophages of breast cancer patients, *Int. J. Immunopharmacol.* **4**:445.

Cantarow, W. D., Cheung, H. T., and Sundharades, G., 1978, Effects of prostaglandins on the spreading, adhesion, and migration of mouse peritoneal macrophages, *Prostaglandins* **16**:39.

Chang, J., Wigley, F., and Newcombe, D., 1980, Neutral protease activation of peritoneal macrophage prostaglandin synthesis. *Proc. Natl. Acad. Sci. USA* **77**:4736.

Chang, J., Liu, M. C., and Newcombe, D. S., 1982, Identification of two monohydroxyeicosatetraenoic acids synthesized by human pulmonary macrophages, *Am. Rev. Respir. Dis.* **126**:457.

Cook, J. A., Wise, W. C., and Halushka, P. V., 1981, Thromboxane A_2 and prostacyclin production by lipopolysaccharide-stimulated peritoneal macrophages, *J. Reticuloendothel. Soc.* **30**: 445.

Davies, P., Bonney, R. J., Humes, J. L., and Kuehl, F. A., 1980, The synthesis of arachidonic acid oxygenation products by various mononuclear phagocyte populations, in: *Mononuclear Phagocytes: Functional Aspects*, Part II (R. van Furth, ed.), pp. 1317–1345, Nijhoff, The Hague.

Debatin, K. M., Leser, H.-G., Northoff, H., and Gemsa, D., 1982, Depressed prostaglandin E (PGE) and interleukin-1 (IL-1) production from peritoneal exudate cells (PEC) of immunized rats following an i.p. antigen challenge, *Immunobiology* **159**:113.

Deimann, W., Seitz, M., and Gemsa, D., 1981, Release of prostaglandin E (PGE) from spleen macrophages and relationship to suppression of T lymphocyte stimulation during tumor growth in mice, *Immunobiology* **159**:102.

Demenkoff, J. H., Ansfield, M. J., Kaltreider, H. B., and Adam, E., 1980, Alveolar macrophage suppression of canine bronchoalveolar lymphocytes: The role of prostaglandin E_2 in the inhibition of mitogen responses, *J. Immunol.* **124**:1365.

Doig, M. V., and Ford-Hutchinson, A. W., 1980, The production and characterization of products of the lipoxygenase enzyme system released by rat peritoneal macrophages, *Prostaglandins* **20**:1007.

Droller, M. J., Lindgren, J. A., Claessen, H.-E., and Perlmann, P., 1979, Production of prostaglandin

E$_2$ by bladder tumor cells in tissue culture and a possible mechanism of lymphocyte inhibition, *Cell. Immunol.* **47**:261.

Ellner, J. J., and Spagnuolo, P. J., 1979, Suppression of antigen and mitogen-induced human T lymphocyte DNA synthesis by bacterial lipopolysaccharide: Mediation by monocyte activation and production of prostaglandins, *J. Immunol.* **123**:2689.

Farram, E., and Nelson, D. S., 1980, Mechanism of action of mouse macrophages as antitumor effector cells: Role of arginase, *Cell. Immunol.* **55**:283.

Ferber, E., Kroner, E., Schmidt, B., Fischer, H., Peskar, B. A., and Anders, C., 1980, Dynamics of membrane fatty acids during lymphocyte stimulation by mitogens, in: *Membrane Fluidity: Biophysical Techniques and Cellular Regulation* (M. Kates and A. Kuksis, eds.), pp. 239–263, Humana Press, Clifton, N.J.

Ferraris, V. A., DeRubertis, F. R., Hudson, T. H., and Wolfe, L., 1974, Release of prostaglandins by mitogen and antigen-stimulated leukocytes in culture, *J. Clin. Invest.* **54**:378.

Ferreira, S. H., 1979, Prostaglandins in: *Chemical Messengers in the Inflammatory Process* (J. C. Houck, ed.), pp. 113–151, Elsevier/North-Holland, Amsterdam.

Feuerstein, N., and Ramwell, P. W., 1981, OKY-1581, a potential selective thromboxane synthetase inhibitor, *Eur. J. Pharmacol.* **69**:533.

Feuerstein, N., Bash, J. A., Woody, J. N., and Ramwell, P. W., 1981, Leukotriene C stimulates prostaglandin release from rat peritoneal macrophages, *Biochem. Biophys. Res. Commun.* **100**:1085.

Fitzpatrick, F. A., Stringfellow, D. A., Maclouf, J., and Rigaud, M., 1979, Glass capillary gas chromatography with electron capture detection: Separation of prostaglandins, *J. Chromatogr.* **177**:51.

Flower, R. J., and Blackwell, G. J., 1976, The importance of phospholipase A$_2$ in prostaglandin biosynthesis, *Biochem. Pharmacol.* **25**:285.

Foster, S. J., 1980, Cyclic nucleotides, possible intracellular mediators of macrophage activation and secretory processes, *Agents Actions* **10**:556.

Friedman, S. A., Remold-O'Donnell, E., and Piessens, W. F., 1979, Enhanced PGE production by MAF-treated peritoneal exudate macrophages, *Cell. Immunol.* **42**:213.

Gallin, J. I., Sandler, J. A., Clyman, R. I., Manganiello, V. C., and Vaughan, M., 1978, Agents that increase cyclic AMP inhibit accumulation of cGMP and depress human monocyte locomotion, *J. Immunol.* **120**:492.

Garrigues, H. J., Romero, P., Hellstrom, I., and Hellstrom, K. E., 1981, Adherent cells (macrophages) in tumor-bearing mice suppress MLC responses, *Cell. Immunol.* **60**:109.

Gartner, S. M., Belisle, E. H., and Strausser, H. R., 1981, Peritoneal macrophages of lupus model mice (NZB/W and BSXB/MPJ) do not produce prostaglandins in response to immune complex stimulation, 1981, *Fed. Proc.* **40**(3/2):975.

Gemsa, D., Seitz, M., Kramer, W., Till, G., and Resch, K., 1978, The effects of phagocytosis, dextran sulfate, and cell damage on PGE$_1$ sensitivity and PGE$_1$ production by macrophages, *J. Immunol.* **120**:1187.

Gemsa, D., Seitz, M., Kramer, W., Grimm, W., Till, G., and Resch, K., 1979a, Ionophore A23187 raises cyclic AMP levels in macrophages by stimulating prostaglandin E formation, *Exp. Cell Res.* **118**:55.

Gemsa, D., Seitz, M., Menzel, J., Grimm, W., Kramer, W., and Till, G., 1979b, Phagocytosis-induced release of prostaglandins by macrophages, *Monogr. Allergy* **14**:194.

Gemsa, D., Kramer, W., Brenner, M., Till, G., and Resch, K., 1980, Induction of prostaglandin E release from macrophages by colchicine, *J. Immunol.* **124**:376.

Gemsa, D., Deimann, W., Leser, H. G., Seitz, M., and Resch, K., 1981, Suppression of T lymphocyte stimulation in tumor bearing mice: Participation of macrophages releasing prostaglandin E (PGE), *Fed. Proc.* **40**(3/2):1040.

Glatt, M., Kalin, H., Wagner, K., and Brune, K., 1977, Prostaglandin release from macrophages: An assay system for anti-inflammatory drugs in *in vitro*, *Agents Actions* **7**:321.

Goldyne, M. E., 1977, Prostaglandins and the modulation of immunological responses, *Int. J. Dermatol.* **16**:701.

Goldyne, M. E., and Stobo, J. D., 1979, Synthesis of prostaglandins E$_2$ and E$_1$ by subpopulations of human peripheral blood monocytes, *Prostaglandins* **18**:687.

Goldyne, M. E., and Stobo, J. D., 1980, Prostaglandin E_2 as a modulator of macrophage–T lymphocyte interactions, *J. Invest. Dermatol.* **74**:297.

Goldyne, M. E., and Stobo, J. D., 1981, Immunoregulatory role of prostaglandins and related lipids, *CRC Crit. Rev. Immunol.* **2**:189.

Goodwin, J. S., 1981, Prostaglandins and host defense in cancer, *Med. Clin. North Am.* **65**:829.

Goodwin, J. S., Bankhurst, A. D., and Messner, R. P., 1977a, Suppression of human T-cell mitogenesis by prostaglandins: Evidence of a prostaglandin producing suppressor cell, *J. Exp. Med.* **146**:1719.

Goodwin, J. S., Messner, R. P., Bankhurst, A. D., Peake, G. T., Saiki, J. H., and Williams, R. C., 1977b, Prostaglandin-producing suppressor cells in Hodgkins disease, *N. Engl. J. Med.* **297**:963.

Goodwin, J. S., Messner, R. P., and Peake, G. T., 1978, Prostaglandin suppression of mitogen-stimulated lymphocytes *in vitro*: Changes with mitogen dose and preincubation, *J. Clin. Invest.* **62**:753.

Goodwin, J. S., Wiik, A., Lewis, M., Bankhurst, A. D., and Williams, R. C., 1979a, High-affinity binding sites for prostaglandin E on human lymphocytes, *Cell. Immunol.* **43**:150.

Goodwin, J. S., DeHoratius, R., Israel, H., Peake, G. T., and Messner, R. P., 1979b, Suppressor cell function in sarcoidosis, *Ann. Intern. Med.* **90**:169.

Gordon, D., Bray, M. A., and Morley, J., 1976, Control of lymphokine secretion by prostaglandins, *Nature (London)* **262**:401.

Grimm, W., Seitz, M., Kircher, H., and Gemsa, D., 1978, Prostaglandin synthesis in spleen cell cultures of mice injected with *Corynebacterium parvum*, *Cell. Immunol.* **40**:419.

Gryglewski, R. J., Ranczenko, R., Korbut, R., Grodzinska, L., and Ocetkiewicz, A., 1975, Corticosteroids inhibit prostaglandin release from mesenteric blood vessels of rabbit and from perfused lungs of sensitized guinea pigs, *Prostaglandins* **10**:343.

Henney, C. S., Bourne, H. R., and Lichtenstein, L. M., 1972, The role of cyclic 3',5' adenosine monophosphate in the specific cytolytic activity of lymphocytes, *J. Immunol.* **108**:1526.

Higgs, G. A., Vane, J. R., Hart, F. D., and Wojtulewski, J. A., 1974, Effects of antiinflammatory drugs on prostaglandins in rheumatoid arthritis, in: *Prostaglandin Synthetase Inhibitors* (H. J. Robinson and J. R. Vane, eds.), pp. 165–173, Raven Press, New York.

Hsueh, W., and Kuhn, C. S., 1979, Prostaglandin secretion in rabbit alveolar macrophages and its relationship to phagocytosis, *Chest* **75**(Suppl.):249.

Hsueh, W., Kuhn, C., and Needleman, P., 1979, Relationship of prostaglandin secretion by rabbit alveolar macrophages to phagocytosis and lysosomal enzyme release, *Biochem. J.* **184**:345.

Hsueh, W., Desai, U., Gonzalez-Crussi, F., Lamb, R., and Chu, A., 1981a, Two phospholipase pools for prostaglandin synthesis in macrophages, *Nature (London)* **290**:710.

Hsueh, W., Desai, U., and Gonzalez-Crussi, F., 1981b, Evidence for the existence of two phospholipase (PLASE) sites for prostaglandin synthesis in rabbit alveolar macrophages (RAM), *Fed. Proc.* **40**:797.

Humes, J. L., Bonney, R. J., Pelus, L., Dahlgren, M. E., Sadowski, S., Kuehl, F. A., and Davies, P., 1977, Macrophages synthesize and release prostaglandins in response to inflammatory stimuli, *Nature (London)* **269**:149.

Humes, J. L., Davies, P., Bonney, R. J., and Kuehl, F. A., Jr., 1978, Phorbol myristate acetate stimulates the release of arachidonic acid and its cyclooxygenase products by macrophages, *Fed. Proc.* **27**:1318.

Humes, J. L., Burger, S., Galavage, M., Kuehl, F. A., Wightman, P. D., Dahlgren, M. E., Davies, P., and Bonney, R. J., 1980, The diminished production of arachidonic acid oxygenation products by elicited mouse peritoneal macrophages: Possible mechanisms, *J. Immunol.* **124**:2110.

Humes, J. L., Sadowski, S., Galavage, M., Goldenberg, M., Subers, E., Bonney, R. J., and Kuehl, F. A., 1982, Evidence for two sources of arachidonic acid for oxidative metabolism by mouse peritoneal macrophages, *J. Biol. Chem.* **257**:1591.

Keller, R., 1979, Suppression of natural antitumor defense mechanisms by phorbol esters, *Nature (London)* **282**:729.

Keller, R., Keist, R., Adolf, W., Opferkuch, H. J., Schmidt, R., and Hecker, E., 1982, Tumor-promoting diterpene esters prevent macrophage activation and suppress macrophage tumoricidal capacity, *Exp. Cell Biol.* **50**:121.

Kennedy, D. A., Sullivan, T. J., Sylvester, P., and Parker, C. W., 1979, Diacylglycerol metabolism in mast cells: A potential role in membrane fusion and arachidonic acid release, *J. Exp. Med.* **150**:1039.

Kennedy, M. S., and Stobo, J. D., 1980, Modulation of macrophage cyclic AMP by self-synthesized prostaglandins, *Clin. Res.* **28**:351a.

Kennedy, M. S., and Stobo, J. D., 1981, Prostaglandin E_2 and thromboxane A_2: Dual feedback regulators of macrophages, *Clin. Res.* **29**:171a.

Kennedy, M. S., Stobo, J. D., and Goldyne, M. E., 1980, *In vitro* synthesis of prostaglandins and related lipids by populations of human peripheral blood mononuclear cells, *Prostaglandins* **20**:135.

Koopman, W. J., Gillis, M. H., and David, J. R., 1973, Prevention of MIF activity by agents known to increase cellular cyclic AMP, *J. Immunol.* **110**:1609.

Kunkel, S. L., Plewa, M., Kaercher, K., and Armstrong, G., 1982, Synthesis and potential immuno-modulating activity of various cyclooxygenase compounds produced by macrophages, *Fed. Proc.* **41**:485.

Kurland, J. I., and Bockman, R. S., 1978, Prostaglandin E production by human blood monocytes and mouse peritoneal macrophages, *J. Exp. Med.* **147**:952.

Kurland, J., and Moore, M. A. S., 1977, Modulation of hemopoiesis by prostaglandins, *Exp. Hematol.* **5**:357.

Kurland, J., Bockman, R. S., Broxmeyer, H. E., and Moore, M. A. S., 1978a, Limitation of excessive myelopoiesis by the intrinsic modulation of macrophage-derived prostaglandin E, *Science* **199**:552.

Kurland, J., Broxmeyer, H. E., Pelus, L. M., Bockman, R. S., and Moore, M. A. S., 1978b, Role for monocyte-macrophage derived colony stimulating factor and prostaglandin E in the positive and negative feedback control of myeloid stem cell proliferation, *Blood* **52**:388.

Kurland, J. I., Pelus, L. M., Ralph, P., Bockman, R. S., and Moore, M. A. S., 1979, Induction of prostaglandin E synthesis in normal and neoplastic macrophages: Role for colony-stimulating factor(s) distinct from effects on myeloid progenitor cell proliferation, *Proc. Natl. Acad. Sci. USA* **76**:2326.

Lichtenstein, L. M., Gillespie, E., Bourne, H. R., and Henney, C. S., 1972, The effects of a series of prostaglandins on *in vitro* models of the allergic response and cellular immunity, *Prostaglandins* **2**:519.

Lim, L. M., Hunt, N. H., Evans, T., and Weidemann, M. J., 1981, Rapid changes in the activities of the enzymes of cyclic AMP metabolism after addition of A23187 to macrophages, *Biochem. Biophys. Res. Commun.* **103**:745.

McCarthy, K., Harper, T., Murphy, R. C., Musson, R. A., and Henson, P. M., 1981, A possible mechanism for the regulation of macrophage acid hydrolase production and secretion, *J. Cell Biol.* **91**:400a.

McCarthy, M. E., and Zwilling, B. S., 1981, Differential effects of prostaglandins on the antitumor activity of normal and BCG-activated macrophages, *Cell. Immunol.* **60**:91.

McMillan, R. M., Hasselbacher, P., Hahn, J. L., and Harris, E. D., Jr., 1981, Interactions of murine macrophages with monosodium urate crystals: Stimulation of lysosomal enzyme release and prostaglandin synthesis, *Rheumatology* **8**:555.

Mason, R. J., Stossel, T. P., and Vaughan, M., 1972, Lipids of alveolar macrophages, Poly-morphonuclear leukocytes, and their phagocytic vesicles, *J. Clin. Invest.* **51**:2399.

Mattingly, J. A., and Kemp, J. D., 1979, Suppression of secondary plaque-forming cell responses by rat splenic adherent cells: Evidence for dependence on prostaglandin production, *Cell. Immunol.* **48**:195.

Melmon, K. L., Bourne, H. R., Weinstein, Y., Shearer, G. M., Kram, J., and Bauminger, S., 1974, Hemolytic plaque formation by leukocytes *in vitro*, *J. Clin. Invest.* **53**:13.

Meltzer, M. S., and Wahl, L. M., 1979, Synergistic interaction of lymphokines and bacterial lipopolysaccharides for macrophage tumor cytotoxicity and secretion of prostaglandin E_2, *Fed. Proc.* **38**:933.

Metzger, Z., Hoffeld, J. T., and Oppenheim, J. J., 1980, Macrophage-mediated suppression. 1.

Evidence for participation of both hydrogen peroxide and prostaglandins in suppression of murine lymphocyte proliferation, *J. Immunol.* **124**:983.

Metzger, Z., Hoffeld, J. T., and Oppenheim, J. J., 1981, Regulation by PGE$_2$ of the production of oxygen intermediates by LPS-activated macrophages, *J. Immunol.* **127**:1109.

Moore, R. N., Unbaschek, R., Wahl, L. M., and Mergenhagen, S. E., 1979, Prostaglandin regulation of colony-stimulating factor production by lipopolysaccharide-stimulated murine leukocytes, *Infect. Immun.* **26**:408.

Moore, R. N., Vogel, S. N., Wahl, L. M., and Mergenhagen, S. E., 1980, Factors influencing lipopolysaccharide-induced interferon production, in: *Microbiology 1980* (D. Schlessinger, ed.), pp. 131–134, American Society for Microbiology, Washington, D.C.

Morley, J., Bray, M. A., Jones, R. W., Nugteren, D. H., and van Dorp, D. A., 1979, Prostaglandin and thromboxane production by human and guinea-pig macrophages and leucocytes, *Prostaglandins* **17**:729.

Mullink, H., and Von Blomberg, M., 1980, Influence of anti-inflammatory drugs on the interaction of lymphocytes and macrophages, *Agents Actions* **10**:512.

Murota, S.-I, Kawamura, M., and Morita, I., 1978, Transformation of arachidonic acid into thromboxane B$_2$ by the homogenates of activated macrophages, *Biochim. Biophys. Acta* **528**:507.

Muscoplat, C. C., Klausner, D. J., Brunner, C. J., Sloane, E. D., and Johnson, D. W., 1979, Regulation of mitogen- and antigen-stimulated lymphocyte blastogenesis by prostaglandins, *Fed. Proc.* **38**:933.

Myatt, L., Bray, M. A., Gordon, D. A., and Morley, J., 1975, Macrophages on intrauterine contraceptive devices produce prostaglandins, *Nature (London)* **257**:227.

Novogrodsky, A., Rubin, A. L., and Stenzel, K. H., 1979, Selective suppression by adherent cells, prostaglandin, and cyclic AMP analogues of blastogenesis induced by different mitogens, *J. Immunol.* **122**:1.

Oehler, J. R., Herberman, R. B., and Holden, H. T., 1978, Modulation of immunity by macrophages, *Pharmacol. Ther.* **2**:551.

Oropeza-Rendon, R. L., Speth, V., and Fischer, H., 1980, Action of prostaglandin E$_1$ and F$_{2\alpha}$ on the pinocytic activity of horseradish peroxidase in bone-marrow derived macrophages, *Eur. J. Cell Biol.* **22**:761.

Panayi, G. S., and Corrigal, V., 1979, Lymphocyte studies in rheumatoid. IV. Evidence for a prostaglandin producing suppressor cell, *Agents Actions Suppl.* **4**:213.

Passwell, J. H., Dayer, J.-M., and Merler, E., 1979, Increased prostaglandin production by human monocytes after membrane receptor activation, *J. Immunol.* **123**:115.

Passwell, J. H., Dayer, J.-M., Gass, K., and Edelson, P. J., 1980, Regulation by F$_c$ fragments of the secretion of collagenase, PGE$_2$, and lysozyme by mouse peritoneal macrophages, *J. Immunol.* **125**:910.

Pelus, L. M., and Bockman, R. S., 1979, Increased prostaglandin synthesis by macrophages from tumor-bearing mice, *J. Immunol.* **123**:2118.

Pelus, L. M., Broxmeyer, H. C., Kurland, J. E., and Moore, M. A. S., 1979, Regulation of macrophage and granulocyte proliferation, *J. Exp. Med.* **150**:277.

Pelus, L. M., Saletan, S., Silver, R. T., and Moore, M. A. S., 1982, Expression of Ia antigens on normal and chronic myeloid leukemic human granulocyte-macrophage colony-forming cells (CFU-GM) is associated with the regulation of cell proliferation by prostaglandin E, *Blood* **59**:284.

Picker, L. J., Raff, H. V., Goldyne, M. E., and Stobo, J. D., 1980, Metabolic heterogeneity among human monocytes and its modulation by PGE$_2$, *J. Immunol.* **124**:2557.

Plant, M., 1979, The role of cyclic AMP in modulating cytotoxic T lymphocytes, *J. Immunol.* **123**:692.

Prosser, F. H., Nichols, S. V., and Nochols, W. K., 1979, Enhancement and suppression of macrophage responses to bacterial factors by prostaglandin E$_1$, *Fed. Proc.* **38**:962.

Rabinovitch, H., Durand, J., Rigaud, M., Mendy, F., and Breton, J.-C., 1981, Transformation of arachidonic acid into monohydroxy-eicosatetraenoic acids by mouse peritoneal macrophages, *Lipids* **16**:518.

Rapoport, B., Pillarisetty, R. J., Herman, E. A., and Congco, E. G., 1977, Evidence for prostaglandin production by human lymphocytes during culture with human thyroid cells in monolayer: A possible role for prostaglandins in the pathogenesis of Grave's disease, *Biochem. Biophys. Res. Commun.* **77**:1245.

Razin, E., Razin, M., and Lohmann-Matthes, M. L., 1980, The role of prostaglandins in the development of macrophages from bone marrow cells, *J. Reticuloendothel. Soc.* **27**:377.

Razin, E., Rivnay, B., and Globerson, A., 1981, Prostaglandins as modulators of macrophage development from bone marrow, *J. Reticuloendothel. Soc.* **30**:239.

Remold-O'Oonnell, E., 1974, Stimulation and desensitization of macrophage adenylate cyclase by prostaglandins and catecholamines, *J. Biol. Chem.* **249**:3615.

Rigaud, M., Durane, J., and Breton, J. C., 1979, Transformation of arachidonic acid into 12-hydroxy-5,8,10,14-eicosatetraenoic acid by mouse peritoneal macrophages, *Biochim. Biophys. Acta* **573**:408.

Robinson, D. R., and Levine, L. 1974, Prostaglandin concentrations in synovial fluid in rheumatic diseases: Action of indomethacin and aspirin, in: *Prostaglandin Synthetase Inhibitors* (H. J. Robinson and J. R. Vane, eds.), pp. 223–228, Raven Press, New York.

Rosenstein, M. M., and Strausser, H. R., 1980, Macrophage-induced T cell mitogen suppression with age, *J. Reticuloendothel. Soc.* **27**:159.

Roubin, R., Mencia-Huerta, J.-M., and Benveniste, J., 1982, Release of platelet-activating factor (PAF-acether) and leukotrienes C and D from inflammatory macrophages, *Eur. J. Immunol.* **12**:141.

Rouzer, C. A., Scott, W. A., Kempe, J., and Cohn, Z. A., 1980a, Prostaglandin synthesis by macrophages requires a specific receptor–ligand interaction, *Proc. Natl. Acad. Sci. USA* **77**:4279.

Rouzer, C. A., Scott, W. A., Cohn, Z. A., Blackburn, P., and Manning, J. M., 1980b, Mouse peritoneal macrophages release leukotriene C in response to a phagocytic stimulus, *Proc. Natl. Acad. Sci. USA* **77**:4928.

Rouzer, C. A., Scott, W. A., Griffith, O. W., Hamill, A. L., and Cohn, Z. A., 1981, Depletion of glutathione selectively inhibits synthesis of leukotriene C by macrophages, *Proc. Natl. Acad. Sci. USA* **78**:2532.

Rouzer, C. A., Scott, W. A., Hamill, A. L., and Cohn, Z. A., 1982a, Synthesis of leukotriene C and other arachidonic acid metabolites by mouse pulmonary macrophages, *J. Exp. Med.* **155**:720.

Rouzer, C. A., Scott, W. A., Hamill, A. L., Liu, F.-T., Katz, D. H., and Cohn, Z. A., 1982b, IgE immune complexes stimulate arachidonic acid release by mouse peritoneal macrophages, *Proc. Natl. Acad. Sci. USA* **79**:5656.

Russell, S. W., and Pace, J. L., 1982, T-cell hybridoma production of lymphokine activity that interferes with PGE$_2$-mediated negative regulation of macrophage activation, *J. Reticuloendothel. Soc.* **32**:71.

Schaumburg, B. P., 1973, Binding of prostaglandin E$_1$ to rat thymocytes, *Biochim. Biophys. Acta* **326**:127.

Schmidt-Gayk, H. E., Jacobs, K. H., and Hackenthal, E., 1975, Cyclic AMP and phagocytosis in alveolar macrophages: Influence of hormones and dibutyryl cyclic AMP, *J. Reticuloendothel. Soc.* **17**:251.

Schnyder, J., Dewald, B., and Baggiolini, M., 1981, Effects of cyclooxygenase inhibitors and prostaglandin E$_2$ on macrophage activation *in vitro*, *Prostaglandins* **22**:411.

Schultz, R. M., 1980a, Macrophage activation by interferons, in: *Lymphokine Reports*, Volume 1 (E. Pick, ed.), pp. 63–97, Academic Press, New York.

Schultz, R. M., 1980b, E-type prostaglandins and interferons: Yin-yang modulation of macrophage tumoricidal activity, *Med. Hypotheses* **6**:831.

Schultz, R. M., and Jackson, W. T., 1981, Effects of inhibitors and products of arachidonic acid metabolism on macrophage-mediated cytotoxicity induced by interferon and lipopolysaccharide, in: *Mediation of Cellular Immunity in Cancer by Immune Modifiers* (M. A. Chirigos, ed.), pp. 89–99, Raven Press, New York.

Schultz, R. M., Pavlidis, N. A., Stylos, W. A., and Chirigos, M. A., 1978, Regulation of macrophage tumoricidal function: A role for prostaglandin of E series, *Science* **202**:320.

Schultz, R. M., Stoychkov, J. N., Pavlidis, N., Chirigos, M. A., and Olkowski, Z. L., 1979a, Role of E-type prostaglandins in the regulation of interferon-treated macrophage cytotoxic activity, *J. Reticuloendothel. Soc.* **26**:93.

Schultz, R. M., Pavlidis, N. A., Stoychkov, J. N., and Chirigos, M. A., 1979b, Prevention of macrophage tumoricidal activity by agents known to increase cellular cyclic AMP, *Cell. Immunol.* **42**:71.

Schultz, R. M., Chirigos, M. A., and Olkowski, Z. L., 1980, Stimulation and inhibition of neoplastic cell growth by tumor promoter-treated macrophages, *Cell. Immunol.* **54**:98.

Scott, W. A., Zrike, J. M., Hamill, A. L., Kempe, J., and Cohn, Z. A., 1980, Regulation of arachidonic acid metabolites in macrophages, *J. Exp. Med.* **152**:324.

Scott, W. A., Pawlowski, N. A., Murray, H. W., Andreach, M., Zrike, J., and Cohn, Z. A., 1982, Regulation of arachidonic acid metabolism by macrophage activation, *J. Exp. Med.* **155**:1148.

Scott, W. A., Rouzer, C. A., and Cohn, Z. A., 1983, Leukotriene C release by macrophages, *Fed. Proc.* **42**:129.

Shaw, J. O., Russell, S. W., Printz, M. P., and Skidgel, R. A., 1979, Macrophage-mediated tumor cell killing: Lack of dependence on the cyclooxygenase pathway of prostaglandin synthesis, *J. Immunol.* **123**:50.

Smith, J. W., Steiner, A. L., and Parker, C. W., 1971, Human lymphocyte metabolism: Effects of cyclic and noncyclic nucleotides on stimulation by phytohemagglutinin, *J. Clin. Invest.* **50**:442.

Snyder, D. S., Beller, D. I., and Unanue, E. R., 1982, Prostaglandins modulate macrophage Ia expression, *Nature (London)* **299**:163.

Spagnuolo, P. J., Ellner, J. J., Hassid, A., and Dunn, M. J., 1980, A role for thromboxanes in the surface activation of human monocytes, *Clin. Res.* **28**:509a.

Steeg, P. S., Johnson, H. M., and Oppenheim, J. J., 1982, Regulation of murine macrophage Ia antigen expression by an immune interferon-like lymphokine: Inhibitory effect of endotoxin, *J. Immunol.* **129**:2402.

Stobo, J. D., Kennedy, M. S., and Goldyne, M. E., 1979, Prostaglandin E modulation of the mitogenic response of human T cells: Differential response of T cell subpopulations, *J. Clin. Invest.* **64**:1188.

Stockman, G. D., and Mumford, D. M., 1974, The effect of prostaglandins on the *in vitro* blastogenic response of human peripheral blood lymphocytes, *Exp. Hematol.* **2**:65.

Stossel, T. P., Mason, R. J., and Smith, A. L., 1974, Lipid peroxidation by human bood phagocytes, *J. Clin. Invest.* **54**:628.

Stringfellow, D. A., 1978, Prostaglandin restoration of the interferon response of hyporeactive animals, *Science* **201**:376.

Stringfellow, D. A., Fitzpatrick, F. A., Sun, F. F., and McGuire, J. C., 1978, Prostacyclin biosynthesis in activated, stimulated, and normal mouse peritoneal cell populations, *Prostaglandins* **16**:901.

Strom, T. B., Carpenter, C. B., Garovoy, M. R., Austen, K. F., Merrill, J. P., and Kaliner, M., 1973, The modulating influence of cyclic nucleotides upon lymphocyte-mediated cytotoxicity, *J. Exp. Med.* **138**:381.

Sturge, R. A., Yates, D. B., Gordon, D., Franco, M., Paul, W., Bray, M. A., and Morley, J., 1978, Prostaglandin production in arthritis, *Ann. Rheum. Dis.* **37**:315.

Sykes, J. A., and Maddox, I. S., 1972, Prostaglandin production by experimental tumors and effects of anti-inflammatory compounds, *Nature New Biol.* **237**:59.

Taffet, S. M., and Russell, S. W., 1981, Macrophage-mediated tumor cell killing: Regulation of expression of cytolytic activity by prostaglandin E, *J. Immunol.* **126**:424.

Taffet, S. M., Pace, J. L., and Russell, S. W., 1981, Lymphokine maintains macrophage activation for tumor cell killing by interfering with the negative regulatory effect of prostaglandin E, *J. Immunol.* **127**:121.

Tracey, D. E., and Adkinson, N. F., 1980, Prostaglandin synthesis inhibitors potentiate the BCG-induced augmentation of natural killer cell activity, *J. Immunol.* **125**:136.

Tracey, D. E., Davis, J. W., and Taggart, M. T., 1982, Independent secretion of prostaglandins and interferons by stimulated macrophages, *Int. J. Immunopharmacol.* **4**:348.

Unanue, E. R., 1978, The regulation of lymphocyte functions by the macrophage, *Immunol. Rev.* **40**:227.

Unanue, E. R., 1981, The regulatory role of macrophages in antigenic stimulation. Part two: Symbiotic relationship between lymphocyte and macrophages, *Adv. Immunol.* **31**:1.

Valone, F. H., Franklin, M., and Goetzl, E. J., 1979, Generation of a human polymorphonuclear leukocyte chemotactic factor by the lipoxygenase pathway of alveolar macrophages, *Clin. Res.* **27**:476A.

Vassalli, J., Hamilton, J., and Reich, E., 1976, Macrophage plasminogen activator: Modulation of enzyme production by anti-inflammatory steroids, mitotic inhibitors, and cyclic nucleotides, *Cell* **8**:271.

Verma, D. S., Spitzer, G., Zander, A. R., McCredie, K. B., and Dicke, K. A., 1981, Prostaglandin E_1-mediated augmentation of human granulocyte-macrophage progenitor cell growth *in vitro*, Leuk. Res. **5**:65.

Wahl, L. M., Olsen, C. E., Sandberg, A. L., and Mergenhagen, S. E., 1977, Prostaglandin regulation of macrophage collagenase production, *Proc. Natl. Acad. Sci. USA* **74**:4955.

Webb, D. R., and Nowowiejski, I., 1978, Mitogen-induced changes in lymphocyte prostaglandin levels: A signal for the induction of suppressor cell activity, *Cell. Immunol.* **41**:72.

Weidemann, M. J., Peskar, B. A., Wrogemann, K., Rietschel, E. T., Staudinger, H., and Fischer, H., 1978, Prostaglandin and thromboxane synthesis in a pure macrophage population and the inhibition, by E-type prostaglandins, of chemiluminescence, *FEBS Letts.* **89**:136.

Wightman, P. D., Humes, J. L., Davies, P., and Bonney, R. J., 1980, Characterization of two phospholipase A_2 (PLA_2) activities in resident mouse peritoneal macrophages, *Fed. Proc.* **39**:1897.

Yamamoto, M., Taki, N. A., Rapoport, B., and Hinds, W. E., 1979, Modulation by thymus-derived (T) cells of thyroid cell-stimulated prostaglandin E release by human peripheral blood mononuclear cells, *Proc. Natl. Acad. Sci. USA* **76**:6627.

Yaron, M., Yaron, I., Gurari-Rotman, D., Revel, M., Lindner, H. R., and Zor, U., 1977, Stimulation of prostaglandin E production in cultured human fibroblasts by poly I·poly C and human interferon, *Nature (London)* **267**:457.

Yoneda, T., and Mundy, G. R., 1979, Prostaglandins are necessary for osteoclast activating factor production by activated peripheral blood leukocytes, *J. Exp. Med.* **149**:279.

Zurier, R. B., Dukor, P., and Weissman, G., 1971, Effect of cyclic AMP and colchicine on hydrolase release from phagocytes, *Clin. Res.* **19**:453.

8

Immunopharmacologic Regulation of the Mononuclear Phagocyte System

THOMAS E. SCHINDLER, JOHN R. SADLIK,
and JOHN W. HADDEN

1. INTRODUCTION

The mononuclear phagocyte system (MPS) is centrally important in both specific and nonspecific immune responses. Once regarded primarily as scavenger cells with remarkable phagocytic capacity, macrophages are now recognized as effector cells that function in the induction, amplification, expression, and regulation of humoral and cellular immunity. Through numerous, diverse secretory products, mononuclear phagocytes contribute to inflammatory reactions and delayed-type hypersensitivity, participate in tissue repair and wound healing, and regulate proliferation and differentiation of various tissues. Cells of this system are responsible for processing antigen and presenting immunogen to lymphocytes. Activated macrophages are capable of intracellular destruction of microbial pathogens and extracellular lysis of tumor cells. Thus, mononuclear phagocytes are considered vital to host defenses against a wide variety of pathogens and contribute to immunosurveillance against neoplasia.

As the wide variety of macrophage functions are being elucidated, immunologists are becoming more interested in developing immunotherapeutic approaches aimed at manipulating the MPS. A growing list of natural agents and synthetic compounds have recently been under investigation as potential therapies against microbial infections and cancer and as new approaches to the treatment of autoimmune diseases and immunodeficiencies. Many of the most

THOMAS E. SCHINDLER • Xytronyx, Inc., Chicago, Illinois 60616.   JOHN R. SADLIK • Department of Hematology–Oncology, Ohio State University, Columbus, Ohio 43210. JOHN W. HADDEN • Departments of Microbiology, Immunology, and Internal Medicine, University of South Florida College of Medicine, Tampa, Florida 33260.

155

promising immunostimulants appear to exert their antimicrobial or antitumor effects by inducing or enhancing one or more of the functions of activated macrophages. In this review we will discuss how some of the chemically defined immunostimulants interact with the MPS to promote host defense mechanisms against disease.

2. DIVERSITY OF THE MPS

The MPS is comprised of three basic, developmental stages: bone marrow stem cells, monoblasts, and promonocytes; bone marrow monocytes and peripheral blood monocytes; and macrophages residing in diverse tissues, organs, and cavities (van Furth *et al.*, 1975). Tissue macrophages populate the lungs, lymph nodes, bone marrow and bone tissue, serous cavities, liver, nervous system, spleen, and connective tissue. Recruitment, proliferation, and differentiation of mononuclear phagocytes are regulated by colony-stimulating factors (CSF) and differentiation factors, some of which are produced by macrophages (Stanley, 1979; Sachs, 1978). In addition to the distinct maturational stages and adaptive differences acquired at various tissue sites, macrophages may exhibit different degrees of activation, depending on the level of stimulation induced by inflammation or immune activation.

Mononuclear phagocytes are capable of expressing a wide diversity of functions (Table 1). They participate in inflammatory reactions through their secretory products and receptors, which interact with the complement and clotting systems, platelets, sinovial fibroblasts, connective tissue, and the vasculature. In the aftermath of acute reactions they are involved in wound healing and tissue repair. They are important effector cells in host defenses against intracellular bacteria, viruses, certain fungi, and protozoans. Recent cancer research has focused on the role of macrophages in immunosurveillance and immune rejection of neoplasia (Adams and Snyderman, 1979). Mononuclear phagocytes can act as effector cells that spontaneously lyse tumor cells. They appear to regulate NK cells. Mononuclear phagocytes can operate in the induction of immune reactions by trapping, processing, and presenting antigen to T and B cells. Lymphocyte proliferation and effector functions are amplified by monokines and modulated by suppressor factors, prostaglandins, and other inhibitory products secreted by macrophages. The far-ranging, functional versatility of the MPS indicates that therapeutic manipulation of this system may favorably alter the clinical course of many different diseases and disorders.

The basic properties of mononuclear phagocytes that enable them to perform so many roles are: chemotaxis, phagocytosis, antigen presentation, secretion of various mediators, and acquisition of microbicidal and antitumor effector functions. The capacity for directional mobility in response to chemotactic stimuli is important for rapid infiltration of inflammatory sites. Phagocytosis is necessary for microbicidal activity, degradation and processing of antigen, bone resorption, and disposal of senescent cells. A subpopulation of macrophages expresses membrane Ia antigens that regulate the proliferation, helper function,

TABLE 1. FUNCTIONAL DIVERSITY OF THE MPS

Inflammatory responses
  Fever
  Immediate-type hypersensitivity
  Clotting
  Platelet activation
Cell-mediated immunity
  Delayed-type hypersensitivity
  Contact dermatitis
  Granuloma formation
Regulation
  Induction and modulation of T- and B-cell responses
  Regulation of NK cells
  Monocytopoiesis and granulopoiesis
Tissue growth and repair
  Wound healing
  Fibroblast proliferation
  Bone resorption
  Disposal of senescent cells
  Tissue remodeling
Effector cell function
  Intracellular destruction of pathogens
  Extracellular inhibition and lysis of neoplastic and virus-infected cells

and suppressor activity of T cells (Benacerraf, 1981). Macrophages are important secretory cells and may release four classes of mediators (Unanue, 1981; Nathan *et al.*, 1980):

1. Enzymes that affect extracellular proteins and connective tissue, including neutral proteases (plasminogen activator, collagenase, and elastase) and acid hydrolases (proteinases, ribonucleases, phosphatases, glucosidases, and sulfatases);
2. Products involved in host defense mechanisms—complement components, interferon, lysozyme, and endogenous pyrogen;
3. Regulatory factors that modulate proliferation and activity of other cells, such as lymphocyte activation factor (LAF or IL-1), CSF, fibroblast growth factor, and inhibitor of DNA synthesis;
4. Low-molecular-weight compounds that mediate macrophage effector functions (hydrogen peroxide and reactive metabolites of oxygen) and regulatory or inflammatory effects (prostaglandins, leukotrienes, thymidine, and cyclic nucleotides).

Modulation of the secretory activities of mononuclear phagocytes may have profound effects on many different homeostatic, inflammatory, and immunologic processes.

3. MACROPHAGE ACTIVATION

Mononuclear phagocytes capable of inhibiting or killing either intracellular pathogens or neoplastic cells are called "activated macrophages." Early studies of the role of macrophages in host resistance demonstrated that infection by intracellular pathogens leads to the development of activated macrophages accumulated at the site of infection. The microbicidal capacity of activated macrophages is nonspecific, transient, and regulated by T lymphocytes (Mackaness, 1964, 1969; Blanden and Langman, 1972). Infection with various intracellular pathogens results in nonspecific resistance against challenge with unrelated bacteria, protozoans, fungi, and viruses (Hibbs *et al.*, 1980; Hadden and England, 1979). This acquired, nonspecific immunity requires the continued presence of the sensitizing antigens and responsive lymphocytes which promote the microbicidal activity of macrophages. In response to microbial components and inflammatory stimuli, mononuclear phagocytes infiltrate the site of infection where they are functionally modified by sensitized lymphocytes (North, 1970). The local population of activated macrophages is replenished by responsive mononuclear phagocytes that infiltrate the inflammatory site from the peripheral circulation (Ando *et al.*, 1972). Continued expression of microbicidal activity persists as long as the inducing antigens are present to stimulate immune lymphocytes which provide activation stimuli (Ando and Dannenberg, 1972). The emergence of microbicidal activity and delayed hypersensitivity is preceded by the proliferation of newly arrived mononuclear phagocytes (North, 1969, 1970; Shima *et al.*, 1972; Dannenberg *et al.*, 1972). Products of sensitized T lymphocytes are implicated in the induction of macrophage proliferation (Hadden *et al.*, 1975a; Sadlik *et al.*, 1983).

In vitro studies have indicated that lymphocytes secrete lymphokines that promote the development of cellular immunity. Culture supernatants of antigen- or mitogen-stimulated lymphocytes contain distinct factors that are capable of inducing chemotactic movement, proliferation, and activation of mononuclear phagocytes (Hadden *et al.*, 1981). Nonspecific, acquired immunity is thought to develop *in vivo* by the combined effects of lymphokines that mobilize [chemotactic factor (CF)], trap [migration inhibitory factor (MIF)], expand (CSF), and activate [macrophage-activating factor (MAF) and immune interferon (IFN)] the population of macrophages at the site of infection.

Reactive products of inflammation also contribute to nonspecific resistance. CSF, kinins and their split products, fibrinogen, complement components, haptoglobulin, C-reactive protein, α_2-macroglobulin, and "phlogokines" modulate inflammatory macrophages and enhance activation (Fauve *et al.*, 1981; Giroud *et al.*, 1981; Fauve, this volume). In addition to providing specific antigenic stimulation of lymphocytes, components of microbial cell walls have been shown to induce the proliferation of mononuclear phagocytes and to directly stimulate microbicidal activity (see Section 4.1). The stimuli provided by environmental microorganisms or immunoadjuvants may be sufficient to mobilize macrophages, in the absence of T-cell mediators, and establish nonspecific resistance (Meltzer, 1976; Nickol and Bonventri, 1977; Stinnett and Majeski, 1980).

A number of studies have shown that chronic infection with intracellular pathogens may also enhance host resistance to tumors (Hibbs *et al.*, 1980). The development of activated macrophages capable of the intracellular stasis or lysis of microbial pathogens coincides with enhanced macrophage capacity to inhibit the growth and survival of tumor cells. The requirements for induction of tu-moricidal macrophages appear to be very similar to the process of activation of microbicidal capacity: (1) persistence of microbial antigens and stimulating components, such as endotoxin; (2) induction and maintenance of activation by lymphokines and inflammatory mediators; and (3) infiltration of new, responsive mononuclear phagocytes into the tumor site.

The process of activation, by which a monocyte develops into a cytotoxic or microbicidal effector cell, requires a series of stimuli that promote successively higher levels of activity (Cohn, 1978; Adams *et al.*, 1982; Meltzer *et al.*, 1982a). Discrete activation levels, ranging from relative inactivity to heightened cytotoxic activity, are represented by: (1) "resident" macrophages or fresh peripheral blood monocytes; (2) macrophages "elicited" by nonspecific, nonimmunogenic stimuli (e.g., casein, thioglycollate, mineral oil); and (3) macrophages "activated" by lymphokines. Macrophages elicited by sterile inflammation can be distinguished from resident, peritoneal macrophages by altered morphology, enhanced phagocytosis, heightened secretory activity, and stimulated metabolism (Cohn, 1978). Elicited macrophages are not sufficiently activated, however, to kill intracellular pathogens or tumor cells. Microbicidal and tumoricidal capacities are acquired by macrophages activated *in vivo* by infection or vaccination (e.g., *Listeria* or BCG) or *in vitro* by antigen- or mitogen-induced lymphokines. Multiple influences, such as endotoxin and lymphokine (Meltzer, 1981) or endotoxin and IFN (Kleinschmidt and Schultz, 1982), can interact synergistically to achieve the activated state. Whether the activation process represents differentiation stages of one population of cells or involves specialization of separate subpopulations is not clear. Many of the synthetic agents that stimulate the MPS induce inflammatory or fully activated macrophages, probably by mimicking or modulating the natural activation signals or by altering the cellular responses to these signals.

4. IMMUNOPHARMACOLOGIC MANIPULATION OF THE MPS

An important objective in the development of immunotherapy is to selectively modify those properties of mononuclear phagocytes that are critical to host defense mechanisms. The evaluation of agents that modulate the MPS is dependent on qualitative and quantitative assessment of macrophage activities. *In vitro* studies permit the identification of the cellular targets of direct drug action, facilitate the exploration of dose–response relationships for specific cellular functions, and elucidate the biochemical aspects of drug action. The significance of such studies is indicated by *in vivo* studies that confirm direct drug effects and reveal their indirect impact on the complex inflammatory and immune networks that undergird host defenses. The development of effective therapies depend on understanding how the modified macrophage property—effector function, regulatory influence, or secretory product—contributes to defense mechanisms, and whether or not immunopharmacologic modulation can predictably improve host recovery and survival. In addition to their potential value as new therapies, immunopharmacologic agents are useful for probing the roles of mononuclear phagocytes in hemopoiesis, inflammation, and immuno-regulation.

4.1. NATURAL IMMUNOSTIMULANTS

4.1.1. Components of Mycobacteria

As discussed above, intracellular pathogens are potent stimulators of mono-nuclear phagocytes and lymphocytes. The effectiveness of Freund's complete adjuvant is dependent on the immunostimulating capacity of mycobacteria. Two classes of chemically defined components of mycobacterial cell walls (Table 2), which exhibit adjuvant activity, are the synthetic peptidoglycan derivatives, such as muramyl dipeptide (MDP, for N-acetylmuramyl-L-alanyl-D-isogluta-mine.), and trehalose esters, such as cord factor (Lederer, 1980; Lemaire *et al.*, this volume). In addition to enhancement of humoral immunity to T-dependent and T-independent antigens, MDP induces delayed-type hypersensitivity, elic-its nonspecific resistance to bacterial infections, and increases phagocytic clear-ance. Trehalose dimycolates also stimulate resistance against microbial infec-

TABLE 2. CHEMICALLY DEFINED IMMUNOSTIMULANTS OF THE MPS

Category	Examples
Natural agents	
Microbial components	
Peptidoglycans	Muramyl dipeptide
Glycolipids	Trehalose dimycolates
Polysaccharides	Glucan
Antibiotics	Bestatin
Endogenous mediators	
Peptides	Tuftsin
Proteins	IFN, CSF
Synthetic agents	
IFN inducers	
Polyanions	Pyran copolymer, MVE-2
Polynucleotides	Poly(rI:rC)
Fluorenones	Tilorone
Pyrimidines	6-Aryl pyrimidinoles
Immunoadjuvants	
Cyanaziridine	Azimexone
Lipoidal amines	CP-46,665-1
Phospholipids	Alkyl-lysophospholipids
Immunopotentiators	
Phenylimidothiazole	Levamisole
Nucleoside derivatives	Isoprinosine, NPT 15392

tions. Some of the *in vivo* effects of peptidoglycans, such as antibacterial resistance and delayed hypersensitivity, can be dissociated by chemical modification. Adjuvant therapies employing MDP encapsulated in liposomes, MDP linked to mycolic acids, or MDP combined with trehalose dimycolates have achieved regression of established tumors (Uemiya *et al.*, 1979; McLaughlin *et al.*, 1980; Yarkoni *et al.*, 1981; Fidler *et al.*, 1982).

Numerous *in vitro* studies have been carried out to elucidate the effects of MDP on macrophages. Direct effects of MDP on mononuclear phagocytes include: enhancement of spreading and adherence, inhibition of macrophage migration (Yamamoto *et al.*, 1978), augmentation of superoxide anion generation (Pabst and Johnston, 1980), heightened secretory activity (Wahl *et al.*, 1979), and stimulation of microbicidal (Hadden *et al.*, 1979) and tumoricidal capacity (Juy and Chedid, 1975).

Many of the immunostimulatory effects of MDP appear to be mediated by macrophage secretory products. Secretion of IL-1 and CSF presumably contribute to adjuvant effects by expanding populations of lymphocytes and mononuclear phagocytes, which interact in the development of humoral and cellular immunity. Secretion of CSF (Staber *et al.*, 1978) and IL-1 (Oppenheim *et al.*, 1980) can be detected in macrophage cultures shortly after the addition of MDP. Supernatants of peritoneal exudate macrophages, elicited by sterile inflammation and cultured for 10 hr with MDP, stimulate macrophage proliferation (Schindler *et al.*, 1982). MDP induces secretion of IL-1 within 1 hr of contact with elicited macrophages (Tenu *et al.* 1980). Tumoricidal activity is also enhanced in cultures soon after stimulation with MDP (Adams and Dean, 1982; Sone and Fidler, 1980; Tenu *et al.*, 1980). In these studies MDP provides the additional stimulus needed to fully activate cytotoxic effectors which have been primed *in vivo* by adjuvant or conditioned *in vitro* by lymphokines. Adams has proposed that the first signal, such as MAF, augments the binding of tumor cells by macrophages; MAF-primed macrophages then respond to the second signal, such as MDP or LPS, which triggers the release of cytolytic serine protease (Adams and Dean, 1982).

The mechanism of action of MDP on macrophage secretory functions— although not clearly delineated—may be mediated by cGMP. Elevated levels of cGMP can be detected within minutes of stimulating peritoneal exudate cells with MDP (Hadden *et al.*, 1978). cGMP or inducers of cGMP stimulate secretion of IL-1 by peritoneal macrophages (Diamatstein and Ulmer, 1976; Oppenheim *et al.*, 1979). That cGMP may be involved in relaying MDP stimulation of macrophage secretion is suggested by other studies implicating cGMP in the mechanism of enzyme release by neutrophils (Zurier *et al.*, 1974; Ignarro and Cech, 1976), mast cells (Kaliner *et al.*, 1972), and NK cells (Katz *et al.*, 1982).

4.1.2. Glucan

Polysaccharides isolated from fungal cell walls markedly stimulate the MPS. Glucan, a β(1–3)polyglucose isolated from yeast cell walls (zymosan), induces proliferation of peritoneal exudate cells and peripheral leukocytes and produces hypertrophy of the spleen, liver, and lungs (Riggi and DiLuzio, 1961; Burgaleta and Golde, 1977). Hyperplasia of the macrophage populations in these tissues is accompanied by increased phagocytic clearance (Wooles and DiLuzio, 1964; DiLuzio and Morrow, 1971), enhanced humoral and cellular immunity (Wooles and DiLuzio, 1963, 1964), and nonspecific resistance to viral, fungal, bacterial and parasitic infections (Williams and DiLuzio, 1980; Williams *et al.*, 1978; Kokoshis *et al.*, 1978; Cook *et al.*, 1980). Glucan has been shown to be effective as an antitumor adjuvant in animal models of allogeneic and syngeneic tumors (DiLuzio *et al.*, 1976). Clinical trials have indicated that intralesional treatment often achieves regression of tumor nodules. Dense infiltration of the glucan-treated lesions by macrophages that have engulfed glucan appears to mediate antitumor effects (Mansell *et al.*, 1978). Glucan treatment elicits macrophages that exhibit tumoristatic and tumoricidal capacity *in vitro* (Schultz *et al.*, 1978a). The effective activation of macrophages by glucan treatment of nude mice, indicates that T-cell lymphokines are not required for the induction of tumoricidal macrophages (Schultz *et al.*, 1978a; Cook *et al.*, 1978). Other β(1–3)glucans, such as scleroglucan and lentinan, are not as potent as glucan for macrophage activation, and require competent T lymphocytes for expression of antitumor effects (Maeda and Chihara, 1973). Although glucan may be a more potent macrophage stimulator than other polysaccharides, its antitumor activity is considerably weaker than other immunoadjuvants, such as *C. parvum* (Bomford and Moreno, 1981; Fisher and Gebhardt, 1978).

One or more of the secretory products of glucan-stimulated macrophages may be involved in the expression of tumoricidal and microbicidal activities. Serum lysozyme levels increase concomitantly with enhanced phagocytic clearance and hypertrophy of the major reticuloendothelial organs in glucan-treated rats (DiLuzio, 1979). DiLuzio suggests that glucan stimulates macrophage secretion of lysozyme, which makes tumor cells more suspectible to binding and lysis. Since glucans activate the alternative pathway of complement, C3a and C3b may contribute to antitumor effects (Glovsky *et al.*, 1976; Hamuro *et al.*, 1978). C3b stimulates macrophage secretory functions and activates tumoricidal capacity (Schorlemmer *et al.*, 1977; Ferluga *et al.*, 1978). Activated macrophages not only produce C3, but are able to cleave C3, releasing C3a, which is lytic for transformed cells (Ferluga *et al.*, 1976, 1978). Macrophage stimulation via activation of the complement system represents another T-independent route of induction of nonspecific resistance to infection and neoplasia. Glucan may generate other acute-phase reactants *in vivo*, such as the kinins and CSF, which can enhance macrophage cytolytic and microbicidal activity (Fauve *et al.*, 1981; Giroud *et al.*, 1981; Handman and Burgess, 1979).

Glucan administration stimulates monocytopoiesis and granulopoiesis. Production of CSF by macrophages of glucan-treated animals results in increased numbers of macrophages in the peritoneum, spleen, bone marrow, and periphery (Burgaleta and Golde, 1977; Patchen and Lotzova, 1980). Although stimulation of hemopoiesis may be dissociated from glucan's antitumor effects (Suit *et al.*, 1978), the former activity of glucan might be useful for reconstituting bone marrow and peripheral leukocytes following cytoreductive therapy (Patchen and Lotzova, 1980). The capacity of glucan to depress NK activity and prevent rejection of parental bone marrow grafts by F_1 recipients, also indicates therapeutic applications in clinical bone marrow transplantation (Lotzova and Gutterman, 1979).

4.1.3. Bestatin

Another immunostimulant derived from microorganisms is bestatin [(2S,3R)3-amino-2-hydroxyl-4-phenylbutanoyl)-L-leucine], a specific inhibitor of aminopeptidases, isolated from *Streptomyces olivoreticuli* (Umezawa *et al.*, 1976). Bestatin is bound by aminopeptidases on the surfaces of macrophages and to a lesser extent by lymphocytes (Muller *et al.*, 1982). Enhancement of B- and T-lymphocyte proliferation is mediated by bestatin-stimulated macrophages (Umezawa, 1981). *In vivo* treatment of young adult mice induces tumoristatic macrophages (Florentin *et al.*, 1981). Macrophages may also contribute to *in vivo* enhancement of humoral immune responses (Florentin *et al.*, 1981). Long-term administration of bestatin to aged mice restores humoral responses and augments tumoristatic activity of macrophages (Bruley-Rosset *et al.*, 1979). Preferential binding to macrophages and subsequent stimulation may explain the decreased incidence of spontaneous tumors in aged mice in this study.

4.1.4. Endogenous Mediators

4.1.4a. Tuftsin. Endogenous mediators represent another category of immunostimulators important to our understanding of how the MPS participates in nonspecific resistance and immunoregulation. Tuftsin, an endogenous tetrapeptide (L-Thr-L-Lys-L-Pro-L-Arg), is released *in vivo* upon cleavage of IgG (Najjar and Nishioka, 1970). It binds to polymorphonuclear leukocytes (PMNs) and macrophages, stimulating phagocytic activity, leukotaxis, bactericidal capacity, cytotoxic effector function, and immunogenic presentation (Nishioka *et al.*, 1981; Tzehoval *et al.*, 1979). *In vivo* antitumor activity cannot be attributed solely to the direct activation of macrophage tumoricidal capacity, since NK, T-cell, and antibody-dependent cytotoxic activities are also enhanced by tuftsin (Florentin *et al.*, 1978, 1981; Phillips *et al.*, 1981). Immunoregulatory influences on T, B, and NK cells may be mediated by tuftsin-stimulated accessory macrophages. The secretory and effector functions of macrophages and leukocytes which specifically bind tuftsin, may be modulated by activation of oxidative metabolism and increased levels of intracellular cGMP (Spirer *et al.*, 1975; Stabinsky *et al.*, 1980). Investigation of the mechanism of action of tuftsin has elucidated the process by which Fc-receptor-bound immunoglobulin (Fc-Ig) stimulates phagocytosis. It is thought that two enzymes, one of which is located on the leukocyte cell surface, cleave Fc-Ig, releasing the tetrapeptide and thus triggering phagocytosis (Najjar and Nishioka, 1970; Tzehoval *et al.*, 1979). Receptor-bound tuftsin also potentiates the immunogenic function of antigen-presenting cells, which regulate antigen-induced T-cell proliferation, specific antibody production and memory (Tzehoval *et al.*, 1978, 1979). The adjuvant activity of tuftsin may result from an amplification of the naturally occurring process of immunization.

4.1.4b. IFN. Nonspecific resistance to microbial infections and neoplasia can be induced by the actions of IFN on the MPS and also mediated by macrophage production of IFN. Viruses, double-stranded RNA, polysaccharides, bacteria, endotoxin, polyanions and other synthetic IFN-inducers stimulate macrophages to produce IFN (DeClercq and Merigan, 1970; Schultz *et al.*, 1977; Havell and Spitalny, 1980). IFN and IFN inducers stimulate macrophage spreading, phagocytosis, and tumoricidal capacity (Rabinovitch *et al.*, 1977; Schultz *et al.*, 1977, 1978b; Hamburg *et al.*, 1980). These findings have led to the view that IFN inducers activate macrophages indirectly by stimulating macrophage production of IFN, which in turn activates cytolytic macrophages. Evidence for this mechanism of macrophage activation comes from studies indicating that:

1. Anti-IFN antiserum abrogates the *in vitro* activation of macrophage cytotoxicity by endotoxin, pyran copolymer, and poly(rI:rC) (Schultz and Chirigos, 1979)
2. Anti-IFN also nullifies the *in vivo* antitumor effects of poly(rI:rC) or statolon, although the protective effects of BCG or pyran are not affected (Gresser *et al.*, 1978)
3. Enhancement of macrophage phagocytic activity, associated with the induction of IFN by virus, is also inhibited by anti-IFN antibody (Rabinovitch and Manejias, 1978)

Schultz and colleagues have extended these studies in their investigation of the active component in lymphokine preparations that induces macrophage tumoricidal capacity (Schultz *et al.*, 1978c). Antiviral and macrophage-activating moieties in lymphokine preparations share similar physicochemical properties, and they are both neutralized by anti-IFN-γ antibody (Kleinschmidt and Schultz, 1982). Other investigators have demonstrated that IFN can be separated from another distinct component in lymphokine preparations, which induces macrophage tumoricidal activity (Meltzer *et al.*, 1982b; Kniep *et al.*, 1981). These results indicate that IFN-γ, produced by lymphocytes in response to antigenic or mitogenic stimulation, is one mechanism of lymphokine-mediated macrophage activation.

IFN may be an important mediator of macrophage regulatory effects on humoral and cellular immunity. IFN suppresses antibody responses to T-dependent and T-independent antigens, decreases antigen- and mitogen-induced proliferation, and inhibits delayed-type hypersensitivity (Stiehm *et al.*, 1982). Thus, some of the immunosuppressive effects of IFN inducers may be mediated by macrophage-produced IFN. Enhancement and maintenance of NK activity by macrophage-produced IFN may be a normal control mechanism for natural resistance to neoplasia and viral infection. This is suggested by the ability of agents toxic for macrophages, such as silica and carrageenan, to block both spontaneous NK activity and its boosting by either poly(rI:rC) (Djeu *et al.*, 1979) or BCG (Tracey, 1979). Host response to viral infection involves the development of marrow-dependent NK cells, which are regulated by macrophages (Chapes *et al.*, 1981). Monocytes also participate in natural immunity against viruses as IFN producers and effectors of spontaneous lysis of virus-infected target cells (Chapes and Tompkins, 1979; Stanwick *et al.*, 1982).

4.1.4c. CSF. The CSFs represent a family of glycoproteins whose main function was thought to be the regulation of growth and differentiation of bone marrow progenitor cells, resulting in the production of mature macrophages and granulocytes (Metcalf and Moore, 1971). It is becoming increasingly evident, however, that CSFs are also potent regulators of mature macrophage effector functions. The growth-promoting activity of CSFs is not only limited to the bone marrow compartment, as CSF will also induce the proliferation of mature macrophages found in the periphery and at sites of inflammation (Hadden *et al.*, 1978). In addition to expanding populations of effector cells of the MPS, CSFs modulate macrophage function by inducing the release of secretory products associated with activation. CSFs are also capable of directly activating macrophages to become microbicidal (Handman and Burgess, 1979) and tumoristatic (Wing *et al.*, 1982).

At present at least two distinct types of CSFs acting on the macrophage have been identified (Stanley, 1979). They differ with respect to physical properties, target cell specificity, receptor affinity, and biologic and immunologic activity. One type of CSF induces bone marrow cells to form colonies of granulocytes and macrophages (Burgess *et al.*, 1977). This type of CSF, obtained from a number of sources including T lymphocytes, macrophages, and various tissues, has been traditionally called GM-CSF. Two subtypes of GM-CSF have been identified. Purified GM-CSF is capable of directly activating macrophages to kill ingested trypanosomes (Handman and Burgess, 1979). Many of the immunostimulants discussed herein stimulate macrophages to produce GM-CSF, which may contribute to some of the biologic effects observed.

Type 1 CSF (CSF-1)—also referred to as macrophage growth factor (MGF) (Stanley *et al.*, 1976) or the lymphokine MMF (Hadden *et al.*, 1975a; Sadlik *et al.*, 1983)—is functionally, structurally, and antigenically distinct from GM-CSF (Stanley, 1979). Bone marrow cells, when cultured with pure CSF-1, produce colonies composed of macrophages. CSF-1 was first isolated from mouse fibroblasts (Stanley and Heard, 1977), and has recently been purified from human urine (Das *et al.*, 1981; Motoyoshi *et al.*, 1982) and the supernatants of antigen-stimulated lymphocytes (Sadlik *et al.*, 1983). It has also been found in human serum and the supernatants of human T-cell hybridomas (Le *et al.*, 1983).

Although CSF-1 is capable of acting on bone marrow cells, its principal activity may be the regulation of mature macrophage function. Receptors specific for CSF-1 have been found on all cells of the MPS including blood monocytes and tissue macrophages (Byrnes *et al.*, 1981). CSF-1 is capable of inducing marked proliferation of mature alveolar and peritoneal macrophages (Hadden *et al.*, 1978; Sadlik *et al.*, 1983). CSF-1 is also capable of inducing macrophages to release GM-CSF (Motoyoshi *et al.*, 1982), thereby indirectly promoting the production of granulocytes and macrophages from the bone marrow.

CSF-1 may influence macrophage activation by triggering the release of a number of macrophage secretory products, including prostaglandins (Kurland *et al.*, 1978), thromboxane B_2, and plasminogen activator (Hamilton *et al.*, 1980). CSF-1 is required for lymphokine-induced production of IL-1 (Moore *et al.*, 1980). CSF-1 is also capable of acting as an IFN inducer (Moore *et al.*, 1981). CSF-1 activates tumoristatic macrophages by a mechanism distinct from MAF.

The tumoristatic activity may be due to a secretory product, since macrophages cultured in the presence of CSF-1 elaborate a factor cytotoxic for transformed fibroblasts (Sadlik, unpublished observation).

The CSFs constitute a class of MPS stimulators capable of promoting growth and differentiation in the bone marrow and the periphery, resulting in the expansion (or restoration) of effector populations. The CSFs also act as endogenous regulators that modulate macrophage and lymphocyte effector functions and influence the production of mediators of inflammation.

4.2. SYNTHETIC IMMUNOSTIMULANTS

4.2.1. IFN Inducers

Synthetic polyanions, such as polycarboxylates, polysulfates, and polyribonucleotides, are IFN inducers and immunostimulants capable of enhancing host resistance to pathogens and cancer. Two of the polyanionic IFN inducers, pyran (a random copolymer of maleic anhydride and divinyl ether) and poly(rI:rC), have been studied extensively. The synthetic polyanions are similar in their structural properties and biologic activities to endotoxin, a naturally occurring polyanionic lipopolysaccharide (LPS) (DeClercq and Merigan, 1970). LPS and pyran are relatively poor IFN inducers compared to poly(rI:rC) and viral IFN inducers (Morahan, 1981). Macrophages play an important role in determining antiviral, immunomodulatory, and antitumor activities of polyanionic immunostimulators.

4.2.1a. Pyran. Pyran is a powerful stimulator of the MPS. Hepatosplenomegaly, enhanced phagocytic clearance, and elevated numbers of esterase-positive spleen cells result from intravenous administration of pyran (Baird and Kaplan, 1978). Intraperitoneal injection of pyran stimulates an influx of macrophages, capable of inhibiting the replication of intracelluar viruses or bacteria and of suppressing the proliferation of lymphocytes and tumor cells (Morahan and Kaplan, 1976, 1978; Schultz *et al.*, 1976; Baird and Kaplan, 1978). Pyran-activated macrophages also suppress spleen cell NK activity (Santoni *et al.*, 1980). The antiviral and antitumor effects of pyran, both *in vivo* and *in vitro*, appear to be mediated by activated macrophages (Morahan and Kaplan, 1976; Schultz *et al.*, 1978c; Breinig and Morahan, 1980).

Different structural requirements and alternate mechanisms of action contribute to the antiviral or antitumor effects of pyran. *In vivo* antiviral activity, but not antitumor or MPS-stimulating effects, correlates with molecular weight of the pyran preparation. High-molecular-weight fractions (> 21,300) exhibit better antiviral activity, but are also more toxic, than low-molecular-weight fractions (< 15,500). The low-molecular-weight fraction, MVE-2, retains the antitumor and macrophage-activating properties of high-molecular-weight fractions (Munson *et al.*, 1981; Morahan *et al.*, 1978; Dean *et al.*, 1981; Chirigos and Stylos, 1980) and appears to be less toxic in human cancer patients (Hersh *et al.*, 1981; Powell *et al.*, 1981).

Several possible mechanisms of action for the immunomodulatory effects of pyran have been considered. Inhibition of mitogen-induced lymphoproliferation and spontaneous NK activity may be due to increased production of prostaglandins by activated macrophages (Goodwin *et al.*, 1977; Brunda *et al.*, 1980). Enhancement of NK activity, detected relatively early after administration of pyran, has been attributed to IFN induction (Herberman *et al.*, 1981). The role of IFN in macrophage activation has also been implicated in pyran's antitumor activity (Schultz and Chirigos, 1979). Anti-IFN antibody nullifies pyran activation of macrophages *in vitro*, but fails to affect antitumor activity *in vivo* (Gresser *et al.*, 1978). The antiviral effects of pyran do not correlate with IFN protection, since some pyran preparations, which do not induce detectable IFN, provide antiviral protection (Morahan, 1981).

4.2.1b. Poly(rI:rC). Stimulation of the MPS by poly(rI:rC) is indicated by increased phagocytic clearance and the activated morphology of peritoneal macrophages of treated mice (Finter, 1973; Rabinovitch *et al.*, 1977). In addition to adjuvant effects on humoral and cellular immunity (Turner *et al.*, 1970; Chirigos *et al.*, 1981), poly(rI:rC) enhances NK activity and activates macrophage tumoricidal capacity (Alexander and Evans, 1971; Oehler *et al.*, 1978). Antitumor effects of poly(rI:rC) correlate with macrophage activation and IFN production. A number of studies indicate that macrophage-produced IFN mediates both the NK-enhancing and the macrophage-activating effects of poly(rI:rC) (Schultz *et al.*, 1978c; Schultz and Chirigos, 1979; Gidlund *et al.*, 1978; Herberman *et al.*, 1981; Chirigos *et al.*, 1981). Other studies, however, fail to show a correlation between IFN production and antitumor or antiviral activities of poly(rI:rC) (Rhim and Huebner, 1971; Weinstein *et al.*, 1971; DeClercq, 1977; Stebbing *et al.*, 1980). Other mechanisms of action, in addition to IFN production, must be involved in enhancement of nonspecific resistance by poly(rI:rC).

Activation of the complement or coagulation system generates cleavage components that may influence macrophage activation. Complement components have also been shown to have direct, tumoricidal activity (Ferluga *et al.*, 1976, 1978). Similarly, mobilization of macrophages into sites of infection or tumor may be enhanced by monocyte CF, arising from the interaction of polyanions with the complement system (Majeski and Stinnett, 1977).

Polyanions may also directly activate macrophages by interacting with nuclear DNA. Pyran complexes with divalent cations, forming microspheres that presumably enter mononuclear phagocytes by endocytosis and bind to intracellular receptors (Fiel *et al.*, 1976). Binding is dependent on polyanionic structure, as pyran, dextran sulfate, and poly(rI:rC) all compete for receptor binding (Papamatheakis *et al.*, 1978). A direct, nuclear effect of polyanions is indicated by the ability of pyran and poly(rI:rC) to derepress nuclear DNA templates possibly by reversing histone-induced inhibition (Mohr *et al.*, 1972, 1978). The capacity for derepression of nuclear templates is related to molecular weight. This may be relevant to those antiviral activities of polyanions that also depend on molecular weight.

4.2.1c. Tilorone. Tilorone hydrochloride, 2,7-bis[2-(diethylamino)ethoxy]-fluoren-9-one, is an IFN inducer with broad-spectrum antiviral activity (Mayer and Krueger, 1970; Krueger and Mayer, 1970). Tilorone induces relatively high levels of IFN in mice, comparable to poly(rI:rC), but it is less active in other species (Stringfellow, 1980). IFN induction contributes to the antiviral effects of tilorone, but stimulation of the MPS and possibly more direct antiviral effects contribute to protection against pathogens. Tilorone distributes primarily in the liver and spleen, concentrated intracellularly in the nucleus (Regelson, 1981). It enhances phagocytic clearance and hepatic uptake of radiolabeled SRBC (Munson *et al.*, 1972). Stimulation of the MPS may account for antitumor effects and increased resistance to some bacteria (Regelson, 1981). IFN production by stimulated macrophages appears to mediate enhancement of NK activity and contribute to antitumor effects (Gresser *et al.*, 1978; Herberman *et al.*, 1981). Direct activation of macrophages, possibly mediated by macrophage-produced IFN, is suggested by the capacity of tilorone to induce IFN in nude mice and to stimulate macrophages of splenectomized mice (Gibson *et al.*, 1976; Rabinovitch *et al.*, 1977). Like the synthetic polyanions, tilorone interacts with DNA. Intercalation with DNA, inhibition of viral DNA polymerases, and inhibition of protein synthesis may relate to the mechanisms of IFN induction and cause direct antiviral effects; but these actions may also lead to toxicity. Clinical development of tilorone has been restricted by its toxicity in animals and humans, which include cytoplasmic inclusions, corneal lesions, retinopathy, and lymphopenia (Regelson, 1981).

   4.2.1d. Pyriminidoles.   The development of IFN inducers for clinical use has been hampered by their toxicity and hyporeactivity to IFN induction that result from repeated administration. Recent studies with 6-aryl pyriminidoles indicate antiviral and immunomodulatory activity associated with relatively little toxicity (Stringfellow, 1980, 1981). Two of these compounds, 2-amino-5-bromo-6-phenyl-4-pyrimidinol (ABPP)   and   2-amino-5-iodo-6-phenyl-4-pyrimidinol (AIPP), activate cytotoxic macrophages and enhance NK activity. ABPP is a potent IFN inducer. AIPP is a poor IFN inducer, however, which suggests an alternative mechanism of action on macrophages and NK cells. The hyporeactive state can be circumvented by less frequent administration of IFN inducers. Administration of pyriminidoles along with prostaglandins has been shown to restore IFN production in hyporeactive animals (Stringfellow, 1978).

4.2.2. Immunoadjuvants

   Azimexone, a 2-cyanosubstituted aziridine, is a new immunostimulator that modulates T-cell and macrophage functions. Oral or intravenous administration of azimexone enhances cellular and humoral immune responses and induces tumoristatic, peritoneal macrophages (Bicker, 1978; Florentin *et al.*, 1981). The relative antitumor activity, evaluated as an immunotherapy for transplanted tumor or as an adjunct with tumor vaccine, is comparable to the microbial adjuvants BCG and *C. parvum* (Bicker, 1978; Chirigos and Stylos, 1980). Enhanced NK and/or T-cell cytotoxicity also may contribute to the antitumor effects of azimexone in young mice, but only tumoristatic macrophages are induced in chronically treated, aged mice (Florentin *et al.*, 1981). *In vitro* activation of tumoricidal macrophages suggests that azimexone may stimulate macrophages directly, independent of IFN induction (Schultz and Chirigos, 1980). An alternate mechanism of macrophage activation, however, has not yet been determined.

Other synthetic immunoadjuvants capable of directly activating macrophages have been developed recently. The lipoidal amine, CP-46,665-1 (4-aminomethyl-1[2,3-(di-*n*-decyloxy)-*n*-propyl]-4-phenylpiperidine dihydrochloride), and the alkyl-lysophospholipids elicit peritoneal exudate macrophages and accumulate in tissue macrophages (Munder *et al.*, 1979; Berdel *et al.*, 1980; Wolff *et al.*, 1982). CP-46,665-1 does not induce IFN, but does exhibit antitumor effects in mice, which are attributed to activated macrophages (Wolff *et al.*, 1982). The alkyl-lysophospholipids have also demonstrated some effectiveness as antitumor agents in animal models, which may be due in part to induction of tumoristatic macrophages (Munder *et al.*, 1979, 1981).

4.2.3. Immunopotentiators

4.2.3a. Levamisole. Levamisole is a phenylimidothiazole antihelminthic that modifies responses of T cells and mononuclear phagocytes both *in vivo* and *in vitro*. Although levamisole does not directly activate microbicidal or tumoricidal effector cells (Schultz *et al.*, 1976; Kelly, 1978; Hadden *et al.*, 1979), it is capable of potentiating macrophage functions important to nonspecific resistance. Levamisole enhances phagocytosis, chemotaxis, and bactericidal capacity (Hoebecke and Franchi, 1973; Snyderman *et al.*, 1978; Hadden *et al.*, 1979). Augmentation of lymphokine-induced chemotaxis (Snyderman *et al.*, 1978) and enhancement of lymphokine-activated bactericidal capacity (Hadden *et al.*, 1979) illustrate levamisole's action as a macrophage potentiator. Potentiation of macrophage functions is contrasted with the direct, activating effects of immunoadjuvants such as pyran or MDP.

Levamisole appears to be effective in restoring to normal the macrophage functions of the immunodepressed or immature host. Extended treatment with levamisole enhances T-cell responses that have declined in aged mice and stimulates tumoristatic macrophages. These responses may be related to the decline in spontaneous tumors observed in aging mice that received long-term administration of levamisole (Bruley-Rosset *et al.*, 1978, 1981). Levamisole may accelerate maturation of phagocytes in newborn animals resulting in increased nonspecific resistance to bacterial and viral infections (Fisher *et al.*, 1974, 1978). Monocyte chemotaxis, depressed during influenza, can be restored by levamisole (Snyderman *et al.*, 1978). Similarly, levamisole treatment following surgery or radiation therapy has improved monocyte chemotaxis (Smith *et al.*, 1978). Levamisole has shown limited efficacy as an adjuvant to conventional cancer treatments (Chirigos, 1978; Amery, 1978) and as an alternative therapy for certain recurrent and chronic infections (Symeons *et al.*, 1979). Reconstitution of T-cell and/or monocyte functions is thought to contribute to therapeutic benefits.

Possible mechanisms of action to account for levamisole's enhancement of macrophage responses emphasize the imidazole- or sulfur-containing rings of levamisole. The imidazole moiety is implicated in mediating levamisole's stimulatory effect by altering intracellular levels of cyclic nucleotides. Levamisole and imidazole potentiate phagocytic activity of murine peritoneal macrophages (Lima *et al.*, 1974). These agents increase levels of cGMP and decrease cAMP in lymphocytes (Hadden *et al.*, 1975b). Others report that elevated cGMP may enhance monocyte chemotaxis (Sandler *et al.*, 1975a,b). Another possible mechanism of levamisole's action on macrophages implicates its sulfur-containing ring which is cleaved into the thiol, OMPI (Renoux, 1978). It has been suggested that OMPI potentiates leukocyte phagocytic and bactericidal functions by augmenting glutathione metabolism and maintaining microtubule integrity (Symeons *et al.*, 1979).

   4.2.3b.   Isoprinosine.   Isoprinosine is a complex of the *p*-acetoamidobenzoic acid salt of *N,N,*-dimethylamino-2 propanol and inosine (3 : 1 ratio) (Simon and Glasky, 1978; Hadden and Giner-Sorolla, 1981). Like levamisole, this immunostimulator has little direct effect on macrophages. *In vitro*, isoprinosine acts as a potentiator of lymphokine-induced macrophage proliferation and lymphokine-activated bactericidal capacity (Hadden *et al.*, 1979). Isoprinosine enhances the *in vivo* antiviral and antitumor effects of another cytokine, IFN (Chany and Cerutti, 1977; Cerutti *et al.*, 1978). A number of studies have characterized the modulating effects of isoprinosine on T-cell functions and differentiation (Vecchi *et al.*, 1978; Hadden and Giner-Sorolla, 1981). Administration of isoprinosine to young adult mice increases the spleen cell proliferative response to LPS (Florentin *et al.*, 1981). Production of B-cell growth factor by macrophages may contribute to *in vivo* or *in vitro* effects on the proliferation and antibody response of B cells (Hadden and Giner-Sorolla, 1981). Similarly, isoprinosine may modulate NK activity by enhancing macrophage regulation of NK cells (Florentin *et al.*, 1981).

   4.2.3c.   NPT 15392.   NPT 15392, a derivative of hypoxanthine (erythro-9[2-hydroxy,3-nonyl]hypoxanthine), is an immunopotentiator similar in structure and biologic effects to isoprinosine (Hadden and Giner-Sorolla, 1981). *In vitro*, NPT 15392 modulates T-lymphocyte differentiation and proliferation, and suppressor and cytotoxic effector functions. Modulation of T-cell effector, helper, and regulatory functions can account for most of the reported *in vivo* effects of NPT 15392 (Hadden and Wybran, 1980). Similar to levamisole, treatment with NPT 15392 can restore T-cell and T-dependent, B-cell responses of the immunosuppressed host. NPT 15392 *in vitro* also potentiates lymphokine-induced proliferation of macrophages (Hadden *et al.*, 1980). The possible involvement of macrophages in mediating some of the immunomodulatory effects of NPT 15392 is indicated by increased monocyte phagocytosis of zymosan (Hadden and Wybran, 1980).

5.   SUMMARY

   In this review we have examined some of the naturally occurring and synthetic immunostimulants that exhibit a variety of effects on the MPS. Based on the range of activity upon mononuclear phagocytes, MPS stimulators may be classified as adjuvants, endogenous mediators, IFN inducers, or potentiators. Adjuvants, the most potent stimulators of the MPS, are capable of: stimulating monocytopoiesis; mobilizing macrophage populations at sites of inflammation, infection, and tumors; activating macrophage effector functions; enhancing production of mediators and regulatory factors; and facilitating cellular and humoral immunity. Cell wall components of bacteria (MDP, trehalose dimycolates) and fungi (the glucans) as well as synthetic agents, including azimexone, CP-46,665, and the alkyl-lysophospholipids, produce extensive effects on the MPS typical of adjuvants. IFN inducers potently stimulate the MPS; however, many of their effects cannot be attributed solely to IFN. Thus, many of the IFN inducers—polyanions, florenones, and pyrimidinoles—also act like adjuvants. Endogenous mediators, such as tuftsin, IFNs and CSFs, have narrower, more selective effects on the MPS, reflecting their natural roles in immunoregulation, macrophage activation, and monocytopoiesis. Potentiators, such as levamisole, isoprinosine, and NPT 15392, have little direct action on the MPS, but appear to augment macrophage responses to lymphokines, chemotactic factors, and phagocytic stimuli. Future research will permit more refined classification of MPS stimulators and provide better guidelines for effective therapeutic applications aimed at selectively manipulating discrete compartments of the MPS.

REFERENCES

Adams, D. O., and Dean, J. H., 1982, Analysis of macrophage activation and biological response modifier effects by use of objective markers to characterize the stages of activation, in: *NK Cells and Other Natural Effector Cells* (R. B. Herberman, ed.), p. 511, Academic Press, New York.

Adams, D. O., and Snyderman, R., 1979, Do macrophages destroy nascent tumors?, *J. Natl. Cancer Inst.* **62**:1341.

Adams, D. O., Johnson, W. J., and Marino, P. A., 1982, Mechanisms of target recognition and destruction in macrophage-mediated tumor cytotoxicity, *Fed. Proc.* **41**:2212.

Alexander, P., and Evans, R., 1971, Endotoxin and double-stranded RNA render macrophages cytotoxic, *Nature New Biol.* **232**:76.

Amery, W. K., 1978, Overview of levamisole effectiveness in experimental and clinical cancer studies, in: *Immune Modulation and Control of Neoplasia by Adjuvant Therapy* (M. A. Chirigos, ed.), p. 93, Raven Press, New York.

Ando, M., and Dannenberg, A. M., 1972, Macrophage accumulation, division, maturation, and digestive and microbicidal capacities in tuberculous lesions. IV. Macrophage turnover, lysosomal enzymes, and division in healing lesions, *Lab. Invest.* **27**:466.

Ando, M., Dannenberg, A. M., and Shima, K., 1972, Macrophage accumulation, division, maturation, and digestive and microbicidal capacities in tuberculous lesions. II. Rate at which mononuclear cells enter and divide in primary BCG lesions and those of reinfection, *J. Immunol.* **109**:8.

Baird, L. G., and Kaplan, A. M., 1978, Immunoregulatory macrophages from pyran treated mice, in: *Immune Modulation and Control of Neoplasia by Adjuvant Therapy* (M. A. Chirigos, ed.), p. 435, Raven Press, New York.

Benacerraf, B., 1981, Role of MHC gene products in immune regulation, *Science* **212**:1229.

Berdel, W. E., Bausert, W. R., Weltzien, H. U., Modolell, M. R., Widmann, K. H., and Munder, P. G., 1980, The influence of alkyl-lysophospholipids and lysophospholipid-activated macrophages on the development of metastasis of 3-Lewis lung carcinoma, *Eur. J. Cancer* **16**:1199.

Bicker, U., 1978, Immunomodulating effects of BM 12.531 in animals and tolerance in man, *Cancer Treat. Rep.* **62**:1987.

Blanden, R. V., and Langman, R. E., 1972, Cell-mediated immunity to bacterial infection in the mouse: Thymus-derived cells as effectors of acquired resistance to *Listeria monocytogenes, Scand. J. Immunol.* **1**:379.

Bomford, R., and Moreno, C., 1981, Critical overview of the potential of various microbial polysaccharides for cancer immunotherapy, in: *Augmenting Agents in Cancer Therapy* (E. M. Hersh, M. A. Chirigos, and M. J. Mastrangelo, eds.), p. 91, Raven Press, New York.

Breinig, M. C., and Morahan, P. S., 1980, Interferon inducers: Polyanions and others, in: *Interferon and Interferon Inducers: Clinical Applications* (D. A. Stringfellow, ed.), p. 239, Dekker, New York.

Bruley-Rosset, M., Florentin, I., Kiger, N., Davigny, M., and Mathé, G., 1978, Effects of bacillus Calmette-Guerin and levamisole on immune responses in young, adult, and age-immunodepressed mice, *Cancer Treat. Rep.* **62**:1641.

Bruley-Rosset, M., Florentin, I., Kiger, N., Schultz, J., and Mathé, G., 1979, Restoration of impaired immune functions of aged animals by chronic bestatin treatment, *Immunology* **38**:75.

Bruley-Rosset, M., Florentin, I., Kiger, N., Schultz, J. I., and Mathé, G., 1981, Correction of immunodeficiency in aged mice by levamisole and bestatin administration, *Recent Results Cancer Res.* **76**:137.

Brunda, M. J., Herberman, R. B., and Holden, H. T., 1980, Inhibition of murine natural killer cell activity by prostaglandins, *J. Immunol.* **124**:2682.

Burgaleta, C., and Golde, D. W., 1977, Effect of glucan on granulopoiesis and macrophage genesis in mice, *Cancer Res.* **37**:1739.

Burgess, A. W., Camakaris, J., and Metcalf, D., 1977, Purification and properties of colony-stimulating factors from mouse lung-conditioned medium, *J. Biol. Chem.* **252**:1998.

Byrnes, P. V., Guilbert, L. J., and Stanley, E. R., 1981, Distribution of cells bearing receptors for a CSF-1 in murine tissues, *J. Cell Biol.* **91**:848.

Cerutti, I., Chany, C., and Schlumberger, J. F., 1978, Isoprinosine increases the antitumor action of interferon, *Cancer Treatment. Rep.* **62**:1971.

Chany, C., and Cerutti, I., 1977, Enhancement of antiviral protection against encephalomyocarditis virus by a combination of isoprinosine and interferon, *Arch. Virol.* **55**:225.

Chapes, S. K., and Tompkins, W. A. F., 1979, Cytotoxic macrophages in hamsters by vaccinia virus: Selective cytotoxicity for virus-infected targets by macrophages collected late after immunization, *J. Immunol.* **123**:303.

Chapes, S. K., Fan, S. S., Cummins, J. M., and Tompkins, W. A. F., 1981, Activation of natural killer cell cytotoxicity from bone marrow cells cocultivated with immune peritoneal macrophages, *J. Reticuloendothel. Soc.* **29**:341.

Chirigos, M. A. (ed.), 1978, Proceedings of the 4th conference on immune modulation and control of neoplasia by adjuvant therapy, *Cancer Treat. Rep.* **62**:1609–1996.

Chirigos, M. A., and Stylos, W. A., 1980, Immunomodulatory effects of various molecular weight anhydride divinyl ethers and other agents in vitro, *Cancer Res.* **40**:1967.

Chirigos, M. A., Papademetriou, V., Bartocci, A., Read, E., and Levy, H. B., 1981, Immune response modifying activity in mice of polyinosinic:polycytidylic acid stabilized with poly-L-lysine, in carboxymethycellulose (poly-ICLC), *Int. J. Immunopharmacol.* **3**:329.

Cohn, Z. A., 1978, The activation of mononuclear phagocytes: Fact, fancy and future, *J. Immunol.* **121**:813.

Cook, J. A., Taylor, D., Cohen, C., Rodrigue, J., Malshet, V., and DiLuzio, N. R., 1978, Comparative evaluation of the role of macrophages and lymphocytes in mediating the antitumor action of glucan, in: *Immune Modulation and Control of Neoplasia by Adjuvant Therapy* (M. A. Chirigos, ed.), p. 183, Raven Press, New York.

Cook, J. A., Holbrook, T. W., and Parker, T. W., 1980, Visceral leishmaniasis in mice: Protective effects of glucan, *J. Reticuloendothel. Soc.* **27**:567.

Dannenberg, A. M., Ando, M., and Shima, K., 1972, Macrophage accumulation, division, maturation and digestive and microbicidal capacities in tuberculous lesions. III. The turnover of macrophages and its relation to their activation and antimicrobial immunity in primary BCG lesions and those of reinfection, *J. Immunol.* **109**:1109.

Das, S. K., Stanley, E. R., Guilbert, L. J., and Forman, L. W., 1981, Human CSF-1 radioimmunoassay resolution of 3 subclasses of human colony stimulating factors, *Blood* **58**:630.

Dean, J. H., Luster, M. I., Boorman, G. A., Lauer, L. D., Adams, D. O., Padarasingh, M. L., Jerrels, T. R., and Mantovani, A., 1981, Macrophage activation by pyran co-polymers of graded molecular weight: Approaches to quantitative measurement of macrophage activation, in: *Augmenting Agents in Cancer Therapy* (E. M. Hersh, M. A. Chirigos, and M. J. Mastrangelo, eds.), p. 497, Raven Press, New York.

DeClercq, E., 1977, Effect of mouse interferon and polyriboinosinic acid-polyribocytidylic acid on L cell tumor growth in nude mice, *Cancer Res.* **37:**1502.

DeClercq, E., and Merigan, T. C., 1970, Induction of interferon by nonviral agents, *Arch. Intern. Med.* **126:**94.

Diamantstein, J., and Ulmer, 1976, Two distinct lymphocyte-stimulating soluble factors (LAF) released from murine peritoneal cells. I. The cellular source and the effect of cGMP on their release, *Immunology* **30:**741.

Diluzio, N. R., 1979, Lysozyme, glucan-activated macrophages and neoplasia, *J. Reticuloendothel. Soc.* **26:**67.

DiLuzio, N. R., and Morrow, S. H., 1971, Comparative behavior of soluble and particulate antigens and inert colloids in reticuloendothelial-stimulated or depressed mice, *J. Reticuloendothel. Soc.* **9:**273.

DiLuzio, N. R., McNamee, R., Jones, R., Cook, J. A., and Hoffman, E. O., 1976, The employment of glucan and glucan activated macrophages in the enhancement of host resistance to malignancies in experimental animals, in: *The Macrophage in Neoplasia* (M. A. Fink, ed.), p. 181, Academic Press, New York.

Djeu, J. Y., Heinbaugh, J. A. Holden, H. T., and Herberman, R. B., 1979, Role of macrophages in the augmentation of mouse natural killer cell activity by poly I:C and interferon, *J. Immunol.* **122:**182.

Fauve, R. M., Hevin, M. B., and Fontan, E., 1981, Non-specific inflammation and host resistance against pathogens, in: *Advances in Immunopharmacology* (J. W. Hadden, L. Chedid, P. Mullen, and F. Spreafico, eds.), p. 245, Pergamon Press, Elmsford, N.Y.

Ferluga, J., Schorlemmer, H. U., Baptista, L. C., and Allison, A. C., 1976, Cytolytic effects of the complement cleavage product, C3a, *Br. J. Cancer* **34:**624.

Ferluga, J., Schorlemmer, H. U., Baptista, L. C., and Allison, A. C., 1978, Production of the complement cleavage product, C3a, by activated macrophages and its tumorolytic effects, *Clin. Exp. Immunol.* **31:**512.

Fidler, I. J., Farnes, Z., Fogler, W. E., Kirsh, R., Bugelski, P., and Poste, G., 1982, Involvement of macrophages in the eradication of established metastases following intravenous injection of liposomes containing macrophage activators, *Cancer Res.* **42:**496.

Fiel, R. J., Musser, D. A., and Munson, B. R., 1976, Role of divalent cation complex formation in pyran-inhibition of nucleic acid biosyntheses, *J. Natl. Cancer Inst.* **5:**1319.

Finter, N. B., 1973, Interferons and inducers in vivo. I. Antiviral effects in experimental animals, in: *Interferons and Interferon Inducers* (N. B. Finter, ed.), p. 295, North-Holland, Amsterdam.

Fisher, B., and Gebhardt, M., 1978, Comparative effects of *Corynebacterium parvum, Brucella abortus* extract, bacillus Calmette-Guerin, glucan, levamisole, and tilorone with or without cyclophosphamide on tumor growth, macrophage proliferation and macrophage cytotoxicity in a murine mammary tumor model, *Cancer Treat. Rep.* **62:**1919.

Fisher, G. W., Podgore, J. K., Bass, J. W., and Kelley, J. L., 1974, Enhancement of immature defense mechanisms with levamisole in suckling rats, in: *Modulation of Host Immune Resistance in the Prevention or Treatment of Induced Neoplasia* (M. A. Chirigos, ed.), p. 343, U.S. Government Printing Office, Washington D.C.

Fisher, G. W., Cumrine, M. H., Balk, M. W., Chang, S. P., Hokama, Y., Heer, P., and Chou, S. C., 1978, Effect of levamisole on suckling rat spleen cells: Evidence for macrophage regulation, in: *Immune Modulation and Control of Neoplasia by Adjuvant Therapy* (M. A. Chirigos, ed.), p. 75, Raven Press, New York.

Florentin, I., Bruley-Rosset, M., Kiger, N., Imbach, J. L., Winternitz, F., and Mathé, G., 1978, In vivo immunostimulation by tuftsin, *Cancer Immunol. Immunother.* **5:**211.

Florentin, I., Bruley-Rosset, M., Schultz, J., Davigny, M., Kiger, N., and Mathé, G., 1981, Attempt at functional classification of chemically-defined immunomodulators, in: *Advances in Immunophar-*

macology (J. W. Hadden, L. Chedid, P. Mullen, and F. Spreafico, eds.), p. 311, Pergamon Press, Elmsford, N.Y.

Gibson, J., P., Megel, H., Camyre, K. P., and Michael, J. P., 1976, Effect of tilorone on the lymphoid and interferon response of athymic mice, *Proc. Soc. Exp. Biol. Med.* **151**:264.

Gidlund, M. A., Orn, H., Wigzell, A., Senik, A., and Gresser, I., 1978, Enhanced NK activity in mice injected with interferon and interferon inducers, *Nature (London)* **273**:759.

Giroud, J. P., Florentin, I., Pelletier, M., and Nolibe, D., 1981, Influence of an acute non-immunological inflammation on resistance to infection and neoplasia, in: *Advances in Immunopharmacology* (J. W. Hadden, L. Chedid, P. Mullen, and F. Spreafico, eds.), p. 249, Pergamon Press, Elmsford, N.Y.

Glovsky, M., DiLuzio, N. R., Alenty, A., and Ghekiere, L., 1976, Complement activation by glucan, *J. Reticuloendothel. Soc.* **20**:54a.

Goodwin, J. S., Bankhurst, A. D., and Messner, R. P., 1977, Suppression of human T-cell mitogenesis by prostaglandin: Existence of a prostaglandin-producing suppressor cell, *J. Exp. Med.* **146**:1719.

Gresser, I., Maury, C., Bandu, M.-T., Tovey, M., and Maunoury, M.-T., 1978, Role of endogenous interferon in the anti-tumor effect of poly I:C and statolon as demonstrated by the use of anti-mouse interferon serum, *Int. J. Cancer* **21**:72.

Hadden, J. W., and Englard, A., 1979, Molecular aspects of macrophage activation and proliferation, in: *Phagocytosis: Its Physiology and Pathology* (Y. Kokubun and N. Kobayashi, eds.), p. 147, University of Tokyo Press, Tokyo.

Hadden, J. W., and Giner-Sorolla, A., 1981, Isoprinosine and NPT 15392: Modulators of lymphocyte and macrophage development and function, in: *Augmenting Agents in Cancer Therapy* (E. M. Hersh, M. A. Chirigos, and M. J. Mastrangelo, eds.), p. 497, Raven Press, New York.

Hadden, J. W., and Wybran, J., 1980, Immunopotentiators. II. Isoprinosine, NPT 15392 and azimexone: Modulators of lymphocyte development and function, in: *Advances in Immunopharmacology* (J. W. Hadden, L. Chedid, P. Mullen, and F. Spreafico, eds.), p. 457, Pergamon Press, Elmsford, N.Y.

Hadden, J. W., Sadlik, J. R., and Hadden, E. M., 1975a, Macrophage proliferation induced in vitro by a lymphocyte factor, *Nature (London)* **257**:483.

Hadden, J. W., Coffey, R. G., Hadden, E. M., Lopez-Corrales, E., and Sunshine, G. H., 1975b, Effects of levamisole and imidazole on lymphocyte proliferation and cyclic nucleotide levels, *Cell. Immunol.* **20**:98.

Hadden, J. W., Sadlik, J. R., and Hadden, E. M., 1978, The induction of macrophage proliferation in vitro by a lymphocyte-produced factor, *J. Immunol.* **121**:231.

Hadden, J. W., Englard, A., Sadlik, J. R., and Hadden, E. M., 1979, The comparative effects of isoprinosine, levamisole, muramyl dipeptide and SM1213 on lymphocyte and macrophage proliferation and activation in vitro, *Int. J. Immunopharmacol.* **1**:17.

Hadden, J. W., Hadden, E. M., Spira, T., and Giner-Sorolla, A., 1980, NPT 15392: A modulator of in vitro lymphocyte and macrophage functions, *Int. J. Immunopharmacol.* **2**:198.

Hadden, J. W., Sadlik, J. R., and Warfel, A. H., 1981, Characterization of lymphokines acting on the macrophage, in: *The Lymphokines* (J. W. Hadden and W. E. Stewart, eds.), p. 73, Humana Press, New York.

Hamburg, S. I., Cassell, G. H., and Rabinovitch, M., 1980, Relationship between enhanced macrophage phagocytic activity and the induction of interferon by Newcastle disease virus in mice, *J. Immunol.* **124**:1360.

Hamilton, J. A., Stanley, E. R., Burgess, A. W., and Shadduck, R. K., 1980, Stimulation of macrophage plasminogen activator activity by CSF, *J. Cell. Physiol.* **103**:435.

Hamura, J., Wagner, H., and Röllinghoff, M., 1978, $\beta(1-3)$Glucans as a probe for T cell specific immune adjuvants. II. Enhanced *in vitro* generation of cytoxic T lymphocytes, *Cell Immunol.* **38**:358.

Handman, E., and Burgess, A. W., 1979, Stimulation by granulocyte-macrophage colony-stimulating factor of *Leishmania* tropical killing by macrophages, *J. Immunol.* **122**:1134.

Havell, E. A., and Spitalny, G. I., 1980, The induction and characterization of interferon from pure cultures of murine macrophages, *Ann. N.Y. Acad. Sci.* **350**:413.

Herberman, R. B., Brunda, M. J., Cannon, G. B., Djeu, J. Y., Nunn-Hargrove, M. E., Jett, J. R., Ortaldo, J. R., Reynolds, C., Riccardi, C., and Santoni, A., 1981, Augmentation of natural killer cell activity by interferon and interferon inducers, in: *Augmenting Agents in Cancer Therapy* (E. M. Hersh, M. A. Chirigos, and M. J. Mastrangelo, eds.), p. 497, Raven Press, New York.

Hersh, E. M., Gutterman, J. U., Alexanian, R., Lotzova, E., and Murphy, S. G., 1981, A seven parameter host defense assay system for evaluating biological response modifiers (BRM) therapy of human cancer, *ABS American Soc. Clinical Oncology* **22**:C156, 372.

Hibbs, J. B., Remington, J. S., and Stewart, C. C., 1980, Modulation of immunity and host resistance by microorganisms, *Pharmacol. Ther.* **8**:37.

Hoebecke, J., and Franchi, G., 1973, Influence of tetramisole and its optical isomers on the mononuclear phagocytic system, *J. Reticuloendothel. Soc.* **14**:317.

Ignarro, L. J., and Cech, S. Y., 1976, Bidirectional regulation of lysosomal enzyme secretion and phagocytosis in human neutrophils by guanosine 3',5'-monophosphate and adenosine 3',5'-monophosphate, *Proc. Soc. Exp. Biol. Med.* **151**:448.

Juy, D., and Chedid, L., 1975, Comparison between macrophage activation and enhancement of non-specific resistance to tumors by mycobacterial immunoadjuvants, *Proc. Natl. Acad. Sci. USA* **72**:4105.

Kaliner, M., Orange, R. P., and Austen, K. F., 1972, Immunological release of histamine and slow reacting substance of anaphylaxis from human lung. IV. Enhancement of cholinergic and alpha adrenergic stimulation, *J. Exp. Med.* **136**:556.

Katz, P., Zaytoun, A. M., and Fauci, A. S., 1982, Mechanism of human cell-mediated cytotoxicity. I. Modulation of natural killer cell activity by cyclic nucleotides, *J. Immunol.* **129**:287.

Kelly, M. T., 1978, Modulation of macrophage function by levamisole, *J. Reticuloendothel. Soc.* **24**:139.

Kleinschmidt, W. J., and Schultz, R. M., 1982, Similarities of murine gamma interferon and the lymphokine that renders macrophages cytotoxic, *J. Interferon Res.* **2**:291.

Kniep, E. M., Domzig, W., Lohmann-Matthes, M.-L., and Kickhofen, B., 1981, Partial purification and chemical characterization of macrophage cytotoxicity factor (MCF, MAF) and its separation from migration inhibitory factor (MIF), *J. Immunol.* **127**:417.

Kokoshis, P. L., Williams, D. L., Cook, J. A., and DiLuzio, N. R., 1978, Increased resistance to *Staphylococcus aureus* infection and enhancement in serum lysozyme activity by glucan, *Science* **199**:1340.

Krueger, R. F., and Mayer, G. D., 1970, Tilorone hydrochloride: An orally active antiviral agent, *Science* **169**:1213.

Kurland, J. I., Bockman, R. S., Broxmeyer, H. E., and Moore, M. A. S., 1978, Limitation of excessive myelopoiesis by the intrinsic modulation of macrophage derived prostaglandin E, *Science* **199**:552.

Le, J., Vilchech, J., Sadlik, J. R., Cheung, M. K., Balazs, I., Sarngadharan, M. G., and Prensky, W., 1983, Lymphokine production by human T cell hybridomas, *J. Immunol.* **130**:1231.

Lederer, E., 1980, Synthetic immunostimulants derived from the bacterial cell wall, *J. Med. Chem.* **23**:819.

Lima, A. O., Javierre, M. G., Dias de Silva, W., and Camara, D. S., 1974, Immunological phagocytosis: Effect of drugs on phosphodiesterase activity, *Experientia* **30**:945.

Lotzova, E., and Gutterman, J. U., 1979, Effect of glucan on natural killer (NK) cell and bone marrow effector cell activities, *J. Immunol.* **123**:607.

Mackaness, G. B., 1964, The immunological basis of acquired cellular resistance, *J. Exp. Med.* **120**:105.

Mackaness, G. B., 1969, The influence of immunologically committed lymphoid cells on macrophage activity *in vivo*, J. Exp. Med. **129**:973.

McLaughlin, C. A., Schwartzman, S. M., Horner, B. L., Jones, G. H., Moffat, J. G., Nestor, J. J., and Tegg, D., 1980, Regression of tumors in guinea pigs after treatment with synthetic muramyl dipeptides and trehalose dimycolate, *Science* **208**:415.

Maeda, Y. Y., and Chihara, G., 1973, The effects of neonatal thymectomy on the antitumor activity of lentinan, carboxymethyl pachymaran and zymosan and their effects on various immune responses, *Int. J. Cancer* **11**:153.

Majeski, J. A., and Stinnett, J. D., 1977, Chemoattractant properties of*Corynebacterium parvum* and pyran copolymer for human monocytes and neutrophils, *J. Natl. Cancer Inst.* **58**:781.

Mansell, P. W. A., Rowden, G., and Hammer, C., 1978, Clinical experiences with the use of glucan, in: *Immune Modulation and Control of Neoplasia by Adjuvant Therapy* (M. A. Chirigos, ed.), p. 255, Raven Press, New York.

Mayer, G. D., and Krueger, R. F., 1970, Tilorone hydrochloride: Mode of action, *Science* **169**:1214.

Meltzer, M. S., 1976, Tumoricidal responses *in vitro* of peritoneal macrophages from conventionally housed and germ-free nude mice, *Cell. Immunol.* **22**:176.

Meltzer, M. S., 1981, Macrophage activation for tumor cytotoxicity: Characterization of priming and trigger signals during lymphokine activation, *J. Immunol.* **127**:179.

Meltzer, M. S., Occhionero, M., and Ruco, L. P., 1982a, Macrophage activation for tumor cytotoxicity: Regulatory mechanisms for induction and control of cytotoxic activity, *Fed. Proc.* **41**:2198.

Meltzer, M. S., Benjamin, W. R., and Farrar, J. J., 1982b, Macrophage activation for tumor cytotoxicity: Induction of macrophage tumoricidal activity by lymphokines from EL-4, a continuous T cell line, *J. Immunol.* **129**:2802.

Metcalf, D., and Moore, M. A. S., 1971, *Hemopoietic Cells*, North-Holland, Amsterdam.

Mohr, S. J., Brown, D. G., and Coffey, D. S., 1972, Size requirement of polyinosinic acid for DNA synthesis, viral resistance and increased survival of leukemic mice, *Nature New Biol.* **240**:250.

Mohr, S. J., Massicot, J. G., and Chirigas, M. A., 1978, Derepression of nuclear template restriction for DNA synthesis by the immunostimulator pyran copolymer, *Cancer Res.* **38**:161.

Moore, R. N., Oppenheim, J. J., Farrar, J. J., Carter, C. S., Waheed, A., and Shadduck, R. K., 1980, Production of lymphocyte-activating factor (interleukin 1) by macrophages activated with colony-stimulating factors, *J. Immunol.* **125**:1302.

Moore, R. N., Hoffeld, J. T., Farrar, J. J., Mergenhagen, S. E., Oppenheim, J. J. and Shadduck, R. K., 1981, Role of CSFs as primary regulators of macrophage functions, in: *Lymphokines*, Volume 3 (E. Pick, ed.), p. 119, Academic Press, New York.

Morahan, P. S., 1981, Anionic polymers and polysaccharides: Overview of interferon inducing ability, antitumor activity and mechanisms of action, in: *Augmenting Agents in Cancer Therapy* (E. M. Hersh, M. A. Chirigos, and M. J. Mastrangelo, eds.), p. 185, Raven Press, New York.

Morahan, P. S., and Kaplan, A. M., 1976, Macrophage activation and anti-tumor activity of biologic and synthetic agents, *Int. J. Cancer* **17**:82.

Morahan, P. S. and Kaplan, A. M., 1978, Antiviral and antitumor functions of activated macrophages, in: *Immune Modulation and Control of Neoplasia by Adjuvant Therapy* (M. A. Chirigos, ed.), p. 447, Raven Press, New York.

Morahan, P. S., Barnes, D. W., and Munson, A. E., 1978, Relationship of molecular weight to antiviral and antitumor activities and toxic effects of maleic anhydride-devinyl ether (MVE) polyanions, *Cancer Treat. Rep.* **62**:1797.

Motoyoshi, K., Suda, T., Kusumoto, K., Tahaku, F., and Muira, Y., 1982, Granulocyte-macrophage colony-stimulating and binding activity of purified human urinary colony-stimulating factor to murine and human bone marrow cells, *Blood* **60**:1378.

Muller, W. E. G., Schuster, D. K., Zahn, R. K., Maidhoff, A., Leyhausen, G., Falke, D., Koren, R., and Umezawa, H., 1982, Properties and specificity of binding sites for the immunomodulator bestatin on the surface of mammalian cells, *Int. J. Immunopharmacol.* **4**:393.

Munder, P. G., Modolell, M., Andreison, R., Weltzien, H. U., and Westphal, O., 1979, Lysophosphatidylcholine (lysolecithin) and its synthetic analogues: Immunomodulating and other biologic effects, *Springer Semin. Immunopathol.* **2**:187.

Munder, P. G., Modolell, M., Bausert, W., Oettgen, H. F., and Westphal, O., 1981, Alkyllysophospholipids in cancer therapy, in: *Augmenting Agents in Cancer Therapy* (E. M. Hersh, M. A. Chirigos, and M. J. Mastrangelo, eds.), p. 441, Raven Press, New York.

Munson, A. E., Munson, J. A., Regelson, W., and Wampler, G. L., 1972, Effect of tilorone hydrochloride and congeners on RES tumors and immune response, *Cancer Res.* **32**:1397.

Munson, A. E., White, K. C., and Klykken, P. C., 1981, Pharmacology of MVE polymers, in: *Augmenting Agents in Cancer Therapy* (E. M. Hersh, M. A. Chirigos, and M. J. Mastrangelo, eds.), p. 329, Raven Press, New York.

Najjar, V. A., and Nishioka, K., 1970, Tuftsin: A natural phagocytosis stimulating peptide, *Nature (London)* **228**:672.

Nathan, C. F., Murray, M. D., and Cohn, Z. A., 1980, The macrophage as an effector cell, *N. Engl. J. Med.* **303**:622.

Nickol, A. D., and Bonventri, P. F., 1977, Anomalous high native resistance of athymic mice to bacterial pathogens, *Infect. Immun.* **18**:636.

Nishioka, K., Amoscato, A. A., and Babcock, G. F., 1981, Tuftsin: A hormone-like tetrapeptide with antimicrobial and antitumor activities, *Life Sci.* **28**:1081.

North, R. J., 1969, The mitotic potential of fixed phagocytes in the liver as revealed during the development of cellular immunity, *J. Exp. Med.* **130**:315.

North, R. J., 1970, The relative importance of blood monocytes and fixed macrophages to the expression of cell-mediated immunity to infection, *J. Exp. Med.* **132**:521.

Oehler, J. R., Lindsay, L. R., Nunn, M. E., Holden, H. T., and Herberman, R. B., 1978, Natural cell-mediated cytotoxicity in rats. II. In vivo augmentation of NK cell activity, *Int. J. Cancer* **21**:210.

Oppenheim, J. J., Mizel, S. B., and Meltzer, M. S., 1979, Biological effects of lymphocyte and macrophage-derived mitogenic "amplification" factors, in: *Biol⌃ ry of the Lymphokines* (S. Cohen, E. Pick, and J. J. Oppenheim, eds.), p. 291, Academic Press, New York.

Oppenheim, J. J., Togawa, A., Chedid, L., and Mizel, S., 1980, Components of mycobacteria and muramyl dipeptide with adjuvant activity induce lymphocyte activating factor, *Cell. Immunol.* **50**:71.

Pabst, M. J., and Johnston, R. B., 1980, Increased production of superoxide anion by macrophages exposed *in vitro* to muramyl dipeptide or lipopolysaccharide, *J. Exp. Med.* **151**:101.

Papamatheakis, J. D., Schultz, R. M., Chirigos, M. A., and Massicot, J. G., 1978, Cell and tissue distribution of ^{14}C-labelled pyran copolymer, *Cancer Treat. Rep.* **62**:1845.

Patchen, M. L., and Lotzova, E., 1980, Modulation of murine hemopoiesis by glucan, *Exp. Hematol.* **8**:409.

Phillips, J. H., Babcock, G. F., and Nishioka, K., 1981, Tuftsin: A naturally occurring immunopotentiating factor. I. *In vitro* enhancement of murine natural cell-mediated cytotoxicity, *J. Immunol.* **126**:915.

Powell, M. L., Hersh, E. M., Gutterman, J. U., Zander, A. R., Granati, R., Alexanian, R., Hartobagyi, G., and Murphy, S. G., 1981, Phase I study of MVE-2 therapy in human cancer, *Proc. AACR & ASCO* **22**:189.

Rabinovitch, M. and Manejias, R. E., 1978, Anti-interferon globulin inhibits macrophage phagocytic enhancement *in vivo* by tilorone or Newcastle disease virus, *Cell. Immunol.* **39:**:402.

Rabinovitch, M., Manejias, R. E., Russo, M., and Abbey, E. E., 1977, Increased spreading of macrophages from mice treated with interferon inducers, *Cell Immunol.* **29**:86.

Regelson, W., 1981, The biological activity of the synthetic polyanion, pyran copolymer (DIVEEMA, MVE, 46015) and the heterocyclic bis DEAE fluorenone derivative tilorone and congeners: Chemical and laboratory effects of these agents as modulators of host resistance, *Pharmacol. Ther.* **15**:1.

Renoux, G., 1978, Modulation of immunity by levamisole, *Pharmacol. Ther.* **2**:397.

Rhim, J. S., and Huebner, R. J., 1971, Comparison of the antitumor effect of IFN and IFN inducers, *Proc. Soc. Exp. Biol. Med.* **136**:524.

Riggi, S. J., and DiLuzio, N. R., 1961, Identification of a reticuloendothelial stimulating agent in zymosan, *Am. J. Physiol.* **200**:297.

Sachs, L., 1978, Control of normal cell differentiation and the phenotypic reversion of malignancy in myeloid leukemia, *Nature (London)* **274**:535.

Sadlik, J. R., Hadden, E. M., and Hadden, J. W., 1983, Lymphokine-induced macrophage proliferation: Purification and characterization of antigen-induced MGF/CSF, in: *Advances in Immunopharmacology II* (J. W. Hadden, L. Chedid, P. Duckor, F. Spreafico, and D. Willoughby, eds.), p. 221, Pergamon Press, Oxford.

Sandler, J. A., Gallin, J. I., and Vaughan, M., 1975a, Effects of serotonin, carbamylcholine and ascorbic acid on leukocyte cyclic GMP and chemotaxis, *J. Cell Biol.* **67**:480.

Sandler, J. A., Clyman, R. I., Manganiello, V. C., and Vaughan, M., 1975b. The effect of serotonin (5-hydroxytrytamine), and derivatives on guanosine 3',5' monophosphate in human monocytes, *J. Clin. Invest.* **55**:431.

Santoni, A., Riccardi, C., Barlozzari, T., and Herberman, R. B., 1980, Suppression of activity of mouse natural killer (NK) cells by activated macrophages from mice treated with pyran copolymer, *Int. J. Cancer* **26**:837.

Schindler, T. E., Chedid, L. A. and Hadden, J. W., 1982, Stimulatory effects of MDP and its butyl ester derivative on macrophage proliferation and activation *in vitro, Int. J. Immunopharmacol.* **4:**382.

Schorlemmer, H. U., Bitter-Suermann, D., and Allison, A. C., 1977, Complement activation by the alternative pathway and macrophage enzyme secretion in the pathogenesis of chronic inflammation, *Immunology* **32:**929.

Schultz, R. M., and Chirigos, M. A., 1979, Selective neutralization by anti-interferon globulin of macrophage activation by L-cell interferon, *Brucella abortus* ether extract, *Salmonella typhimurium* lipopolysaccharide, and polyanions, *Cell. Immunol.* **48:**52.

Schultz, R. M., and Chirigos, M. A., 1980, Macrophage activation for nonspecific tumor cytotoxicity, *Adv. Pharmacol. Chemother.* **17:**157.

Schultz, R. M., Papamatheakis, J. D., Stylos, W. A., and Chirigos, M. A., 1976, Augmentation of specific macrophage-mediated cytotoxicity: Correlation with agents which enhance antitumor resistance, *Cell. Immunol.* **25:**309.

Schultz, R. M., Papamatheakis, J. D., and Chirigos, M. A., 1977, Interferon: An inducer of macrophage activation by polyanions, *Science* **197:**674.

Schultz, R. M., Papamatheakis, J. D., and Chirigos, M. A., 1978a, Tumoricidal effect *in vitro* of peritoneal macrophages from mice treated with glucan, in: *Immune Modulation and Control of Neoplasia by Adjuvant Therapy* (M. A. Chirigos, ed.), p. 241, Raven Press, New York.

Schultz, R. M., Chirigos, M. A., and Heine, U. J., 1978b, Functional and morphologic characteristics of interferon-treated macrophages, *Cell. Immunol.* **35:**84.

Schultz, R. M., Papamatheakis, J. E., and Chirigos, M. A., 1978c, Correlation between antitumor activity and macrophage activation by polyanions, in: *Immune Modulation and Control of Neoplasia by Adjuvant Therapy* (M. A. Chirigos, ed.), p. 459, Raven Press, New York.

Simon, L. N., and Glasky, A. J., 1978, Isoprinosine: An overview, *Cancer Treat. Rep.* **62:**1963.

Shima, K., Dannenberg, A. M., Ando, M., Chandrasekhar, S., Seluzicki, J. A., and Fabrikant, J. I., 1972, Macrophage accumulation, division, maturation, and digestive and microbicidal capacities in tuberculous lesions. I. Studies involving their incorporation of tritiated thymidine and their content of lysosomal enzymes and bacilli, *Am. J. Pathol.* **67:**159.

Smith, R. B., de Kernion, J., Lincoln, B., Skinner, D. G., and Kaufman, J. J., 1978, Preliminary report of the use of levamisole in the treatment of bladder cancer, *Cancer Treat. Rep.* **62:**1709.

Snyderman, R., Pike, M. C., and Daniels, C. A., 1978, Levamisole and human monocyte chemotaxis: Reversal of an influenza-induced chemotactic defect in: *Immunomodulation and Control of Neoplasia by Adjuvant Therapy* (M. A. Chirigos, ed.), p. 29, Raven Press, New York.

Sone, S., and Fidler, I. J., 1980, Synergistic activation by lymphokines and muramyl dipeptide of tumoricidal properties in rat alveolar macrophages, *J. Immunol.* **125:**2454.

Spirer, Z., Zakuth, V., Golander, A., Bogair, N., and Fridkin, M., 1975, The effect of tuftsin on the nitrous blue tetrazolium reduction of normal human polymorphonuclear leukocytes, *J. Clin. Invest.* **55:**198.

Staber, F. G., Gisler, R. H., Schumann, G., Tarcsay, L., Schlafli, E., and Dukor, P., 1978, Modulation of myelopoiesis by different cell wall components: Induction of colony-stimulating activity (by pure preparations, low-molecular weight degradation products, and a synthetic low-molecular analog of bacterial cell-wall components) *in vitro, Cell. Immunol.* **37:**174.

Stabinsky, Y., Bar-Shavit, A., Fridkin, W., and Goldman, R., 1980, On the mechanism of action of the phagocytosis-stimulating peptide tuftsin, *Mol. Cell. Biochem.* **30:**71.

Stanley, E. R., 1979, Colony stimulating factor radioimmunoassay: Detection of a CSF subclass stimulating macrophage production, *Proc. Natl. Acad. Sci. USA* **76:**2969.

Stanley, E. R., 1981, Colony-stimulating factors, in: *The Lymphokines* (J. W. Hadden and W. E. Stewart, eds.), p. 101, Humana Press, Clifton, N.J.

Stanley, E. R., and Heard, P. M., 1977, Factors regulating macrophage production and growth, *J. Biol. Chem.* **12:**4305.

Stanley, E. R., Cifone, M., Heard, P. M., and Defendi, V., 1976, Factor regulating macrophage production and growth: Identity of colony stimulating factor and macrophage growth factor, *J. Exp. Med.* **143:**631.

Stanley, E. R., Chen, D.-M., and Lin, H.-S., 1978, Induction of macrophage proliferation by a purified colony stimulating factor, *Nature (London)* **274:**168.

Stanwick, T. L., Campbell, D. E., and Nahmias, A. J., 1982, Cytotoxic properties of human monocyte macrophages for human fibroblasts infected with herpes simplex virus: Interferon production and augmentation, *Cell. Immunol.* **70**:132.

Stebbing, N., Lindley, I. J. D., and Dawson, K. M., 1980, Variations in the contribution of induced
interferon and adjuvanticity to the antiviral effect of different polyinosinic acid-polycytidylic
acid for formulations in mice infected with encephalomyocarditis virus, *Infect. Immun.* **29**:960.

Stiehm, E. R., Kronenberg, L. H., Rosenblatt, H. M., Bryson, Y., and Merigan, T. C., 1982, Interferon: Immunobiology and clinical significance, *Ann. Intern. Med.* **96**:80.

Stinnett, J. D., and Majeski, J. A., 1980, Macrophage activation and mobilization in nude mice by
Corynebacterium parvum and pyran: A functional and histologic study, *J. Surg. Oncol.* **14**:327.

Stringfellow, D. A., 1978, Prostaglandin restoration of the interferon response of hyporeactive
animals, *Science* **201**:376.

Stringellow, D. A., 1980, Interferon inducers: Theory and experimental application, in: *Interferon and
Interferon Inducers* (D. A. Stringfellow, ed.), p. 145, Dekker, New York.

Stringfellow, D. A., 1981, 6-Aryl pyrimidinoles: Interferon inducers—immunomodulators—antiviral and antineoplastic agents, in: *Augmenting Agents in Cancer Therapy* (E. M. Hersh, M. A.
Chirigos, and M. J. Mastrangelo, eds.), p. 215, Raven Press, New York.

Stylos, W. A., Chirigos, M. A., Papademetriou, V., and Lauer, L., 1980, The immunomodulatory
effect of BM 12.531 (azimexon) on normal or tumored mice: *In vitro* and *in vivo* studies, *Int. J.
Immunopharmacol.* **2**:113.

Suit, H. D., Elman, A., Sedlacek, R., and Silobrcic, V., 1978, Comparative evaluation of tumor-
inhibitory activity of glucan and *Corynebacterium parvum* in a mouse fibrosarcoma model, in:
Immune Modulation and Control of Neoplasia by Adjuvant Therapy (M. A. Chirigos, ed.), p. 235,
Raven Press, New York.

Symeons, J., Rosenthal, M., DeBravander, M., and Goldstein, G., 1979, Immunoregulation with
levamisole, *Springer Semin. Immunopathol.* **2**:196.

Tenu, J. P., Lederer, E., and Petit, J. F., 1980, Stimulation of thymocyte mitogenic protein secretion
and of cytostatic activity of mouse peritoneal macrophages by trehalose dimycolate and
muramyl dipeptide, *Eur. J. Immunol.* **10**:647.

Tracey, D. E., 1979, The requirement for macrophages in the augmentation of natural killer cell
activity by BCG, *J. Immunol.* **123**:840.

Turner, W., Chan, S. P., and Chirigos, M. A., 1970, Stimulation of humoral and cellular antibody
formation in mice by poly Ir:Cr, *Proc. Soc. Exp. Biol. Med.* **133**:334.

Tzehoval, E., Segal, S., Stabinsky, Y., Fridkin, M., Spirer, Z., and Feldman, M., 1978, Tuftsin (an Ig-
associated tetrapeptide) triggers the immunogenic function of macrophages: Implications for
activation of programmed cells, *Proc. Natl. Acad. Sci. USA* **75**:3400.

Tzehoval, E., Segal, S., Stabinsky, Y., Fridkin, M., Spirer, Z., and Feldman, M., 1979, Immunostimulation by an Ig-derived tetrapeptide, tuftsin, *Springer Semin. Immunopathol.* **2**:2005.

Uemiya, M., Sugimura, K., Kusama, T., Saiki, I., Mikio, Y., Azuma, I., and Yamamura, Y., 1979,
Adjuvant activity of 6-O-mycoloyl derivatives of N-acetyl muramyl L-seryl-D-isoglutamine and
related compounds in mice and guinea pigs, *Infect. Immun.* **24**:83.

Umezawa, H., 1981, Screening of small molecular microbial products modulating immune response
and bestatin, *Recent Results Cancer Res.* **76**:209.

Umezawa, H., Aoyagi, T., Suda, H., Hamada, M., and Takeuchi, T., 1976. Bestatin, a new aminopeptidase B inhibitor produced by actinomycetes, *J. Antibiot.* **29**:97.

Unanue, E. R., 1981, The regulatory role of macrophages in antigenic stimulation. Part two: symbiotic relationship between lymphocytes and macrophages, *Adv. Immunol.* **31**:1.

van Furth, R., Langervoort, H. L., and Schaberg, A., 1975, Mononuclear phagocytes in human
pathology—proposal for an approach to improved clarification, in: *Mononuclear Phagocytes* (R.
van Furth, ed.), p. 1, Davis, Philadelphia.

Vecchi, A., Sironi, M., and Spreafico, F., 1978, Priminary characterization in mice of the effect of
isoprinosine on the immune system, *Cancer Treat. Rep.* **62**:1975.

Wahl, S. M., Wahl, L. M., McCarthy, J. B., Chedid, L., and Mergenhagen, S. E., 1979, Macrophage
activation by mycobacterial water-soluble compounds and synthetic muramyl dipeptide, *J. Immunol.* **122**:2226.

Weinstein, A. J., Grazday, A. F., Sims, H. Z., and Levy, H. B., 1971, Lack of correlation between interferon induction and antitumor effect of poly I-poly C, *Nature New Biol.* **231**:53.

Williams, D. L., and DiLuzio, N. R., 1980, Glucan-induced modification of viral hepatitis, *Science* **208**:67.

Williams, D. L., Cooke, J. H., Hoffman, E. D., and DiLuzio, N. R., 1978, Protective effects of glucan in experimentally-induced candidiasis, *J. Reticuloendothel. Soc.* **23**:479.

Wing, E. T., Waheed, A., Shadduck, R. K., Nagle, L. S., and Stephenson, K., 1982, Effect of colony stimulating factor on murine macrophages, *J. Clin. Invest.* **69**:270.

Wolff, J. S., Hemsworth, G. R., Kraska, A. R., Hoffman, W. W., Figdor, S. K., Fisher, D. O., Jakowski, A. M., Niblack, J. F., and Jensen, K. E., 1982, CP-46.665-1: A novel lipoidal amine with antimetastatic and immunomodulatory properties, *Cancer Immunol. Immunother.* **12**:97.

Wooles, W. R., and DiLuzio, N. R., 1963, Reticuloendothelial function and the immune response, *Science* **142**:1078.

Wooles, W. R., and DiLuzio, N. R., 1964, The phagocytic and proliferative response of the reticuloendothelial system following glucan administration, *J. Reticuloendothel. Soc.* **1**:160.

Yamamoto, Y., Nagao, S., Tanaka, A., Koga, T., and Kaoru, O., 1978, Inhibition of macrophage migration by synthetic muramyl dipeptide, *Biochem. Biophys. Res. Commun.* **80**:923.

Yarkoni, E., Lederer, E., and Rapp, H. J., 1981, Immunotherapy of experimental cancer with a mixture of synthetic muramyl dipeptide and trehalose dimycolate, *Infect. Immun.* **32**:273.

Zurier, R. B., Weissmann, G., Hoffstein, S., Kammerman, S., and Tai, H. H., 1974, Mechanisms of lysosomal enzyme release from human leukocytes. II. Effects of cAMP and cGMP, autonomic agonists, and agents which affect microtubule function, *J. Clin. Invest.* **53**:297.

9

Effects of Microbially Derived Products on Mononuclear Phagocytes

GENEVIÈVE LEMAIRE, JEAN-PIERRE TENU, JEAN-FRANÇOIS PETIT, and EDGAR LEDERER

1. INTRODUCTION

The cell wall, the outer layer of the microbial cell, is the zone of contact between the microorganism and the external world; it is thus not surprising that many cell wall constituents are recognized by the immune system. The epitopes, on the external side of the cell wall, elicit specific responses; other cell wall components stimulate immunity in a nonspecific way—adjuvants, which modulate the intensity and the nature of the specific response; mitogens, inducers of interferon; and macrophage activators, which induce a state of increased host resistance to a variety of pathogens and neoplasms.

The concept of activated macrophages was introduced by Mackaness (1962) who showed that macrophages harvested from animals that had resisted an infection by *Listeria monocytogenes*, exhibited an enhanced ability to kill *in vitro L. monocytogenes* and an unrelated intracellular bacterium, *Salmonella typhimurium*. This concept of cross-resistance to infections mediated by activated macrophages was then extended to phylogenetically unrelated organisms: infection with *Toxoplasma gondii*, for example, confers resistance to bacteria (*L. monocytogenes, S. typhimurium, Brucella abortus, Mycobacterium leprae*, and *Nocardia asteroides*), fungi (*Cryptococcus, Aspergillus*), protozoans (*Toxoplasma, Besnoitia, Trypanosoma cruzi*), and viruses (Remington, 1982). Activated macrophages also acquire extracellular killing capacity for tumor cells (Hibbs *et al.*, 1971, 1972; Krahenbuhl and Remington, 1974). It was then shown that macrophages could be activated, not only during persistent intracellular infection, by lymphokines

GENEVIÈVE LEMAIRE, JEAN-PIERRE TENU, JEAN-FRANÇOIS PETIT, and EDGAR LEDERER • Institut de Biochimie, Université Paris-Sud, 91405 Orsay, France.

produced by T lymphocytes when they meet the sensitizing antigen, but also by an array of substances, among which components of microbial cell walls play a dominant role (Alexander and Evans, 1971; Juy and Chedid, 1975; Yarkoni *et al.*, 1977; Schultz *et al.*, 1977a,c). The search for exogenous stimulants able to activate macrophages has been conducted with the hope that the ability to stimulate nonspecific resistance with chemically defined substances will allow a better understanding of some mechanisms of cellular immunity and perhaps their effective manipulation.

We will first review the alterations induced in the activity of mononuclear phagocytes by defined components of the bacterial cell wall: (1) lipopolysaccharides of the external membrane of gram-negative bacteria, (2) products derived from the peptidoglycan, and (3) trehalose diesters, glycolipids from the cell wall of bacteria of the CMN group (*Corynebacterium, Mycobacterium, Nocardia*). Then we will summarize the data published on two classes of products especially studied for their antitumor action: glucans obtained from fungal cell walls, and synthetic polynucleotides. Finally, we will briefly mention the potentialities of some secondary metabolites released by microorganisms.

For each class of substances, we will examine three aspects of their action on mononuclear phagocytes: (1) the alterations induced *in vitro* on cells of the monocyte-macrophage lineage, (2) the specific properties of macrophages originating from animals treated *in vivo*, and (3) the *in vivo* effects on some phenomena in which macrophages may be implicated as effector cells (particle clearance, nonspecific resistance to infections, and resistance to tumors).

After reviewing the large number of structural and functional alterations that occur in mononuclear phagocytes in response to microbially derived products, we shall try to evaluate the relative efficiency of the different substances and to determine if some of them are able to conduct macrophages through all the steps of the activation process.

This review is intended to give a detailed picture of the influence on mononuclear phagocytes of well-defined microbial fractions or of their synthetic counterparts. It seems useful, however, to mention briefly the "old-fashioned" whole bacterial preparations that are still used for various experimental and clinical purposes.

The main products currently investigated in cancer immunotherapy in man are *Propionibacterium acnes*, previously called *Corynebacterium parvum* (Halpern, 1975; Hersh *et al.*, 1981), penicillin-treated streptococci (OK432 or Picibanil) (see for instance Moriyasu *et al.*, 1982), BCG or *Nocardia rubra* cell wall skeleton, on the surface of oil droplets emulsified in saline (for reviews see Yamamura *et al.*, 1981; Yamamura and Azuma, 1982), and MER, a methanol extraction residue of BCG (Weiss *et al.*, 1975; Hersh *et al.*, 1981).

P. acnes is used as a reference in laboratory assays to evaluate nonspecific resistance (see for instance Krahenbuhl *et al.*, 1981; Mahmoud *et al.*, 1979). It was one of the first nonliving agents used to obtain activated mouse peritoneal macrophages (Halpern *et al.*, 1966; Basic *et al.*, 1975) and is still in current use for that purpose (see for instance Sorrell *et al.*, 1978; Scott *et al.*, 1982). Attempts to obtain better defined or less toxic preparations from *P. acnes* are reviewed by Tuttle and Cantrell (1981).

Killed BCG cells are used as standards in antiinfectious (Parant *et al.*, 1977) and antitumor assays (Leclerc *et al.*, 1976); by i.p. injection, they elicit in the peritoneal cavity of mice activated macrophages that suppress the growth of simultaneously injected tumor cells (Freedman *et al.*, 1980).

Nocardia opaca is an important source of immunostimulants (Ciorbaru *et al.*, 1975,1976). Delipidated cells (NOC-NDCM, *Nocardia* delipidated-cell mitogen) exert a potent mitogenic activity on B lymphocytes of various species, including man (Brochier *et al.*, 1976; Guglielmi *et al.*, 1982; Barot-Ciorbaru *et al.*, 1982). Delipidated cells and soluble extracts (NWSM, *Nocardia* water-soluble mitogen) have antitumor activity when administered intralesionally in rat and mouse tumors (Barot-Ciorbaru *et al.*, 1981b). A fraction, devoid of peptidoglycan fragments, NWSMP (*Nocardia* water-soluble mitogen pellet), induces circulating type I interferon in mice, including nude and irradiated animals, thus pointing toward macrophages as the target cells (Barot-Ciorbaru *et al.*, 1978, 1981a).

Vaccination of laboratory animals with attenuated strains of *B. abortus* increases their resistance to infections and tumors; this led to assays of killed and detoxified *B. abortus* cells: such preparations have antitumor properties *in vivo* and induce activated macrophages (for recent reviews see Dazord *et al.*, 1982; Youngner and Feingold, 1982). EBP (extract of bacterial phospholipid), phospholipid extracts from *L. monocytogenes* or *S. typhimurium*, protect mice against various infectious agents including *L. monocytogenes* (Fauve and Hevin, 1974). Killed or penicillin-treated streptococci have also been used to obtain activated macrophages (Saito and Tomioka, 1979; Tomioka and Saito, 1980; Lemaire *et al.*, 1982).

2. LIPOPOLYSACCHARIDES

2.1. PREPARATION AND STRUCTURE

Lipopolysaccharides (LPS) are constant constituents of the outer part of the gram-negative bacterial cell wall. They are usually prepared by extracting whole bacterial cells or cell envelopes with aqueous phenol and are recovered from the aqueous phase by high-speed centrifugation (Westphal and Jann, 1965). Peptides and phospholipids are present only in minor amounts in phenol–water-extracted LPS (1–3%); in contrast, LPS extracted with TCA or butanol contains a polypeptide component (see Section 2.5) and phospholipids.

The structure and properties of LPS from various species have been reviewed by Galanos *et al.* (1977) and Westphal *et al.* (1983).

Chemically, LPS from wild-type strains consist of three distinct regions (Fig. 1):

1. The outer region is hydrophilic; it is composed of heteropolysaccharide chains that contain repeating oligosaccharide units (*O*-specific antigenic units). A large diversity of sugars has been found in the *O*-specific chains, allowing a classification of LPS into chemotypes. The primary structure and the spatial configuration of these *O*-specific chains determine the serological specificities of the organism.
2. The central region, the core, is an acidic oligosaccharide. It is similar for large

groups of bacteria (only five distinct core structures have been identified, for example, in *Enterobacteriaceae*) and, in the vast majority of cases, is terminated by a 2-keto-3-deoxyoctulosonic acid (KDO).

3. The inner region is a hydrophobic lipid called lipid A. The lipid A unit of *Salmonella* is built up of glucosaminyl β1'→6 glucosamine disaccharides substituted in 1 and 4' by phosphate groups that may form pyrophosphate bridges with adjacent glucosamine disaccharides (Fig. 2). The C-6' OH group is the attachment site, through a KDO residue, of the polysaccharide chain to the lipid A. The other hydroxyl groups of the diglucosaminyl residues are esterified by long-chain fatty acids and the amino groups are substituted by 3-hydroxy fatty acids, which represent characteristic lipid A markers. The chain length of the hydroxy acid is characteristic for a particular bacterial group (in Enterobacteriaceae, 3-hydroxymyristic acid is present).

Free lipid A can be prepared from LPS by mild acid hydrolysis (which cleaves the ketosidic linkage between the polysaccharide and the lipid A). Free lipid A is a water-insoluble material; soluble preparations can be made by complexing lipid A with a carrier such as bovine serum albumin or after electrodialysis and subsequent neutralization with triethylamine or NaOH (Galanos and Lüderitz, 1975). Core-defective mutants have been obtained from various *Salmonella* and *E. coli* strains: a lipid A-trisaccharide can be isolated from the most deficient strain (Re) of *Salmonella*. The phenol–chloroform–petroleum ether method is convenient for the isolation of LPS from R mutants (Galanos *et al.*, 1969). Several groups are working on partial or total synthesis of lipid A (Shiba, 1982; Charon and Szabo, 1983; Szabo *et al.*, 1983).

Thus, thousands of LPS exist, differing in chemical structure (at least in the polysaccharide moiety). When a particular species is considered, several causes of heterogeneity exist: the nature and the length of all the O chains may not be identical (with different degrees of polymerization of the repeating unit and various substitutions in nonequimolar ratios); in lipid A, ester-bound phosphate residues (at C-4') may not be present in equimolar amounts and phosphate groups may be substituted (in *Salmonella*, the C-4' phosphate group is partly substituted with L-4-aminoarabinoside); furthermore, 3-hydroxy fatty acids may be partially 3-*O*-acylated. In the case of free lipid A, further causes of heterogeneity exist: partial degradation, presence of polyamines and cations, aggregates of different sizes (different salt forms of free lipid A exhibit large differences in their sedimentation coefficient).

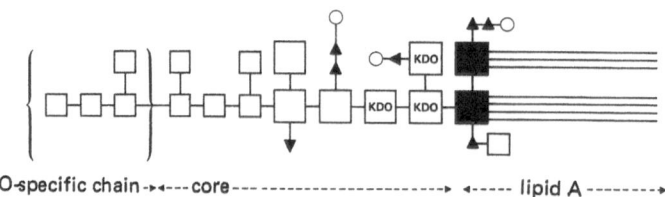

O-specific chain →◄--- core ---------------------→ ◄----- lipid A --------→

FIGURE 1. Schematic representation of the general structure of lipopolysaccharides. □, monosaccharide; ■, glucosamine; ▲, phosphate; ○, ethanolamine; —, long-chain (hydroxy) fatty acid.

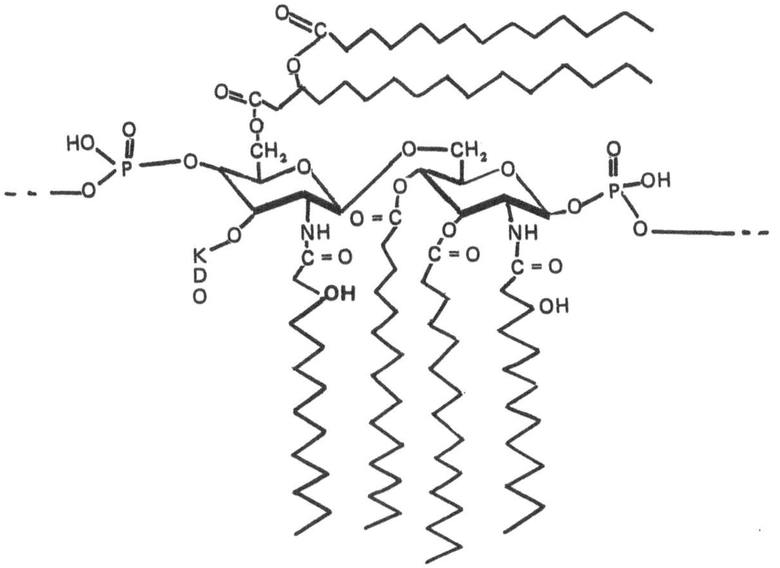

FIGURE 2.   General structure of lipid A.*

In this review, we will focus on the effects of LPS† on mononuclear pha-gocytes (macrophages, monocytes, and their bone marrow progenitors)—direct or indirect modifications of the activity of these cells and the consequences of these modifications. However, it must be kept in mind that possible targets of LPS are extremely numerous, since cells sensitive to LPS include besides mono-nuclear phagocytes, PMN, platelets, B and T lymphocytes, fibroblasts, and hepatocytes. The action of LPS on some of these cells induces the release of soluble mediators that alter the activity of a series of secondary targets. LPS can also interact directly with some serum components (activation of complement and of kinin-generating system, chelation of iron) (for reviews see Bradley, 1979; Morrison and Ryan, 1979).

2.2.   *IN VITRO* EFFECTS OF LPS ON MONONUCLEAR PHAGOCYTES

2.2.1.   Effects on the Proliferative Capacity

LPS exerts direct and indirect effects on the proliferation of the cells of the mononuclear phagocyte system. The indirect effects are mediated by a soluble

---

*Since the completion of the manuscript, it has been shown that the D-glucosamine disaccharide is substituted by KDO on position 6' instead of 3'. For recent structural work on lipid A, see Rietschel *et al.* (1984).

†The term LPS is used in this review although purity and homogeneity of all the preparations may not be identical.

factor, colony-stimulating factor (CSF), produced by monocytes and macrophages when they are stimulated by LPS (see Table 3). CSF stimulates proliferation and differentiation of bone marrow cells into granulocytes and macrophages; it also stimulates the proliferation of macrophages and macrophage precursors from various locations in the body.

Direct inhibitory effects can be observed when LPS is added to cells undergoing a proliferative response (macrophage tumor cell lines or exudate macrophages cultured in the presence of CSF for example). As shown in Table 1A, many macrophage cell lines are extremely sensitive to growth inhibition by LPS. This may be a consequence of induced terminal differentiation: the production of lysozyme is not affected and the production of CSF is induced or enhanced. LPS also inhibits macrophage colony formation in thiogycollate-elicited macrophages cultured in the presence of optimal or supraoptimal concentrations of CSF and incorporation of thymidine in oil-induced guinea pig macrophages (Table 1A). In contrast, in some cases LPS seems to provide the necessary stimulus for macrophages to enter the cell cycle: it increases the number of starch-elicited macrophages able to proliferate *in vitro*, and of resident macrophages responsive in the presence of CSF; it has an enhancing effect on the cloning response of thioglycollate-elicited macrophages maintained in suboptimal doses of CSF (Table 1B).

2.2.2. Changes Induced in the Morphology, the Enzymatic Equipment, and the General Metabolism

Extensive changes in macrophage morphology have been reported following *in vitro* stimulation with LPS: larger size, marked spreading, membrane ruffling, enhanced pseudopod formation (Mørland and Kaplan, 1977; Nozawa *et al.*, 1980b; Pabst and Johnston, 1980). LPS increases attachment of monocytes to plastic surfaces (the number of adherent cells after 1 hr was doubled in the presence of 20 μg/ml LPS) (Ellner and Spagnuolo, 1979).

At high concentrations, LPS has a cytotoxic effect on macrophages *in vitro*. The lethal dose seems to depend on the type of macrophage studied, the presence of serum, and the age of the culture (Wiener and Levanon, 1968); in most cases, no cytotoxicity was detected unless doses greater than 50 μg/ml were used (Doe and Henson, 1979; Peavy *et al.*, 1978). As macrophages are extremely sensitive to the presence of LPS (many responses are elicited by concentrations of LPS in the range of nanograms/ml—see Table 3), cytotoxicity is observed only in extreme cases.

In fact, LPS is stimulatory for many metabolic processes in macrophages. The stimulation may be evidenced following global parameters such as the rate of protein synthesis (Wiener and Levanon, 1968), RNA content (Stadler and de Weck, 1980), glucose utilization [the glucose consumption is increased six-fold when resident macrophages are incubated 3 days with 50 μg/ml LPS (Ryan *et al.*, 1979)], or glucosamine incorporation (Wilton *et al.*, 1975; Tanaka *et al.*, 1982). Some cellular enzymatic activities, however, seem more specifically enhanced: lactate dehydrogenase (Allison *et al.*, 1973; Miyama *et al.*, 1980), aminopeptidase

TABLE 1. MODULATION OF MACROPHAGE PROLIFERATION BY LPS[a]

A. Growth inhibition

Cells	LPS[b] Origin	ng/ml	Growth inhibition	CSF produced or added	References
Tumor cell lines					
P388D₁	S. typhosa (w)	10	0%		Ralph and Nakoinz (1977)
J774		100	50%		
WEHI 3		4	50%	Constitutive	Raschke et al. (1978)
RAW 264		0.5	50%		
WR 19		100	50%		Ralph et al. (1977)
PU5–1.8		1	40%	0	
		1000	90%	+	
Macrophages[c]					
TG-elicited	E. coli O26B6 (w)	1000	90% (No. of cells)	20% L.CM	Nozawa et al. (1980b)
TG-elicited	E. coli K235 (w)	1000	50% (clone formation)	5% L.CM	Moore et al. (1980a)
Oil-elicited (guinea pig)	E. coli O127B8	1000	60% ([³H]-TdR incorporation)		Tanaka et al. (1982)

B. Stimulation of cell proliferation

Cells[c]	LPS[b] Origin	ng/ml	Proliferative response	CSF	References
Starch-elicited	E. coli O127B8	1000	³H-TdR-labeled cells increase from 1 to 20%	0	Dienstman and Defendi (1978)
		1000	No effect	30% L.CM	
Resident		1000	³H-TdR-labeled cells increase from 0.1 to 7%	30% L.CM	
TG-elicited	E. coli K235 (w)	0.01	Cloning increases 1.7-fold	200 U/ml CSF	Moore et al. (1980a)

[a]Abbreviations: L.CM, conditioned medium of L cells; TG, thioglycollate broth.
[b]LPS (w) prepared by the phenol–water method of Westphal and Jann (1965).
[c]Mouse peritoneal macrophages were used except where otherwise stated.

(Allison *et al.*, 1973), transglutaminase [enhanced three-fold in oil-elicited guinea pig macrophages, after 20 hr with 1 μg/ml LPS (Leu *et al.*, 1982)], ornithine decarboxylase [transiently increased (Nichols and Prosser, 1980)—see Section 4.3], and some lysosomal enzymes. When LPS has been assayed for its effects on lysosomal enzymes, the major and more frequently reported change was a marked stimulation of acid phosphatase activity, by 160% (Mørland, 1979), 200% (Allison *et al.*, 1973), or even 360% (Miyama *et al.*, 1980). All other lysosomal enzymes were not increased in parallel [cathepsin D, e.g., was modified after phagocytosis of latex or carbon particles but not after LPS endocytosis (Mørland and Mørland, 1978)]. Conflicting results have been published on the degree of stimulation of β-glucuronidase (compare Allison *et al.*, 1973, and Mørland, 1979) and of *N*-acetylglucosaminidase (NAG) (compare Mørland and Kaplan, 1977, and Allison *et al.*, 1973). LPS induces a selective release of some lysosomal enzymes: acid phosphatase (Wiener and Levanon, 1968; Allison *et al.*, 1973), NAG (Allison *et al.*, 1973; Doe *et al.*, 1977; Bentley *et al.*, 1981), and β-glucuronidase (Doe *et al.*, 1977). Ia$^+$ macrophages are able to participate in cell contact-dependent lymphocyte activation. LPS has no significant effect on macrophage Ia antigen expression, but inhibits its induction and maintenance by interferon (Steeg *et al.*, 1982).

2.2.3. Alterations of the Functional Properties of Macrophages

2.2.3a.   Migration, Endocytosis, and Antimicrobial Activity.   LPS inhibits the *in vitro* migration of oil-elicited guinea pig macrophages from capillary tubes (Fox and Rajaraman, 1979; Nagao *et al.*, 1982).

The endocytic capacities of macrophages are in general stimulated after incubation with LPS. LPS enhances the pinocytosis of horseradish peroxidase in guinea pig macrophages (Schubert and David, 1980); it transiently stimulates latex ingestion (twofold after 24 hr) by PU5-1.8 cells (Ito *et al.*, 1979); it promotes a complement-mediated phagocytosis of erythrocytes: unstimulated macrophages do not internalize significantly via the C3 receptors, but when pretreated for 72 hr with LPS, they internalize 40% of the attached particles (Mørland and Kaplan, 1977). Fc-mediated phagocytosis, in contrast, is not stimulated by LPS: according to Mørland and Kaplan (1977), it is unaffected, but Vogel *et al.* (1979) reported an inhibition (by 40%).

LPS has been reported to stimulate the anti-*Listeria* activity of oil-induced guinea pig macrophages (Sheagren *et al.*, 1975; Hadden *et al.*, 1979) and the fungicidal activity of mouse resident macrophages (killing of *Candida parapsilosis* was increased eightfold by LPS 1 μg/ml) (Nozawa *et al.*, 1980a).

2.2.3b.   Antitumor Activity.   In contrast to the rare data published on LPS as an *in vitro* stimulant of the antimicrobial activity of macrophages, there is an abundant literature on LPS as a stimulant of antitumor activity. Depending on the experimental system used, three modes of action of LPS have been described. (1) LPS can directly activate noncytotoxic macrophages to become cytotoxic; (2) the presence of LPS can reduce the decrease of cytolytic activity observed when cytotoxic macrophages are cultured *in vitro* or restore this activity; and (3) LPS has a synergistic effect with lymphokines to induce cytotoxicity *in vitro*.

Several reports describe the direct *in vitro* activation of noncytotoxic macrophages to cytotoxicity by LPS (Table 2A): macrophages become cytotoxic for allogeneic or syngeneic tumor cells. However, in other cases, the activation by LPS was not possible (see for example Expts. 3a, 4a, 8b, and 9a in Table 2A); in fact, macrophages from untreated animals seem relatively unresponsive (except perhaps immediately after collection, Expt. 8a); macrophages from inflammatory exudates or harvested from infected animals are more easily activated (compare Expts. 4a–c and Expts. 9a and b in Table 2A). Even with inflammatory macrophages a direct activation may be difficult: according to Shaw *et al.* (1979), for example, exposure to LPS up to 10 μg/ml failed to induce cytolytic activity in thioglycollate-elicited macrophages. Activated macrophages rapidly lose their cytolytic activity when isolated *in vitro*. The presence of LPS may prevent or reduce this decrease and even restore the cytotoxicity (Table 2B); however, LPS does not prevent the loss of cytotoxicity of macrophages activated *in vitro* by lymphokines (Expt. 15). Some discrepancies exist about the activation stage of macrophages treated by lymphokines alone or LPS alone but there is a general agreement that a combined treatment by lymphokines and LPS induces a strong cytotoxicity and that the two stimulants act in synergy (Table 2C): in the presence of lymphokines or after a pretreatment, the doses of LPS required to activate macrophages to cytotoxicity are reduced 50- to 100-fold.

In conclusion, LPS is an *in vitro* amplification signal for the cytotoxicity of macrophages; its efficiency depends on the other activation signals received by macrophages: cells stimulated *in vivo* or *in vitro* by lymphokines are easily induced by LPS to develop tumoricidal activity; in contrast, macrophages cultured *in vitro* become refractory (they no longer develop a cytotoxic activity in response to LPS but cannot be considered simply as unresponsive to LPS since other functional properties are still modulated). In normal or inflammatory exudates, the number of cells able to express cytotoxicity may be low; thus, the antitumor activity observed depends on the experimental conditions used, especially the effector/target ratio and population density.

2.2.4. Alterations Induced in the Secretory Activity of Macrophages

Macrophages release into the extracellular medium a great variety of mediators able to modify the activity of other cell populations or of macrophages themselves. The mediators fall into three categories: derivatives of arachidonic acid, metabolites of oxygen, proteins and enzymes. The addition of LPS modifies the rate of production of all these mediators (Table 3). In many cases, the treatment by LPS is an absolute requirement to measure a detectable production, in other cases LPS is stimulatory, and in a few cases LPS has inhibitory effects.

LPS primes resident macrophages or J774.1 cells to respond with increased O_2^- production after stimulation with PMA or opsonized zymosan: the amount (n moles) of O_2^- released is increased sevenfold after a preincubation of resident macrophages with 1 μg/ml LPS (Pabst and Johnston, 1980).

TABLE 2. IN VITRO STIMULATION OF ANTITUMOR ACTIVITY OF MACROPHAGES BY LPS

A. Direct activation to cytotoxicity

	Macrophages[a]	Treatment			Target[c]	E/T	Assay	Effect[d]	References
		LPS[b]	μg/ml	Time					
1	Resident	DBA/2 Lipid A	50	1 hr	2SL2	20	Cell number	GI 0 → 90%	Evans and Alexander (1976)
2	Resident	C3HeB/Fe *S. enteritidis* (w)	2	Assay	P815	10	[3H]-TdR incorp.	GI 0 → 70%	Chedid et al. (1976)
3a	Thioglycollate	BALB/c *E. coli* O111B4 (w)	10	Assay	P815	10	51Cr release	SR 0 → 0%	Russell et al. (1977)
b	Regressing sarcoma		0.01					SR 45 → 80%	
c	Progressing sarcoma		0.01					SR 0 → 65%	
4a	Resident	C3H/HeN *E. coli* O128B12 (w)	10	Assay	3T12	3	Visual	0	Weinberg et al. (1978)
b	Proteose peptone		0.5					+	
c	BCG		0.001					+	
d	Cloned macrophages		0.05					+	
5	Thioglycollate	C57BL *S. minnesota* R595	10	24 hr	P815	20	51Cr release	SR 0 → 65%	Doe and Henson (1978)
6a	BCG	C3H/HeJ *E. coli* K235 (w)	2	4 hr	1023	10	[3H]-TdR release	SR 8 → 48%	Ruco and Meltzer (1978b)
b	Con A		2					SR 5 → 35%	
7	Human monocytes cultured 5 days	*E. coli* O26B6 (b)	10	8 hr	SK-BR-3	20	[3H]-TdR release	SR 0 → 24%	Cameron and Churchill (1980)
8a	Resident	C3H/HeN *E. coli* O111B4 (w)	0.1	4 hr	P815	10	51Cr release	SR 0 → 40%	Taffet et al. (1981)
b	Resident		0.1	24 hr				SR 0 → 5%	
9a	Resident	C57BL *E. coli* O111B4	10	18 hr	RLδ1	36	51Cr release	SR 0 → 7%	Taramelli and Varesio (1981)
b	Proteose peptone							SR 0 → 35%	
10	Resident	BALB/c *E. coli* O55B5	10		P815	10	No. of cells	GI 0 → 46%	Schultz and Jackson (1981)
11	Starch	C3H/HeN *E. coli* O127B8 (w)	0.002	4 hr	C3H/HeD	3	Adherent cells	C 10 → 90%	Drysdale and Shin (1981)
12	Human alveolar macrophages	*E. coli* O55135	5	24 hr	A375	5	Adherent cells	C 0 → 46%	Sone et al. (1982)

B. Prevention of the *in vitro* decrease of cytotoxicity or restoration

	Macrophages[a]		LPS[b]	Treatment		Target[c]	E/T	Assay	Effect[d]	References
	Origin	In vitro		ng/ml	Time					
13	Rat peritoneal	48 hr	E. coli	15 × 10⁴	Assay	L929	2	⁸⁶Rb incorp.	GI 0 → 40%	Reed and Lucas (1975)
14	Regressing sarcoma	24 hr	E. coli O1114 (w)	10	Assay	P815	10	⁵¹Cr release	SR 0 → 75%	Russell et al. (1977)
15	Lymphokine-treated	16 hr	E. coli K235 (w)	50	4 hr	1023	20	[³H]-TdR release	SR 4 → 6%	Ruco and Meltzer (1978a)
16	Tumor explanted	24 hr	E. coli O1114 (w)	10	16 hr	P815		⁵¹Cr release	SR 4 → 75%	Shaw et al. (1979)
17	TDM[e]-elicited	—	S. enteritidis (w)	5 × 10⁴	48 hr	P815	20	[³H]-TdR incorp.	GI 78 → 97%	Tenu et al. (1980)
18	BCG-elicited	18 hr	E. coli O26136 (w)	20	15 min	P815	2.5	⁵¹Cr release	SR 4 → 49%	Adams and Marino (1981)

C. Synergistic effects of LPS and lymphokines

	Macrophages[a]	LPS[b]	Treatment		Target[c]	E/T	Assay	Effect[d]	References
			ng/ml	Time					
19a	PBS	C3H/HeJ	E. coli K235 (w)	5 × 10⁴	8 hr	1023	20	[³H]-TdR release	SR 8 → 34%	Ruco and Meltzer (1978a)
b		C3H/HeN		25					SR 23 → 55%	
20	Proteose peptone	C3H/HeN	E. coli O128B12 (w)	10	Assay	3T12	3	[³H]-TdR release	SR 0 → 48%	Weinberg et al. (1978)
21	Fetal serum	BALB/c	E. coli O111B4 (w)	5	4 hr	P815	1	⁵¹Cr release	SR 1 → 51%	Russell et al. (1980)
22	Proteose peptone	C57BL	E. coli O111B4 (w)	10	18 hr	RL♂1	36	⁵¹Cr release	SR 5 → 30%	Taramelli and Varesio (1981)
23	Resident	C3H/HeN	E. coli O111B4 (w)	5	4 hr	P815	9	⁵¹Cr release	SR 0 → 80%	Taffett et al. (1981)

[a] Mouse peritoneal macrophages were used except where otherwise stated.
[b] LPS (w) prepared by the phenol–water method of Westphal and Jann (1965); (b) prepared by extraction with butanol or TCA.
[c] Targets: 2 SL2, lymphoma derived from a thymoma of the DBA2 mouse; P815, mastocytoma of the DBA2 mouse; 3T12, spontaneously transformed tumorigenic fibroblasts of the BALB/c mouse; 1023, methylcholanthrene-induced lymphoma of the C3H/He mouse; SK-BR-3, derived from a human adenocarcinoma of the breast; RL♂1, radiation-induced lymphoma of the BALB/c mouse; C3H/HeD, lymphosarcoma of the C3H mouse; A 375, human melanoma cell line; L929, transformed mouse fibroblasts.
[d] GI, percent of growth inhibition; SR, specific release; C, cytotoxicity = loss of labeled adherent cells. The results are expressed as the antitumor activity of untreated macrophages compared to the activity of LPS-treated macrophages.
[e] TDM = trehalose dimycolate, see p. 212.

TABLE 3. FACTORS RELEASED AFTER TREATMENT OF MONOCYTES OR MACROPHAGES BY LPS

Name	Bioassay	Production Cells	LPS treatment μg/ml	LPS treatment Time	Other inducers/comments	References
Lymphocyte-activating factor[a] (LAF)	Incorporation of [3H]-TdR in thymocytes	Macrophages elicited by thioglycollate, pyran, PHA, LPS, or BCG	50	72 hr	See Oppenheim *et al.* (1979)	Meltzer and Oppenheim (1977)
B-cell-activating factor[a] (BAF)	Antibody response to SRBC in the absence of T cells	Human monocytes	0.1	24 hr	MDP	Wood and Cameron (1978)
	Production of MIF by immune T lymphocytes	Oil-induced macrophages (guinea pig)	20	1 hr	MDP; see Iribe *et al.* (1982)	Yamamoto *et al.* (1978)
Endogenous pyrogen[a] (EP)	Febrile response in rabbit	Starch-elicited rabbit peritoneal exudate cells	0.1	1 hr	See Dinarello (1982)	Pacak and Siegert (1982)
Mononuclear cell factor[a] (MCF)	Production of PGE and collagenase by synovial cells	Human monocytes	20	72 hr	Con A, Fc fragments	Krane *et al.* (1982)
Fibroblast-activating factor[a] (FAF)	Fibroblast proliferation	Oil-induced macrophages (guinea pig)	30	1 hr	MDP	Wahl *et al.* (1980)
Serum amyloid A[a] (SAA) inducer	SAA concentration	Thioglycollate-elicited macrophages	10	3 hr		Sipe *et al.* (1979)
Colony-stimulating factor (CSF)	Colonies in bone marrow cells cultured *in vitro*	Resident	0.01	6 hr		Eaves and Bruce (1974)

	Biological activity assay	Cell type	Concentration	Time	Comments	Reference
Interferon type I	Protection of L cells against vesicular stomatitis virus	Resident	100	24 hr		Maehara and Ho (1977)
Cytotoxin	Growth inhibition of leukemia cells	Human monocytes treated by lymphokines	0.1	7 hr		Nissen-Meyer and Hammerstrom (1982)
	Cytotoxicity to L929 cells	BCG-elicited	1×10^{-4}	2 hr	= Tumor-necrotizing factor	Männel et al. (1980)
	Inhibition of migration of tumor cells	Freund's complete adjuvant-elicited	2	8 hr		Young et al. (1980)
Collagenase	Degradation of collagen	Oil-induced macrophages (guinea pig)	30	48 hr	MDP inducer	Wahl et al. (1974, 1980)
	Production of collagenase by chondrocytes	Oil-induced macrophages (rabbit)	30	20 hr		Deshmukh-Phadke et al. (1978)
Macrophage insulin-like activity (MILA)	Glucose oxidation	Caseinate-induced macrophages (rat)	100	24 hr		Filkins (1980)
Glucocorticoid-antagonizing factor (GAF)	Inducibility of PEPCK[b] by cortisol	Resident	100	17 hr		Moore et al. (1976)
Factor B[c]	Hemolytic assay	Resident	25	24 hr		Miyama et al. (1980)
Procoagulant activity (PCA)	Shortening of the clotting time of plasma	Hepatic macrophages (rabbit)	0.01	8 hr	Membrane enzyme	Maier and Ulevitch (1981)
Arginase	Degradation of arginine	Resident	25	24 hr		Currie (1978)
Fibronectin[c]	Immunoassay	Oil-induced macrophages (guinea pig)	30	24 hr	MDP inducer	Tsukamoto et al. (1981)
LPL-suppressing[d] mediator	Adipocyte lipoprotein lipase	Thioglycollate	10	26 hr		Kawakami and Cerami (1981)

[a]Biological activity exhibited by purified IL-1 according to Simon and Willoughby (1982).
[b]PEPCK, phosphoenol pyruvate carboxinase.
[c]Factor B and fibronectin are produced by untreated macrophages; LPS stimulates production.
[d]LPL, lipoprotein lipase.

LPS stimulates the production of PGE by resident mouse peritoneal macrophages (Kurland and Bockman, 1978; Moore *et al.*, 1979; Pelus and Bockman, 1979; Humes *et al.*, 1982), by oil-elicited guinea pig macrophages (Wahl *et al.*, 1977), and by human monocytes (Passwell *et al.*, 1979; Oppenheim *et al.*, 1980a). Splenic and peritoneal macrophages from tumor-bearing animals produce higher amounts of PGE than resident cells; this production is further increased by LPS (Pelus and Bockman, 1979), which also stimulates the synthesis of PGI_2 (Pelus and Bockman, 1979; Cook *et al.*, 1981; Taffet *et al.*, 1982) and thromboxane (Cook *et al.*, 1981). It has no effect on the level of leukotriene C_4 (Humes *et al.*, 1982). The magnitude of the increase of PGE secretion produced by exposure of monocytes or macrophages to stimuli such as Fc fragments, Con A, or PHA greatly exceeds the effect observed after addition of LPS.

Unstimulated macrophages have an intense secretory activity: they produce large amounts of lysozyme, complement components of the classical and alternative pathways. This "basal" secretory activity is relatively unsensitive to LPS: it requires high doses of LPS to reduce to 50% the secretion of lysozyme (Passwell *et al.*, 1980; Miyama *et al.*, 1980; Drapier *et al.*, 1982).

The addition of LPS, however, initiates the synthesis and (or) the release of various soluble mediators of protein nature, the monokines (Table 3). The extreme diversity of secondary targets affected by mediators released by macrophages must be emphasized. If we take into account all the observations made with mononuclear phagocytes of various origins, normal or elicited, LPS-treated macrophages have been described to release: (1) soluble factors able to modify the activity of thymocytes, T and B lymphocytes, fibroblasts, synovial cells, chondrocytes, adipocytes, hepatocytes, transformed cells, and of macrophages themselves and their precursors; (2) mediators responsible for fever and inflammation; (3) enzymes that affect extracellular and connective tissue proteins; (4) proteins directly involved in defense processes.

Our knowledge about the mode of production of these factors and the mechanism of their induction by LPS is limited. Since most of them are undetectable in medium conditioned by resident macrophages, their production requires an induction. In many cases, there is a wide variety of inducers, LPS being one (see for example the list of LAF inducers in Oppenheim *et al.*, 1979). Significant activity appears in culture supernatants after a lag period and the release generally reaches a plateau after 24 or 48 hr; however, it is not known if this arrest is due to a regulation (repression or production of an inhibitor) or to *in vitro* conditions. It is currently understood that these factors are not preformed but synthesized upon stimulation, even if in some cases the experimental proofs are not strong: the addition of cycloheximide at the same time as LPS has been shown to block the appearance of interferon, CSF, pyrogen, and collagenase but it increases the level of extracellular LAF [either by a superinduction phenomenon (Unanue and Kiely, 1977) or by a stimulation due to cell damage (Gery *et al.*, 1981)]. The release of a mediator is not necessarily coupled to its synthesis: in some experimental conditions (e.g., in resident macrophages a few hours after culturing or after LPS treatment) high levels of intracellular LAF can be detected in the absence of excretion (Unanue and Kiely, 1977; Gery *et al.*, 1981).

Some secretions are negatively regulated by LPS. Inflammatory macrophages, elicited by injection of nondigestible substances (thioglycollate broth, killed group C streptococci, asbestos, pyran, etc.), produce and release high levels of neutral proteases such as plasminogen activator and elastase. The release of plasminogen activator is inhibited by LPS (Chapman *et al.*, 1979; Werb *et al.*, 1980; Drapier *et al.*, 1982): in thioglycollate-elicited macrophages, 50 ng/ml LPS reduced by 80% the extracellular plasminogen activator activity and by 60% the intracellular activity, the secretion of lysozyme being only reduced by 20% (Drapier *et al.*, 1982). This inhibition of plasminogen activator, in LPS-treated macrophages, can be observed in parallel with the stimulation of other functions: enhancement of LAF production and inhibition of plasminogen activator have been demonstrated in the same culture (Bouchahda and Lemaire, unpublished results); Chapman *et al.* (1979) proposed that an inverse correlation exists, between modulation by LPS of tumoricidal potential and plasminogen activator secretion, in *Toxoplasma*-activated macrophages.

In conclusion, these *in vitro* studies indicate that LPS appears able to modify extensively the interactions of macrophages with their environment: migration is inhibited and production of plasminogen activator is blocked; in contrast, the capacities of endocytosis are enhanced, the antimicrobial and antitumor activities are stimulated, and, furthermore, the release of various monokines is induced.

2.3. PROPERTIES OF LPS-ELICITED MACROPHAGES

When LPS is injected i.p. (20–100 μg/mouse), it induces an inflammatory response: total peritoneal cell counts rise two- to threefold above normal levels and peritoneal macrophages harvested 3–4 days after treatment exhibit some original characteristics. There is an increase in cell size, in the number of acid phosphatase-positive granules, in the number and length of mitochondria, and an enlargement of the Golgi zone (Cohn *et al.*, 1966); spreading is important (Rabinovitch *et al.*, 1977) and membrane ruffling extensive (Mørland and Kaplan, 1977). Macrophages from LPS-treated animals contain larger quantities of acid hydrolases [acid phosphatase, NAG, β-glucuronidase, cathepsin (Cohn and Benson, 1965; Mørland and Kaplan, 1977)]; the largest increase is that of acid phosphatase (400%), but levels of 5'-nucleotidase (Edelson, 1980) and of cAMP phosphodiesterase activities (Zendegui and Klein, 1982) are reduced. LPS-induced macrophages could be distinguished from resident macrophages by qualitative and quantitative differences in the electrophoretic pattern of exterior plasma membrane polypeptides (Yin *et al.*, 1980).

LPS-elicited macrophages do not produce significantly more plasminogen activator than resident macrophages but they can do so after a second stimulus such as phagocytosis (Gordon *et al.*, 1974); according to Klimetzek and Sorg (1979), they produce neither plasminogen activator nor fibrinolysis inhibitors; they do not release elastase and their overall capacity to degrade extracellular matrix is limited (Werb *et al.*, 1980). They secrete four times less hemolytically active C5 than resident cells (Ooi *et al.*, 1980). However, when mice are treated with 100 μg LPS (i.v.), the release of factor B and lysozyme during cultivation is increased twofold (Miyama *et al.*, 1980). Macrophages from LPS-treated mice (100 μg i.p. 7 days earlier) are able to produce LAF when cultured *in vitro* [especially if they are restimulated *in vitro* by LPS (Meltzer and Oppenheim, 1977)]. They are primed to release high quantities of O_2^- upon PMA triggering (Johnston *et al.*, 1978) or after stimulation by *Candida* (Sasada and Johnston, 1980).

The capacity of macrophages to phagocytize erythrocytes is increased after LPS treatment of the animals, especially the endocytosis mediated by the C3 receptor (Mørland and Kaplan, 1977). According to Griffin *et al.* (1975), 30–50% of the cells in an LPS-elicited population ingest via the complement receptor. Macrophages harvested from mice treated 6 hr previously with LPS (25 μg i.v.) phagocytize bacteria more efficiently than normal macrophages (Jenkin and Palmer, 1960). LPS-elicited macrophages kill *C. albicans* more efficiently than do resident cells (Sasada and Johnston, 1980).

In contrast, it is not clear whether macrophages from LPS-injected mice are cytotoxic to tumor cells *in vitro*. According to Ruco and Meltzer (1978b), macrophages from mice treated i.p. with 1 μg LPS 2 days previously are not cytotoxic and do not develop cytotoxic activity after any treatment *in vitro* (PPD, LPS, Con A, or lymphokines); however Evans and Alexander (1976) and Juy and Chedid (1975) rendered macrophages nonspecifically cytotoxic by injecting endotoxin i.p. When tested *in vitro*, maximal cytotoxic activity was observed for macrophages recovered 7 days after injection.

In conclusion, LPS-induced macrophages differ from macrophages of untreated animals by membrane protein patterns, lysosomal activities, secretory capacities, C3-mediated phagocytosis, and cytotoxicity. They differ from other inflammatory macrophages (such as thioglycollate-elicited macrophages) since they do not produce plasminogen activator or elastase. They exhibit properties that do not seem inducible by LPS *in vitro*: increase of lysozyme secretion, NAG activity, and Fc-mediated phagocytosis. The response of peritoneal cells to *in vivo* stimulation by LPS is certainly complex and cannot be compared to a direct *in vitro* stimulation, especially when macrophages are harvested 4–7 days after treatment. However, the injection of LPS, as the *in vitro* stimulation, yields a macrophage population (probably quite heterogeneous) that possesses some properties of activated macrophages.

2.4. *IN VIVO* EFFECTS OF LPS MEDIATED BY CELLS OF THE MONONUCLEAR PHAGOCYTE SYSTEM

2.4.1. Clearance of Particles and Cells from the Bloodstream

In mice and rabbits pretreated with LPS, a markedly enhanced clearance of colloidal carbon particles follows a short period of decreased activity (Biozzi *et al.*, 1955). More recently, Waters and Ferraresi (1980) reported that a parenteral injection of 25 μg LPS caused a clearance rate increase of 245%, 24 hr after injection (twice that of a 2-mg dose of MDP); LPS, in contrast to MDP, increases spleen and liver size. The removal of bacteria from the peritoneal cavity of mice is rapidly increased following the injection of small doses of LPS (2–10 μg i.v.) (Jenkin and Palmer, 1960). The blood clearance of viable *Klebsiella pneumoniae* is more rapid in LPS-treated animals (Chedid *et al.*, 1976).

2.4.2. Increase of Nonspecific Resistance to Infections

Mice pretreated 24 hr earlier with LPS (1 μg i.v.) are completely protected against a challenge with 4×10^4 *K. pneumoniae*. No protection is observed in the case of LPS-hyporesponsive mice (C3H/HeJ) (Chedid *et al.*, 1976). The spectrum of resistance to infections induced by LPS is very broad: it includes intracellular pathogens (*Salmonella, Brucella, Mycobacterium tuberculosis*, and *L. monocytogenes*). LPS-treated mice are able to control the growth of *L. monocytogenes*: destruction of bacteria by splenic and hepatic macrophages is increased (Fauve and Hevin, 1971); increased resistance is expressed despite a depressed acquired immunity (Galelli *et al.*, 1981).

2.4.3. Antitumor Effects

Parenteral injection of LPS causes hemorrhagic necrosis and regression of solid tumors: early observations about the antitumor effects of "bacterial toxins" were reviewed by Nauts *et al.* (1953). More recently, LPS has been shown to be effective in protecting mice from various tumors (Butler and Nowotny, 1979) and in inducing regression of subcutaneous and intradermal tumors (Parr *et al.*, 1973) or ascites tumors (Dye and North, 1980).

TNF (tumor-necrotizing factor), a soluble mediator found, within 4 hr after injecting LPS, in the serum of mice infected with BCG or pretreated with *C. parvum* or other agents known to activate macrophages, may be one effector mechanism of tumor necrosis. (1) TNF-positive serum is as effective as endotoxin in causing necrosis of some transplanted tumors. (2) TNF displays antitumor activity when incubated with tumor cells *in vitro* (Carswell *et al.*, 1975); TNF-positive sera are also effective against parasites *in vitro* (Taverne *et al.*, 1981) and against *K. pneumoniae* and *L. monocytogenes in vivo* (Parant *et al.*, 1980b). (3) A rabbit antiserum, directed against TNF, neutralized a macrophage-derived cytotoxin induced *in vitro* by LPS (Männel *et al.*, 1981). It has yet to be shown that TNF is liberated in tumor-bearing animals.

However, LPS-dependent necrosis and regression may be separate events: regression, but not necrosis, seems dependent on the immunogenicity of the tumor and on the generation of a mechanism of T-cell-mediated immunity [regression is prevented by treatment with antilymphocyte globulin and abolished in irradiated or thymectomized animals (Parr *et al.*, 1973; Berendt *et al.*, 1978)]. Thus, North (1981) proposed that macrophages have to be activated by lymphocytes to be able to respond to LPS in a way that leads to tumor destruction: activated macrophages may be generated in response to growth of an immunogenic tumor or after an intratumoral injection of *C. parvum*.

2.4.4. Soluble Factors in Post-LPS Sera

Besides TNF, several soluble factors that are produced *in vitro* by LPS-treated macrophages, are also found in post-LPS sera. Six hours after injection of LPS, sera contain CSF and support the formation of colonies in bone marrow cells cloned in soft agar (Apte *et al.*, 1976). Interferon titers increase 2 hr after injection of LPS and then rapidly decline (Stinebring and Youngner, 1964). Ninety minutes after LPS administration, serum amyloid A (SAA) inducer is present in serum and 2 or 3 hr later, SAA concentration in serum begins to rise (Sipe *et al.*, 1979); i.v. injection of LPS produces, 4 hr later, a significant depression of phosphoenolpyruvate carboxykinase (PEPCK) induction due to cortisol; this effect is attributed to a factor, produced by macrophages, that, by blocking the induction of PEPCK (a key enzyme in gluconeogenesis) may explain the change observed in carbohydrate metabolism in LPS-treated animals (Moore *et al.*, 1976). A transferable factor that causes a suppression of lipoprotein lipase activity in adipose tissue has also been described (Kawakami and Cerami, 1981).

LPS has, thus, a triple effect on the mononuclear phagocyte system: it promotes the development of macrophages from their precursors in the bone marrow, it stimulates the activity of existing macrophages (phagocytosis and killing), and induces the production by macrophages of soluble mediators that affect diverse target cells.

2.5. ACTIVITIES OF LIPID A

The lipid moiety—lipid A—seems essential for the activity of LPS·Lipid A, obtained by mild acid hydrolysis or extracted from core-deficient mutants, is able to reproduce all the *in vitro* and *in vivo* effects described for LPS. Furthermore, when the lipid moiety of the LPS molecule is complexed with polymyxin B, LPS is inactive (Table 4).

Free polysaccharides obtained from LPS are found inactive in most assays; however, a polysaccharide fraction was found active in bone marrow colony stimulation and radioprotection (Nowotny *et al.*, 1975; Behling and Nowotny, 1982). Mitogen and adjuvant properties have also been reported recently for the carbohydrate region.

Phenol extraction (but not butanol treatment) removes from endotoxin a protein called lipid A-associated protein (LAP), which is mitogenic. LAP is active in all mice, including C3H/HeJ mice (Betz and Morrison, 1977); it stimulates several macrophage functions such as cytotoxicity (Doe *et al.*, 1978) and arginase synthesis (Ryan *et al.*, 1980).

3. PEPTIDOGLYCAN DERIVATIVES

The peptidoglycan, which is the basal layer of the bacterial cell wall, is a rigid macromolecule surrounding the cytoplasmic membrane. It is formed by the polymerization of a disaccharide tetrapeptide subunit (e.g., *N*-acetylglucosaminyl-β1→4*N*-acetylmuramyl-L-Ala-γ-D-isoGln-meso-DAP-D-Ala); in the intact

TABLE 4. EFFECTS OF LPS ON MONONUCLEAR PHAGOCYTES REPRODUCED BY FREE LIPID A AND R595 GLYCOLIPID OR BLOCKED BY POLYMYXIN B

In vivo effects
  Pyrogenicity:
    Free lipid A is pyrogenic (Galanos *et al.*, 1972)
  Generation of serum CSF and proliferation of splenic granulocyte-macrophage progenitor cells
    Free lipid A and R595 glycolipid are active, free polysaccharide is inactive (Apte *et al.*, 1976)
  Antitumor activity:
    Free lipid A and R595 glycolipid are active against established tumors (Parr *et al.*, 1973)
In vitro effects
  Toxicity:
    Free lipid A and SL 1102 glycolipid are toxic, free polysaccharide and native protoplasmic polysaccharide from *E. coli* O111B4 are nontoxic (Peavy *et al.*, 1978)
  Inhibition of proliferation:
    Blocked by polymyxin B (Moore *et al.*, 1980a)
  Stimulation of pinocytosis:
    Free lipid A is active; the effect is abolished by polymyxin B (Schubert and David, 1980)
  Induction of interferon:
    R595 glycolipid is active (Fleit and Rabinovitch, 1981; see also Neumann, 1982)
  Induction of collagenase:
    Free lipid A and R595 glycolipid are active, the lipid free-polysaccharide fraction is inactive (Wahl *et al.*, 1974)
  Induction of procoagulant activity:
    R595 glycolipid is active (Maier and Ulevitch, 1981)
  Stimulation of factor B production:
    Abolished by alkali or acid treatment of LPS (Miyama *et al.*, 1980)
  Stimulation of cytotoxicity to tumor cells:
    Free lipid A and R595 glycolipid are active, native protoplasmic polysaccharide from *E. coli* O113 is inactive; the effect is abolished by polymyxin B (Doe *et al.*, 1978; see also Alexander and Evans, 1971; Weinberg *et al.*, 1978)

---

peptidoglycan, disaccharides form linear chains whereas peptides are linked by interpeptide linkages (see Schleifer and Kandler, 1972).

The recognition of the immunomodulating properties of peptidoglycans and peptidoglycan fragments is the result of the work aimed at identifying the structure responsible for the adjuvant activity of the mycobacterial cells in Freund's adjuvant (see for instance Adam *et al.*, 1981). Simple active molecules were soon produced by organic synthesis followed by a vast array of analogs and derivatives. These can be classified into four categories: (1) simple muramyl peptides, (2) lipophilic derivatives of muramyl peptides, (3) carrier-coupled muramyl peptides, and (4) desmuramyl peptides and derived peptidolipids.

3.1. SYNTHETIC MURAMYL PEPTIDES

3.1.1. Simple Muramyl Peptides

The smallest immunoactive synthetic muramyl peptide is *N*-acetyl-muramyl-L-alanyl-D-isoglutamine or MDP (Fig. 3) (Ellouz *et al.*, 1974; Adam *et*

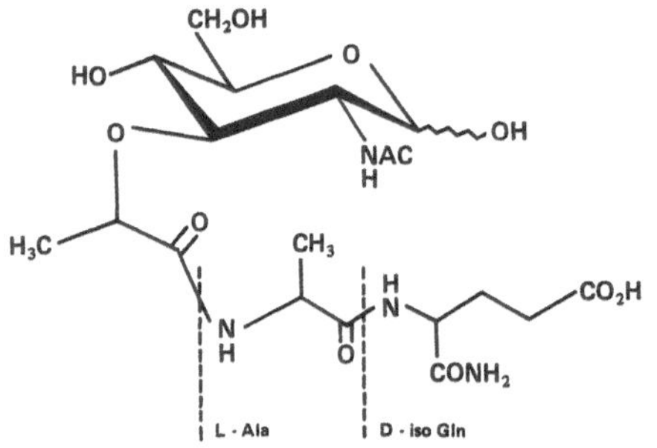

FIGURE 3.   Muramyl dipeptide.

al., 1975; Kotani *et al.*, 1975; Merser *et al.*, 1975). Several hundred analogs and derivatives of MDP have been synthesized and cannot be presented here (for a review see Adam *et al.*, 1981). The products discussed in this chapter are described in Table 5.

3.1.2.   Lipophilic Derivatives

To recover some properties of insoluble peptidoglycans and to replace oil vehicles, lipophilic derivatives have been prepared. Substitutions can be made on the 6-OH of the muramyl residue with naturally occurring α-branched β-hydroxylated mycolic acids (Yamamura *et al.*, 1976; Azuma *et al.*, 1978; Uemiya *et al.*, 1979), with linear or branched fatty acids (Takada *et al.*, 1979), or with ubiquinone derivatives (Azuma *et al.*, 1979). Lipophilic substituents can also be introduced at the C-terminal end of the peptide chain [MDP-L-Ala-glyceryl-mycolate (Parant *et al.*, 1980a)]. These lipophilic derivatives exhibit stronger macrophage-stimulating effects than MDP. In a series of straight-chain fatty esters, prepared by esterification of the carboxyl of *N*-acetylmuramyl-L-Ala-D-Gln, the butyl ester "murabutide" (see Table 5) is especially interesting since, contrary to MDP, it is not pyrogenic (Lefrancier *et al.*, 1982; Chedid *et al.*, 1982). MDP-L-Ala coupled to dimalmitoyl phosphatidylethanolamine (MTP-PE) was developed for inclusion into liposomes (Schroit and Fidler, 1982).

3.1.3.   Carrier-Coupled Muramyl Peptides

MDP has been coupled to proteins and peptides (Reichert *et al.*, 1980). MDP and its DD analog (where L-Ala is replaced by D-Ala) have been coupled to poly(DL-Ala-L-Lys) (Chedid *et al.*, 1979).

3.1.4.   Desmuramyl Peptides and Derived Peptidolipids

Peptidoglycan derivatives can be immunologically active in the absence of muramic acid (Migliore-Samour *et al.*, 1980): *N*-lauroylation of an adjuvant-inactive cell wall tetrapeptide isolated from a *Streptomyces* gives a compound, LTP (see Table 5), that produces delayed hypersensitivity to ovalbumin and protects mice against *L. monocytogenes*.

The "desmuramyl" derivative of MDP-L-Ala-glyceryl-mycolate, i.e., L-

TABLE 5. MDP, ANALOGS, AND DERIVATIVES

	Abbreviations	Comments
MurNAc-L-Ala-D-isoGln	MDP	
MurNAc-D-Ala-D-isoGln	MDP-D-D	Inactive
MurNAc-L-Ala-D-Glu	MDP-A	
Desmethyl MurNAc-L-Ala-D-isoGln	Nor-MDP	
MurNAc-L-Ser-D-isoGln	MDP(Ser)	
MurNAc-L-α-aminobutyryl-D-isoGln	MDP(Abu)	
MurNAc-L-Ala-D-Gln-O-n-butyl	Murabutide	Nonpyrogenic
MurNAc-L-Ala-D-isoGln-L-Lys	MDP-L-Lys	
MurNAc-L-Ala-γ-D-Glu-meso-DAP-D-Ala-D-Ala	MPP	
MDP coupled to multi-poly(DL-Ala)poly(L-Lys)	MDP-A-L	
MDP-D-D coupled to multi-poly(DL-Ala)poly(L-Lys)	MDP-D-D-A-L	
Lipophilic derivatives		
6-O-mycoloyl-MurNAc-L-Ala-D-isoGln	6-O-mycolyl-MDP	
6-O-stearoyl-MurNAc-L-Ala-D-isoGln	(L-18)-MDP	
6-O-(2-tetradecyl-hexadecanoyl)-MurNAc-L-Ala-D-isoGln	(B-30)-MDP	
6-O-quinonyl (QS 10)-MurNAc-L-Val-D-isoGln-O-methylester	Quinonyl-MDP-66	
MurNAc-L-Ala-D-isoGln-L-Ala-glycerol mycolate	MDP-L-Ala-glycerol mycolate	
Desmuramyl peptides		
L-Ala-D-isoGln-L-Ala-glycerol mycolate	Triglymyc	
N^2[N-[N-(N-lauroyl-L-alanyl)-γ-D-glutamyl]N^6-(glycyl)-DD-LL-diamino-2,6-pimelamic acid (lauroyl tetrapeptide)	LTP	Nonadjuvant
LACTYL-L-Ala-D-Glu-meso-DAP-D-Ala	FK 156	
Capryloyl-D-Glu-meso-DAP		
Stearoyl-D-Glu-meso-DAP		

Ala-D-isoGln-L-Ala-glyceryl-mycolate ("triglymyc"), is as active as the MurNAc derivative in stimulating nonspecific resistance to infections; it is, however, inactive as an adjuvant in guinea pigs (Parant *et al.*, 1980a).

More recently, the lactyl-tetrapeptide FK156 (see Table 5) has been found active; when caprylylated or stearoylated, the dipeptide γ-D-Glu-meso-DAP was also found active, even as an adjuvant (Kitaura *et al.*, 1982).

3.2. *IN VITRO* EFFECTS OF MDP AND DERIVATIVES ON MACROPHAGES

Mononuclear phagocytes were earlier thought to be the main target of peptidoglycan derivatives. As work progressed on the mechanism of adjuvant activity, it appeared that B and T lymphocytes are the targets (for a review see Leclerc and Chedid, 1982); macrophages seem, however, involved in adjuvant activity through secretion of soluble factors (Février *et al.*, 1978). Muramyl peptides are also able to enhance various properties of PMNs (Osada *et al.*, 1982b) and to stimulate NK activity (Sharma *et al.*, 1981).

3.2.1. Morphological and Biochemical Changes Induced in Macrophages

Addition of MDP (Wahl *et al.*, 1979) or adjuvant-active analogs (Tanaka *et al.*, 1980; Nagao *et al.*, 1981) to oil-induced guinea pig peritoneal macrophages increases their spreading and adherence to culture vessels. But when MDP is applied to nonadherent macrophages in migration assays, no spreading is observed (Nagao *et al.*, 1982). MDP and murabutide are weakly mitogenic for macrophages; however, under certain circumstances (Schindler *et al.*, 1982), they inhibit thymidine incorporation (Tanaka, 1982) and can even antagonize the action of macrophage mitogenic factor (Hadden *et al.*, 1979).

Adjuvant-active muramyl peptides increase [^{14}C]-D-glucosamine incorporation into thioglycollate-induced peritoneal guinea pig macrophages; (B-30)-MDP (see Table 5) is more active than MDP and (L-18)-MDP (Takada *et al.*, 1979). According to Imai *et al.* (1980), MDP also increases glucose metabolism through the hexose monophosphate shunt, as measured by the release of $^{14}CO_2$ from [1-^{14}C]glucose.

3.2.2. Changes in the Functional Properties of Macrophages

3.2.2a. Endocytosis. MDP added *in vitro* considerably increases the phagocytosis of *L. monocytogenes* by oil-induced guinea pig peritoneal macrophages (Hadden *et al.*, 1979), whereas it is inactive on the phagocytosis of erythrocytes by mouse peritoneal macrophages (Löwy *et al.*, 1977). LTP increases the phagocytosis of opsonized erythrocytes by resident mouse peritoneal macrophages (Werner *et al.*, 1982).

3.2.2b. Migration. In the presence of muramyl peptides, the kinesis of oil-induced guinea pig peritoneal macrophages is diminished as judged by a decrease of their spreading out of a capillary tube (Yamamoto *et al.*, 1978; Adam *et al.*, 1978; Nagao *et al.*, 1979, 1982). There is a correlation between the adjuvant activity of a given muramyl peptide and its action on kinesis. Cell walls, peptidoglycan monomers, and muramyl peptides are chemotactic for human monocytes (Ogawa *et al.*, 1982, 1983). This chemotactic activity is not in contradiction with the inhibition of kinesis described above: a product can be chemotactic in a gradient and, at high concentration, inhibit kinesis.

3.2.2c.   Antimicrobial Activities.   Hadden *et al.* (1979) have shown that MDP added *in vitro* to oil-induced guinea pig macrophages increases considerably the phagocytosis (see above) and the killing of *L. monocytogenes*. Nozawa *et al.* (1980a) reported an increased killing of *C. parapsilosis* by resident mouse peritoneal macrophages, but only at high doses of MDP (100 μg/ml), the effect being rather small.

3.2.2d.   Antitumor Activity.   Incubation of resident mouse peritoneal macrophages with muramyl peptides increases to a small extent their cytostatic activity (Juy and Chedid, 1975; Matter, 1979; Tenu *et al.*, 1980) but increases significantly the cytostatic activity of thioglycollate-elicited macrophages (Juy and Chedid, 1975; Tenu *et al.*, 1980); the adjuvant-inactive MDP-D-D-A-L is as efficient as MDP (Galelli *et al.*, 1980); the activity reached after stimulation *in vitro* by muramyl peptides is, however, far lower than that of macrophages elicited by BCG (Germain *et al.*, 1975) or trehalose dimycolate (TDM) (Lepoivre *et al.*, 1982). Muramyl peptides can also prevent the loss of cytostatic activity during *in vitro* cultivation of macrophages elicited by TDM (Tenu *et al.*, 1980).

Muramyl peptides are able to enhance the cytolytic activity of macrophages that infiltrate murine sarcoma virus-induced tumors and of macrophage cell lines (Taniyama and Holden, 1979); these authors found MDP inactive on macrophages or cell lines of C57BL/6 genetic background, an observation that they correlated with the nonresponsiveness of B lymphocytes of C57BL/6 mice to the mitogenic activity of MDP (Damais *et al.*, 1977). MDP increases significantly the cytotoxic activity of rat peritoneal macrophages (Reisser *et al.*, 1982).

Consistent levels of cytotoxicity are obtained when alveolar macrophages of rat and mouse are incubated in the presence of 50 μg/ml MDP (Fidler *et al.*, 1981; Sone and Fidler, 1980, 1981). In the presence of MAF, the dose of MDP can be lowered to 0.1 μg/ml (Sone and Fidler, 1980). By encapsulating MDP into phosphatidylcholine:phosphatidylserine (PC:PS, 7:3) multilamellar liposomes, Fidler *et al.* (1981) were able to obtain a 2-fold increase of cytotoxicity with a 1000-fold lower dose of MDP. This kind of liposome is phagocytized by the macrophages (Schroit and Fidler, 1982), lending support to the possibility that muramyl peptides do not act through external receptor sites (see Section 4.2.). The experiments of Fidler *et al.* were performed on C57BL/6 macrophages: the apparent contradiction with the results of Taniyama and Holden (1979) might be due to a higher sensitivity of alveolar macrophages to MDP. Sone and Tsubura (1982) were able to increase the cytolytic activity of human alveolar macrophages with free and liposome-encapsulated MDP.

3.2.3. Action on the Secretory Properties of Macrophages

3.2.3a. Interleukins and Cytokines. Peptidoglycan and petidoglycan-derived products, when added to cultures of monocytes or macrophages, induce the release in the culture medium of a series of "activities" that have been related to protein mediators.

The most studied has been LAF. Human monocytes release LAF when cultivated in the presence of MDP (Oppenheim *et al.*, 1980b; Damais *et al.*, 1982), WSA [a water-soluble complex of peptidoglycan and arabinogalactan (Adam *et al.*, 1972)], or 6-*O*-stearoyl-MDP (Oppenheim *et al.*, 1980b) or the nonpyrogenic murabutide (Damais *et al.*, 1982). Resident mouse peritoneal macrophages cannot be induced to secrete LAF by MDP or a muramyl pentapeptide (MPP) (Tenu *et al.*, 1980), but the situation is different with elicited macrophages: peritoneal macrophages from mice pretreated with BCG secrete LAF when treated with MDP (Oppenheim *et al.*, 1980b); the production of LAF by mouse peritoneal macrophages elicited by thioglycollate medium or TDM is increased several times by MDP or MPP (Tenu *et al.*, 1980). This is also the case of the macrophage cell line P388D$_1$ (Oppenheim *et al.*, 1980b); the effect on P388D$_1$ is increased by the presence of nonadherent spleen cells or human peripheral cells. LAF can also be released by oil-elicited rabbit peritoneal macrophages treated with MDP or murabutide (Damais *et al.*, 1982).

Most muramyl peptides are pyrogenic: this activity has been related to their ability to induce the release of endogenous pyrogen (EP) from mononuclear phagocytes (Dinarello *et al.*, 1978; Dinarello, 1982), although a direct central action cannot be excluded since these substances are active by the intracerebroventricular route and in rabbits made leukopenic by mustard treatment (Riveau *et al.*, 1980). EP has been found in the culture medium of human monocytes or oil-elicited rabbit peritoneal macrophages incubated with MDP or MDP-A-L (Damais *et al.*, 1982). In contrast, murabutide, which is not pyrogenic, does not induce the release of EP, although it induces the release of LAF (Damais *et al.*, 1982). When used at very low doses, MDP-A-L, which is strongly pyrogenic, induces the release of EP, without production of LAF (Damais *et al.*, 1982). These experiments strongly argue in favor of LAF and EP being different molecules, although it has been proposed that they could be two different activities carried by the same molecule (Rosenwasser and Dinarello, 1981).

Other activities can be induced by peptidoglycans or muramyl peptides: Staber *et al.* (1978) obtained the production of a colony-stimulating activity (CSF) by MDP acting on splenic or peritoneal mouse macrophages. MDP or WSA induced the release by oil-induced guinea pig peritoneal macrophages of a substance capable of initiating fibroblast proliferation (Wahl *et al.*, 1979). Wood and Staruch (1980) found a BAF activity (stimulation of the IgM plaque response of T-cell-deficient murine splenocytes to heterologous erythrocytes) after incubation of human monocytes with MDP: it coeluted with a LAF activity. Oil-induced guinea pig peritoneal macrophages, treated by MDP, release a helper activity for the antigenic stimulation of T lymphocytes to produce MIF (migration inhibition factor) (Iribe *et al.*, 1981) and synthesize factors comitogenic with PHA for lymph node T lymphocytes (Iribe *et al.*, 1982).

3.2.3b.   Enzymes and Prostaglandins.   MDP or WSA induce the secretion by oil-elicited guinea pig macrophages of collagenase (Wahl *et al.*, 1979). This induction is dependent on the synthesis of prostaglandins by macrophages: a correlation between prostaglandin and collagenase production was noted in response to varying concentrations of MDP (Wahl *et al.*, 1980). In contrast, WSA or MPP (but not MDP) inhibits the release and the cellular activity of plasminogen activator in inflammatory mouse peritoneal macrophages (Drapier *et al.*, 1982).

An increased production of PGE_1 and PGE_2 induced by incubation with MDP was observed by Parant *et al.* (1980c) with oil-induced rabbit peritoneal macrophages.

3.2.3c.   Activated Oxygen Species.   After 4 hr of culture in the presence of MDP, the ability of mouse peritoneal macrophages to release O_2^- upon stimulation by PMA was more than doubled. (B-30)-MDP is twice as active than MDP (Pabst *et al.*, 1980). The same phenomenon was observed with the macrophage cell line J774.1 (Pabst and Johnston, 1980). MDP also prevents the loss during *in vitro* culture of the capacity to release O_2^- of human monocytes (Pabst *et al.*, 1982).

3.3.   PROPERTIES OF MACROPHAGES FROM ANIMALS TREATED *IN VIVO* WITH PEPTIDOGLYCAN-DERIVED PRODUCTS

Muramyl peptides (Parant *et al.*, 1979; Yapo *et al.*, 1982) or a disaccharide pentapeptide (Tomasič *et al.*, 1980) when injected i.p. in saline are eliminated rapidly through the kidney: this is certainly one of the reasons why, to obtain antitumor macrophages or to achieve an antiinfectious activity *in vivo*, it is necessary to use high doses and/or repeated or continuous administration.

Juy and Chedid (1975) were the first to report that a peptidoglycan-derived product injected *in vivo* could increase the *in vitro* antitumor activity of macrophages: i.p. injection of 30 µg WSA increases the cytostatic activity against the P815 mastocytoma of mouse peritoneal macrophages; 30 µg MDP is not active. However, Matter (1979) was able, by repeated i.p. injections of 1 or 10 mg MDP/mouse, to activate peritoneal macrophages for cytostatic activity against Meth-A sarcoma cells. Reisser *et al.* (1982) obtained rat peritoneal macrophages cytotoxic for a syngeneic tumor 2 hr after i.p. injection of 100 µg MDP but not later.

With an s.c. injection of 25–100 µg MDP 18 hr before harvesting, Cummings *et al.* (1980) were able to obtain peritoneal macrophages that released five times more O_2^- upon PMA triggering and killed twice the number of ingested *C. albicans* than peritoneal macrophages from untreated mice; these macrophages showed increased spreading, protein content, LDH and β-N-acetylglucosaminidase activity.

To avoid repeated injection or high doses, muramyl peptides can be delivered in liposomes. By the use of an appropriate lipid composition, namely PC:PS 7:3 (Fidler *et al.*, 1980; Schroit and Fidler, 1982), for the multilamellar liposomes into which they encapsulate immunostimulants, Fidler and co-workers were able to target part of them toward the lung capillary bed and eventually to integrate their content into monocytes, which migrate into alveoli and become alveolar macrophages (Poste *et al.*, 1982). Whereas i.v. injection of as much as 200 μg MDP in saline did not render mouse alveolar macrophages cytotoxic for tumor cells, this could be achieved with 2.5 μg when encapsulated into liposomes (Fidler *et al.*, 1981).

3.4. *IN VIVO* EFFECTS OF PEPTIDOGLYCAN-DERIVED PRODUCTS ON MONONUCLEAR PHAGOCYTES

3.4.1. Clearance of Particles and Cells from the Bloodstream

MDP and analogs having antiinfectious activity increase the clearance of colloidal carbon when administered 24 hr before the challenge in mice and rats but not in guinea pigs (Waters and Ferraresi, 1980; Fraser-Smith *et al.*, 1982). The MDP analogs found active are also adjuvants in saline (Tanaka *et al.*, 1979). Increase of carbon clearance in mice has also been observed with a lactyltetrapeptide and the caprylol and stearoyl derivatives of the dipeptide γ-D-Glu-meso-DAP (Kitaura *et al.*, 1982). Parant *et al.* (1978b) have shown that MDP increases the clearance of living *K. pneumoniae* injected i.v. to mice. MDP and four analogs that increase carbon clearance in mice also increase the clearance from the lung of ^{125}I-iododeoxyuridine-labeled cells of the B16 melanoma injected i.v. (Proctor *et al.*, 1982).

3.4.2. Increase of Nonspecific Resistance to Infection

Injection of 100 μg MDP or oral administration of 2 mg protects mice against an infectious challenge with *K. pneumoniae* 24 hr later (Chedid *et al.*, 1977; for a review see Parant, 1979); even neonatal mice, insensitive to LPS, are protected (Parant *et al.*, 1978b). MDP is also active in T-cell-depleted and immunosuppressed mice (Parant, 1979). Various analogs are active such as MDP-A, MDP-L-Lys (Parant *et al.*, 1978b), the DAP-containing MPP (Yapo *et al.*, 1982), and the nonpyrogenic murabutide (Chedid *et al.*, 1982). MDP-A-L is very active and its activity extends toward *Pseudomonas aeruginosa* and *L. monocytogenes*. The inactive MDP-D-D becomes active when conjugated to A-L (Chedid *et al.*, 1979). Humphries *et al.* (1980) obtained a good protection against *Streptococcus pneumoniae* with MDP. In a series of 18 analogs of MDP, a correlation was found between antiinfectious activity against *P. aeruginosa* and *C. albicans* and ability to increase carbon clearance; the greatest protection was obtained with nor-MDP and MDP(Abu) (Fraser-Smith *et al.*, 1982).

Acylation on the 6-OH of muramic acid with mycolic acids resulted in a decreased activity against *E. coli* relative to MDP, but substitution with straight-chain fatty acids improved the activity with an optimum for (L-18)-MDP (Matsumoto *et al.*, 1981); (L-18)-MDP can stimulate the resistance of immunocompromised mice (aged, irradiated, or cyclophosphamide-treated) (Osada *et al.*, 1982a); it is also active against *P. aeruginosa*, *S. aureus*, and *C. albicans* (Osada *et al.*, 1982a). MDP-L-Ala-glycerol-mycolate and its nonpyrogenic desmuramyl derivative are more active than MDP against *K. pneumoniae;* their activity extends to *P. aeruginosa* (Parant *et al.*, 1980a). The capryloyl and stearoyl derivatives of the dipeptide γ-D-Glu-meso-DAP are as active as MDP against *E. coli* (Kitaura *et al.*, 1982).

No protection was usually observed with simple muramyl peptides against intracellular microorganisms such as *L. monocytogenes* (Parant *et al.*, 1979; Humphries *et al.*, 1980). However, using repeated injections (every day for 4 days before challenge) and higher doses (1.5 mg/mouse), Fraser-Smith and Matthews (1981) found nor-MDP and MDP(Abu) active against *L. monocytogenes* injected i.p. MDP injected at a high dose (2 days before challenge) or delivered continuously by an Alzet minipump (7 days starting 2 days before challenge) protects Swiss mice against *T. cruzi* (Kierszenbaum and Ferraresi, 1979); Krahenbuhl *et al.* (1981) could obtain some degree of protection against *T. gondii* in CBA mice (but not in the more susceptible C57BL/6) by s.c. injection of 1.3 mg MDP the day before challenge.

Some lipophilic derivatives seem more active than water-soluble products to protect against intracellular bacteria. LTP, and various analogs, which are nonpyrogenic, are active against *K. pneumoniae* and also against *L. monocytogenes* (Migliore-Samour *et al.*, 1980; Floc'h *et al.*, 1981; Werner *et al.*, 1982). L-Ala-D-isoGln-L-Ala-glycerol-mycolate is also active against *L. monocytogenes* when incorporated into liposomes (Parant *et al.*, 1980a).

From the data collected above, it is difficult to assess the degree of participation of the mononuclear phagocytes in the antiinfectious activity of peptidoglycan derivatives. However, if we take the anti-*Listeria* activity as a criterion for the direct participation of mononuclear phagocytes, some derivatives, such as LTP and its analogs, seem able to activate macrophages more than other compounds. One can tentatively conclude that peptidoglycan derivatives act either through direct activation of mononuclear phagocytes (high doses, lipophilic derivatives) or through other mechanisms in which less drastic changes in mononuclear phagocytes than activation for microbicidal activity against intracellular microorganisms might play a role.

3.4.3. Resistance to Tumors

Hydrosoluble peptidoglycan derivatives do not have antitumor activities *in vivo*. Some lipophilic derivatives are able to induce suppression, i.e., to inhibit the growth of tumor cells injected simultaneously: Azuma *et al.* (1978) described such an activity for 6-O-mycoloyl-, nocardomycoloyl-, or corynomycoloyl-MDP attached to oil droplets, against a methylcholanthrene-induced fibrosarcoma; quinonyl-MDP-66 is active in saline (Saiki *et al.*, 1981). Kitaura *et al.* (1982) found a similar activity for stearoyl-γ-D-Glu-meso-DAP suspended in a solution of methylcellulose. Four intratumoral injections of 400 μg quinonyl-MDP-66 in 10% squalene were able to induce the regression of the line 10 hepatocarcinoma of the strain 2 guinea pig growing intradermally and of its metastases (Yamamura and Azuma, 1982; Saiki *et al.*, 1982). The cells involved in this antitumor activity have not been identified.

In contrast, the role of the activation of host macrophages in the eradication of metastases of the B16 melanoma in the lung of C57BL/6 mice following the administration of MDP encapsulated into PC:PS 7:3 liposomes has been clearly established: MDP encapsulated into liposomes that are not retained in the lung are inactive; treatment of tumor-bearing animals with agents that impair macrophage functions makes encapsulated MDP inefficient; i.v. injection of thioglycollate-elicited peritoneal macrophages activated *in vitro*, by MDP in liposomes, prevents significantly the growth of metastases in the lung (Fidler *et al.*, 1982). T cells are not involved as thymectomized/irradiated and nude mice are protected (Fidler, 1981).

3.4.4. Pyrogenicity

Upon stimulation, monocytes secrete about 100 times more EP than neutrophils (Dinarello, 1982). It is thus safe to assume that most of the circulating EP originates from monocytes or macrophages. Following i.v. administration of MDP, plasma transfer demonstrated the presence of circulating EP (Dinarello *et al.*, 1978; Riveau *et al.*, 1980), whereas none was present after the administration of murabutide (Chedid *et al.*, 1982).

It is interesting that i.v. administration of MDP is followed by a drop in the number of all populations of circulating leukocytes, whereas no such leukopenia is observed after murabutide.

4. MECHANISMS OF ACTION OF LPS AND MURAMYL PEPTIDES *IN VITRO*

4.1. MONOCYTES AND MACROPHAGES AS PRIMARY TARGETS

In vitro experiments with peritoneal cells usually do not exclude a 1% contamination by lymphocytes, which produce macrophage-stimulating factors. However, there is considerable evidence that muramyl peptides and LPS may directly stimulate macrophages. The arguments are of several types. (1) In some assays, contaminations were unlikely due to the experimental conditions used [LPS and MDP, e.g., increase production of O_2^- in macrophages from nude mice (Pabst and Johnston, 1980) and cytotoxicity in macrophages from irradiated mice (Doe and Henson, 1978)]. (2) In many cases, the addition of nonadherent cells did not enhance the response of adherent cells (Pabst and Johnston, 1980; Sipe *et al.*, 1979; Männel *et al.*, 1980). (3) Many effects of LPS and muramyl peptides are too rapid to be mediated by factors released by other cells [a significant effect of LPS can be observed within 30 min for priming of O_2^- production (Pabst and Johnston, 1980)]. (4) Muramyl peptides and LPS stimulate cloned macrophages or tumor cell lines (data summarized in Table 6).

TABLE 6. EFFECTS OF LPS AND MDP ON MACROPHAGE CELL LINES, BONE MARROW-DERIVED MACROPHAGES, OR CLONED MACROPHAGES

Effect	Cells	References
Growth inhibition	See Table 1	Ralph et al. (1978)
Production of CSF	PU5-1.8,J774,P388D$_1$	Fleit and Rabinovitch (1981)
Production of interferon	Bone marrow-derived macrophages	Neumann (1982)
	J774 2,IC 21	
Production of LAF	P388D$_1$,J774,WEHI 3,PU5-1.8	Lachman et al. (1977)
	P388D$_1$	Oppenheim et al. (1980)
Production of a cytotoxin	PU5-1.8,cloned macrophages	Männel et al. (1980)
Induction of ornithine decarboxylase	J774 1	Nichols and Prosser (1980)
Production of PGE	SK2,WEHI 3,J774,RAW 264	Kurland and Bockman (1978)
Priming for O$_2^-$ release	J774 1	Pabst and Johnston (1980)
Stimulation of phagocytosis	PU5-1.8	Ito et al. 1979
Stimulation of cytotoxicity against tumor cells	PU5-1.8	Taniyama and Holden (1980)
	PU5-1.8,P388D$_1$,J774,RAW 264	Taniyama and Holden (1979, 1980)
	RAW 264	Russell et al. (1980)
Stimulation of ADCC	Cloned macrophages	Weinberg et al. (1978)
	RAW 264, J774, PU5	Ralph and Nakoinz (1981)

Nevertheless, lymphocytes may mediate some effects of LPS on macrophages. Wilton *et al.* (1975) demonstrated a critical role for B lymphocytes in the stimulation of macrophage uptake of glucosamine in the presence of LPS. More recently, Ryan and Yoke (1981) showed that LPS-treated B lymphocytes are able to stimulate macrophage metabolism (glucose consumption) and secretion (arginase). According to Levy *et al.* (1981), LPS-triggered T-enriched cells induced a monocyte procoagulant activity (PCA) in the absence of free LPS probably by contact-mediated collaboration.

4.2.   INTERACTIONS OF MURAMYL PEPTIDES AND LPS WITH MACROPHAGES

A study of the rate of endocytosis of [^{3}H]-MPP or of a fluorescent MDP-neoglycoprotein (obtained by coupling *p*-aminophenyl-MDP to fluoresceinated BSA) did not reveal any specific interactions between muramyl peptides and mouse peritoneal macrophages that could account for a ligand-mediated endocytosis (Tenu *et al.*, 1982): muramyl peptides seem to enter mononuclear phagocytes by simple liquid pinocytosis. Since the increase of IL-1 secretion induced by MDP, for example, is a saturable, concentration-dependent phenomenon, the existence of receptors inside the macrophage is suggested. It has been shown that macrophages take up vesicles as intact particles (Schroit and Fidler, 1982); thus, since immunomodulators (MAF or MDP) encapsulated into liposomes are 1000-fold more efficient in enhancing tumoricidal capabilities of macrophages than the free drugs (Fidler *et al.*, 1981), we suggest that it is the rate of entry into macrophages by liquid pinocytosis that limits the efficiency of soluble immunomodulators.

Plasma membrane receptors for LPS have been found on erythrocytes, platelets, granulocytes, lymphocytes, mast cells, and hepatocytes. Haeffner-Cavaillon *et al.* (1982) have shown the presence of a lectinlike receptor for LPS on the membrane of rabbit peritoneal macrophages: the binding of tritium-labeled pertussis endotoxin was inhibited by one of the two polysaccharides present in this endotoxin but not by lipid A. The selective binding of LPS, through its polysaccharide moiety, could enhance its rate of pinocytosis.

4.3.   BIOCHEMICAL EVENTS FOLLOWING MACROPHAGE–IMMUNOMODULATOR INTERACTION

Prostaglandins, especially PGE, have been implicated as second messengers of LPS and MDP action. Wahl *et al.* (1979) and McCarthy *et al.* (1980) have shown that MDP- and LPS-induced production of collagenase is preceded by synthesis of PGE and increase in intracellular levels of cAMP. Indomethacin inhibits prostaglandin synthesis as well as cAMP and collagenase production. Inhibition by indomethacin is overcome by addition of exogenous PGE; dibutyryl cAMP or cholera toxin can restore collagenase production (but not prostaglandin synthesis) in LPS- or MDP-stimulated macrophages; however, the addition of PGE, dibutyryl cAMP, or cholera toxin is ineffective in the absence of immunomodulators. Thus, two sequences of events are necessary to trigger collagenase synthesis: (1) The immunomodulator induces PGE synthesis that, in turn, increases cAMP level; the elevation of cAMP initiates collagenase production. (2) LPS or MDP induce another sequence of undefined events as indicated by the inability of PGE to trigger collagenase synthesis in the absence of LPS.

In the same way, PGE does not negatively regulate cytolytic activity unless it is added to macrophages in conjunction with a modulator, despite the fact that exposure to PGE is sufficient to increase intracellular levels of cAMP within minutes: thus, more than activation of adenylate cyclase and induction of a generalized cAMP response is needed (Russell *et al.*, 1981). In a study of the production of LAF by LPS-stimulated J774.1 cells, Kikutani *et al.* (1981) proposed that the elevation of cAMP induces the phosphorylation of nonhistone nuclear proteins. Nichols and Prosser (1980) suggested that a transient rise in ornithine decarboxylase (a protein that modulates the activity of RNA polymerase I) is promoted by the increase of cAMP.

Is the production of PGE an obligatory intermediate of MDP and LPS action? The use of indomethacin has distinguished at least three cases (Table 7): some effects are dependent on prostaglandin synthesis (collagenase production, plasminogen activator inhibition), others are independent (FAF and EP production), and some events are inhibited by the production of prostaglandin (CSF and interferon production).

TABLE 7. EFFECTS OF INDOMETHACIN ON MDP- OR LPS-MEDIATED CHANGES OF MACROPHAGE PROPERTIES

Indomethacin suppresses:
    Elevation of prostaglandin levels (Wahl *et al.*, 1979; McCarthy *et al.*, 1980; Parant *et al.*, 1980c)
    Inhibition of lymphocyte functions (Ellner and Spagnuolo, 1979)
    Induction of collagenase (Wahl *et al.*, 1977)
    Inhibition of plasminogen activator release (Drapier and Petit, unpublished results)
    Induction of cytotoxicity in noncytotoxic macrophages (Drysdale and Shin, 1981; Snider *et al.*, 1982)
    Inhibitory effects on Ia$^+$ antigen expression in the presence of interferon (Steeg *et al.*, 1982)
Indomethacin enhances:
    CSF production (Moore *et al.*, 1979)
    Interferon production (Moore *et al.*, 1980b)
    LAF production induced by murabutide (Damais *et al.*, 1982)
Indomethacin is without effect on:
    Inhibition of phagocytosis (Vogel *et al.*, 1979)
    Endogenous pyrogen release (Parant *et al.*, 1980c; Damais *et al.*, 1982)
    FAF release (Wahl and Wahl, 1981)
    Inhibition of clonal proliferation (Moore *et al.*, 1980a)
    Inhibition of thymidine uptake (Tanaka, 1982)
    Induction of listericidal activity (Hadden *et al.*, 1979)
    Induction of tumor cytotoxicity by BCG-elicited macrophages (Meltzer, 1981)
    Return of cytolytic activity in tumor macrophages cultured *in vitro* (Shaw *et al.*, 1979)

As an alternative mechanism of MDP action, Hadden (1978) has observed that MDP increases macrophage levels of cGMP and has suggested that this indomethacin-insensitive process may relate to actions of MDP as an inducer of macrophage proliferation and activation since other agents that stimulate these processes also act to increase cGMP.

Exposure of cultured tumor macrophages to LPS (100 ng/ml) causes a rapid resurgence of cytolytic activity (see Table 2B) that is preceded by a transient perturbation of the plasma membrane (detected by electron spin resonance techniques). No similar changes occur in membranes of thioglycollate-elicited macrophages or of $P388D_1$ cells incubated with the same concentration of LPS (Esser and Russell, 1979).

5.   TREHALOSE DIESTERS

5.1.   STRUCTURE AND PHYSICOCHEMICAL PROPERTIES

Mycobacteria, corynebacteria, and nocardiae synthesize as a part of their cell wall trehalose diesters (6,6'-diesters of α,α-D-trehalose) in which trehalose is

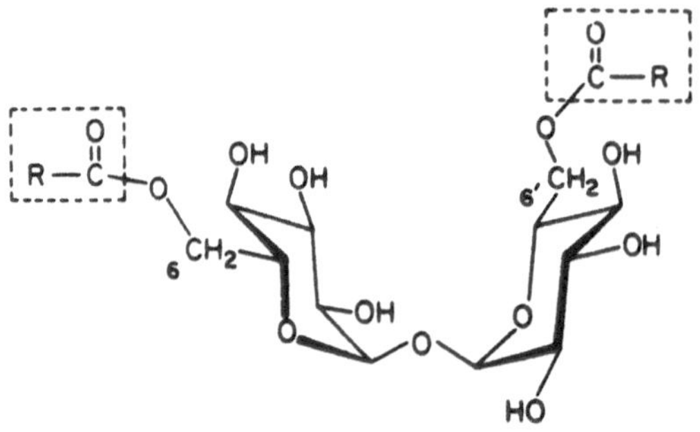

Total carbon number	Structure of R-C-OH $\overset{O}{\underset{\|}{}}$
$\sim C_{180}$ (cord factor = TDM = P_3)	Mycobacterial mycolic acids, i.e. : $CH_3(CH_2)_{19}CH-CH(CH_2)_{14}CH-CH-(CH_2)_{17}\overset{OH}{\underset{\|}{C}}H-CH-CO_2H$ with CH_2, CH_2, $C_{24}H_{49}$
1	$C_{84}H_{164}O_3$
C_{76}	Synthetic racemic $CH_3(CH_2)_{14}\overset{OH}{\underset{\|}{C}}-CH-CO_2H$ with H, $C_{14}H_{29}$
2	$C_{32}H_{64}O_3$

FIGURE 4.   Trehalose 6,6'-diesters.

esterified by long-chain β-hydroxy α-branched fatty acids called mycolic acids (Fig. 4). The size of the esterifying acids ranges from C_{28} in corynebacteria to about C_{90} in mycobacteria (for reviews see Asselineau and Asselineau, 1978; Lederer, 1979, 1980, 1982; Goren, 1982). Lower homologs have been synthesized (Polonsky et al., 1978) (they are designated by their total number of carbon atoms).

Most studies reported here have been made with TDM* isolated from the human virulent mycobacterial strains Brévannes and Peurois and the bovine attenuated BCG strain AN5. The trehalose diester produced by M. smegmatis contains two double bonds and can be used to obtain a tritiated derivative of high specific radioactivity (9 Ci/mmole) (Tenu, unpublished results).

Trehalose diesters are insoluble in water and must be used either as water/oil emulsions or as aqueous suspensions.

5.1.1. Emulsions of TDM (TDM/o)

Mineral oil such as Bayol F and Drakeol, peanut oil, squalene, or squalane with various amounts of Tween 80 have been used. The average size of oil droplets increases with increasing oil concentration and decreases with increasing Tween concentration: it also depends on the method, grinding or sonication, used to prepare the emulsion (Yarkoni and Rapp, 1977).

5.1.2. Aqueous Suspensions of TDM (TDM/w)

Kato (1970) proposed a method to prepare stable aqueous suspensions of TDM that can be kept several months at 4°C and diluted in saline (50 μg/ml) before use. Such TDM suspensions contain liposomelike particles: freeze-fracture electron microscopy revealed that the TDM particles have a concentric multilamellar structure with an intralamellar distance of 90 Å, thus containing little free water. From laser quasi-elastic light-scattering data the average diameter of the particles is 1.4 μm (Lepoivre et al., 1982). Phase-transition temperatures vary from 18 to 32°C, according to the size of the esterifying fatty acid (Durand et al., 1979a).

In contrast, when sonicated in an aqueous phase, TDM forms long cylindrical micelles (123 ± 16 Å in diameter), but which are inactive in vivo (Retzinger et al., 1982).

5.2. *IN VITRO* EFFECTS OF TDM ON MACROPHAGES

TDM/w particles ([³H]-TDM from M. smegmatis) are rapidly endocytized by thioglycollate-elicited macrophages (one-third of TDM/w added to the culture medium is endocytized after 20 hr compared to 0.2% for a soluble molecule such

---

*Mycobacterial trehalose diesters [i.e., trehalose dimycolates (TDM)] have also been named cord factor, or P_3.

as sucrose). Internalized TDM is retained in the cells up to 24 hr (Tenu, unpublished results), and thus might provide a permanent stimulus. However, the addition of TDM/w to macrophage monolayers does not elicit any cytostatic activity against tumor cells in resident peritoneal macrophages of mice (Tenu *et al.*, 1980) or rats (Reisser *et al.*, 1984). A moderate cytostatic activity is detected in thioglycollate-elicited macrophages treated by TDM/w (Tenu *et al.*, 1980).

Yarkoni *et al.* (1977) reported that TDM/o does not induce *in vitro* the increase of acid phosphatase activity and the stimulation of *L. monocytogenes* phagocytosis it produces when injected *in vivo*.

5.3. PROPERTIES OF MACROPHAGES FROM TDM-TREATED ANIMALS

5.3.1. Changes in Acid Phosphatase Activity and Antimicrobial Properties

Peritoneal macrophages harvested from mice that received 20–40 μg TDM/o 3 days previously exhibit a twofold increased acid phosphatase activity that persists at least 15 days. They also present an increased ability to phagocytize *L. monocytogenes* (Yarkoni *et al.*, 1977).

5.3.2. Antitumor Activity

When mice receive 50 μg TDM/w i.p. 7 days before harvesting the cells, the TDM-elicited macrophages inhibit *in vitro* the growth of P815 cells even at an effector/target ratio as low as 1.5. Macrophages elicited with the synthetic analog C_{76} also have a clear cytostatic effect (less than after treatment with TDM). The cytostasis takes place rapidly: DNA synthesis stops 2 hr after the beginning of cocultivation (Lepoivre *et al.*, 1982). TDM-elicited macrophages induce a specific release of [^{51}Cr] or [^{3}H]proline from prelabeled P815 cells (Orbach-Arbouys *et al.*, 1983). Similarly, Reisser *et al.* (1984) have shown that peritoneal macrophages harvested from TDM/w-treated rats were cytolytic for syngeneic intestinal tumor cells. Alveolar macrophages harvested from mice pretreated 1, 3, and 6 days earlier with 100 μg TDM/w i.v., exhibit a significant cytostatic activity against P815 tumor cells (Lepoivre, Nolibe, and Petit, unpublished results).

5.3.3. Biochemical Characteristics of TDM-Elicited Macrophages

Various biochemical parameters have been compared in mouse peritoneal resident macrophages and TDM/w-elicited macrophages, in an attempt to identify biochemical correlates of macrophage antitumor functional state. Results of these comparative studies are summarized in Table 8. Four parameters clearly distinguish TDM-elicited macrophages from noncytostatic macrophages. (1) There is a 10-fold reduction in alkaline phosphodiesterase activity (Lepoivre *et al.*, 1982). Morahan *et al.* (1980) proposed that a depressed level of alkaline phosphodiesterase was a correlate of antitumor activity in mouse peritoneal macrophages. Furthermore, such a modification of the level of an enzymatic

TABLE 8. COMPARISON OF SOME BIOCHEMICAL MARKERS IN TDM-ELICITED MACROPHAGES AND OTHER MACROPHAGE POPULATIONS[a]

Properties	TDM/w-elicited macrophages	Resident macrophages	Thioglycollate-elicited macrophages
Cytostatic efficiency (α)[b]	32	0	0
Cellular enzymatic activities[c]			
Alkaline phosphodiesterase	0.09 ± 0.02	0.9 ± 0.3	1.4 ± 0.5
β-Galactosidase	0.55 ± 0.15	1.5 ± 0.5	1.2 ± 0.3
Plasminogen activator	2.1 ± 1.5	0.6 ± 0.9	19.1 ± 7.7
Secretion			
H_2O_2[d]	0.95 ± 0.45	0	0.11 ± 0.04
Thromboxane B_2[e]	29 ± 6	9 ± 1	
6-Keto-$PGF_{1\alpha}$[e]	12 ± 4	127 ± 30	
Glycoproteins[f]			
Cellular	10.7	1.5	1.9
Secreted	6	2.4	0.5

[a] Data from Lepoivre et al. (1982), Lemaire et al. (1982), and Drapier et al. (1983 and unpublished results).
[b] For definition see Fig. 5.
[c] Specific activities measured in cell lysates prepared from macrophages cultured 4 hr and expressed as μmoles of product generated/hr per mg cellular protein.
[d] H_2O_2 (nmoles/min per 10^6 macrophages) released, upon PMA triggering, by macrophages cultured 4 hr.
[e] Released from [^{14}C]-20:4-prelabeled macrophages (cpm/μg cellular protein).
[f] [^3H]-2-D-mannose incorporated into proteins after 2 days [dpm ($\times 10^{-3}$)/μg cellular protein].

activity indicates that the peritoneal population has been renewed or modified at least by 90%, after TDM injection. (2) There is a 30-fold increase in the thromboxane B_2/6-keto-$PGF_{1\alpha}$ ratio (Drapier *et al.*, 1983). The overall amount of arachidonate metabolites released upon zymosan triggering is almost as great in TDM-elicited macrophages as in resident cells but arachidonic acid is converted into PGE_2 and thromboxane rather than into PGI_2. A similar profile was observed by Scott *et al.* (1982) for *C. parvum*-elicited macrophages. (3) The capacity to release O_2^- and H_2O_2 upon pharmacological triggering differs (Lepoivre *et al.*, 1982). Resident macrophages and thioglycollate-elicited macrophages do not release H_2O_2 after addition of PMA. TDM-elicited macrophages release large amounts of H_2O_2 (1 nmole H_2O_2/min per 10^6 cells). The release of H_2O_2 continues for at least 2 hr, yielding a concentration up to 50 μM in the macrophage environment. (4) There is a high rate of incorporation of mannose into glycoproteins: in TDM-elicited macrophages, the level of cellular mannosylated proteins is elevated 8-fold in comparison to resident cells. Their secretion is increased 3-fold (Grand-Perret and Lemaire, unpublished results).

In contrast, the cellular plasminogen activator activity is not significantly modified (Lepoivre *et al.*, 1982); TDM-elicited macrophages do not secrete spontaneously high amounts of LAF but their capacity to secrete LAF is considerably increased by *in vitro* addition of muramyl peptides (Tenu *et al.*, 1980).

5.4. *IN VIVO* EFFECTS OF TDM

5.4.1. Granuloma Formation

The intensity of the granulomatous reaction induced in lungs of mice by TDM/o i.v. depends on the size of the oil droplets (Yarkoni and Rapp, 1977). The synthetic C_{76} ester is not granulomagenic (Yarkoni *et al.*, 1978).

5.4.2. Nonspecific Resistance to Infections

Mice pretreated with TDM (emulsified in Bayol F 0.4%, Tween 0.04%) are protected against an i.p. challenge with *S. typhimurium* (50% of survivors) (Yarkoni and Bekierkunst, 1976). C_{76} (emulsified in Bayol F), injected i.v. 14 days before challenge, protects 70% of the mice against *L. monocytogenes* (Parant *et al.*, 1978a). An injection of TDM/w, under the same conditions, increases the percentage of survivors from 8% to 81% (Parant *et al.*, 1977).

TDM/w induces resistance of mice against *Schistosoma mansoni* (Olds *et al.*, 1980) and *Babesia microti* (Clark, 1979).

5.4.3. Resistance to Tumors

TDM (emulsified in Bayol F or in peanut oil) shows a marked antitumor activity against L1210 leukemia (Leclerc *et al.*, 1976). Injection of TDM/w (50 μg i.p.) protects to some extent mice against the grafting 7 days later of P815 cells or L1210 cells (Orbach-Arbouys *et al.*, 1983); C_{76} is less active.

TDM/o is as active as living BCG for suppressing urethan-induced lung adenomas (Bekierkunst *et al.*, 1971). Regressions of established tumors after TDM/o treatment have been described: regression of a murine fibrosarcoma after intralesional injection of TDM/o or C_{76} (Yarkoni *et al.*, 1978) and of a rat ascitic tumor by i.p. injection of TDM/o or some lower synthetic analogs (Pimm *et al.*, 1979).

5.5. MECHANISM OF ACTION

5.5.1. Interaction with Proteins and Phospholipids

Studying the structure–activity relationship of glycolipids, Kato *et al.* (1978) proposed that the absence of toxicity of the short-chain esters is explained by their neutralization by serum albumin. It has been suggested by Retzinger *et al.* (1981) that properties of trehalose diesters in oil emulsions did not involve recognition of specific structures of the glycolipid molecule and that the essential parameter is the hydrophile/lipophile balance (HLB) of the compound: only those with an HLB > 2 are able to concentrate proteins on the surface of oil droplets and are adjuvants (Hunter *et al.*, 1981).

The effects of TDM/o can be reproduced by a monomolecular film formed by the glycolipid on the surface of hydrophobic polystyrene beads. These TDM monolayers adsorb fibrinogen; the adsorption is thought to be required for maximal biological activity (Retzinger *et al.*, 1982). The hypothesis that fibrinogen is a cofactor of TDM activity may explain the finding by Kelly (1977) that TDM/o is chemotactic for oil-elicited guinea pig macrophages in the presence of plasma (but not in the presence of serum).

A stronger interaction with biological membrane components (especially PC) is observed when the glycolipids are in the fluid state rather than in the gel state (Durand *et al.*, 1979b; Lanéelle and Tocanne, 1980).

5.5.2. Modification of the Peritoneal Cell Population after i.p. Injection of TDM

After injection of TDM/w (50 μg i.p.), the number of peritoneal cells first decreases; 2 days after treatment it rises up to 3-fold and is back to normal on day 5 (Tenu, unpublished results). Seven days after TDM administration, more than 45% of peritoneal macrophages have peroxidase-positive granules (vs. 10% in untreated animals). These observations and the 10-fold decrease in the level of macrophage alkaline phosphodiesterase (see Section 5.3.3) suggest an important renewal of the peritoneal macrophage population after TDM injection.

5.5.3. Role of Macrophages

When TDM/w is injected in thymectomized, irradiated mice, the macrophages harvested 7 days later exhibit the same cytostatic activity as TDM-elicited macrophages from normal animals (Orbach-Arbouys *et al.*, 1983). This suggests that T lymphocytes are not necessary for the activation of peritoneal macrophages by TDM/w. When mice are treated with cobra venom factor (a C3b-like glycoprotein), TDM/w no longer induces a protection of the animals against L1210 and the peritoneal macrophages are not cytostatic *in vitro* (Orbach and Tenu, unpublished results). Macrophage activation thus seems to be an important component of the antitumor activity of TDM.

The relative inability of TDM/w to activate macrophages *in vitro* raises two questions. Are there macrophage subpopulations especially responsive to TDM? Is the activation mediated by soluble factors [complement components as suggested by Ramanathan *et al.* (1980) or fibrinogen-derived peptides as suggested by Retzinger *et al.* (1982)]?

5.6. SYNERGY WITH OTHER PRODUCTS

The capacity of several immunostimulants to act in synergy has mainly been studied in experiments of regression of the line 10 hepatocarcinoma of the strain 2 guinea pig growing intradermally and of its metastases (Zbar *et al.*, 1974). In this system, living BCG can be replaced by crude cell walls attached to oil droplets (Ribi *et al.*, 1976). Deproteinized delipidated cell walls (covalent skeleton) are inactive but their activity can be restored by TDM (Azuma *et al.*, 1974). In the presence of oil, a combination of TDM with an Re endotoxin of *S. typhimurium* is active (Ribi *et al.*, 1976); the endotoxin can be replaced by two nontoxic subfractions (Qureshi *et al.*, 1982). Complete cures can be obtained using combinations of defined immunomodulators: TDM plus nor-MDP or MDP(Abu) (McLaughlin *et al.*, 1980) or TDM plus MDP (Yarkoni *et al.*, 1981).

6. SYNTHETIC POLYNUCLEOTIDES

6.1. PREPARATION AND CHARACTERISTICS

Synthetic polynucleotides are prepared by the action of polynucleotide phosphorylase on nucleotide diphosphates. The poly(I:C) or poly(A:U) complexes are spontaneously formed when polymerized single strands, from opposite base pairs, are mixed.

Rapid hydrolysis of poly(I:C) by an enzyme found in primate serum appears responsible for its absence of antitumor and antiviral activity in man. A stabilized complex of poly(I:C) with poly(L-Lys) [poly(ICLC)] is significantly more resistant to hydrolysis (Krown *et al.*, 1981). Poly(A:U) is active in man (Lacour *et al.*, 1980).

Only double-stranded complexes are active as immune stimulants (Johnson, 1979). Polymers with high molecular weights (> 20 S) are more efficient (Niblack and McCreary, 1971). Poly(I:C) is toxic and pyrogenic; however, polymers with mismatched bases preserve the ability to induce interferon but do not elicit undesirable effects (Carter *et al.*, 1981). Incorporation of poly(I:C) into liposomes might reduce toxicity (Magee, 1978).

Schell (1971) has shown that poly(I:C) is adsorbed on the surface of mammalian cells; the double-strand complex does not enter the cell as an entity, poly(C) remaining at the cell surface while part of the poly(I) enters the cell.

6.2. EFFECT ON MACROPHAGES *IN VITRO*

The ability of poly(A:U) to amplify antibody response is probably due to its action on macrophages: when thioglycollate-elicited peritoneal exudate cells are incubated *in vitro* with antigen plus poly(A:U), washed, and reinjected into syngeneic mice, an important boost in circulating antibodies is observed (Johnson and Johnson, 1971). Adherent cells are essential for the effect of poly(A:U) in mixed lymphocyte culture (Narayanan *et al.*, 1978).

Macrophages (adherent spleen cells and PU5-1.8 cells) (Djeu *et al.*, 1979) or bone marrow-derived macrophages (Havell and Spitalny, 1980; Fleit and Rabinovitch, 1981) produce interferon in response to poly(I:C) and poly(A:U). Interferon produced by macrophages probably mediates the poly(I:C) effect on NK cells: *in vitro*, inactivation or depletion of macrophages by silica, carrageenan, or rayon adherence, effectively inhibited poly(I:C) boosting of fresh spleen cells for NK activity (Djeu *et al.*, 1979).

Alexander and Evans (1971) were the first to point out that dsRNAs, poly(I:C), and poly(A:U) could render mouse peritoneal macrophages cytotoxic for tumor cells. Their observations have been confirmed by several authors (Johnson, 1979; Schultz *et al.*, 1977b; Taramelli and Varesio, 1981). According to Taramelli and Varesio (1981), poly(I:C) is a more powerful inducer of cytolytic macrophages than LPS or MAF. (1) Poly(I:C), in contrast to MAF, shows no requirement for LPS to activate macrophages. (2) Poly(I:C) but not MAF or LPS is able to induce strong cytolytic activity in resident macrophages. (3) Poly(I:C) (at high concentration) has the ability to overcome the defect of macrophages from C3H/HeJ mice, which do not respond to MAF or LPS. (4) In kinetic studies, it appears that poly(I:C), in contrast to MAF or LPS, activates macrophages in a short time (2-hr pulse). Incubation of murine peritoneal macrophages with poly(A:U) augments their cytotoxic activity against syngeneic leukemia cells and the metabolism of glucose through the hexose monophosphate pathway (Johnson, 1982).

6.3. PROPERTIES OF MACROPHAGES HARVESTED FROM ANIMALS TREATED *IN VIVO*

Intravenous injection of poly(I:C) induces an increased spreading of mouse peritoneal macrophages (Rabinovitch *et al.*, 1977) and an augmentation of their ability to phagocytize opsonized erythrocytes (Hamburg *et al.*, 1978).

Mouse peritoneal macrophages harvested 7 days after injection of poly(I:C) exhibit *in vitro* a cytostatic activity against an M109 syngeneic alveolar carcinoma (Schultz *et al.*, 1977a). Maximal *in vitro* cytostatic activity against an MBL-2 target is observed with macrophages harvested 1 day after injection of poly(ICLC) (Bartocci *et al.*, 1982).

6.4. *IN VIVO* EFFECTS

Macrophages seem to be the origin for most of poly(I:C)-induced circulating interferon: Jullien *et al.* (1974) demonstrated that serum interferon produced after i.v. administration of poly(I:C) originates from radioresistant cells derived from the hemopoietic system; inoculation of mice with silica or carrageenan before i.p. injection of poly(I:C) decreases the level of circulating interferon (Djeu *et al.*, 1979); it also depresses the augmentation of NK activity in the spleen.

Macrophages may also be responsible for the antibacterial effect of poly(A:U) in experimental murine brucellosis: administration of this poly-nucleotide close to the time of injection of *B. abortus* reduces markedly the number of these organisms in the spleen and liver of CBA/H mice 10-days later (Madraso and Cheers, 1978a,b). Poly(A:U) is as effective against *Brucella* in athymic *nu/nu* mice as in normal mice and no antibodies were found in pro-tected animals (Renoux *et al.*, 1972; Cheers and Cone, 1974).

7. POLYSACCHARIDES

Polysaccharides with antitumor activity have been isolated from bacteria, fungi, lichens, yeast, and plants (for reviews see Whistler *et al.*, 1976; Aszalos, 1981). The properties of lentinan, a β(1→3)glucan from *Lentinus edodes*, which has been extensively studied in animals and clinical experiments, are described in Chapter 11 of this volume. We will thus restrict our discussion to the mac-rophage-dependent effects of some purified polysaccharides: β(1→3)glucans, mannans, and mannozym from the *Saccharomyces cerevisiae* cell wall, schizo-phyllan from the culture broth of *Schizophyllum commune*, and levan from *Aero-bacter levan.*

7.1. β(1→3)GLUCANS FROM *S. CEREVISIAE*

7.1.1. Preparation

Mannan fractions are obtained from hot water extract of yeast cells and glucans by alkaline extraction of the residue. The preparation of a particulate, water-insoluble glucan has been described by DiLuzio *et al.* (1979). Soluble glucans obtained by acid hydrolysis of particulate glucan are active at high dosage only, but, contrary to the insoluble glucan, they do not induce hepato-splenomegaly (DiLuzio *et al.*, 1979).

7.1.2. Properties of Macrophages Harvested from Animals Treated *in Vivo*

Macrophages from glucan-treated animals are different from resident macrophages in size, chemotactic mobility, spreading, adherence, and surface morphology (Burgaleta *et al.*, 1978). They release high amounts of arachidonic acid derivatives (Way *et al.*, 1982) and produce increased CSF compared to controls (Burgaleta and Golde, 1977).

Glucan-elicited macrophages exhibit cytostatic activity against syngeneic M109 lung carcinoma cells (Schultz *et al.*, 1977a), against mammary carcinoma and RI leukemia cells (Cook *et al.*, 1978; Bomford and Moreno, 1981), and against MBL-2 allogeneic tumor targets (Schultz *et al.*, 1978). They reduce the *in vitro* multiplication of *Leishmania donovani* (Cook *et al.*, 1982).

7.1.3. *In Vivo* Effects

Glucan has been shown to increase both the number and the activity of cells of the monocyte-macrophage system. A 2-fold increase in peripheral leukocytes along with an increase in the total macrophage count of the spleen, bone marrow, and peritoneal cavity were observed in glucan-treated mice. One week after injection of glucan, there is a 10-fold increase in colony-forming cells in the spleen and a 2-fold increase in the bone marrow and the peritoneal cavity (Burgaleta and Golde, 1977).

The i.v. administration of glucan enhances the clearance of colloidal carbon in rats (Kohoshis *et al.*, 1978). It promotes a hyperphagocytic state associated with Kupffer cell activation, and granuloma formation (Way *et al.*, 1982).

Glucan-treated animals are protected against *S. aureus* (DiLuzio and Williams, 1978), Venezuelan equine encephalomyelitis virus, and Rift Valley fever virus (Reynolds *et al.*, 1980). Destruction of *M. leprae*, growing in the footpad of mice, is enhanced by i.v. glucan treatment (Delville and Jacques, 1980). Injection of methylpalmitate, which is reported to reverse macrophage activation, negates the beneficial effect of glucan administration in mice challenged by *E. coli* (Williams *et al.*, 1982). The administration of glucan to mice and rats inhibits the growth of tumor cells of many types (for reviews see Whistler *et al.*, 1976; Arrigoni-Martelli, 1981). The protective effect is thought to be mainly mediated by glucan-activated macrophages: (1) the inhibition of melanoma B16 proliferation occurs both in normal and in athymic mice (Cook *et al.*, 1978); (2) the depression of lung nodule formation due to i.v. administration of $\beta(1\to3)$-linked glucans resists 800-R whole body irradiation (Bomford and Olivetto, 1974).

7.2. MANNANS, MANNOZYM, SCHIZOPHYLLAN, AND LEVAN

7.2.1. Origin and Structure

Yeast mannan consists of an α-D$(1\to6)$-linked backbone with side chains containing α-D$(1\to3)$ and α-D$(1\to2)$ linkages. Wild-type strains possess a high degree of branching compared to some mutants (Matsumoto *et al.*, 1982). The extracellular linear mannan produced by *Rhodotorula rubra* contains $\beta(1\rightarrow3)$ and $\beta(1\rightarrow4)$ links (M_r 65,000–120,000) (Elinov *et al.*, 1982).

Mannozym is a glucomannan from *S. cerevisiae* (Bartocci *et al.*, 1982).

Schizophyllan is isolated from the culture broth of the fungus *Schizophyllum commune*: it is a β-D$(1\rightarrow3)$glucan having a β-D-glucopyranosyl group linked $1\rightarrow6$ to every third or fourth residue of the main chain (Mitani *et al.*, 1982).

Levan, a polyfructose with mostly $\beta(2\rightarrow6)$ links, is extracted from the cell wall of *A. levan* (Bomford and Moreno, 1981).

7.2.2. *In Vitro* and *in Vivo* Effects on Macrophages

R. rubra mannans added *in vitro* to macrophages stimulate chemotaxis, attachment to glass, and phagocytic and degradative activities. Injected *in vivo* they elicit macrophages with analogous properties (Elinov *et al.*, 1982). Macrophages from polysaccharide-treated animals limit *in vitro* the growth of tumor cells (Table 9).

Polysaccharides have strong antitumor activity when administered *in vivo*. However, there are few data documenting the participation of macrophages. Mannans, for example, are highly active *in vivo*: at a dose of 150 mg/kg during 10 successive days, mannan from *S. cerevisiae* gives a complete protection (96% survivors) against sarcoma 80 and Ehrlich carcinoma and definite regression of the same tumors (Matsumoto *et al.*, 1982); however, no data are available concerning the macrophages harvested from these animals, and cytostatic activity induced *in vitro* by mannan is low (Table 9). The activity of schizophyllan seems mediated, in part, by macrophages: studies by electron microscopic auto-

TABLE 9. *IN VITRO* ANTITUMOR PROPERTIES OF POLYSACCHARIDE-TREATED MACROPHAGES[a]

Polysaccharide	Treatment	Target	% GI	References
Mannan	*In vitro* 4 mg/ml resident macrophages	Ehrlich carcinoma, E/T = 10	27%	Matsumoto *et al.* (1982)
Glucan	*In vivo* 25 mg/kg i.p. day −7	M109 (S), E/T = 10	35%	Schultz *et al.* (1977c)
	5 mg/kg i.p. day −6	MBL2 (A), E/T = 10	95%	Schultz *et al.* (1978)
Schizophyllan	100 mg/kg day −7	Lewis carcinoma (S)		Izumi *et al.* (1982)
Levan	50 mg/kg i.p. day −6	MBL2 (A), E/T = 10	81%	Bartocci *et al.* (1982)
Mannozym	4 mg/kg i.p. day −3	MBL2 (A), E/T = 10	95%	Bartocci *et al.* (1982)

[a]M109, spontaneous lung carcinoma of the BALB/c mouse; MBL2, lymphoblastic leukemia cells; (S), tumor cells and macrophages are syngeneic; (A), tumor cells and macrophages are allogeneic.

radiography show that tritiated schizophyllan is concentrated in macrophages surrounding tumor cells in mice responsive to the action of the polysaccharide (Mizuhira *et al.*, 1982a,b), and schizophyllan-elicited macrophages are cytostatic *in vitro* (Table 9).

8. SECONDARY METABOLITES

8.1. CYCLOMUNINE

The hexacyclodepsipeptide cyclomunine, a metabolite of *Fusarium equiseti*, increases *in vitro* various parameters of resident rat peritoneal macrophages such as D-glucosamine incorporation, neutral protease release, ability to produce O_2^- upon phagocytosis of zymosan, cytotoxic activity against DHD-K12 tumor cells, or ability to kill *Schistosoma mansoni* larvae in the presence of immune serum. Injection (i.v. or i.p.) of cyclomunine induces, in the peritoneal cavity, macrophages activated for antitumor or bactericidal activity (Joseph *et al.*, 1981).

8.2. BESTATIN

The dipeptide bestatin, an inhibitor of aminopeptidase B produced by an actinomycete (Umezawa, 1980), is also able to increase *in vitro* various macrophage functions such as the ability to release activated oxygen or cytotoxic activity against tumor cells (Schorlemmer *et al.*, 1982a). *In vitro* activated macrophages injected simultaneously with tumor cells have an antitumor effect. Bestatin injected i.p. induces cytotoxic macrophages in the peritoneal cavity (Schorlemmer *et al.*, 1982b).

9. CONCLUSIONS

Most of the immunomodulators presented in this review are able to interact *in vitro* with macrophages and two of them, LPS and MDP, have been found active on several macrophage tumor cell lines. The changes induced *in vitro*, in macrophage functional properties, by all these products of such diverse molecular weight and chemical structure seem, however, similar. In the case of LPS and muramyl peptides, enough data are available for comparison: both immunomodulators inhibit macrophage migration, have an antiproliferative action, but stimulate spreading, adherence, and glucosamine incorporation; they both enhance the production of LAF, EP, CSF, collagenase, and prostaglandins and prime macrophage for O_2^- release. However, MDP, in contrast to LPS, does not seem able to induce the production of interferon (see Leclerc and Chedid 1982; for exception to this statement, see Chapter 1 of this volume). Quantitative comparisons of the efficiency of the two immunomodulators are more difficult because they have been tested only in a few parallel experiments. In most assays, LPS appears 100-fold more active, on a weight basis, than MDP or derivatives: inhibition of migration (Nagao *et al.*, 1982), inhibition of plasminogen activator release (Drapier *et al.*, 1982), priming for O_2^- production (Pabst and Johnston, 1980); changes are also more rapid and more pronounced with LPS (Pabst and Johnston, 1980; Wood and Staruch, 1980). However, in some cases, active doses, kinetics of action, and magnitude of the effects are similar for LPS and MDP: for example, Wahl *et al.* (1980) observed maximal PGE and collagenase production after treatment with 10 μg/ml MDP and 30 μg/ml LPS. Thus, the relative efficiency of LPS and MDP seems to vary depending on the parameter measured: this may reflect real differences in the specificity of the two compounds or may be explained if some species of macrophages (oil-induced guinea pig macrophages, alveolar macrophages) respond comparatively better to MDP than other populations.

Macrophages are extremely plastic cells: changes in their morphology and metabolism are not automatically linked to the appearance of an activated state, with antimicrobial and antitumor activities. It is important to recognize whether exogenous immunomodulators do in fact activate macrophages. Reports about *in vitro* activation of macrophages to cytotoxicity are indeed conflicting (Table 2A), and comparisons of the results obtained with various immunomodulators are hazardous because the compounds have been tested in different systems: (1) E/T ratios used in *in vitro* antitumor activity assays vary from 1 to 50. (2) Some targets are more resistant to macrophages than others. (3) Three types of assays are used, which measure different parameters: growth inhibition, loss of cellular integrity, reduction of the number of adherent target cells. (4) The mode of expression of the results may also be misleading: the percent of growth inhibition, often used to evaluate cytostasis, does not accurately reflect the relative potentialities of various macrophage populations (Fig. 5). From Table 10 it ap-

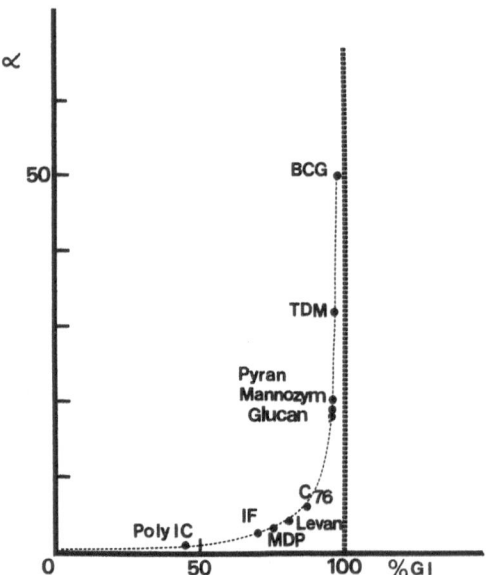

FIGURE 5. Cytostatic efficiency (α), a new parameter to evaluate *in vitro* cytostatic activity (Tenu, unpublished).

The percentage of growth inhibition (GI) is given as $[(R - X)/R] \times 100$, where R is the increase of target cell number when cultivated on control macrophages and X is the increase of target cell number when cultivated on stimulated macrophages. The cytostatic efficiency α is given as $(R/X) - 1$. At the end of the coculture, the increase in target cell number cocultivated with control macrophages is (α + 1)-fold higher than that observed in the presence of stimulated macrophages. When both numbers are identical, α = 0. For strong cytostatic activities, % GI is very close to 100, its limit value, whereas the increase of α is not limited. A plot of α versus % GI shows that α discriminates among strongly activated macrophage populations. The data are from Table 11.

TABLE 10. COMPARISON OF THE ANTITUMOR ACTIVITY INDUCED IN RESIDENT MACROPHAGES BY VARIOUS IMMUNOMODULATORS

Macrophages	Immunomodulator	Effect[a]	References
Peritoneal macrophages (mouse)	MDP	α = 0.5–2	Juy and Chedid (1975), Matter (1979), Tenu et al. (1980)
	TDM	α = 0.7	Tenu et al. (1980)
	Poly(I:C)	α = 2.3	Schultz et al. (1977a)
		SR = 30%	Taramelli and Varesio (1981)
	LPS	SR = 40%	Taffet et al. (1981); see also Table 2A
	Pyran	α = 3–4	Schultz et al. (1977a)
	Interferon	α = 10	Schultz et al. (1977b)
Peritoneal macrophages (rat)	MDP	SR = 18%	Reisser et al. (1982)
	TDM	SR = 0%	Reisser et al. (1984)
Alveolar macrophages (mouse)	MDP	SR = 33%	Fidler et al. (1981)
	MDP in liposomes	SR = 60%	
Alveolar macrophages (rat)	MDP	SR = 30%	Sone and Fidler (1981)
	MDP in liposomes	SR = 60–70%	
Alveolar macrophages (human)	MDP	SR = 15–35%	Sone and Tsubara (1982)
	MDP in liposomes	SR = 37–47%	
	LPS	SR = 38–59%	

[a]α = cytostatic efficiency (see Fig. 5); SR = specific release.

pears that poly(I:C) and LPS are stimulatory, even for mouse resident peritoneal macrophages (whether interferon is involved as an intermediate is not clear). Other immunomodulators require more receptive macrophages, adequate presentation (liposomes for instance), or the presence of lymphokines. Both LPS and MDP act in synergy with lymphokines: the active dose can be lowered to the nanogram range for LPS and to the microgram range for MDP. Since LPS is efficient at very low concentrations, especially when used at the same time as lymphokines, its absence must be carefully checked before concluding that a drug or a lymphokine preparation is active (Weinberg *et al.*, 1978; Wood and Cameron, 1978; Fox and Rajaraman, 1980; Lachman and Metzgar, 1980). At least two factors seem to limit the efficiency of immunomodulators *in vitro*: the number of responsive macrophages in a given population [1/10 according to the data of Meltzer *et al.* (1980) in untreated mouse peritoneal macrophages] and a negative feedback probably exerted by prostaglandins (Taffet *et al.*, 1981).

In Table 11 are compared the *in vitro* antitumor activities of macrophages elicited *in vivo* by various immunomodulators. A comparison of Tables 10 and 11 clearly shows that some immunomodulators are relatively more effective *in vivo* (TDM, pyran) and others more active *in vitro* [poly(I:C)]. Correlations between the macrophage cytotoxicity measured *in vitro* and the increase of life span of tumor-bearing mice observed, for example, after pretreatment with glucan and poly(I:C), with TDM and its synthetic analog C_{76}, or with MDP encapsulated in liposomes support a role of macrophages in control of tumor development.

Another possibility to evaluate the ability of a drug to activate macrophages is to examine the drug's capacity to protect animals against a challenge with intracellular bacteria or parasites. As shown in Table 12, several purified immunomodulators of microbial origin and synthetic molecules increase the survival time of animals infected with *L. monocytogenes*, *T. gondii*, or *T. cruzi*, pathogens efficiently killed by activated macrophages only.

Several kinds of advantages can *a priori* be expected from the use of purified or synthetic immunomodulators: reproducible chemical and physical properties, less toxicity, increased specificity, and, thus, better efficiency. In fact, most of the synthetic or purified immunomodulators are not devoid of toxicity but, in some instances, it is possible to suppress undesirable side effects by chemical modifications, without loss of activity: a derivative of MDP, murabutide (see Table 5), is not pyrogenic, does not induce leukopenia (Damais *et al.*, 1982), but has retained the adjuvant and antiinfectious activities of MDP.

Contrary to expectation, even a simple molecule such as MDP has a large array of target cells and elicits a great number of seemingly unrelated effects. It has been possible to dissociate some of these activities by synthesizing ad hoc analogs. MDP(Ser), for instance, is still adjuvant but has no antiinfectious activity (Audibert *et al.*, 1980); in contrast, "triglymyc" (see Table 5) is not adjuvant but stimulates nonspecific resistance to infections (Parant *et al.*, 1980a).

As far as efficiency is concerned, adequate targeting and/or chemical modifications can render to synthetic molecules some of the properties of complex natural products they have lost: appropriate targeting and presentation of MDP in liposomes (Fidler *et al.*, 1982) returns to this molecule the antitumor properties

TABLE 11. COMPARISON OF THE ANTITUMOR ACTIVITY OF MACROPHAGES ELICITED BY VARIOUS IMMUNOMODULATORS[a]

Macrophages	Eliciting agent	Antitumor activity in vitro	Target	In vivo effects	References
Peritoneal macrophages (mouse)	MDP	α = 3	Fibrosarcoma (A)	No effect	Matter (1979)
	LPS	α = 0	P815 (S)	No effect	Leclerc et al. (1976)
	TDM	α = 6–9	P815 (S)	See Parr et al. (1973)	Juy and Chedid (1975)
	C_{76}	α = 32	P815 (S)	P815 growth reduced	Orbach-Arbouys et al. (1983)
	Poly(I:C)	α = 6	M109 (S)	25% increase in life span	Lepoivre et al. (1982)
	Poly(ICLC)	α = 0.8	MBL2 (A)		Schultz et al. (1977c)
	Glucan	α = 3	MBL2 (A)		Bartocci et al. (1982)
		α = 19	M109 (S)	20% increase in life span	Schultz et al. (1978)
	Levan	α = 0.5	MBL2 (A)		Schultz et al. (1977c)
	Mannozym	α = 4	MBL2 (A)		Bartocci et al. (1982)
		α = 19	MBL2 (A)		Bartocci et al. (1982)
	BCG	α = 49	P815 (S)	See Creau-Goldberg and Salomon (1980)	Germain et al. (1975)
	Interferon	α = 2.3	MBL2 (A)		Stoychkov et al. (1979)
	Pyran	α = 20	MBL2 (A)		Stoychkov et al. (1979)
		α = 2.3	M109 (S)	60% increase in life span	Schultz et al. (1977c)
Alveolar macrophages (mouse)	MDP	SR = 0%	B16 (S)	No effect	Fidler et al. (1981)
	MDP in liposomes	SR = 41%	B16 (S)	Eradication of lung metastases	Fidler et al. (1981)

[a] α, cytostatic efficiency (see Fig. 5); SR, specific release; B16, melanoma of the C57BL/6 mouse; (S), tumor cells and macrophages are syngeneic; (A), tumor cells and macrophages are allogeneic. For each immunomodulator, optimal data are given.

TABLE 12. PROTECTION AGAINST INTRACELLULAR PATHOGENS INDUCED BY IMMUNOMODULATORS

Immunomodulator	Treatment	Protection against	References
LPS	1 μg (i.v.) day −1	*Listeria monocytogenes* (i.v.)	Galelli et al. (1981)
	200 μg (i.p.) day −5	*Listeria monocytogenes* (i.v.)	Fauve and Delaunay (1966)
MDP	0.5 mg (i.p.) day −2	*Trypanosoma cruzi* (trypomastigotes, i.p.)	Kierszenbaum and Ferraresi (1979)
	1.3 mg (s.c.) day −1	*Toxoplasma gondii* (tachyzoites, i.p.)	Krahenbuhl et al. (1981)
Nor-MDP, MDP(Abu)	1.5 mg (i.p.) day −4 to day −1	*Listeria monocytogenes* (i.p.)	Fraser-Smith et al. (1981)
MDP-A-L	10 μg (i.v.) day −4	*Listeria monocytogenes* (i.v.)	Chedid et al. (1979)
LTP	40 μg (i.p.) day −1	*Listeria monocytogenes* (i.v.)	Floc'h et al. (1981)
TDM/o	150 μg (i.v.) day −4	*Listeria monocytogenes* (i.v.)	Parant et al. (1978a)
TDM/w	150 μg (i.v.) day −14	*Listeria monocytogenes* (i.v.)	Parant et al. (1977)
Poly(A:U)	500 μg (i.p.) 1 hr after challenge	*Brucella abortus* (i.v.)	Cheers and Cone (1974)
Glucan		*Mycobacterium leprae* (in the footpad)	Delville and Jacques (1980)

of mycobacterial cells. Quinonyl-MDP-66 is as effective as crude BCG cell for curing the hepatocarcinoma of the line 10 guinea pig (Yamamura and Azuma, 1982; Saiki *et al.*, 1982). Further potentialities of microbially derived products as immunomodulators will no doubt be revealed by future work, especially synthesis of new analogs and derivatives and improved modes of presentation.

REFERENCES

Adam, A., Ciorbaru, R., Petit, J.-F., and Lederer, E., 1972, Isolation and properties of a macromolecular, water-soluble, immunoadjuvant fraction from the cell wall of *Mycobacterium smegmatis, Proc. Natl. Acad. Sci. USA* **69**:851.

Adam, A., Ellouz, F., Ciorbaru, R., Petit, J.-F., and Lederer, E., 1975, Peptidoglycan adjuvants: Minimal structure required for activity, *Z. Immunitaetsforsch.* **149**:341.

Adam, A., Souvannavong, V., and Lederer, E., 1978, Nonspecific MIF-like activity induced by the synthetic immunoadjuvant N-acetylmuramyl-L-alanyl-D-isoglutamine (MDP), *Biochem. Biophys. Res. Commun.* **85**:684.

Adam, A., Petit, J.-F., Lefrancier, P., and Lederer, E., 1981, Muramyl peptides: Chemical structure, biological activity and mechanism of action, *Mol. Cell. Biochem.* **41**:27.

Adams, D. O., and Marino, P. A., 1981, Evidence of a multistep mechanism of cytolysis by BCG-activated macrophages: The interrelationship between the capacity for cytolysis, target binding and secretion of cytolytic factor, *J. Immunol.* **126**:981.

Alexander, P., and Evans, R., 1971, Endotoxin and double stranded RNA render macrophages cytotoxic, *Nature New Biol.* **232**:76.

Allison, A. C., Davies, P., and Page, R. C., 1973, Effects of endotoxin on macrophages and other lymphoreticular cells, in: *Bacterial Lipopolysaccharides* (E. H. Kass and S. M. Wolff, eds.), pp. 204–211, University of Chicago Press, Chicago.

Apte, R. N., Galanos, C., and Pluznik, D. H., 1976, Lipid A, the active part of bacterial endotoxins in inducing serum colony stimulating activity and proliferation of splenic granulocyte/macrophage progenitor cells, *J. Cell. Physiol.* **87**:71.

Arrigoni-Martelli, E., 1981, Developments in drugs enhancing the immune responses, *Meth. Find. Exp. Clin. Pharmacol.* **3**:247.

Asselineau, C., and Asselineau, J., 1978, Trehalose containing glycolipids, *Prog. Chem. Fats Other Lipids* **16**:59.

Aszalos, A., 1981, Immunomodulators of microbial origin, in: *Antitumor Compounds of Natural Origin: Chemistry and Biochemistry* (A. Aszalos, ed.), pp. 155–190, CRC Press, Boca Raton, Fla.

Audibert, F., Parant, M., Damais, C., Lefrancier, P., Derrien, M., Choay, J., and Chedid, L., 1980, Dissociation of immunostimulant activities of muramyl dipeptide (MDP) by linking amino-acids or peptides to the glutaminyl residue, *Biochem. Biophys. Res. Commun.* **96**:915.

Azuma, I., Ribi, E., Meyer, T., and Zbar, B., 1974, Biologically active components from mycobacterial cell walls: Isolation and composition of cell wall skeleton and component P3, *J. Natl. Cancer Inst.* **52**:95.

Azuma, I., Sugimura, K., Yamawaki, M., Uemiya, M., Kusumoto, S., Okada, O., Shiba, T., and Yamamura, Y., 1978, Adjuvant activity of synthetic 6-O-"mycoloyl"-N-acetyl muramyl-L-alanyl-D-isoglutamine and related compounds, *Infect. Immun.* **20**:600.

Azuma, I., Yamawaki, M., Uemiya, M., Saiki, I., Panio, Y., Kobayashi, S., Fukuda, T., Imaeda, I., and Yamamura, Y., 1979, Adjuvant and antitumor activities of quinonyl-N-acetylmuramyl-dipeptides, *Gann* **76**:847.

Barot-Ciorbaru, R., Wietzerbin, J., Petit, J.-F., Chedid, L., Falcoff, E., and Lederer, E., 1978, Induction of interferon synthesis in mice by fractions from *Nocardia, Infect. Immun.* **19**:353.

Barot-Ciorbaru, R., Catinot, L., Wietzerbin, J., Petit, J.-F., Chedid, L., and Falcoff, E., 1981a, Involvement of a radioresistant cell in production of circulating interferon induced by *Nocardia* fractions in mice, *J. Reticuloendothel. Soc.* **30**:247.

Barot-Ciorbaru, R., Petit, J.-F., Chassoux, D. R., and Salomon, J.-C., 1981b, Antitumor activity of intralesionally administered *Nocardia opaca* preparations in rat and mouse tumors: A comparison with BCG and *Corynebacterium parvum*, *Int. J. Immunopharmacol.* **3**:115.

Barot-Ciorbaru, R., Boschetti, E., Falcoff, E., Chedid, L., and Petit, J.-F., 1982, Delipidated cells, cell wall, peptidoglycan and soluble fractions of *Nocardiae* as immunomodulators. Affinity chromatography behaviour of NWSM induced interferon (IF), 5th European Immunology Meeting, Istanbul, p. 305.

Bartocci, A., Read, E. L., Welker, R. D., Schilck, E., Papademetriou, V., and Chirigos, M. A., 1982, Enhancing activity of various immunoaugmenting agents on the delayed-type hypersensitivity response in mice, *Cancer Res.* **42**:3514.

Basic, I., Milas, L., Grdina, D. J., and Withers, H. R., 1975, *In vitro* destruction of tumor cells by macrophages from mice treated with *Corynebacterium parvum*, *J. Natl. Cancer Inst.* **55**:589.

Behling, U. H., and Nowotny, A., 1982, Immunostimulation by LPS and its derivatives, in: *Immunomodulation by Bacteria and Their Products* (H. Friedman, T. W. Klein, and A. Szentivanyi, eds.), pp. 165–179, Plenum Press, New York.

Bekierkunst, A., Levij, I. S., Yarkoni, E., Vilkas, E., and Lederer, E., 1971, Suppression of urethane-induced lung adenomas in mice treated with trehalose 6-6'-dimycolate (cord factor) and living B.C.G., *Science* **174**:1240.

Bentley, C., Zimmer, B., and Hadding, V., 1981, The macrophage as a source of complement components, in: *Lymphokines*, Volume 4 (E. Pick, ed.), pp. 197–230, Academic Press, New York.

Berendt, M. J., North, R. J., and Kirstein, D. P., 1978, The immunological basis of endotoxin induced tumor regression: Requirement for T-cell mediated immunity, *J. Exp. Med.* **148**:1550.

Betz, S. J., and Morrison, D. C., 1977, Chemical and biologic properties of a protein rich fraction of bacterial lipopolysaccharides. I. The *in vitro* murine lymphocyte response, *J. Immunol.* **119**:1475.

Biozzi, G., Benacerraf, B., and Halpern, B. N., 1955, The effect of *Salmonella typhi* and its endotoxin on the phagocytic activity of the reticuloendothelial system in mice, *Br. J. Pathol.* **36**:226.

Bomford, R., and Moreno, C., 1981, Critical overviews of the potential of various microbial polysaccharides for cancer immunotherapy, in: *Augmenting Agents in Cancer Therapy* (E. M. Hersh, M. A. Chirigos, and M. J. Mastrangelo, eds.), pp. 91–99, Raven Press, New York.

Bomford, R., and Olivetto, M., 1974, The mechanism of inhibition by *Corynebacterium parvum* of the growth of lung nodules from intravenously injected tumour cells, *Int. J. Cancer* **14**:226.

Bradley, S. G., 1979, Cellular and molecular mechanisms of action of bacterial endotoxins, *Annu. Rev. Microbiol.* **33**:67.

Brochier, J., Bona, C., Ciorbaru, R., Revillard, J. -P., and Chedid, L., 1976, A human T-independent B lymphocyte mitogen extracted from *Nocardia opaca*, *J. Immunol.* **117**:1434.

Burgaleta, C., and Golde, D. W., 1977, Effect of glucan on granulopoiesis and macrophage genesis in mice, *Cancer Res.* **37**:17.

Burgaleta, C., Territo, M. C., Quan, S. G., and Golde, D. W., 1978, Glucan activated macrophages: Functional characteristics and surface morphology, *J. Reticuloendothel. Soc.* **23**:195.

Butler, R. C., and Nowotny, A., 1979, Combined immunostimulation in the prevention of tumor take in mice using endotoxins, their derivatives and other immune adjuvants, *Cancer Immunol. Immunother.* **6**:255.

Cameron, D. J., and Churchill, W. H., 1980, Cytotoxicity of human macrophages for tumor cells: Enhancement by bacterial lipopolysaccharides (LPS), *J. Immunol.* **124**:708.

Carswell, E. A., Old, L. J., Kassel, R. L., Green, S., Fiore, N., and Williamson, B., 1975, An endotoxin-induced serum factor that causes necrosis of tumors, *Proc. Natl. Acad. Sci. USA* **72**:3666.

Carter, W. A., Strayer, D. R., Gillespie, D. H., Brodsky, I., Greene, J. J., and Ts'o, P. O. P., 1981, Poly I:C with mismatched bases, prospects for cancer therapy, in: *Augmenting Agents in Cancer Therapy* (E. M. Hersh, M. A. Chirigos, and M. J. Mastrangelo, eds.), pp. 177–183, Raven Press, New York.

Chapman, H. A., Vavrin, Z., and Hibbs, J. B., 1979, Modulation of plasminogen activator secretion by activated macrophages: Influence of serum factors and correlation with tumoricidal potential, *Proc. Natl. Acad. Sci. USA* **76**:3899.

Charon, D., and Szabo, L., 1983, Synthesis of O-{-deoxy-2-[(3R)-3-hydroxytetradecanamino] 2D-glycopyranosyl-4-phosphate}n(1—6)-2 deoxy -2-[(3 R)-3-hydroxytetradecanamido]-D-glucose: The disaccharide route, *Carbohydr. Res.* **11**:C13.

Chedid, L., Parant, M., Damais, C., Parant, F., Juy, D., and Carelli, A., 1976, Failure of endotoxin to increase non-specific resistance to infection of lipopolysaccharide low responder mice, *Infect. Immun.* **13**:722.

Chedid, L., Parant, M., Parant, F., Lefrancier, P., Choay, J., and Lederer, E., 1977, Enhancement of non-specific immunity to *Klebsiella pneumoniae* infection by a synthetic immunoadjuvant (N-acetylmuramyl-L-alanyl-D-isoglutamine) and several analogs, *Proc. Natl. Acad. Sci. USA* **74**:2089.

Chedid, L., Parant, M., Parant, F., Audibert, F., Lefrancier, P., Choay, J., and Sela, M., 1979, Enhancement of certain biological activities of muramyl dipeptide derivatives after conjugation to a multi-poly-(DL-alanyl)-poly(L-lysine) carrier, *Proc. Natl. Acad. Sci. USA* **76**:6557.

Chedid, L., Parant, M. A., Audibert, F. M., Riveau, G. J., Parant, F. J., Lederer, E., Choay, J. P., and Lefrancier, P. L., 1982, Biological activity of a new synthetic muramyl peptide adjuvant devoid of pyrogenicity, *Infect. Immun.* **35**:417.

Cheers, C., and Cone, R. E., 1974, Effect of polyadenine:polyuridine on brucellosis in conventional and congenitally athymic mice, *J. Immunol.* **112**:1535.

Ciorbaru, R., Adam, A., Petit, J.-F., Lederer, E., Bona, C., and Chedid, L., 1975, Isolation of mitogenic and adjuvant fractions from various species of *Nocardiae*, *Infect. Immun.* **11**:275.

Ciorbaru, R., Petit, J.-F., Lederer, E., Zissman, E., Bona, C., and Chedid, L., 1976, Presence and subcellular localization of two distinct mitogenic fractions in the cells of *Nocardia rubra* and *Nocardia opaca*: Preparation of soluble mitogenic peptidoglycan fractions, *Infect. Immun.* **13**:1084.

Clark, I. A., 1979, Protection of mice against *Babesia microti* with cord factor, COAM, zymosan, glucan, *Salmonella*, and *Listeria*, *Parasite Immunol.* **1**:179.

Cohn, Z. A., and Benson, B., 1965, The differentiation of mononuclear phagocytes: Morphology, cytochemistry and biochemistry, *J. Exp. Med.* **121**:153.

Cohn, Z. A., Hirsch, J. G., and Fedorko, M. E., 1966, The *in vitro* differentiation of mononuclear phagocytes. IV. The ultrastructure of macrophage differentiation in the peritoneal cavity and in culture, *J. Exp. Med.* **123**:747.

Cook, J. A., Taylor, D. Cohen, C., Rodrigue, J., Malshet, V., and DiLuzio, N. R., 1978, Comparative Evaluation of the role of macrophages and lymphocytes in mediating the antitumor action of glucan, in: *Immune Modulation and Control of Neoplasia by Adjuvant Therapy* (M. A. Chirigos, ed.), pp. 183–194, Raven Press, New York.

Cook, J. A., Wise, W. C., and Halushka, P. V., 1981, Thromboxane A_2 and prostacyclin production by lipopolysaccharide stimulated peritoneal macrophages, *J. Reticuloendothel. Soc.* **30**:445.

Cook, J. A., Holbrook, T. W., and Dougherty, W. J., 1982, Protective effect of glucan against visceral leishmaniasis in hamsters, *Infect. Immun.* **37**:1261.

Creau-Goldberg, N., and Salomon, J.-C., 1980, Immunotherapy of primary methylcholanthrene induced mouse tumours by intratumoural BCG, *Br. J. Cancer* **41**:541.

Cummings, N. P., Pabst, M. J., and Johnston, R. B., 1980, Activation of macrophages for enhanced release of superoxide anion and greater killing of *Candida albicans* by injection of muramyl dipeptide, *J. Exp. Med.* **152**:1659.

Currie, G. A., 1978, Activated macrophages kill tumors cells by releasing arginase, *Nature (London)* **273**:758.

Damais, C., Parant, M., and Chedid, L., 1977, Non-specific activation of murine spleen cells *in vitro* by a synthetic immunoadjuvant (N-acetyl-muramyl L-alanyl-D-isoglutamine), *Cell. Immunol.* **34**:49.

Damais, C., Riveau, G., Parant, M., Gerota, J., and Chedid, L., 1982, Production of lymphocyte activating factor in the absence of endogenous pyyogen by rabbit or human leukocytes stimulated by a muramyl dipeptide derivative, *Int. J. Immunopharmacol.* **4**:451.

Dazord, L., Martin, A., Collet, B., Le Garrec, Y., David, C., and Toujas, L., 1982, Modifications of the biological response against tumours by *Brucella abortus*, *Hum. Cancer Immunol.* **13**:1.

Delville, J., and Jacques, P. J., 1980, Therapeutic effect of intravenously administered yeast glucan in mice locally injected by *Mycobacterium leprae*, *Adv. Exp. Med. Biol.* **121A**:245.

Deshmukh-Phadke, K., Lawrence, M., and Nanda, S., 1978, Synthesis of collagenase and neutral proteases by articular chondrocytes: Stimulation by a macrophage-derived factor, *Biochem. Biophys. Res. Commun.* **85**:490.

Dienstman, S. R., and Defendi, V., 1978, Necessary and sufficient conditions for recruitment of macrophages into the cell cycle, *Exp. Cell Res.* **115**:191.

DiLuzio, N. R., and Williams, D. L., 1978, Protective effect of glucan against systemic *Staphylococcus aureus* septicemia in normal and leukemic mice, *Infect. Immun.* **30**:804.

DiLuzio, N. R., Williams, D. L., McNamee, R. B., Edwards, R. E., and Kitahama, A., 1979, Comparative tumor inhibitory and anti-bacterial activity of soluble and particulate glucan, *Int. J. Cancer* **24**:773.

Dinarello, C. A., 1982, Leucocytic pyrogen, in: *Lymphokines*, Volume 7 (E. Pick, ed.), pp. 23–74, Academic Press, New York.

Dinarello, C. A., Elin, R. J., Chedid, L., and Wolff, S. M., 1978, The pyrogenicity of the synthetic adjuvant muramyl dipeptide and two structural analogues, *J. Infect. Dis.* **138**:760.

Djeu, J. Y., Heinbauch, J. A., Holden, H. T., and Herberman, R. B., 1979, Role of macrophages in the augmentation of mouse NK cell activity by polyI:C and interferon, *J. Immunol.* **122**:188.

Doe, W. F., and Henson, P. M., 1978, Macrophage stimulation by bacterial lipopolysaccharides. I. Cytolytic effect on tumor target cells, *J. Exp. Med.* **148**:544.

Doe, W., Yang, D., and Henson, P., 1977, Bacterial lipopolysaccharide (LPS)-induced macrophage stimulation: Selective lysosomal enzyme release, *Fed. Proc.* **36**:1263a.

Doe, W. F., Yang, S. T., Morrison, D. C., Betz, S. J., and Henson, P. M., 1978, Macrophage stimulation by bacterial lipopolysaccharides. II. Evidence for differentiation signals delivered by lipid A and by a protein rich fraction of lipopolysaccharides, *J. Exp. Med.* **148**:557.

Drapier, J.-C., Lemaire, G., and Petit, J.-F., 1982, Regulation of plasminogen activator secretion in mouse peritoneal macrophages. II. Inhibition by immunomodulators of bacterial origin, *Int. J. Immunopharmacol.* **21**:34.

Drapier, J.-C., Roubin, R., Petit, J.-F., and Benveniste, J., 1983, Lipid mediator synthesis in peritoneal macrophages from mice injected with immunostimulants, *Biochim. Biophys. Acta* **751**:90.

Drysdale, B. E., and Shin, H. S., 1981, Activation of macrophages for tumor cell cytotoxicity; Identification of indomethacin sensitive and insensitive pathways, *J. Immunol.* **127**:760.

Durand, E., Gillois, M., Tocane, J.-F., and Laneelle, G., 1979a, Property and activity of mycolate esters of methyl glucoside and trehalose, *Eur. J. Biochem.* **94**:109.

Durand, E., Welby, M., Laneelle, G., and Tocane, J.-F., 1979b, Phase behavior of cord factor and related glycolipid toxins: A monolayer study, *Eur. J. Biochem.* **93**:103.

Dye, E. S., and North, R. J., 1980, Macrophage accumulation in murine ascites tumors. I. Cytoxan-induced dominance of macrophages over tumor cells and the antitumor effect of endotoxin, *J. Immunol.* **125**:1650.

Eaves, A. C., and Bruce, W. R., 1974, *In vitro* production of colony stimulating activity. I. Exposure of mouse peritoneal cells to endotoxin, *Cell Tissue Kinet.* **7**:19.

Edelson, P. J., 1980, Macrophage ecto-enzymes: Their identification, metabolism and control, in: *Mononuclear Phagocytes: Functional Aspects* (R. van Furth, ed.), pp. 665–681, Nijhoff, The Hague.

Elinov, N. P., Kashkina, M. A., Arkadieva, G. Y., and Freidlin, I. S., 1982, Comparison of different properties of mononuclear phagocytes activated with yeast polysaccharides, *Int. J. Immunopharmacol.* **4**:266a.

Ellner, J. J., and Spagnuolo, P. J., 1979, Suppression of antigen and mitogen induced human T lymphocyte DNA synthesis by bacterial lipopolysaccharide: Mediation by monocyte activation and production of prostaglandins, *J. Immunol.* **123**:2689.

Ellouz, F., Adam, A., Ciorbaru, R., and Lederer, E., 1974, Minimal structural requirements for adjuvant activity of bacterial peptidoglycan derivatives, *Biochem. Biophys. Res. Commun.* **59**:1317.

Esser, A. F., and Russell, S. W., 1979, Membrane perturbation of macrophages stimulated by bacterial lipopolysaccharide, *Biochem. Biophys. Res. Commun.* **87**:532.

Evans, R., and Alexander, P., 1976, Mechanisms of extracellular killing of nucleated mammalian cells by macrophages, in: *Immunobiology of the Macrophage* (D. S. Nelson, ed.), pp. 535–576, Academic Press, New York.

Fauve, R. M., and Delaunay, A., 1966, Résistance cellulaire à l'infection microbienne, *Ann. Inst. Pasteur Paris* **110**(Suppl. 3):95.

Fauve, R. M., and Hevin, M. B., 1971, Pouvoir bactéricide des macrophages spléniques et hépatiques de souris envers *Listeria monocytogenes:* Influence du traitement préalable des animaux par des glucocorticoides, une endotoxine, *Corynebacterium parvum* et l'acide polyinosinique polycytidylique (poly I:C), *Ann. Inst. Pasteur Paris* **120**:399.

Fauve, R. M., and Hevin, M. B., 1974, Immunostimulation with bacterial phospholipid extracts, *Proc. Natl. Acad. Sci. USA* **71**:573.

Février, M., Birrien, J. L., Leclerc, C., Chedid, L., and Liacopoulos, P., 1978, The macrophage, target cell of the synthetic adjuvant muramyl dipeptide, *Eur. J. Immunol.* **8**:558.

Fidler, I. J., 1981, The *in situ* induction of tumoricidal activity in alveolar macrophages by liposome containing muramyl dipeptide is a thymus-independent process, *J. Immunol.* **127**:1719.

Fidler, I. J., Raz, A., Fogler, W. E., Kirsh, R., Bugelski, P., and Poste, G., 1980, Design of liposomes to improve delivery of macrophage-augmenting agents to alveolar macrophages, *Cancer Res.* **40**:4460.

Fidler, I. J., Sone, S., Fogler, W. E., and Barnes, Z. L., 1981, Eradication of spontaneous metastases and activation of alveolar macrophages by intravenous injections of liposomes containing muramyl dipeptide, *Proc. Natl. Acad. Sci. USA* **78**:1680.

Fidler, I. J., Barnes, Z., Fogler, W. E., Kirsh, R., Bugelski, P., and Poste, G., 1982, Involvement of macrophages in the eradication of established metastases following intravenous injection of liposomes containing macrophage activators, *Cancer Res.* **42**:496.

Filkins, J. P., 1980, Endotoxin-enhanced secretion of macrophage insulin-like activity, *J. Reticuloendothel. Soc.* **27**:507.

Fleit, H. B., and Rabinovitch, M., 1981, Production of interferon by *in vitro* derived bone marrow macrophages, *Cell. Immunol.* **57**:495.

Floc'h, F., Bouchaudon, J., Werner, G. H., Migliore-Samour, D., and Jollès, P., 1981, Augmentation par des lipopeptides immunostimulants de la résistance de la souris à l'infection par *Listeria monocytogenes*, *Ann. Immunol. (Paris)* **132D**:265.

Fox, R. A., and Rajaraman, K., 1980, Endotoxin and macrophage-migration inhibition, *Cell. Immunol.* **53**:333.

Fraser-Smith, E. B., and Matthews, T. R., 1981, Protective effect of muramyl dipeptide analogs against infections of *Pseudomonas aeruginosa* or *Candida albicans, Infect. Immun.* **34**:676.

Fraser-Smith, E. B., Waters, R. V., and Matthews, T. R., 1982, Correlation between *in vivo* anti-*Pseudomonas* and anti-*Candida* activities and clearance of carbon by the reticuloendothelial system for various muramyl dipeptide analogs, using normal and immunosuppressed mice, *Infect. Immun.* **35**:105.

Freedman, V. H., Calvelli, T. A., Silagl, S., and Silverstein, S. C., 1980, Macrophages elicited with heat-killed bacillus Calmette-Guérin protect C57BL/6J mice against a syngeneic melanoma, *J. Exp. Med.* **152**:657.

Galanos, C., and Lüderitz, O., 1975, Electrodialysis of lipopolysaccharides and their conversion to uniform salt forms, *Eur. J. Biochem.* **54**:603.

Galanos, C., Lüderitz, O., and Westphal, O., 1969, A new method for the extraction of R lipopolysaccharides, *Eur. J. Biochem.* **9**:245.

Galanos, C., Rietschel, E. T., Lüderitz, O., and Westphal, O., 1972, Biological activities of lipid A complexed with bovine serum albumin, *Eur. J. Biochem.* **31**:230.

Galanos, C., Lüderitz, O., Rietschel, E. T., and Westphal, O., 1977, Newer aspects of the chemistry and biology of bacterial lipopolysaccharide, with special reference to their lipid A component', in: *Biochemistry of Lipids II*, Volume 14 (T. W. Goodwin, ed.), p. 239, University Park Press, Baltimore.

Galelli, A., Le Garrec, Y., Chedid, L., Lefrancier, P., Derrien, M., and Level, M., 1980, Macrophage stimulation *in vitro* by an inactive muramyl dipeptide derivative after conjugation to a multipoly(DL-alanyl)-poly(L-lysine) carrier, *Infect. Immun.* **28**:1.

Galelli, A., Le Garrec, Y., and Chedid, C., 1981, Increased resistance and depressed delayed-type hypersensitivity to *Listeria monocytogenes* induced by pretreatment with lipopolysaccharide, *Infect. Immun.* **31**:88.

Germain, R. N., Williams, R. M., and Benacerraf, B., 1975, Specific and nonspecific antitumor immunity. II. Macrophage-mediated nonspecific effector activity induced by BCG and similar agents, *J. Natl. Cancer Inst.* **54**:709.

Gery, I., Davies, P., Derr, J., Krett, N., and Barranger, J. A., 1981, Relationship between production and release of lymphocyte activating factor (interleukin I) by murine macrophages. I. Effects of various agents, *Cell. Immunol.* **64**:293.

Gordon, S., Unkeless, J. C., and Cohn, Z. A., 1974, Induction of macrophage plasminogen activator by endotoxin stimulation and phagocytosis: Evidence for a two-stage process, *J. Exp. Med.* **140**:995.

Goren, M., 1982, Immunoreactive substances of *mycobacteria*, *Am. Rev. Respir. Dis.* **125**:50.

Griffin, F. M., Bianco, C., and Silverstein, S. C., 1975, Characterization of the macrophage receptor for complement and demonstration of its functional independence from the receptor for the Fc portion of immunoglobulin G, *J. Exp. Med.* **141**:1269.

Guglielmi, P., Preud'homme, J. L., Ciorbaru-Barot, R., and Seligman, M., 1982, Mitogen-induced maturation of chronic lymphocytic leukemia B lymphocytes, *J. Clin. Immunol.* **2**:186.

Hadden, J., 1978, The action of immunopotentiators *in vitro* on lymphocyte and macrophage activation, in: *The Pharmacology of Immunoregulation* (G. H. Werner and F. Floch, eds.), p. 369, Academic Press, New York.

Hadden, J., England, A., Sadlik, J. R., and Hadden, E. M., 1979, The comparative effects of isoprinosine, levamisole, muramyl dipeptide and SM 1213 on lymphocyte and macrophage proliferation and activation *in vitro*, *Int. J. Immunopharmacol.* **1**:17.

Haeffner-Cavaillon, N., Chaby, R., Cavaillon, J. M., and Szabo, L., 1982, Lipopolysaccharide receptor on rabbit peritoneal macrophages: Binding characteristics, *J. Immunol.* **128**:1950.

Halpern, B., 1975, *Corynebacterium parvum: Applications in Experimental and Clinical Oncology*, Plenum Press, New York.

Halpern, B. N., Biozzi, G., Stiffel, C., and Mouton, D., 1966, Inhibition of tumour growth by administration of killed *Corynebacterium parvum*, *Nature (London)* **212**:853.

Hamburg, S. I., Manejias, R. E., and Rabinovitch, M., 1978, Macrophage activation: Increased ingestion of IgG-coated erythrocytes after administration of interferon inducers to mice, *J. Exp. Med.* **147**:593.

Havell, E. A., and Spitalny, G. L., 1980, The induction and characterization of interferon from pure cultures of murine macrophages, *Ann. N.Y. Acad. Sci.* **350**:413.

Hersh, E. M., Murphy, S. G., Quesada, J. R., Gutterman, J. U., Gschwind, C. R., and Morgan, J., 1981, Effect of immunotherapy with *Corynebacterium parvum* and methanol extraction residue of BCG administered intravenously on host defense function in cancer patients, *J. Natl. Cancer Inst.* **66**:993.

Hibbs, J. B., Lambert, L. H., and Remington, J. S., 1971, Resistance to murine tumors conferred by chronic infection with intracellular protozoa, *Toxoplasma gondii* and *Besnoitia jellisoni*, *J. Infect. Dis.* **124**:587.

Hibbs, J. B., Lambert, L. H., and Remington, J. S., 1972, Possible role of macrophage mediated non specific cytotoxicity in tumor resistance, *Nature New Biol.* **235**:48.

Humes, J. L., Sadowski, S., Galavage, M., Goldenberg, M., Subers, E., Bonney, R. J., and Kuehl, F. A., 1982, Evidence for two sources of arachidonic acid for oxidative metabolism by mouse peritoneal macrophages, *J. Biol. Chem.* **257**:1591.

Humphries, R. C., Henika, P. R., Ferraresi, R. W., and Krahenbuhl, J. L., 1980, Effects of treatment with muramyldipeptide and certain of its analogs on resistance to *Listeria monocytogenes* in mice, *Infect. Immun.* **30**:462.

Hunter, R., Strickland, F., and Kezdy, F., 1981, The adjuvant activity of nonionic block polymer surfactant: The role of hydrophile–lipophile balance, *J. Immunol.* **127**:1244.

Imai, K., Tomioka, M., Nagao, S., Kushima, K., and Tanaka, A., 1980, Biochemical evidence for activation of guinea pig macrophages by muramyl dipeptide, *Biomed. Res.* **1**:300.

Iribe, H., Koga, T., Onoue, K., Kotani, S., Kusumoto, S., and Shiba, T., 1981, Macrophage-stimulating effect of a synthetic muramyl dipeptide and its adjuvant active and inactive analogs for the production of T-cell activating monokines, *Cell. Immunol.* **64**:73.

Iribe, H., Koga, T., and Onoue, K., 1982, Production of T cell activating monokine of guinea pig macrophages induced by MDP and partial characterization of the monokine, *J. Immunol.* **129**:1029.

Ito, M., Ralph, P., and Moore, M. A. S., 1979, In vitro stimulation of phagocytosis in a macrophage cell line measured by a convenient radiolabelled latex bead assay, *Cell. Immunol.* **46**:48.

Izumi, T., Kikuchi, M., Mitani, M., Matsuo, T., Yamashima, T., and Tsubura, E., 1982, Response modifying activity of schizophyllan, in: *Immunomodulation by Microbial Products and Related Synthetic Compounds* (Y. Yamamura, S. Kotani, I. Azuma, A. Koda, and T. Shiba, eds.), pp. 407–410, Excerpta Medica, Amsterdam.

Jenkin, C., and Palmer, D. L., 1960, Changes in the titer of serum opsonins and phagocytic properties of mouse peritoneal macrophages following injection of endotoxin, *J. Exp. Med.* **112**:419.

Johnson, A. G., 1979, Modulation of the immune system by synthetic polynucleotides, *Springer Semin. Immunopathol.* **2**:157.

Johnson, A. G., 1982, The immunopharmacology of polyadenylic-polyuridylic acid complexes: A synthetic immunomodulator, in: *Immunomodulation by Microbial Products and Related Synthetic Compounds* (Y. Yamamura, S. Kotani, I. Azuma, A. Koda, and T. Shiba, eds.), pp. 128–133, Excerpta Medica, Amsterdam.

Johnson, H. G., and Johnson, A. G., 1971, Regulation of the immune system by synthetic polynucleotides. II. Action on peritoneal exudate cells, *J. Exp. Med.* **133**:649.

Johnston, R. B., Godzick, C. A., and Cohn, Z. A., 1978, Increased superotide anion production by immunologically activated and chemically elicited macrophages, *J. Exp. Med.* **148**:115.

Joseph, M., Simon-Lavoine, N., and Capron, A., 1981, The stimulation of rat and mouse macrophages by cyclomunine after in vitro and in vivo administration, *Int. J. Immunopharmacol.* **3**:67.

Jullien, P., De Maeyer-Guignard, J., and De Maeyer, E., 1974, Interferon synthesis in X-irradiated animals. V. Origin of mouse interferon induced by polyinosinic-polycytidylic acid and encephalomyocarditis virus, *Infect. Immun.* **10**:1023.

Juy, D., and Chedid, L., 1975, Comparison between macrophage activation and enhancement of nonspecific resistance to tumors by mycobacterial immunoadjuvants, *Proc. Natl. Acad. Sci. USA* **72**:4105.

Kato, M., 1970, Site II specific inhibition of mitochondrial oxidative phosphorylation by trehalose-6-6'-dimycolate (cord factor) of *Mycobacterium tuberculosis, Arch. Biochem. Biophys.* **140**:379.

Kato, M., Tamura, T., Silve, G., and Asselineau, J., 1978, Chemical structure and biological activity of cord factor analogs: Comparative study of esters of methylglucoside and non-hydroxylated fatty acids, *Eur. J. Biochem.* **87**:497.

Kawakami, M. G., and Cerami, A., 1981, Studies on endotoxin decrease in lipoprotein lipase activity, *J. Exp. Med.* **154**:631.

Kelly, M. T., 1977, Plasma-dependent chemotaxis of macrophages towards BCG cell walls and the mycobacterial glycolipid P3, *Infect. Immun.* **15**:180.

Kierszenbaum, F., and Ferraresi, R. W., 1979, Enhancement of host resistance against *Trypanosoma cruzi* infection by the immunoregulatory agent muramyl dipeptide, *Infect. Immun.* **25**:273.

Kikutani, H., Kishimoto, T., Sakaguchi, N., Nishizawa, Y., Ralph, P., and Yamamura, Y., 1981, Activation of cyclic AMP-dependent protein kinase activation during LPS stimulation of macrophage tumor cell line J 774.1, *Int. J. Immunopharmacol.* **3**:57.

Kitaura, Y., Nakaguchi, O., Takeno, H., Okada, S., Yonishi, S., Hemmi, K., Mori, J., Senoh, H., Mine, Y., and Hashimoto, M., 1982, N^2-(γ-D-glutamyl)-meso-2(L),2'(D)-diaminopimelic acid as the minimal prerequisite structure of FK-156: Its acyl derivatives with potent immunostimulating activity, *J. Med. Chem.* **25**:335.

Klimetzek, V., and Sorg, C., 1979, The production of fibrinolysis inhibitors as a parameter of the activation state in murine macrophages, *Eur. J. Immunol.* **9**:613.

Kohoshis, P. L., Williams, D. L., Cook, J. A., and DiLuzio, N. R., 1978, Increased resistance to *Staphylococcus aureus* and enhancement in serum lysozyme activity by glucan, *Science* **199**:1340.

Kotani, S., Watanabe, Y., Kinoshita, F., Shimono, T., and Morisahi, I., 1975, Immunoadjuvant activities of synthetic N-acetyl-muramyl-peptides or amino-acids, *Biken J.* **18**:105.

Krahenbuhl, J. L., and Remington, J. S., 1974, The role of activated macrophages in specific and nonspecific cytostasis of tumor cells, *J. Immunol.* **113**:507.

Krahenbuhl, J. L., Sharma, S. D., Ferraresi, R. W., and Remington, J. S., 1981, Effects of muramyl dipeptide treatment on resistance to infection with *Toxoplasma gondii* in mice, *Infect. Immun.* **31**:716.

Krane, S. M., Goldring, S. R., and Dayer, J. M., 1982, Interactions among lymphocytes, monocytes, and other synovial cells in the rheumatoid synovium, in: *Lymphokines*, Volume 7 (E. Pick, ed.), pp. 75–136, Academic Press, New York.

Krown, S. E., Kerr, D., Stewart, W. E., Pollack, M. S., Cunningham-Rundles, S., Hirshaut, Y., Pinsky, C. M., Levy, H. B., and Oettgen, H. F., 1981, Phase I trial of poly ICLC in patients with advanced cancer, in: *Augmenting Agents in Cancer Therapy* (E. M. Hersh, M. A. Chirigos, and M. J. Mastrangelo, eds.), pp. 165–176, Raven Press, New York.

Kurland, J., and Bockman, R., 1978, Prostaglandin E production by human blood monocytes and mouse peritoneal macrophages, *J. Exp. Med.* **147**:952.

Lachman, L. B., and Metzgar, R. S., 1980, Purification and characterization of human lymphocyte activating factor, in: *Biochemical Characterization of Lymphokines* (A. L. de Weck, F. Kristensen, and M. Landy, eds.), pp. 405–409, Academic Press, New York.

Lachman, L. B., Hacker, M. P., Blyden, G. T., and Handschumacher, R. E., 1977, Preparation of lymphocyte activating factor from continuous macrophage cell lines, *Cell. Immunol.* **34**:416.

Lacour, J., Lacour, F., Spira, A., Michelson, M., Petit, J. Y., Delage, G., Sarrazin, D., Contesso, V., and Wooder, J., 1980, Adjuvant treatment with polyadenylic-polyuridylic acid (poly A:U) in operable breast cancer, *Lancet* **2**:161.

Laneelle, G., and Tocanne, J.-F., 1980, Evidence for penetration in liposomes and in mitochondrial membranes of a fluorescent analog of cord factor, *Eur. J. Biochem.* **109**:177.

Leclerc, C., and Chedid, L., 1982, Macrophage activation by synthetic muramyl peptides, in: *Lymphokines* Volume 7 (E. Pick, ed.), pp. 1–21, Academic Press, New York.

Leclerc, C., Lamensans, A., Chedid, L., Drapier, J. C., Petit, J.-F., Wietzerbin, J., and Lederer, E., 1976, Non-specific immunoprevention of L1210 leukemia by cord factor (6,6'-dimycolate of trehalose) administered in a metabolizable oil, *Cancer Immunol. Immunother.* **1**:227.

Lederer, E., 1979, Cord factor and related synthetic trehalose diesters, *Springer Semin. Immunopathol.* **2**:133.

Lederer, E., 1980, Immunostimulation: Recent progress in the study of natural and synthetic immunomodulators derived from the bacterial cell wall, in: *Immunology 80* (M. Fougereau and J. Dausset, eds.), pp. 1195–1211, Academic Press, New York.

Lederer, E., 1982, Recent progress in the study of natural and synthetic immunomodulators derived from the bacterial cell walls, in: *Immunomodulation by Microbial Products and Related Synthetic Compounds* (Y. Yamamura, S. Kotani, I. Azuma, A. Koda, and T. Shiba, eds.), pp. 3–16, Excerpta Medica, Amsterdam.

Lefrancier, P., Derrien, M., Jamet, X., Choay, J., Lederer, E., Audibert, F., Parant, M., Parant, F., and Chedid, L., 1982, Apyrogenic adjuvant-active N-acetylmuramyl-dipeptides, *J. Med. Chem.* **25**:87.

Lemaire, G., Drapier, J. C., Tenu, J.-P., Bouchahda, A., Lepoivre, M., and Petit, J.-F., 1982, Stimulation of several properties of macrophages after injection of a suspension of killed streptococci, *J. Reticuloendothel. Soc.* **32**:87.

Lepoivre, M., Tenu, J.-P., Lemaire, G., and Petit, J.-F., 1982, Antitumor activity and hydrogen peroxide release by macrophages elicited by trehalose diesters, *J. Immunol.* **129**:860.

Leu, R. W., Herriot, M. J., Moore, P. E., Orr, G. R., and Birckbichler, P. J., 1982, Enhanced transglutaminase activity associated with macrophage activation: Possible role in Fc mediated phagocytosis, *J. Immunol.* **127**:357.

Levy, G. A., Schwartz, B. S., and Edgington, T. S., 1981, The kinetics and metabolic requirements for direct lymphocyte induction of human procoagulant monokines by bacterial lipopolysaccharide, *J. Immunol.* **127**:357.

Löwy, I., Bona, C., and Chedid, L., 1977, Target cells for the activity of a synthetic adjuvant: Muramyl dipeptide, *Cell. Immunol.* **29**:195.

McCarthy, J. B., Wahl, S. M., Rees, J. C., Olsen, C. E., Sandberg, A. L., and Wahl, L. M., 1980, Mediation of macrophage collagenase production by 3'-5' cyclic adenosine monophosphate, *J. Immunol.* **124**:2405.

Mackaness, G. B., 1962, Cellular resistance to infection, *J. Exp. Med.* **116**:381.

McLaughlin, C. A., Schwartzman, S. M., Horner, B. L., Jones, G. H., Moffatt, J. G., Nestor, J. J., Jr., and Tegg, D., 1980, Regression of tumors in guinea pigs after treatment with synthetic muramyl dipeptides and trehalose dimycolate, *Science* **208**:415.

Madraso, E. D., and Cheers, C., 1978a, Polyadenylic and polyuridylic acid (poly A:U) and experimental murine brucellosis. I. Effect of single and double stranded polynucleotides on *Brucella abortus in vivo* and *in vitro*, *Immunology* **35**:69.

Madraso, E. D., and Cheers, C., 1978b, II. Macrophages as target of poly A:U in experimental brucellosis, *Immunology* **35**:77.

Maehara, N., and Ho, M., 1977, Cellular origin of interferon induced by bacterial lipopolysaccharide, *Infect. Immun.* **15**:78.

Magee, W. E., 1978, Incorporation of poly I:C into liposomes also may prove efficacious in reducing toxicity and increasing interferon level, *Ann. N.Y. Acad. Sci.* **308**:308.

Mahmoud, A. A., Peters, P. A. S., Civil, R. H., and Remington, J. S., 1979, *In vitro* killing of schistosomula of *Schistosoma mansoni* by BCG and C. *parvum* activated macrophages, *J. Immunol.* **122**:1655.

Maier, R. V., and Ulevitch, R. J., 1981, The induction of a unique procoagulant activity in rabbit hepatic macrophages by bacterial lipopolysaccharide, *J. Immunol.* **127**:1596.

Männel, D. N., Moore, R. N., and Mergenhagen, S. E., 1980, Macrophages as a source of tumoricidal activity (tumor necrotizing factor), *Infect. Immun.* **30**:523.

Männel, D. N., Falk, W., and Meltzer, M. S., 1981, Inhibition of nonspecific tumoricide activity by activated macrophages with antiserum against a soluble cytotoxic factor, *Infect. Immun.* **33**:156.

Matsumoto, T., Ogawa, H., Kusama, T., Nagase, O., Sawaki, N., Inage, M., Kusumoto, S., Shiba, T., and Azuma, I., 1981, Stimulation of non-specific resistance to infection induced by 6-O-acyl muramyl dipeptide analogs in mice, *Infect. Immun.* **32**:748.

Matsumoto, T., Mikami, T., Nagase, T., Susuki, M., and Suzuki, S., 1982, Relationship between glucan structure and antitumor activity of the mannans of *Saccharomyces cerevisiae*, in: *Immunomodulation by Microbial Products and Related Synthetic Compounds* (Y. Yamamura, S. Kotani, I. Azuma, A. Koda, and T. Shiba, eds.), pp. 427–430, Excerpta Medica, Amsterdam.

Matter, A., 1979, The effects of muramyl dipeptide (MDP) in cell-mediated immunity: A comparison between *in vitro* and *in vivo* systems, *Cancer Immunol. Immunother.* **6**:201.

Meltzer, M. S., 1981, Tumor cytotoxicity by lymphokine-activated macrophages: Development of macrophage tumoricidal activity requires a sequence of reactions, in: *Lymphokines*, Volume 3 (E. Pick, ed.), pp. 319–343, Academic Press, New York.

Meltzer, M. S., and Oppenheim, J. J., 1977, Bidirectional amplification of macrophage–lymphocyte interactions: Enhanced lymphocyte activation factor production by activated adherent mouse peritoneal cells, *J. Immunol.* **118**:77.

Meltzer, M. S., Ruco, L. P., and Leonard, E. J., 1980, Macrophage activation for tumor cytotoxicity: Mechanisms of macrophage activation by lymphokines, *Adv. Exp. Med. Biol.* **121B**:381.

Merser, C., Sinay, P., and Adam, A., 1975, Total synthesis and adjuvant activity of bacterial peptidoglycan derivatives, *Biochem. Biophys. Res. Commun.* **66**:1316.

Migliore-Samour, D., Bouchaudon, J., Floc'h, F., Zerial, A., Ninet, L., Werner, G. H., and Jollès, P., 1980, A short lipopeptide, representative of a new family of immunological adjuvants devoid of sugar, *Life Sci.* **26**:883.

Mitani, M., Arika, T., and Kikuchi, M., 1982, Antitumor activity of schizophyllan against syngeneic murine tumor and its potentiation of the therapeutic response induced by antitumor agent or chemically modified tumor vaccines, in: *Immunomodulation by Microbial Products and Related Synthetic Compounds* (Y. Yamamura, S. Kotani, I. Azuma, A. Koda, and T. Shiba, eds.), pp. 411–414, Excerpta Medica, Amsterdam.

Miyama, A., Kawamoto, Y., Ichikawa, H., Okamoto, K., Hara, S., and Inoue, T., 1980, Complement proteins and macrophages. II. The secretion of factor B by lipopolysaccharide-stimulated macrophages, *Microbiol. Immunol.* **24**:1223.

Mizuhira, V., Shiihashi, M., Yokofujita, J., Amemiya, K., Hase, T., and Asano, T., 1982a, Autoradiographical study of schizophyllan administered to normal and S 180 grafted mice, in: *Immunomodulation by Microbial Products and Related Synthetic Compounds* (Y. Yamamura, S. Kotani, I. Azuma, A. Koda, and T. Shiba, eds.), pp. 415–418, Excerpta Medica, Amsterdam.

Mizuhira, V., Shiihashi, M., Yokofujita, J., Amemiya, K., Hase, T., and Asano, T., 1982b, The fate of schizophyllan administered to BC-47 grafted rats and lung cancer patients, in: *Immunomodulation by Microbial Products and Related Compounds* (Y. Yamamura, S. Kotani, I. Azuma, A. Koda, and T. Shiba, eds.), pp. 419–422, Excerpta Medica, Amsterdam.

Moore, R. N., Goodrum, K. J., and Berry, J. L., 1976, Mediation of an endotoxic effect by macrophages, *J. Reticuloendothel. Soc.* **19**:187.

Moore, R. N., Urbaschek, R., Wahl, L. M., and Mergenhagen, S. E., 1979, Prostaglandin regulation of colony-stimulating factor production by lipopolysaccharide-stimulated murine leukocytes, *Infect. Immun.* **26**:408.

Moore, R. N., Steeg, P. S., Mannel, D. N., and Mergenhagen, S. E., 1980a, Role of lipopolysaccharide in regulating colony-stimulating factor dependent macrophage proliferation in vitro, *Infect. Immun.* **30**:797.

Moore, R. N., Vogel, S. N., Wahl, L. M., and Mergenhagen, S. E., 1980b, Factors influencing lipopolysaccharide-induced interferon production, in *Microbiology—1980* (D. Schlessinger, ed.), pp. 131–134, American Society for Microbiology, Washington, D.C.

Morahan, P. S., Edelson, P. J., and Gass, K., 1980, Changes in macrophage ectoenzymes associated with antitumor activity, *J. Immunol.* **125**:1312.

Moriyasu, F., Miwa, H., and Orita, K., 1982, Immunochemotherapy of gastric cancer patients with OK-432, in: *Immunomodulation by Microbial Products and Related Synthetic Compounds* (Y. Yamamura, S. Kotani, I. Azuma, A. Koda, and T. Shiba, eds.), pp. 442–445, Excerpta Medica, Amsterdam.

Mørland, B., 1979, Studies on the selective induction of lysosomal enzyme activities in mouse peritoneal macrophages, *J. Reticuloendothel. Soc.* **26**:749.

Mørland, B., and Kaplan, G., 1977, Macrophage activation *in vivo* and *in vitro*, *Exp. Cell Res.* **108**:279.

Mørland, B., and Mørland, J., 1978, Selective induction of lysosomal enzyme activities in mouse peritoneal macrophages, *J. Reticuloendothel. Soc.* **23**:469.

Morrison, D. C., and Ryan, J. L., 1979, Bacterial endotoxins and host immune responses, *Adv. Immunol.* **28**:293.

Nagao, S., Tanaka, A., Yamamoto, Y., Koga, T., Onoue, K., Shiba, T., Kusumoto, K., and Kotani, S., 1979, Inhibition of macrophage migration by muramyl peptides, *Infect. Immun.* **24**:308.

Nagao, S., Miki, T., and Tanaka, A., 1981, Macrophage activation by muramyl dipeptide (MDP) without lymphocyte participation, *Microbiol. Immunol.* **25**:41.

Nagao, S., Tanaka, A., Onozaki, K., and Hashimoto, T., 1982, Differences between macrophage migration inhibition by lymphokines and muramyl dipeptide (MDP) or lipopolysaccharide (LPS): Migration enhancement by lymphokines, *Cell. Immunol.* **71**:1.

Narayanan, P. R., Kloehn, D. B., and Sundharadas, G., 1978, Immune response to alloantigens *in vitro*, amplification of the development of cytotoxic lymphocytes by lipopolysaccharide and polyadenylic:polyuridylic acid, *J. Immunol.* **121**:2502.

Nauts, H. C., Fowler, G. A., and Bogatko, F. H., 1953, Review of the influence of bacterial infection and of bacterial products (Coley's toxins) on malignant tumors in man, *Acta Med. Scand.* **45**(Suppl. 276):2.

Neumann, C., 1982, Mononuclear phagocytes as producers of interferon, in: *Lymphokines*, Volume 7 (E. Pick, ed.), pp. 165–201., Academic Press, New York.

Niblack, J. F., and McCreary, M. B., 1971, Relationship of biological activities of polyIpolyC to homopolymer molecular weight, *Nature New Biol.* **233**:52.

Nichols, N. K., and Prosser, F. H., 1980, Induction of ornithine decarboxylase in macrophages by bacterial lipopolysaccharides (LPS) and mycobacterial cell wall material, *Life Sci.* **27**:913.

Nissen-Meyer, J., and Hammerstrom, J., 1982, Physicochemical characterization of cytostatic factors released from human monocytes, *Infect. Immun.* **38**:67.

North, R. B., 1981, Bacterial endotoxin as an immunotherapeutic agent: Basic data on mechanisms of action, in: *Augmenting Agents in Cancer Therapy* (E. M. Hersh, M. A. Chirigos, and M. J. Mastrangelo, eds.), pp. 113–124, Raven Press, New York.

Nowotny, A., Behling, U. H., and Chang, H. L., 1975, Relation of structure to function in bacterial endotoxins. VIII. Biological activities in a polysaccharide-rich fraction, *J. Immunol.* **115**:199.

Nozawa, R. T., Sekiguchi, R., and Yokota, T., 1980a, Stimulation by conditioned medium of L929 fibroblasts, *E. coli* lipopolysaccharide, and muramyl dipeptide of candidacidal activity of mouse macrophages, *Cell. Immunol.* **53**:116.

Nozawa, R. T., Yanaki, N., and Yokota, T., 1980b, Cell growth and antimicrobial activity of mouse peritoneal macrophages in response to glucocorticoids, choleragen and lipopolysaccharide, *Microbiol. Immunol.* **24**:1199.

Ogawa, T., Kotani, S., Fukuda, K., Tsukamoto, Y., Mori, M., Kusumoto, S., and Shiba, S., 1982, Stimulation of migration of human monocytes by bacterial cell walls and muramyl peptides, *Infect. Immun.* **38**:817.

Ogawa, T., Kotani, S., Kusumoto, S., and Shiba, T., 1983, Possible chemotaxis of human monocytes by N-acetylmuramyl-L-alanyl-D-isoglutamine, *Infect. Immun.* **39**:449.

Olds, G. R., Chedid, L., Lederer, E., and Mahmoud, A. A. F., 1980, Induction of resistance to *Schistosoma mansoni* by natural cord factor and synthetic lower homologs, *J. Infect. Dis.* **141**:473.

Ooi, Y. M., Harris, D. E., Edelson, P. J., and Colten, H. R., 1980, Post-translational control of complement (C5) production by resident and stimulated mouse macrophages, *J. Immunol.* **124**:2077.

Oppenheim, J. J., Mizel, S. B., and Meltzer, M. S., 1979, Biological effects of lymphocyte and macrophage-derived mitogenic "amplification" factors, in: *Biology of the Lymphokines* (S. Cohen, E. Pick, and J. J. Oppenheim, eds.), pp. 291–323, Academic Press, New York.

Oppenheim, J. J., Koopman, W. J., Wahl, L. M., and Dougherty, S. F., 1980a, Prostaglandin E$_2$ rather than lymphocyte-activating factor produced by activated human mononuclear cells stimulates increases in murine thymocyte cAMP *Cell. Immunol.* **49**:64.

Oppenheim, J. J., Togawa, A., Chedid, L., and Mizel, S., 1980b, Components of mycobacteria and muramyl dipeptide with adjuvant activity induce lymphocyte activating factor, *Cell. Immunol.* **50**:71.

Orbach-Arbouys, S., Tenu, J.-P., and Petit, J.-F., 1983, Enhancement of *in vitro* and *in vivo* antitumor activity by cord factor (6-6'-dimycolate of trehalose) administered suspended in saline, *Int. Arch. Allergy Appl. Immunol.* **71**:67.

Osada, Y., Mitsuyama, M., Uno, T., Matsumoto, K., Otani, T., Sato, M., Ogawa, H., and Nomoto, K., 1982a, Effect of (L18)-MDP(Ala), a synthetic muramyl dipeptide derivative, on non-specific resistance of mice to microbial infection, *Infect. Immun.* **37**:292.

Osada, Y., Otani, T., Sato, M., Uno, T., Matsumoto, K., and Ogawa, H., 1982b, Polymorphonuclear leucocytes activation by a synthetic muramyl dipeptide analog, *Infect. Immun.* **38**:848.

Pabst, M. J., and Johnston, R. B., 1980, Increased production of superoxide anion by macrophages exposed *in vitro* to muramyl dipeptide or lipopolysaccharide, *J. Exp. Med.* **151**:101.

Pabst, M. J., Cummings, N. P., Shiba, T., Kusumoto, S., and Kotani, S., 1980, Lipophilic derivative of muramyl dipeptide is more active than muramyl dipeptide in priming macrophages to release superoxide anion, *Infect. Immun.* **29**:617.

Pabst, M. J., Hedegaard, H. B., and Johnston, R. B., 1982, Cultured human monocytes require exposure to bacterial products to maintain an optimal oxygen radical response, *J. Immunol.* **128**:123.

Pacak, F., and Siegert, R., 1982, Chemical characterization of a rabbit leukocytic pyrogen, *Eur. J. Biochem.* **127**:375.

Parant, M., 1979, Biologic properties of a new synthetic adjuvant, muramyl dipeptide (MDP), *Springer Semin. Immunopathol.* **2**:101.

Parant, M., Parant, F., Chedid, L., Drapier, J. C., Petit, J.-F., Wietzerbin, J., and Lederer, E., 1977, Enhancement of nonspecific immunity to bacterial infection by cord factor (6,6'-trehalose dimycolate), *J. Infect. Dis.* **135**:771.

Parant, M., Audibert, F., Parant, F., Chedid, L. Soler, E., Polonsky, J., and Lederer, E., 1978a, Nonspecific immunostimulant activities of synthetic trehalose-6,6'-diesters, *Infect. Immun.* **20**:12.

Parant, M., Parant, F., and Chedid, L., 1978b, Enhancement of the neonate's nonspecific immunity to *Klebsiella* infection by muramyl dipeptide, a synthetic immunoadjuvant, *Proc. Natl. Acad. Sci. USA* **75**:3395.

Parant, M., Parant, F., Chedid, L., Yapo, A., Petit, J.-F., and Lederer, E., 1979, Fate of the synthetic immunoadjuvant, muramyl dipeptide (^{14}C)-labelled in the mouse, *Int. J. Immunopharmacol.* **1**:35.

Parant, M., Audibert, F., Chedid, L., Level, M., Lefrancier, P., Choay, J., and Lederer, E., 1980a,

Immunostimulant activities of a lipophilic muramyl dipeptide derivative and of desmuramyl peptidolipid analogs, *Infect. Immun.* **27**:825.

Parant, M., Parant, F., and Chedid, L., 1980b, Enhancement of resistance to infections by endotoxin-induced serum factor from *Mycobacterium bovis* BCG infected mice, *Infect. Immun.* **28**:654.

Parant, M., Riveau, G., Parant, F., Dinarello, C. A., Wolff, S. M., and Chedid, L., 1980c, Effect of indomethacin on increased resistance to bacterial infection and on febrile response induced by muramyl dipeptide, *J. Infect. Dis.* **142**:707.

Parr, I., Wheeler, E., and Alexander, P., 1973, Similarities of the antitumor actions of endotoxin lipid A and double-stranded RNA, *Br. J. Cancer* **27**:370.

Passwell, J. H., Dayer, J. M., and Merler, E., 1979, Increased prostaglandin production by human monocytes after membrane receptor activation, *J. Immunol.* **123**:115.

Passwell, J. H., Dayer, J. M., Gass, K., and Edelson, P. J., 1980, Regulation by Fc fragments of the secretion of collagenase, PGE_2 and lysozyme by mouse peritoneal macrophages, *J. Immunol.* **125**:910.

Peavy, D. L., Baughn, R. E., and Musher, D. M., 1978, Strain-dependent cytotoxic effects of endotoxin for mouse peritoneal macrophages, *Infect. Immun.* **21**:310.

Pelus, L. M., and Bockman, R. S., 1979, Increased prostaglandin synthesis by macrophages from tumor bearing mice, *J. Immunol.* **123**:2118.

Pimm, M. V., Baldwin, R. W., Polonsky, J., and Lederer, E., 1979, Immunotherapy of an ascitic hepatoma with cord factor (trehalose 6,6'-dimycolate) and synthetic analogs, *Int. J. Cancer* **24**:780.

Polonsky, J., Soler, E., and Varenne, J., 1978, Sur la synthèse du cord factor et de ses analogues, *Carbohydr. Res.* **65**:295.

Poste, G., Bucana, C., Raz, A., Bugelski, P., Kirsh, R., and Fidler, I. J., 1982, Analysis of the fate of systemically administered liposomes and implications for their use in drug delivery, *Cancer Res.* **42**:1412.

Proctor, J. W., Waters, R. V., Jones, G. H., Gorecka-Tisers, A., and Yamamura, Y., 1982, Vascular clearance of embolic tumor cells and colloidal carbon and the levels of serum lysozyme following muramyl dipeptide administration, *Oncodev. Biol. Med.* **3**:179.

Qureshi, N., Takayama, K., and Ribi, E., 1982, Purification and structural determination of nontoxic lipid A obtained from the lipopolysaccharide of *Salmonella typhimurium*, *J. Biol. Chem.* **257**:11808.

Rabinovitch, M., Manejias, R. E., Russo, M., and Abbey, E. E., 1977, Increased spreading of macrophages from mice treated with interferon inducers, *Cell. Immunol.* **29**:86.

Ralph, P., and Nakoinz, I., 1977, Direct toxic effects of immunopotentiators on monocytic, myelomonocytic, and histiocytic or macrophage tumor cells in culture, *Cancer Res.* **37**:546.

Ralph, P., and Nakoinz, I., 1981, Differences in antibody-dependent cellular cytotoxicity and activated killing of tumor cells by macrophage cell lines, *Cancer Res.* **41**:3546.

Ralph, P., Broxmeyer, H. E., and Nakoinz, I., 1977, Immunomodulators induce granulocyte/macrophage colony-stimulating activity and block proliferation in a monocyte tumor cell line, *J. Exp. Med.* **146**:611.

Ralph, P., Broxmeyer, H. E., Moore, M. A. S., and Nakoinz, I., 1978, Induction of myeloid colony stimulating activity in murine monocyte tumor cell lines by macrophage activators and in a T-cell line by concanavalin A, *Cancer Res.* **38**:1414.

Ramanathan, V. D., Curtis, J., and Turk, J. L., 1980, Activation of the alternative pathway of complement by mycobacteria and cord factor, *Infect. Immun.* **29**:30.

Raschke, W. C., Baird, S., Ralph, P., and Nakoinz, I., 1978, Functional macrophage cell lines transformed by Abelson leukemia virus, *Cell* **15**:261.

Reed, W. P., and Lucas, Z. J., 1975, Cytotoxic activity of lymphocytes. V. Role of soluble toxin in macrophage inhibited cultures of tumor cells, *J. Immunol.* **115**:395.

Reichert, C. M., Carelli, C., Jolivet, M., Audibert, F., Lefrancier, P., and Chedid, L., 1980, Synthesis of conjugates containing N-acetylmuramyl-L-alanyl-D-isoglutaminyl (MDP): Their use as hapten-carrier systems, *Mol. Immunol.* **17**:357.

Reisser, D., Jeannin, J. F., and Martin, F., 1982, Activation antitumorale des macrophages, péritonéaux de rats par le muramyl dipeptide *in vitro*, *C. R. Acad. Sci. Paris* **295**:485.

Reisser, D., Jeannin, J. F., and Martin, F., 1984, Effet *in vivo* et *in vitro* du dimycolate de tréhalose

(TDM) sur l'activité tumoricide des macrophages péritoneáux de rat, *C. R. Acad. Sci. Paris* **298**:181.

Remington, J. S., 1982, Role of the activated macrophage in resistance to infection, in: *Microbiology—1982* (D. Schlessinger, ed.), pp. 374–377, American Society for Microbiology, Washington, D.C.

Renoux, G., Renoux, M., and Branche, R., 1972, Stimulation of antibacterial vaccination in mice by polyadenylic:polyuridylic complex, *Infect. Immun.* **6**:199.

Retzinger, G. S., Meredith, S. C., Takayama, K., Hunter, R. L., and Kezdy, F. J., 1981, The role of surface in the biological activities of trehalose 6,6'-dimycolate, *J. Biol. Chem.* **256**:8208.

Retzinger, G. S., Meredith, S. C., Hunter, R. L., Takayama, K., and Kezdy, F. J., 1982, Identification of the physiologically active state of the mycobacterial glycolipid trehalose 6,6'-dimycolate and the role of fibrinogen in the biologic activities of trehalose 6,6'-dimycolate monolayers, *J. Immunol.* **129**:735.

Reynolds, J. A., Kastelo, M. D., Harrington, D. G., Crabbs, C. L., Peters, C. J., Jemski, J. V., Scott, G. H., and DiLuzio, N. R., 1980, Glucan-induced enhancement of host resistance to selected infectious diseases, *Infect. Immun.* **30**:51.

Ribi, E., Milner, K. C., Granger, D. L., Kelly, M. T., Yamamoto, K.-I., Brehmer, W., Parker, R., Smith, R. F., and Strain, M. S., 1976, Immunotherapy with nonviable microbial components, *Ann. N.Y. Acad. Sci.* **277**:228.

Riveau, G., Masek, K., Parant, M., and Chedid, L., 1980, Central pyrogenic activity of muramyl dipeptide, *J. Exp. Med.* **152**:869.

Rosenwasser, L. J., and Dinarello, C. A., 1981, Ability of human leucocyte pyrogen to enhance phytohemagglutinin induced murine thymocyte proliferation, *Cell. Immunol.* **63**:134.

Ruco, L. P., and Meltzer, M. S., 1978a, Macrophage activation for tumor cytotoxicity: Development of macrophage cytotoxic activity requires completion of a sequence of short-lived intermediate reactions, *J. Immunol.* **121**:2035.

Ruco, L. P., and Meltzer, M. S., 1978b, Macrophage activation for tumor cytotoxicity: Tumoricidal activity by macrophages from C3H/HeJ mice requires at least two activation stimuli, *Cell. Immunol.* **41**:35.

Russell, S. W., Doe, W. F., and McIntosh, A. T., 1977, Functional characterization of a stable noncytolytic stage of macrophage activation in tumors, *J. Exp. Med.* **146**:1511.

Russell, S. W., Gillepsie, G. Y., and Pace, J. I., 1980, Comparison of responses to activating agents by mouse peritoneal macrophages and cells of the macrophage line RAW 264, *J. Reticuloendothel. Soc.* **27**:607.

Russell, S. W., Taffet, S. M., and Pace, J. L., 1981, The roles of lymphokine and prostaglandin in the regulation of mouse macrophage activation for tumor cell killing, *Prog. Cancer Res. Ther.* **19**:49.

Ryan, J. L., and Yoke, W. B., 1981, Lymphocyte mediation of lipopolysaccharide-stimulated macrophage metabolism, *J. Immunol.* **127**:912.

Ryan, J. L., Glode, L. M., and Rosenstreich, D. L., 1979, Lack of responsiveness of C3H/HeJ macrophages to lipopolysaccharide: The cellular basis of LPS-stimulated metabolism, *J. Immunol.* **122**:932.

Ryan, J. L., Yoke, W. B., and Morrison, D. C., 1980, Stimulation of peritoneal cell arginase by bacterial lipopolysaccharides, *Am. J. Pathol.* **99**:451.

Saiki, I., Tanio, Y., Yamawaki, M., Uemiya, M., Kobayashi, S., Fukuda T., Yukimasa, H., Yamamura, Y., and Azuma, I., 1981, Adjuvant activities of quinonyl-N-acetyl-muramyl dipeptides in mice and guinea pigs, *Infect. Immun.* **31**:114.

Saiki, I., Tanio, Y., Azuma, I., Yamawaki, M., Uemiya, M., Kobayashi, S., Fukuda, T., Yukimasa, H., Imada, I., Okamoto, K., Yajima, A., and Yamamura, Y., 1982, Adjuvant and antitumor activities of quinonyl-N-acetyl muramylpeptides in mice and guinea pigs, in: *Immunomodulation by Microbial Products and Related Synthetic Compounds* (Y. Yamamura, S. Kotani, I. Azuma, A. Koda, and T. Shiba, eds.), pp. 391–394, Excerpta Medica, Amsterdam.

Saito, H., and Tomioka, H., 1979, Enhanced hydrogen peroxide release from macrophages stimulated with streptococcal preparation OK 432, *Infect. Immun.* **26**:779.

Sasada, M., and Johnston, R. B., 1980, Macrophage microbicidal activity: Correlation between phagocytosis associated oxidative metabolism and the killing of *Candida* by macrophages, *J. Exp. Med.* **152**:85.

Schell, P. L., 1971, Uptake of polynucleotides by intact mammalian cells. VIII. Synthetic homo-ribopolynucleotides, *Biochim. Biophys. Acta* **240**:472.

Schindler, T., Chedid, L., and Hadden, J., 1982, Stimulatory effects of MDP and its butyl ester derivative on macrophage proliferation and activation *in vitro, Int. J. Immunopharmacol.* **4**:382.

Schleifer, K. H., and Kandler, O., 1972, Peptidoglycan types of bacterial cell walls and their taxonomic implications, *Bacteriol. Rev.* **36**:407.

Schorlemmer, H. U., Bosslet, K., and Sedlacek, H. H., 1982a, Activation of macrophages for killing of tumor cells by the immunomodulator bestatin, *Int. J. Immunopharmacol.* **4**:278.

Schorlemmer, H. U., Luben, G. H. A., and Sedlacek, H. H., 1982b, Stimulatory effect of bestatin on the functions of mononuclear phagocytes, *Int. J. Immunopharmacol.* **4**:279.

Schroit, A. J., and Fidler, I. J., 1982, Effects of liposome structure and lipid composition on the activation of the tumoricidal properties of macrophages by liposomes containing muramyl dipeptide, *Cancer Res.* **42**:161.

Schubert, R. D., and David, J. R., 1980, Stimulation of guinea pig macrophage pinocytosis by lipopolysaccharides (LPS): Evidence that LPS acts directly on the macrophages, *Cell. Immunol.* **55**:166.

Schultz, R. M., and Jackson, W. T., 1981, Effects of inhibitors and products of arachidonic acid metabolism on macrophage mediated cytotoxicity induced by interferon and lipopolysaccharide, in: *Mediation of Cellular Immunity by Immune Modifiers* (M. A. Chirigos, M. Mitchell, M. J. Mastrangelo, and M. Krim, eds.), pp. 89–99, Raven Press, New York.

Schultz, R. M., Papamatheakis, J. D., and Chirigos, M. A., 1977a, Direct activation *in vitro* of mouse peritoneal macrophages by pyran copolymer (NSC 46015), *Cell. Immunol.* **29**:403.

Schultz, R. M., Papamatheakis, J. D., and Chirigos, M. A., 1977b, Interferon: An inducer of macrophage activation by polyanions, *Science* **197**:674.

Schultz, R. M., Papamatheakis, J. D., Luetzeler, J., and Chirigos, M. A., 1977c, Association of macrophage activation with antitumor activity by synthetic and biological agents, *Cancer Res.* **37**:3338.

Schultz, R. M., Pavlidis, N. A., Chirigos, M. A., and Weiss, J. F., 1978, Effects of whole body X-irradiation and cyclophosphamide treatment on induction of macrophage tumoricidal function in mice, *Cell. Immunol.* **38**:302.

Scott, W. A., Pawlowski, N. A., Murray, H. W., Andreach, M., Zrike, J., and Cohn, Z. A., 1982, Regulation of arachidonic acid metabolism by macrophage activation, *J. Exp. Med.* **155**:1148.

Sharma, S. D., Tsai, V., Krahenbuhl, J. L., and Remington, J. S., 1981, Augmentation of mouse natural killer cell activity by muramyl dipeptide and its analogs, *Cell. Immunol.* **62**:101.

Shaw, J. O., Russ ll, S. W., Printz, M. P., and Skidgel, R. A., 1979, Macrophage mediated tumor cell killing: Lack of dependence on the cyclooxygenase pathway of prostaglandin synthesis, *J. Immunol.* **123**:50.

Sheagren, J. N., Simon, H. B., Tuazon, C. V., and Mehrotra, P. P., 1975, Cell-mediated immunity *in vitro*, in: *Mononuclear Phagocytes in Immunity, Infection and Pathology* (R. van Furth, ed.), pp. 653–659, Blackwell, Oxford.

Shiba, T., 1982, Synthetic approach to elucidation for chemical structure and biological activity of lipid A, in: *Immunomodulation by Microbial Products and Related Synthetic Compounds* (Y. Yamamura, S. Kotani, I. Azuma, A. Koda, and T. Shiba, eds.), pp. 94–102, Excerpta Medica, Amsterdam.

Simon, P. L., and Willoughby, W. F., 1982, Biochemical and biological characterization of rabbit interleukin-1 (IL-1), in: *Lymphokines*, Volume 6 (S. B. Mizel, ed.), pp. 47–63, Academic Press, New York.

Sipe, J. D., Vogel, S. N., Ryan, J. L., McAdam, K. P. W. J., and Rosenstreich, D. L., 1979, Detection of a mediator derived from endotoxin-stimulated macrophages that induces the acute phase serum amyloid A response in mice, *J. Exp. Med.* **150**:597.

Snider, M. E., Fertel, R. H., and Zwillig, B. S., 1982, Prostaglandin regulation of macrophage function: Effect of endogenous and exogenous prostaglandins, *Cell. Immunol.* **74**:234.

Sone, S., and Fidler, I. J., 1980, Synergistic activation by lymphokines and muramyl dipeptides of tumoricidal properties in rat alveolar macrophages, *J. Immunol.* **125**:2454.

Sone, S., and Fidler, I. J., 1981, *In vitro* activation of tumoricidal properties in rat alveolar macrophages by synthetic muramyl dipeptide encapsulated in liposomes, *Cell. Immunol.* **57**:42.

Sone, S., and Tsubura, E., 1982, Human alveolar macrophages: Potentiation of their tumoricidal activity by liposome encapsulated muramyl dipeptide, *J. Immunol.* **129**:1313.

Sone, S., Moriguchi, S., Shimizu, E., Ogushi, F., and Tsubura, E., 1982, *In vitro* generation of tumoricidal properties in human alveolar macrophages following interaction with endotoxin, *Cancer Res.* **42**:2227.

Sorrell, T. C., Lehrer, R. I., and Cline, M. J., 1978, Mechanism of nonspecific macrophage-mediated cytotoxicity: Evidence for lack of dependence upon oxygen, *J. Immunol.* **120**:347.

Staber, F. G., Gisler, R. H., Schumann, G., Tarcsay, L., and Schlafli, E., 1978, Modulation of myelopoiesis by different bacterial cell wall components: Induction of colony-stimulating activity (by pure preparations, low-molecular-weight degradation products, and a synthetic low-molecular analog cell-wall component) *in vitro*, *Cell. Immunol.* **37**:174.

Stadler, B. M., and de Weck, A. L., 1980, Flow-cytometric analysis of mouse peritoneal macrophages, *Cell. Immunol.* **54**:36.

Steeg, P. S., Johnson, H. M., and Oppenheim, J. J., 1982, Regulation of murine macrophage Ia antigen expression by an immune interferon like lymphokine: Inhibitory effect of endotoxin, *J. Immunol.* **129**:2402.

Stinebring, W. R., and Youngner, J. S., 1964, Patterns of interferon appearance in mice injected with bacteria or bacterial endotoxin, *Nature (London)* **204**:712.

Stoychkov, J. N., Schultz, R. M., Chirigos, M. A., Pavlidis, N. A., and Goldin, A., 1979, Effect of adriamycin and cyclophosphamide treatment on induction of macrophage cytotoxic function in mice, *Cancer Res.* **39**:3014.

Szabo, P., Sarfati, R., Diolez, C., and Szabo, L., 1983, Synthesis of *O*-{2-deoxy-2-[(3*R*)-3-hydroxytetradecanamido]-D-glucopyranosyl-4-phosphate- (1 6)-2-deoxy2-(3R)-3-hydroxytetradecanamido -D-glucose: The monosaccharide route, *Carbohydr. Res.* **111**:C9.

Taffet, S. M., Pace, J. L., and Russell, S. W., 1981, Lymphokine maintains macrophage activation for tumor cell killing by interfering with the negative regulatory effect of prostaglandin E, *J. Immunol.* **127**:121.

Taffet, S. M., Eurell, T. E., and Russell, S. W., 1982, Regulation of macrophage-mediated tumor cell killing by prostaglandins: Comparison of the effects of PGE_2 and PGI_2, *Prostaglandins* **24**:763.

Takada, H., Tsujimoto, M., Kato, K., Kotani, S., Kusumoto, S., Inage, M., Shiba, T., Yano, I., Kawata, S., and Yokogawa, K., 1979, Macrophage activation by bacterial cell walls and related synthetic compounds, *Infect. Immun.* **25**:48.

Tanaka, A., 1982, Macrophage activation by muramyl dipeptide (MDP), in: *Immunomodulation by Microbial Products and Related Synthetic Compounds* (Y. Yamamura, S. Kotani, I. Azuma, A. Koda, and T. Shiba, eds.), pp. 72–83, Excerpta Medica, Amsterdam.

Tanaka, A., Nagao, S., Kotani, S., Shiba, T., and Kusumoto, S., 1979, Stimulation of the reticuloendothelial system of mice by muramyl dipeptide, *Infect. Immun.* **24**:302.

Tanaka, A., Nagao, S., Imai, K., and Mori, R., 1980, Macrophage activation by muramyl dipeptide as measured by macrophage spreading and attachment, *Microbiol. Immunol.* **24**:547.

Tanaka, A., Nagao, S., Ikegami, S., Shiba, T., and Kotani, S., 1982, The suppression of macrophage DNA synthesis by MDP, a probable correlate of macrophage activation, in: *Immunomodulation by Microbial Products and Related Synthetic Compounds* (Y. Yamamura, S. Kotani, I. Azuma, A. Koda, and T. Shiba, eds.), pp. 201–204, Excerpta Medica, Amsterdam.

Taniyama, T., and Holden, H. T., 1979, Direct augmentation of cytolytic activity of tumor-derived macrophages and macrophage cell lines by muramyl dipeptide, *Cell. Immunol.* **48**:369.

Taniyama, T., and Holden, H. T., 1980, Cytolytic activity against tumor cells by macrophage cell lines and augmentation by macrophage stimulants, *Int. J. Cancer* **26**:61.

Taramelli, D., and Varesio, L., 1981, Activation of murine macrophages. I. Different pattern of activation by poly I:C than by lymphokine or LPS, *J. Immunol.* **127**:58.

Taverne, J., Dockrell, H., and Playfair, H. L., 1981, Endotoxin-induced serum factor kills malarial parasites *in vitro*, *Infect. Immun.* **33**:83.

Tenu, J.-P., Lederer, E., and Petit, J.-F., 1980, Stimulation of thymocyte mitogenic protein secretion and of cytostatic activity of mouse peritoneal macrophages by trehalose dimycolate and muramyl dipeptide, *Eur. J. Immunol.* **10**:647.

Tenu, J.-P., Roche, A.-C., Yapo, A., Kieda, C., Monsigny, M., and Petit, J.-F., 1982, Absence of cell surface receptors for muramylpeptides in mouse peritoneal macrophages, *Biol. Cell.* **44**:157.

Tomasič, J., Ladesič, B., Valinger, Z., and Hrisak, I., 1980, The fate of ^{14}C labelled peptidoglycan monomer and the corresponding pentapeptide in urine, *Biochim. Biophys. Acta* **629**:77.

Tomioka, H., and Saito, H., 1980, Hydrogen peroxide-releasing function of chemically elicited and immunologically activated macrophages: Differential response to wheat germ lectin and concanavalin A, *Infect. Immun.* **29**:469.

Tsukamoto, Y., Helsel, W. E., and Wahl, S. M., 1981, Macrophage production of fibronectin, a chemoattractant for fibroblasts, *J. Immunol.* **127**:673.

Tuttle, R. L., and Cantrell, J., 1981, *C. parvum*—Determinants of biologic activity, *Prog. Cancer Res. Ther.* **16**:53.

Uemiya, M., Saiki, I., Kusama, T., Azuma, I., and Yamamura, Y., 1979, Adjuvant activity of mycoloyl derivatives of N-acetyl-muramyl-L-alanyl-D-isoglutamine in mice and guinea pigs, *Microbiol. Immunol.* **23**:821.

Umezawa, H., 1980, Low-molecular-weight immunomodulators produced by microorganisms, *Biotechnol. Bioeng.* **22**(Suppl. 1):99.

Unanue, E. R., and Kiely, J. M., 1977, Synthesis and secretion of a mitogenic protein by macrophages: Description of a superinduction phenomenon, *J. Immunol.* **119**:925.

Vogel, S. N., Marshall, S. T., and Rosenstreich, D. L., 1979, Analysis of the effects of lipopolysaccharide on macrophages: Differential phagocytic responses of C3H/HeN and C3H/HeJ macrophages *in vitro*, *Infect. Immun.* **25**:328.

Wahl, L. M., Wahl, S. M., Mergenhagen, S. E., and Martin, G. H., 1974, Collagenase production by endotoxin activated macrophages, *Proc. Natl. Acad. Sci. USA* **71**:3598.

Wahl, L. M., Olsen, C. E., Sandberg, A. L., and Mergenhagen, S. E., 1977, Prostaglandin regulation of macrophage collagenase production, *Proc. Natl. Acad. Sci. USA* **74**:4955.

Wahl, L. M., Wahl, S. M., and McCarthy, J. B., 1980, Adjuvant activation of macrophage functions, in: *Macrophage Regulation of Immunity* (E. R. Unanue and A. S. Rosenthal, eds.), pp. 491–504, Academic Press, New York.

Wahl, S. M., and Wahl, L. M., 1981, Modulation of fibroblast growth and function by monokines and lymphokines, in: *Lymphokines*, Volume 2 (E. Pick, ed.), pp. 179–201, Academic Press, New York.

Wahl, S. M., Wahl, L. M., McCarthy, J. B., Chedid, L., and Mergenhagen, S. E., 1979, Macrophage activation by mycobacterial water-soluble components and synthetic muramyl dipeptide, *J. Immunol.* **122**:2226.

Waters, R. V., and Ferraresi, R. W., 1980, Muramyl dipeptide stimulation of particle clearance in several animal species, *J. Reticuloendothel. Soc.* **28**:457.

Way, C. W., Dougherty, W. J., and Cook, J., 1982, Inhibition of glucan induced hepatic granuloma formation by indomethacin or essential fatty acid deficiency, *Int. J. Immunopharmacol.* **4**:269a.

Weinberg, J. B., Chapman, H. A., and Hibbs, J. B., Jr., 1978, Characterization of the effects of endotoxin on macrophage tumor cell killing, *J. Immunol.* **121**:72.

Weiss, D. W., Stupp, Y., Many, N., and Izak, G., 1975, Treatment of acute myelocytic leukemia (AML) patients with the MER tubercle bacillus fraction: A preliminary report, *Transplant. Proc.* **7**(Suppl. 1):545.

Werb, Z., Bainton, D. F., and Jones, P. A., 1980, Degradation of connective tissue matrices by macrophages. III. Morphological and biochemical studies on extracellular, pericellular and intracellular events in matrix proteolysis by macrophages in culture, *J. Exp. Med.* **152**:1537.

Werner, G. H., Floc'h, F., Bouchaudon, J., Zerial, A., Migliore-Samour, D. and Jollès, P., 1982, Low molecular weight synthetic lipopeptides: A new class of immunopotentiating substances, in: *Current Concepts in Human Immunology and Cancer Immunomodulation* (B. Serrou, ed.), pp. 645–652, Elsevier/North-Holland, Amsterdam.

Westphal, O., and Jann, K., 1965, Bacterial lipopolysaccharides: Extraction with phenol-water and further applications of procedure, *Methods Carbohydr. Chem.* **5**:80.

Westphal, O., Jann, K., and Himmelpach, K., 1983, Chemistry and immunochemistry of bacterial lipopolysaccharides as cell wall antigens and endotoxins, *Prog. Allergy* **33**:9.

Whistler, R. L., Bushway, A. A., Singh, P. P., Nakahara, W., and Tokuzen, R., 1976, Noncytotoxic, antitumor polysaccharides, *Adv. Carbohydr. Chem. Biochem.* **32**:235.

Wiener, E., and Levanon, D., 1968, The *in vitro* interaction between bacterial lipopolysaccharides and differentiating monocytes, *Lab. Invest.* **19**:584.

Williams, D., Browder, W., and DiLuzio, N. R., 1982, Prevention of phagocytic depression, sepsis and mortality induced by *E. coli* by glucan administration: Role of the macrophage, *Int. J. Immunopharmacol.* **4**:264a.

Wilton, J. M., Rosenstreich, D. L., and Oppenheim, J. J., 1975, Activation of guinea pig macrophages by bacterial lipopolysaccharide requires bone marrow-derived lymphocytes, *J. Immunol.* **114**:388.

Wood, D. D., and Cameron, P. M., 1978, The relationship between bacterial endotoxin and human B cell activating factor, *J. Immunol.* **121**:53.

Wood, D., and Staruch, M. J., 1980, Biochemical properties and cellular requirements of BAF, in: *Biochemical Characterization of Lymphokines* (A. L. de Weck, F. Kristensen, and M. Landy, eds.), pp. 423–425, Academic Press, New York.

Yamamoto, Y., Nagao, S., Tanaka, A., Koga, T., and Onoue, K., 1978, Inhibition of macrophage migration by synthetic muramyl dipeptide, *Biochem. Biophys. Res. Commun.* **80**:923.

Yamamura, Y., and Azuma, I., 1982, Cancer immunotherapy with cell-wall skeletons of BCG and *Nocardia rubra* and related synthetic compounds, in: *Immunomodulation by Microbial Products and Related Synthetic Compounds* (Y. Yamamura, S. Kotani, I. Azuma, A. Koda, and T. Shiba, eds.), pp. 17–36, Excerpta Medica, Amsterdam.

Yamamura, Y. Azuma, I., Sugimura, K., Yamawaki, M., Kusumoto, S., Okada, S., and Shiba, T., 1976, Adjuvant activity of 6-O-mycoloyl-N-acetylmuramyl-L-alanyl-D-isoglutamine, *Gann* **67**:867.

Yamamura, Y., Yasumoto, K., Ogura, T., and Azuma, I., 1981, *Nocardia rubra*-cell wall skeleton in the therapy of animal and human cancer, *Prog. Cancer Res. Ther.* **16**:71.

Yapo, A., Petit, J.-F., Lederer, E., Parant, M., Parant, F., and Chedid, L., 1982, Fate of two ^{14}C labelled muramyl peptides: Ac-Mur-L-Ala-γ-D-Glu-meso-A$_2$PM and Ac-Mur-L-Ala-γ-D-Glu-*meso*-A$_2$PM-D-Ala-D-Ala in mice: Evaluation of their ability to increase nonspecific resistance to *Klebsiella* infection, *Int. J. Immunopharmacol.* **4**:143.

Yarkoni, E., and Bekierkunst, A., 1976, Nonspecific resistance against infection with *Salmonella typhi* and *Salmonella typhimurium* induced in mice by cord factor (6-6′ trehalose dimycolate) and its analogs, *Infect. Immun.* **14**:1125.

Yarkoni, E., and Rapp, H. J., 1977, Granuloma formation in lungs of mice after intravenous administration of emulsified trehalose-6,6′-dimycolate (cord factor): Reaction intensity depends on size distribution of the oil droplets, *Infect. Immun.* **18**:552.

Yarkoni, E., Wang, L., and Bekierkunst, A., 1977, Stimulation of macrophages by cord factor and by heat-killed and living BCG, *Infect. Immun.* **16**:1.

Yarkoni, E., Rapp, H. J., Polonsky, J., and Lederer, E., 1978, Immunotherapy with an intralesionally administered synthetic cord factor analog, *Int. J. Cancer* **22**:564.

Yarkoni, E., Lederer, E., and Rapp, H. J., 1981, Immunotherapy of experimental cancer with a mixture of synthetic muramyl dipeptide and trehalose dimycolate, *Infect. Immun.* **32**:273.

Yin, H. L., Aleg, S., Bianco, C., and Cohn, Z. A., 1980, Plasma membrane polypeptides of resident and activated mouse peritoneal macrophages, *Proc. Natl. Acad. Sci. USA* **77**:2188.

Young, M. R., Cheung, H. T., and Sundharadas, G., 1980, Selective inhibition of tumor cell migration by culture supernatants derived from normal and lipopolysaccharide activated macrophages, *J. Reticuloendothel. Soc.* **27**:143.

Youngner, J. S., and Feingold, D. S., 1982, Potential for cancer therapy with a *Brucella abortus* preparation (BRU-PEL), *Prog. Cancer Res. Ther.* **16**:205.

Zbar, B., Ribi, E., Meyer, T., Azuma, I., and Rapp, H. J., 1974, Immunotherapy of cancer: Regression of established intradermal tumors after intralesional injection of mycobacterial cell walls attached to oil droplets, *J. Natl. Cancer Inst.* **52**:1571.

Zendegui, J. G., and Klein, T. W., 1982, Reduction in cyclic 3′5′-adenosine monophosphate phosphodiesterase activity in exudate and cultured mouse peritoneal macrophages, *J. Reticuloendothel. Soc.* **31**:455.

10

Stimulation and Depression of the RES by Pharmacological Agents

KURT B. P. FLEMMING

1. INTRODUCTION

This review is concerned with the effects of pharmacological agents on the phagocytosis function of the RES. With regard to applicability in experimental biology and clinical medicine, the classification into stimulants and depressants appears to be expedient. However, from an objective point of view, such a choice is not always justified and sometimes even appears arbitrary. The physical processes and chemical reactions that are affected by pharmacological agents acting on the organism are modified by specific properties of the biological systems in diverse ways, for example, reabsorption, organ distribution, blood circulation as well as systemic and neural reactions and feedback reactions. With respect to the pharmacological agents, the mode of application and the height of the dose response, i.e., the time over which a certain dose is applied, have to be considered. As a result of these factors, a single agent may act in opposite ways if very different doses are administered or if the effect is established at different times following administration, i.e., it can act both as a stimulant and as a depressant.

The "blockade" of the RES often mentioned in the literature is a complex and poorly defined phenomenon that cannot be dealt with in detail here. Also, no attempt will be made to review all of the known RES-modulating agents.

2. STIMULATION OF PHAGOCYTOSIS

2.1. ESTROGENS

Many studies in guinea pigs, mice, and rats of both sexes have shown that natural and synthetic estrogens stimulate the RES as indicated by hypertrophy

---

KURT B. P. FLEMMING • Institute of Biophysics and Radiation Biology, Albert Ludwig University, D-7800 Freiburg, Federal Republic of Germany.

of the liver and spleen, proliferation of liver macrophages, and marked increase of the global phagocytic activity (Nicol, 1935; Nicol and Helmy, 1951; Nicol and Abou-Zirky, 1953; Nicol and Bilbey, 1957; Nicol and Ware, 1960; Nicol *et al.*, 1961, 1965, 1966a,b; Heller *et al.*, 1957; Biozzi *et al.*, 1957a; Trejo *et al.*, 1972a). Comparable results have been reported for man. Diethylstilbestrol (DES) was found to stimulate RES activity in patients with cancer. Moreover, the *in vitro* phagocytosis of human polymorphonuclear blood leukocytes was increased by estradiol and DES (Burger and Leonhardt, 1952).

17β-Estradiol appears to be the principal natural estrogen concerned in the control of RES activity (Nicol *et al.*, 1965), and 17β-estradiol, estradiol benzoate, and DES were found to be the most powerful estrogenic stimulators of macrophage activity (Bilbey and Nicol, 1958).

The strongest synthetic stimulants possess the following features: (1) two *p*-hydroxyphenyl groups attached to adjacent carbon atoms; (2) unsaturation; and (3) absence of hydrogen atoms at the α and β carbon atoms (Nicol *et al.*, 1958).

The most effective RES-stimulating estrogens also show high estrogenicity. However, no direct relationship exists between the estrogenic potency of various preparations of estrogens and their phagocytosis-stimulating capacity (Nicol *et al.*, 1958).

For example, DES and its esters are more potent stimulants of phagocytosis than estradiol benzoate and ethinyl estradiol, although the latter steroids possess estrogenicity greater than 10 times that of DES. The minimal dose of DES required to stimulate RES phagocytosis was about 100 times higher than the dose required for an estrogenic effect (Nicol and Ware, 1960). Heller *et al.* (1957) found 1,3,5-estratriene-3,16-β-diol to be active as an RES stimulant although it had only about 1/1000th of the sex hormone activity of estradiol. However, if the hydroxy group in the 16 position was changed so that there was a 3,16-α-diol, most RES activity was lost. In this connection, it must be mentioned that DES and 17β-estradiol, although being potent stimulants of RES phagocytosis in mice, did not stimulate the granulopoietic activity of the RES in male and female rats (Lázár, 1973a). Therefore, the capacity to stimulate the RES appears to be a property of estrogens that is independent of their classical hormonal actions on sex tissues.

The estrogen-induced enhancement of the global phagocytic RES activity was mostly correlated with an enlargement of the liver and spleen and with marked increase of the number of phagocytizing cells (Heller *et al.*, 1957; Nicol and Bilbey, 1960; Kelly *et al.*, 1962). However, it was found by measuring the uptake of colloidal $Cr^{32}PO_4$ in various organs of estrogen-treated mice that, notwithstanding an enlargement of the liver and spleen, the radioactivity per gram of these organs was markedly reduced (Heller *et al.*, 1957). In further studies using 17β-estradiol (Nothdurft and Flemming, 1971) and DES (Loose and DiLuzio, 1976), an increase of phagocytic activity was observed without a concomitant enlargement of the liver and spleen. Thus, the assumption of Heller *et al.* (1957) was confirmed that the phagocytic increase induced by estrogens cannot be explained by the presence of new cells but by a marked increase in the efficiency of existing RES macrophages. This explanation is supported by studies on estradiol-treated mice showing an increase in DNA synthesis in hepatic macrophages that coincided with the increased vascular carbon clearance rate (Kelly *et al.*, 1962).

An interaction between estrogen-induced proliferation and functional activation of RES macrophages could explain certain effects of combinations of estrogens and stimulating or depressing agents. The phagocytosis-depressing effect of cortisone was reversed by treatment with DES (Nicol and Bilbey, 1957), and the combined administration of estradiol and endotoxin resulted in a greater phagocytic increase than obtained with either one of these stimulants (Dobson and Kelly, 1973). In this connection, it is worth mentioning that, in contrast to other RES-stimulating agents, DES-treated mice did not manifest an enhanced sensitivity to endotoxin, nor did DES alter the endotoxin-detoxifying ability of the liver and spleen (Trejo *et al.*, 1972a).

The effects of estrogens on the activity of the RES are of physiological relevance. Cyclical variations in RES activity were found to occur during the estrous cycle and during pregnancy in the rat and mouse, and RES activity fell after ovariectomy. Two peaks of increased phagocytic activity were associated with the estrous cycle in rodents, one during the follicular phase and the other during the luteal phase (Nicol *et al.*, 1964; Nicol and Vernon-Roberts, 1965). Various investigations in women showed a close correspondence between phagocytic activity of the RES and the known variations in the production of estrogenic hormones during the menstrual cycle and pregnancy (Eufinger, 1932; Brown, 1955, 1956). Moreover, it was shown that, in adult female mice, the phagocytic activity of the RES was higher than in adult males (Galton, 1967, Nothdurft and Flemming, 1971). The sex difference is mainly caused by an increased phagocytic activity of the "responsive" macrophages in female mice and not by a rise in their number (Nothdurft and Flemming, 1971). With respect to the well-known enhanced nonspecific resistance of female mammals and women, it must be mentioned that small "physiological" doses of DES, close to the minimal amount required for the induction of estrus in mice, are sufficient to significantly prolong survival time following bacterial infection (Nicol *et al.*, 1964) and whole body irradiation (Rooks and Dorfman, 1961; Ghys, 1961, 1963).

2.2. CHLOROTRIANISENE

Chlorotrianisene (CTA), previously marketed as Tace or Merbentyl, is a synthetic preestrogen that has shown success in the clinical treatment of prostate carcinoma. CTA itself has no estrogenic activity, but a metabolite exerting weak estrogenic activity is formed during its degradation in the liver (Thompson and Werner, 1953). Following injection in mice of 0.4 mg CTA s.c. or i.p. daily for five consecutive days, a phagocytic stimulation of RES macrophages (carbon clearance) was found that equaled the effects of estrogens (Nicol *et al.*, 1961; Flemming, 1965a). Further studies showed that (1) a single injection of 2 mg CTA was as effective as five fractional injections of 0.4 mg; no weight changes of the liver and spleen were seen. (2) Stimulation of phagocytosis occurred following single doses of 0.2 to 20 mg/20 g body wt, the most effective doses ranging from 2 to 10 mg. (3) The phagocytic index K was significantly increased up to more than 40 days, showing maximum values for a rather long period of about 3 weeks. (4) CTA was effective in both sexes, and even after oral administration (Flemming, 1966a,b, 1974).

Compared to natural and synthetic estrogens, the CTA-induced phagocytic increase was considerably stronger and lasted far longer. A detailed analysis of data obtained from vascular clearance time, changes of organ and body weight, histological observations, and cell counting revealed that the extraordinarily high RES-stimulating effectiveness of CTA is due to a combined activation of both macrophage function and macrophage proliferation (Flemming, 1965a).

For CTA, just as for estrogens, no direct connection appears to exist between estrogenicity and phagocytosis-stimulating capacity. A similar lack of correlation was found for the phagocytosis increase and the radioprotective effectiveness of CTA (Flemming and Langendorff, 1965). The chemical nature of the RES-stimulating CTA metabolite is unknown. The three p-methoxyphenyl groups of CTA might be demethylated in the liver to three p-hydroxyphenyl groups (Schmähl, 1957). This suggestion is supported by our finding that the CTA derivative clomiphene, which contains only one hydroxyphenyl group, also induced a phagocytic increase; however, the effect of clomiphene was much weaker than that of CTA and DES (Flemming, 1966b, 1967).

2.3. FATS AND LIPIDS

A variety of i.v. administered lipids are capable of either stimulating or depressing RES phagocytosis, depending on the specific lipid employed for pretreatment (Stuart et al., 1960; Cooper and West, 1962; Cooper, 1964; DiLuzio and Wooles, 1964; Flemming, 1963a,b; Heller, 1960). Dietary lipids have also been shown to influence the rate of phagocytosis by the RES.

2.3.1. Dietary Fats

Gaillard et al. (1974) observed that, after 6 months on a high-fat diet, rats had an enhanced phagocytic RES activity although the only significant alteration in liver or plasma lipid fractions was a decrease in the liver cholesterol concentration. A stimulating effect of orally administered dietary fats on RES phagocytosis was also found in rats maintained on a choline-deficient diet for 3 weeks (Spratt and Kratzing, 1971). The animals developed very fatty livers, and on a beef fat, corn oil, or safflower oil diet as the lipid source, they showed an accelerated carbon clearance half-time, which was related to the hepatic lipid concentration. The increased phagocytic activity did not occur if coconut oil was used as the lipid source in the choline-deficient diet. Safflower oil, which contained 75% linoleic acid, had a more potent effect on phagocytic activity than the standard diet containing only 16% linoleic acid. From these and further findings, it was suggested that the acceleration of phagocytosis in choline deficiency might be related to peroxidation effects. Following i.v. administration of emulsions of canbra, olive, peanut, rapeseed, and soybean oil, an increased phagocytic activity of the RES was found after 3 days in male rats (Pipy *et al.*, 1975). However, with oral administration, stimulation or depression of phagocytic function was dependent on several factors including the nature of the oil and the physical and chemical structure of the emulsion. According to Pipy *et al.* (1975), the variations in particle size (found in emulsions) make it extremely difficult to draw any comparison between their effects on the phagocytic capacity. The effectiveness of oil emulsions on the phagocytic function of RES macrophages could be related to their physical and chemical properties; the mode of esterification of the fatty acids might be an important factor.

2.3.2. Liver Lipids

A potent RES-stimulating lipid extract from shark livers was shown to be strongly active in stimulating the rate of carbon uptake by the RES and in promoting resistance in mice vaccinated against *Salmonella typhimurium* infection. *In vitro* tests with macrophages indicated that this lipid was very rapidly phagocytized and disappeared in a matter of hours (Heller *et al.*, 1963, 1965). Ringle *et al.* (1966) found that liver lipids from four *elasmobranch* species stimulated carbon clearance in mice. Some of these lipids were approximately as effective as zymosan. Lipids from other sources like elasmobranch testes as well as lipids from marine teleost liver and from frog liver and yolk had no effect. These results suggest that RES-stimulating lipid is widely distributed among elasmobranches and may be restricted to this phylogenetic group.

2.3.3. Triglycerides

In experiments with mice, using the carbon clearance method, Stuart *et al.* (1960) investigated the effect of certain emulsified lipids on the global phagocytic activity of the RES. Glyceryl trioleate (triolein) caused an intense stimulation of phagocytic function, glyceryl monooleate had no effect, and ethyl oleate and ethyl stearate markedly depressed phagocytosis. These findings of a profound effect of certain simple lipids on the sessile cells that remove particulate matter from the bloodstream, were confirmed by a series of further investigations showing that a variety of simple lipids possessed the capacity to modify the global phagocytic activity in the whole animal as well as the uptake or ingestion, respectively, of suspensions of particles, lipid emulsions, and microorganisms into isolated macrophages. Furthermore, it was shown that triolein and ethyl stearate affected mainly the phagocytic cells of the liver and, to a lesser extent, the spleen (Cooper and Stuart, 1961). According to the mode of action, these simple lipids can be subdivided into phagocytosis-stimulating glyceryl esters of fatty acids and phagocytosis-depressing alkyl esters of fatty acids (see Section 3.3). Therefore, a novel and easily controlled means of altering phagocytic function of macrophages *in vitro* and RES activity *in vivo* was given.

Cooper and Stuart (1961), Cooper and West (1962), Stuart and Cooper

(1962), and Stuart (1962) showed that triolein enhanced the blood clearance not only of colloidal carbon but also of ^{51}Cr-labeled endotoxin. Flemming and co-workers (Flemming, 1963a,b; Flemming *et al.*, 1967) found tricaprin and 2-oleodistearin to be as effective as triolein, and all were effective not only in mice but also in rats. Cooper (1964) found further saturated triglycerides to stimulate global RES phagocytosis in mice. His results were very informative because the series of triglycerides used in these experiments ranged from caproic acid (C_6) to stearic acid (C_{18}) and, just as with most other investigators, a standard dose of 10 mg/20 g body wt was administered i.v.

Erucic acid, constituting between 40 and 64% of the total fatty acids of various plant oils, as well as its ethyl ester, ethyl erucate, increased the global phagocytic activity in rats following i.v. injection. Erucic acid was also effective if applied orally whereas ethyl erucate was ineffective in this case (Pipy *et al.*, 1975).

The results of experiments *in vitro* agree well with those of experiments *in vivo*. Cooper and West (1962) compared the effect of triolein on phagocytic activity of peritoneal macrophages following triolein treatment *in vivo* and *in vitro*. *Paralobactrum strain* No. 35 D and other bacterial species were used as test material. Triolein-induced stimulation of macrophage phagocytosis occurred under both experimental conditions. The triolein effect was time- and dose-dependent: maximal effects on 2×10^6 cells were not immediately stimulatory but following prolonged incubation the cells eventually developed significant activity. The most active stimulating triglycerides were triolein and tricaprin. Carr and Williams (1966) demonstrated with peritoneal macrophages *in vitro* that cells stimulated by triolein took up particles more avidly than controls.

With the above-mentioned studies of Cooper (1964), further evidence was presented that triglycerides possessing macrophage-stimulating activity *in vivo* also increase the ability of mouse peritoneal macrophages to phagocytize and destroy microorganisms following exposure *in vitro*. The correlation between the results of these two methods was extremely good. Tricaprin was found to be the most potent substance in this series. It seemed that as the carbon chain length of the fatty acid is increased or decreased from 10, a decrease in stimulatory activity occurred. Tripalmitin (C_{16}) and tristearin (C_{18}) produced a mild hyperactivity only after 72 hr, which was preceded by an early depression of the phagocytic index 4 hr postinjection.

However, as to the evaluation of these results, there were certain variations in the nature of the lipid suspensions (mainly due to differences in particle size and homogeneity, being related to the carbon chain length of the fatty acid) that preclude a strict comparison of activity of these triglycerides. According to Cooper (1964), the particle size might be important for two reasons. First, the organ distribution of radioactivity due to injections of [^{131}I]triolein suspension differed markedly from that found when physiological ^{14}C-labeled lipid emulsions were used (Bragdon and Gordon, 1958). Cooper found that the bulk of the injected radioactivity was retained in the lungs whereas a maximum of 20% localized in the liver and spleen. A marked loss of radioactivity was found within 8 hr postinjection and virtually all had been lost by 24 hr. It was presumed that the lipids were rapidly metabolized in the lungs and liver, and that the ingestion by the macrophage of an energy-rich particle might possibly be sufficient to stimulate phagocytic activity.

Stimulation by simple lipids of macrophage phagocytic activity is very similar to stimulation with the more complex lipids of biological origin, in that hyperactivity is usually evident within 24 hr postinjection. The effective triglycerides directly affect the macrophages of the liver and spleen, for histological studies failed to show changes in other cell systems or organs following their injection in mice (Stuart and Cooper, 1962). This assumption is supported by conclusions from *in vitro* studies that the triolein effect was due to the contact between macrophages and triolein and was independent of the degree of opsonization of the ingested bacterial cells by normal animal sera (Cooper and West, 1962). Studies on peritoneal macrophages demonstrated binding of tritiated glyceryl trioleate to cell surfaces, phagocytosis of droplets, and incorporation into various subcellular components (Carr and Williams, 1966).

However, the basic mechanisms of stimulation that follow the interaction of macrophages and simple lipids are not clear. There are indications that the phagocytic stimulation is related to the chemical properties of the triglycerides. Although there is little chemical similarity between tricaprin and triolein, any interpretation of cell stimulation at a chemical or physicochemical level must account for the similarity of action between these two substances (Stuart, 1970). The mode of esterification may be an important factor; thus, while glyceryl trioleate stimulates activity, the ethyl and cholesterol esters of oleic acid induce a significant depression of carbon clearance activity in mice (Stuart *et al.*, 1960; Stuart, 1962). The results achieved with glyceride esters led to the conclusion that only the triglyceride is active whereas glyceryl monooleate has no effect at all. Moreover, carbon chain length of the fatty acid radical seems to be of considerable importance in determining activity.

However, Cooper (1964) pointed out that any interpretation of triglyceride activity at a chemical level is premature until more is known on the behavior of triglycerides and a more precise relation between particle size and activity has been established. He showed that a relatively homogeneous suspension in which the bulk of particles were less than 5 μm in diameter increased the phagocytic indices of mice to approximately four times those of normal animals, whereas those suspensions in which the majority of particles were greater than 5 μm had far less stimulatory activity. Moreover, it was found that the distribution of a particulate suspension of [^{131}I]triolein was unlike that of other colloids known to be phagocytized (Dobson, 1957), or of other physiological lipid emulsions, or chylomicrons (DiLuzio and Riggi, 1964). Results of further studies have also emphasized particle size as an important factor not only in determining removal rates but also tissue distribution, and illustrated the importance of coordinating tissue levels of the test substance with its removal rate (DiLuzio and Riggi, 1964; Blickens and DiLuzio, 1965).

With respect to the above-mentioned findings in mice of an early depression preceding a mild stimulation following tripalmitin and tristearin, Cooper (1964) argued that these substances act solely as inert colloidal particles, causing changes in RES activity in much the same fashion as large doses of colloidal carbon. As to the experiments with isolated macrophages, the ineffectiveness of tripalmitin and tristearin as well as the inhibition of phagocytosis by relatively large doses of tricaprylin, tricaprin, trilaurin, or triolein was attributed to "overloading" or functional blockade, which could be removed after sufficient time had elapsed for the lipid to be metabolized or excluded from the cell; at this stage the stimulatory effects became evident.

2.3.4. Lysolecithin

Because lysolecithin is released in large amounts in complement-fixed immune reactions and it lowers the surface tension at very low concentrations, Burdzy et al. (1964) investigated its effect on peritoneal macrophages of mice in vivo and in vitro. In both cases, the phagocytic cell function was markedly increased. Larger doses of lysolecithin were toxic.

2.3.5. Choline

Choline chloride (20 mg/kg i.m. twice daily for three consecutive days) was found to increase significantly the rate of blood clearance of colloidal $Cr^{32}PO_4$ in mice (Heller, 1953) and to stimulate the removal of colloidal gold (DiLuzio, 1955) and colloidal carbon (Altura et al., 1965, 1966) in rats. The increased removal rates were correlated with an elevated phagocytic efficiency of the RES due to increased tissue activity of the liver and spleen. Choline-pretreated rats showed, in addition to increased phagocytic activity, significantly higher survival rates after hemorrhagic shock (Altura et al., 1966). However, high doses (200 mg/kg choline chloride) caused a depression in phagocytic efficiency and made rats more susceptible to shock (Altura and Hershey, 1971).

2.4. ZYMOSAN

Yeast and yeastlike microorganisms produce a variety of extracellular and somatic polysaccharides, which can be isolated as polysaccharide–protein complexes or glycopeptides (Sikl et al., 1969). The main constituents of the somatic polysaccharides are those of the cell wall. Detailed studies have investigated the cell wall preparations of Saccharomyces cerevisiae (DiLuzio and Riggi, 1970), Candida albicans (Trnovec et al., 1977), and one kind of the green algae Chlorella (Kojima et al., 1973a,b) all of which were found to stimulate the RES. Zymosan, a cell wall preparation derived from S. cerevisiae, has been amply demonstrated to produce marked hyperplasia and increased phagocytic function of the RES (carbon clearance, erythrophagocytosis) following either single or multiple injections in mice, rats, rabbits, and dogs. The stimulation involved the formation of new RES cells as well as enlargement and hyperactivity of preexisting macrophages (Benacerraf and Sebestyén, 1957; Kelly et al., 1960; Cutler, 1960, 1961; DiLuzio, 1960; Heller, 1960; Kojima, 1960; Kampine et al., 1965). This applies also to lung macrophages, which, following i.v. injection of zymosan, showed proliferation and increased clearance of inhaled fused montmorillonite clay aerosol (Thomas and Chiffelle, 1974). Furthermore, a biphasic increase in the rate of clearance of injected colloidal carbon with peaks at 2 and 73 hr after zymosan injection was seen. Microscopic examination showed that two different processes were responsible for the changed clearance rates at these two periods. At 2 hr the increased rates were due to increased aggregation of carbon in the blood and increased attachment of particles to platelets than in untreated animals; there was no hyperphagocytosis. At 72 hr platelet involvement was reduced below normal levels and clearance was largely achieved by hyperphagocytic Kupffer cells (Tennant and Donald, 1976).

It was shown that the induced RES hyperplasia was not due to the particulate nature of zymosan, and histological studies revealed that zymosan was actively phagocytized by Kupffer cells and within 24–48 hr was broken down or solubilized by RES cells, with release of an agent either primarily or secondarily activating the RES. Chemical analysis showed that zymosan contained polysaccharides, proteins, fats, and inorganic elements (DiCarlo and Fiore, 1958). However, the composition of zymosan is variable, different preparations showing quantitative differences in biological activity (Ransom *et al.*, 1962; Ringle *et al.*, 1966), and lipid (Heller, 1960) as well as polysaccharide and protein fractions have been claimed to contain active material. Later, it was found that the extractable lipid component from yeast cell walls was inactive, as was the polysaccharide mannan. Stimulatory activity was still present in the zymosan residue after removal of free and bound lipids. This active residue was identified as glucan, being responsible for most of the RES-stimulating effects ascribed to zymosan (DiLuzio, 1976; Riggi and DiLuzio, 1961a,b).

2.5. CARBOHYDRATES

2.5.1. Polysaccharides

Glucan, an insoluble, highly purified polysaccharide constituting the inner portion of the cell wall of *S. cerevisiae*, constitutes over 50% of the dry weight of zymosan (DiCarlo and Fiore, 1958; Riggi and DiLuzio, 1961,a,b). The active RES stimulant has been characterized as a polyglucose consisting of a linear chain of glucose residues united by a β1,3glucosidic linkage. A minor component, β1,6glucan, does not affect the RES. The i.v. injection of glucan has been demonstrated to result in intense and specific increase in the phacocytic and proliferative (hepatosplenomegaly, pulmonary hyperplasia) response of the RES in mice, rats, and dogs (Riggi and DiLuzio, 1961a,b; Ashworth *et al.*, 1963; Wooles and DiLuzio, 1964; Kampine *et al.*, 1965). In mice, the peak phagocytic activity occurred 10 days after the last glucan injection and coincided with maximal hepatic and splenic hyperplasia. At 25 days after the cessation of glucan treatment, profound depression of phagocytic activity, associated with a significant reduction in liver weight, was observed. By 30 days RES organ weight and phagocytic activity of mice treated with glucan had essentially returned to control values (Wooles and DiLuzio, 1964). Cells in which glucan particles have been localized seem to be capable of metabolizing the insoluble particle, indicating that the glucan-induced stimulation may not be related to the continuous presence of the glucan particle in the macrophages. *In vivo* and *in vitro* studies carried out to elucidate the relative contribution of humoral and cellular factors in the mechanism of glucan-induced stimulation of the RES showed, among other things, that isolated Kupffer cells from glucan-treated rats manifested a hypophagocytic state. From these and further results, it was concluded that the increase in functional activity of the RES after glucan is not related to an increase in phagocytic capacity of each cell but is due primarily to an increase in the macrophage population, especially the Kupffer cells (DiLuzio *et al.*, 1970). The potent activation of macrophages is also shown by findings that macrophages from glucan-treated animals were larger than those from controls, spread more rapidly and to a greater degree after their attachment to glass, and demonstrated an increase in adherence to glass and augmentation of chemotactic activity (Burgaleta *et al.*, 1978).

Sulfation of glucan influenced its RES-stimulating action in a different way depending on the degree of sulfation. Sulfation of 0.4% of the molecules did not alter RES-stimulating ability or the degree of liver, lung, or spleen hyperplasia. A higher degree of sulfation (11%) resulted in a reduction in the hyperphagocytic state and elimination of hepatic and pulmonary hyperplasia while spleen weights still increased but to a lesser extent than following glucan (DiLuzio and Riggi, 1970).

With respect to the enhanced clearance activity of RES cells following glucan, glucan induced an increased clearance of subsequently injected tumor cells from the lungs of mice. The mechanism responsible for this effect was presumed to be linked to the increased activity of the RES (Stiteler *et al.*, 1978).

Laminarin is a polysaccharide from the alga *Laminaria* and has a chemical structure closely resembling that of glucan, i.e., β1,3glucopyranosidic linkages. Intravenous injection resulted in hyperphagocytosis and hyperplasia of the liver, spleen, and lung. Sulfation of laminarin selectively eliminated pulmonary hyperplasia without modifying the hyperphagocytic state. Laminaribiose, laminaripentose, and water-soluble di- and oligosaccharides isolated from glucan also stimulated phagocytic activity following i.v. injection (Riggi and DiLuzio, 1961b; DiLuzio and Riggi, 1970).

Chlorellan, a RES-stimulating polysaccharide extracted from one kind of the green algae *Chlorella* and containing a polyglucoside of considerably lower molecular weight than laminarin, has also been characterized as β1,3glucan (Kojima *et al.*, 1973a,b). A further glucan was isolated from polysaccharide fractions of *Candida albicans;* its phagocytosis-stimulating effect was in accordance with that of yeast glucan (Trnovec *et al.*, 1977).

Various other polysaccharides (agar, starch, cellulose, methyl cellulose) have been found to exert minor stimulation of RES phagocytosis activity (Blickens and DiLuzio, 1964; Flemming and Graack, 1967). Methyl cellulose was studied in more detail (Blickens and DiLuzio, 1964). Following repeated i.p.

administration in rats, this metabolically inert polymer produced hepatospleno-megaly and a marked stimulation of the global RES activity despite the fact that it is stored in the macrophages.

2.5.2. Oligo- and Monosaccharides

Lactulose, laminaribiose, laminaripentose, melezitose, trehalose, turanose, and glucose show a moderate stimulating effect on RES phagocytosis. Contrary to these carbohydrates, inulin, mannan, cellobiose, maltose, laminaritriose, laminaritetrose, and laminarihexose were uneffective (Blickens and DiLuzio, 1964).

2.6. PROTEINS AND PEPTIDES

2.6.1. Fibronectins

Fibronectins are adhesive glycoproteins (opsonic proteins) of cell surface and blood. Cold-insoluble globulin (CIG) or plasma fibronectin has been shown to be identical to opsonic α_2 surface-binding glycoprotein (Blumenstock et al., 1976, 1978), a protein necessary for normal RES function (Saba and DiLuzio, 1969). CIG opsonizes some types of bacteria for removal by macrophages of the liver and spleen (Molnar et al., 1977). Recent in vitro studies showed that CIG stimulated retention of gelatin-coated latex beads by macrophage monolayers in the absence of heparin (Doran et al., 1980, 1981a,b). Furthermore, opsonic fibronectin (CIG) was demonstrated to be an important serum factor required for maximal in vitro neutrophil phagocytosis of Staphylococcus aureus. Serum depleted of opsonic fibronectin manifested a marked reduction in its ability to support bacterial phagocytosis by neutrophils (Lanser and Saba, 1981). Thus, it was concluded that opsonic fibronectin could be an important protein essential for maximal opsonic activity and phagocytic defense against infection and bacteremia.

2.6.2. Muramyl Dipeptide

Muramyl dipeptide (MDP), a ubiquitous bacterial cell wall constituent, can replace whole mycobacteria in Freund's complete adjuvant for its capacity to stimulate immune responses in experimental animals (see Lemaire et al., this volume). It can also enhance nonspecific immunity of mice to infection. Many bacteria or bacterial products that are immunological adjuvants are known to stimulate phagocytic activity of the RES in vivo. Such an effect was also found for MDP in mice and rats but not in guinea pigs (Tanaka et al., 1979; Waters and Ferraresi, 1980). Following a single parenteral dose to mice, particle clearance stimulation exhibited a log linear dose response lasting 2 to 3 days with maximal effect 1 day following treatment. Oral administration was also effective. Repeated or continuous dosing did not increase the RES stimulation seen following a single treatment. The RES-stimulating ability of MDP might in part explain its protective effects in models of bacterial and parasitic infection in the mouse.

2.6.3. Tuftsin

Tuftsin, a tetrapeptide, was discovered in the course of studies on the physiological role of cytophilic γ-globulins that bind specially to the outer surface of various blood cells (Najjar and Constantopoulos, 1972; Najjar, 1980). Leukophilic γ-globulin stimulates the phagocytic activity of the neutrophilic granulocyte, and is necessary for its survival *in vitro*. The granulocyte possesses the ability to cleave tuftsin from the membrand-bound leukophilic γ-globulin, which is merely a carrier molecule for the tetrapeptide. The freed tuftsin is then capable of exerting a stimulating effect on the phagocytic activity of the cell to the full extent observed with the intact molecule.

Blood neutrophils and tissue macrophages are capable of a basal level of phagocytosis of particulate substances. Upon the addition of tuftsin, their activity increases to a level over twice that of the basal value. The concentration required for approaching maximal activity for both phagocytic cells is about $2–4 \times 10^{-7}$ g/ml. Najjar (1980) concluded that tuftsin stimulates all the known biological activities of the two major phagocytic cells, the granulocyte and the macrophage. In addition to phagocytic stimulation, it also enhances pinocytosis, cell motility, and cell longevity.

2.6.4. Interferon

Interferon is a protein that has antiviral effects and activates macrophages to kill tumor and leukemic cells. A more general activity in the nonspecific host defense against various infectious agents has been discussed. Different preparations of mouse interferon were found to enhance vascular clearance of colloidal carbon in mice (Donahoe and Huang, 1976; Degré and Rollag, 1979). The phagocytosis stimulation was dose-dependent and maximal 24 hr after i.p. injection; moreover, it was confirmed *in vitro* (Huang *et al.*, 1971; Rabinovitch *et al.*, 1980).

2.6.5. Medicaments: Trofopar, Leucotrofina, PVNO

Trofopar and leucotrofina are clinically used complex polypeptides derived from the hepatocyte membrane and from the thymus, respectively. In experiments with rats and mice, both preparations stimulated the phagocytic activity of the RES. Trofopar increased the uptake of colloidal gold in the liver, spleen, bone marrow, and lung. This increase was accompanied by an increased antibody formation (Timar, 1982). Following chronic administration of leucotrofina for 20 days, the carbon clearance rate was significantly increased (Russo and Travaglini, 1978).

Polyvinylpyridin-*N*-oxide (PVNO) checks the induction of quartz dust silicosis, prevents necrosis of alveolar macrophages and collagen formation in alveolar tissue (Schlipköter *et al.*, 1963). Moreover, it protects the membranes of peritoneal macrophages against the toxic effects of SiO_2 (Munder *et al.*, 1966). In mice, PVNO induced a clear and dose-dependent but short-lasting global phagocytic increase, being maximal 24 hr after injection (Flemming and Nothdurft, 1968; Nothdurft and Flemming, 1970). In the liver and spleen, no increases of macrophages occurred but an increased carbon uptake into Kupffer cells was found. There was no indication for a causal connection between phagocytosis stimulation and antisilicogenic action of PVNO.

2.7. IMMUNOSTIMULANTS

2.7.1. Bacteria

Metchnikoff (1901) found that the infection of an animal with microorganisms could increase its resistance against nonrelated pathogenic bacteria. It is well known that the RES can be stimulated by live or attenuated or killed bacteria and by bacterial endotoxins (lipopolysaccharides). The increased nonspecific immunity is considered in part as the result of an activation of the ingestive and bactericidal capacity of the RES macrophages (Thorbecke and Benacerraf, 1962; Mackaness and Blanden, 1967; Biozzi *et al.*, 1957b).

The changes in RES phagocytic activity by infection with viable *Mycobacterium phlei*, *Candida albicans*, or gram-negative bacilli are conditioned by the species and age of the animal, by the rate of blood flow through the liver, and by the characteristics and amounts of the infectious agent (Biozzi *et al.*, 1954; Benacerraf *et al.*, 1957; DiCarlo *et al.*, 1963b; Bird and Sheagren, 1970). The change in phagocytic activity follows, in general, a fairly characteristic pattern. There is first a phase that reaches a maximum 3–5 days after treatment or infection. Phagocytic activity then progressively decreases, reaching a normal level around the day 7–9. In fatal infections the activity of the RES falls to a subnormal level some time before death.

Examples of attenuated or killed bacteria are *Bacillus tuberculosis* (BCG) and *C. parvum*, which are among the most powerful stimulants of the RES. The prolonged enhancement of phagocytosis following *C. parvum* was paralleled by a considerable increase in the weight of the liver and spleen (Biozzi *et al.*, 1957b; Halpern *et al.*, 1963; Warr and Sljivić, 1974). The phagocytosis-stimulating effect of *C. parvum* was also observed in peritoneal macrophages (Miake *et al.*, 1980). Moreover, it is remarkable that the depression of phagocytic function in alcohol-fed rats was partially corrected by injection of *C. parvum* but not by injection of BCG (Thomas *et al.*, 1980).

2.7.2. Endotoxins

Highly purified *endotoxin* or *lipopolysaccharide* (LPS), a toxic principle produced by gram-negative bacteria is firmly bound to their cell wall as a high-molecular-weight complex (Westphal, 1975). A variety of biological effects are elicited by endotoxins. Among other things, a stimulation of the phagocytic RES activity is generally induced (Biozzi *et al.*, 1955; Benacerraf and Sebestyén, 1957; Boehme and Dubos, 1958; Watnick and Gordon, 1964; Filkins and DiLuzio, 1967). In studies of carbon clearance in mice, a complex dose–response relationship was found (Flemming, 1974; Flemming and Nothdurft, 1982). LPS, 50 and 500 µg/kg, produced a biphasic stimulation of phagocytosis with peak values after 2.5 and 48 hr, respectively. On the contrary, after 5000 µg/kg (LD_5) no early stimulation was evoked; between 6 and 24 hr after application of this large dose, pronounced depression of phagocytosis was found, followed by a marked stimulation with maximal values 4 days after injection. Fluctuations in liver weight were not clearly related to the LPS dose, whereas the increase in spleen weight ran parallel to the corresponding K value. The high clearance rates at the time of maximal phagocytic activity were related to enhanced Kupffer cell function in the liver.

Isolated LPS preparations do not always have the same biological reactivity. For example, the phagocytic increase induced by the LPS of the photosynthetic bacterium *Rhodopseudomonas capsulata* was small compared to the potent stimulation following injection of LPS from *Salmonella abortus equi* (Flemming, 1977).

The lipid moiety of LPS, a phospholipid designated as lipid A that is thought to be responsible for the pyrogenic and toxic effects (Galanos *et al.*, 1977), is also a phagocytosis-stimulating agent (Westphal *et al.*, 1958; Cutler, 1960; Nicol *et al.*, 1966c). However, the structural components of LPS that lead to the activation of the RES have not yet been unequivocally determined.

The same applies to bacterial phospholipid extracts that have been shown to increase the blood clearance of *S. typhimurium* in mice. In these experiments, a similar effect was also found for a few pure phospholipids, i.e., phosphatidylinositol, diphospho- and triphosphoinositide (Fauve, 1974). However, it should be mentioned in this connection that the blood clearance of bacteria by the RES is a much more complex process than the clearance of colloidal particles, because the extent of opsonization by antibody and complement affects the efficiency of clearance by the liver and spleen.

2.7.3. Levamisole

Levamisole (l-tetramisole) was found to stimulate the global phagocytic RES activity as measured by the clearance of i.v.-injected colloidal carbon in mice (Hoebeke and Franchi, 1973; Hoebeke, 1976). The effect of levamisole was dose-related, and the optimal effect was obtained with 1.25 mg/kg injected 24 hr before the carbon clearance test. The increased RES activity returned to normal after about 48 hr. No increase in the weight of the liver or spleen was observed, either in the case of single or subchronic treatment. Thus, it was concluded that the increase of phagocytosis was not due to hyperplasia or hypertrophy of the RES but rather to functional activation of the macrophages. Phagocytosis activity was noticeably enhanced by levamisole in the case of a relative deficiency of the RES as found in aged or cortisone-treated animals, in certain strains of animals, and in diseased man (Hoebeke and Franchi, 1973; Verhaegen *et al.*, 1973; van Ginckel and Hoebeke, 1974). Levamisole appeared to restore RES function rather than to stimulate it above normal functional levels of activity.

With respect to the suggestion that the anthelmintic activity of levamisole might be due to the formation of an active metabolite called OMPI [DL-2-

oxo-3-(2-mercaptoethyl)-5-phenylimidazolidine] (Janssen, 1976), it was remarkable that, from sera of levamisol-treated mice, a phagocytosis-stimulating substance had been prepared (van Ginckel and Hoebeke, 1975). The effects of OMPI on the blood clearance of carbon were compared to those of the parent compound levamisole (van Ginckel and de Brabander, 1979). Both compounds stimulated the phagocytic activity of the RES to a similar degree. However, on a molar basis OMPI was approximately 4 times more potent than levamisole, and the phagocytic increase induced by OMPI occurred about 8 hr earlier.

The immunological profile of levamisole was also studied on isolated polymorphonuclear cells or macrophages. The existing literature has been comprehensively reviewed by Symoens and Rosenthal (1977) who summarized the results of studies on phagocytosis in *in vitro* test systems as follows:

> Levamisole increased phagocytosis by polymorphonuclear cells or macrophages when added to these cells or given to donor animals and humans. The effect was most pronounced on hypo-functional cells from patients and weak or absent on cells from normal donors. The drug significantly potentiated Ag-induced stimulation of phagocytosis by macrophages, improved immune phagocytosis of antibody (Ab)-coated particles and increased phagocytic adherence and Ab and complement receptor activity.

2.7.4. Polyanions

Pyran copolymer is a synthetic polyanion exerting antiviral (Regelson and Munson, 1970) and antitumor (Kapila *et al.*, 1971) activity as well as inducing interferon production in both mouse and man. Drummond and Munson (1974) revealed that the mode of pyran depends on the molecular weight of the pyran samples. High-molecular-weight pyran species (> 30,000) depress phagocytic RES activity (see Section 3.4.1) whereas low-molecular-weight species (< 5000) produce phagocytosis stimulation. Munson *et al.* (1968, 1970) studied the effects of pyran on RES activity and immunological responsiveness of mice by intravascular clearance and tissue localization of various test colloids (carbon; ^{131}I-labeled RE lipid test emulsions; ^{51}Cr-labeled SRBC). Pyran was administered i.v. in amounts of 10 to 50 mg/kg for 2 days. Following a preceding depression, a marked stimulation of phagocytosis was observed after 6–10 days. Maximal stimulation coincided with peak increases in liver and spleen weight. These results were confirmed by Kapila *et al.* (1971), who found a time-dependent progressive phagocytic increase following intramuscular pyran injections daily for six consecutive days. The effect on RES macrophages of four other polyanions, i.e., carrageenan, dextran sulfate, polyanethole sulfonate (Liquoid), and suramin, has been studied *in vitro* and *in vivo* (Bloksma *et al.*, 1980. The *in vivo* clearance of carbon in mice that had been injected i.p. with carrageenan (80 mg/kg) and dextran sulfate (24 mg/kg), following a preceding depression (see Section 3.4.1), was stimulated after 72 hr. Small doses of carrageenan (3–30 μg) as well as of polyanethole sulfonate and suramin stimulated yeast cells phagocytosis by peritoneal macrophages *in vitro*.

2.7.5. Dimethyl Dioctadecyl Ammonium Bromide

Dimethyl dioctadecyl ammonium bromide (DDA), a cationic surface lipid, stimulated the vascular clearance of carbon as determined by the phagocytic index K in mice at 24 and 48 hr after injection, and the corrected phagocytic index α was also significantly enhanced 24 and 72 hr after administration (Willers *et al.*, 1979; Bloksma *et al.*, 1983). In mice injected with DDA, *in vitro* phagocytosis by peritoneal macrophages of killed *Lysteria monocytogenes* was also slightly enhanced whereas phagocytosis of viable *L. monocytogenes* was not affected (Hofhuis *et al.*, 1981).

2.7.6. Tilorone and Tilorone Congeners

Tilorone (DEAE-fluorenone), an antiviral agent, induced high levels of circulating interferon and showed *in vivo* RES-stimulating activity (carbon and SRBC clearance) if administered orally (Munson *et al.*, 1972a). Bloksma *et al.* (1983) found an enhanced carbon clearance (K and α values) 24 and 72 hr after i.p. administration; nonspecific resistance of the mice was not enhanced.

Munson *et al.* (1972b) found that five analogs of tilorone HCl demonstrated varying degrees of activity on RES function and various other host defense mechanisms (antitumor and antiviral activity, immunological response). The tilorone congener DBAP-anthroquinone produced the most marked stimulation of the phagocytic activity of the RES 24 and 72 hr after drug injection as well as an increased resistance to *S. aureus*. DEAE-fluorene and PIB-fluorene produced variable stimulation, depending on assay time.

2.7.7. Indoloquinolinone

Indoloquinolinone (IQ) represents a special case. Administration at a relatively nontoxic dose (32 mg/kg per day) to S180J tumor-bearing mice not only caused a significant increase in phagocytic activity in the early stage of therapy in treated as compared to untreated tumor-bearing mice, but also induced a significantly high proportion of tumor regressions. Individuals that eventually became tumor-free tended to have high K values on day 6 and low values on day 42. In contrast, individuals bearing tumors that grew progressively to day 42 tended to have low K values on day 6 and high ones on day 42. Therefore, a strong, early phagocytic response may serve as a prognostic indicator of the subsequent diminution of tumor size in treated mice (Fukushima *et al.*, 1979).

2.7.8. Coenzymes Q

Coenzymes Q (Q_6, Q_9, Q_{10}, identified in liver extracts) greatly enhanced phagocytic activity at doses as low as 750 μg per rat without producing hyperplasia of the RES. Moreover, antibody formation of mice versus SRBC showed a twofold increase (Bliznakov *et al.*, 1970; Heller *et al.*, 1965).

2.8. PLANTS AND SUBSTANCES OF PLANT ORIGIN

2.8.1. *Maytenus laevis* Leaves and Extracts

Certain plant preparations contain a number of agents capable of inducing hyperphagocytic activity in mice and rats. DiCarlo *et al.* (1964a,b) tested desiccated samples of a collection of flowering plants. Suspensions of whole plants, roots, leaves, bark, stems, fruits, and flowers were administered i.v. to mice and a significant increase of phagocytic activity (carbon clearance) was shown by 17 of 32 raw plant preparations and by 4 of 12 plant extracts. Eight of thirteen leaf varieties were active as were half of raw bark varieties. Phagocytic stimulation was also elicited by certain roots, fruits, and stalks, and aboveground growth.

The most potent stimulant appeared to be the leaves of *M. laevis*. A single i.v. dose (50 mg/kg in physiological saline) induced a hyperphagocytic state of the RES that lasted for 3 days, peak stimulation occurring after 2 days. The preparation of these leaves was more potent than zymosan or DES but less potent than endotoxin or live *Mycobacterium phlei* Halpern. Remarkably, no significant hepatosplenomegaly was induced but lung weight was increased for at least 1 week. Histological examination disclosed lung inflammation within 24 hr, sections showing vegetable fibers in the alveoli lying free in the lumen. Some of these fibers were trapped both in the alveoli and in the lymphatic channels around vessels where they seemed to have stimulated a marked leukocytic reaction with the formation of small pneumonialike nodules. Following large doses of *M. laevis* leaves administered by gavage, stimulated phagocytosis was observed for 1–3 days. The hyperphagocytic state of the RES following i.v. injection of pulverized leaves to mice was accompanied by induced resistance to subsequent experimental challenge with pathogenic cocci (DiCarlo *et al.*, 1964b).

These findings were confirmed in mice and in rats; in addition, significant stimulation of phagocytosis induced by *M. laevis* leaves occurred after 2.5 mg/kg and increased with increasing doses reaching a maximum effect 24 hr after injection of 25–50 mg leaf substance (Flemming, 1965b; Graack and Flemming, 1966; Flemming and Graack, 1967). Moreover, radiation resistance was increased in mice showing enhanced RES phagocytic activity due to injection of *M. laevis* leaves (Flemming *et al.*, 1967).

2.8.2. Lignins and Related Substances

Further experiments were carried out to obtain information on the active agent contained in plant material (Flemming, 1965b; Graack and Flemming, 1966; Flemming and Graack, 1967). Various basic constituents of plants such as cellulose, starch, chlorophyll as well as certain kinds of lignins (cuproxam lignin and Björkman lignin) induced a significant but minor increase of phagocytic activity, whereas inulin was ineffective. However, a strong phagocytic increase occurred following injection of suspensions of Scholler–Tornesch (S-T) lignin, a clinically used antidiarrhetic (Porlisan). Studied in greater detail, the RES stimulation was highly significant with doses as low as 0.5 mg/kg. The effect increased with increasing doses up to 100 mg/kg, lasting for 3 days with a maximum on the first day following injection. No weight changes of the liver or spleen occurred.

Leaves often contain tannins, which are converted into phlobaphenes with drying. S-T lignin contains a phlobaphene derived from spruce tannin (Freudenberg, 1933; Brauns and Brauns, 1960; Harborne, 1964). In order to clarify whether phlobaphenes might function in the RES-stimulating effect, phlobaphenes were prepared chemically from S-T lignin, Björkman lignin, and catechin. They had only weak effects equaling that of catechin, i.e., the constituent each has in common. This would mean that the RES-stimulating effects of *M. laevis* leaves and of S-T lignin cannot be attributed to phlobaphenes.

Moreover, it is remarkable that, although lignin is said to be insoluble in alcohol, a methanol extract of S-T lignin induced an increase of phagocytic activity that nearly equaled that of the unextracted specimen of this kind of lignin. However, the respective methanol-extracted specimen was still as active as before extraction. From these results, it must be concluded that neither pure lignin nor condensed phlobaphenes can be the effective agent for the enhancement of phagocytosis.

The only difference between cuproxam lignin and Björkman lignin on the one hand and S-T lignin on the other hand may be that greater care is required for the Scholler–Tornesch processing technique. Thus, in S-T lignin a substance might be preserved that originates from the spruce wood as a primary product, which is destroyed or lost if less careful techniques (Björkman, cuproxam) are applied. Another possibility is that the substance stimulating phagocytosis develops after application of the Scholler–Tornesch procedure. In addition, it must be considered that the hypothetical active agent in S-T lignin may originate from small amounts of plant polysaccharides contained as "impurities" in the S-T lignin.

2.8.3. *Aristolochia clematitis* and Aristolochic Acid

In rabbits and guinea pigs, repeated i.v. administration of highly diluted ethanol extracts from all parts of *A. clematitis* produced marked stimulation of phagocytosis of bacteria by blood leukocytes and peritoneal macrophages *in vitro* as well as by macrophages in infected wounds and ulcers of experimental animals *in vivo* (Möse and Lukas, 1961). These effects were found to be due to aristolochic acid (methoxy-nitro-phenantro-dioxole-carboxylic acid), which was also locally active in rats and following oral administration (Möse, 1963). Aristolochic acid did not increase the number of phagocytizing macrophages. The favorable effects of internal application of aristolochic acid on wounds and ulcers appeared to be mainly due to its stimulating action on macrophage phagocytic activity.

Findings of a stimulation by aristolochic acid of the global phagocytic RES activity in mice remain questionable as such an effect could not be confirmed in our laboratory or by other groups.

3. DEPRESSION OF PHAGOCYTOSIS

3.1. CORTICOSTEROIDS AND RELATED SUBSTANCES

Findings that cortisone depressed the phagocytic activity in mice and rats (Marcus *et al.*, 1953; Heller, 1955; Nicol *et al.*, 1956; Hornnes and Rygaard, 1960) were also confirmed for guinea pigs and rabbits and extended for other glucocorticoids and cortisonelike-acting substances such as hydrocortisone, deoxycorticosterone, corticosterone, prednisone, prednisolone, and 4-hydroxytetramethylmethane (Nicol and Snell, 1955; Reichard *et al.*, 1956; Nicol and Bilbey, 1958; Bilbey and Nicol, 1958; Snell, 1960a,b; Lurie, 1960; Nicol and Druce, 1961; Wierner *et al.*, 1967; Benveniste *et al.*, 1970; Gotjamanos, 1970; Flemming, 1974). The phagocytic depression was due to a marked reduction in the number of Kupffer cells capable of phagocytizing carbon and accompanied by a depression of white blood cells and of γ-globulin level in the serum. Thereby, cortisone deprives the macrophages of much of their innate capacity to inhibit the multiplication of the bacilli in their cytoplasm, and thus markedly lowers resistance (Lurie, 1960). Pointing to evidence for strain and species differences with respect to the susceptibility of hepatocytes for cortisone treatment, Gotjamanos (1970) suggested that these differences might equally apply to the effect produced in Kupffer cells. The amount of carbon taken up by the spleen was not significantly affected by relatively low doses of cortisone, although splenic uptake seemingly occurred more rapidly than normal as a consequence of the reduced phagocytic activity of liver macrophages (Gotjamanos, 1970).

A depressed phagocytosis function of alveolar macrophages was also found in corticosteroid-treated rats (Schorn and Walter, 1975) and guinea pigs (Gudewicz, 1979). In experiments with anesthetized mice treated with cortisone or ACTH, a correlation was found between the posttraumatic depression of RES function, as indicated by the disappearance of ^{51}Cr-labeled heterologous erythrocytes and their uptake in RES organs, and an increase in the plasma corticosteroid level (Schildt and Löw, 1971). It was postulated that the posttraumatic depression of the RES was induced, at least partially, by a release of corticosteroids. The pharmacological relevance of a pathophysiologically induced stimulation of the pituitary–adrenocortical system for the phagocytic activity of the RES has also been demonstrated by the finding of a clear-cut correlation between the endotoxin-induced phagocytosis depression and the endotoxin-induced secretion of corticosteroid hormones by the adrenal cortex (Flemming, 1983).

Worth mentioning are findings that cortisone inhibited the restoration of phagocytic activity after a blocking dose of colloid (Biozzi *et al.*, 1957b), and that pretreatment with cortisone abolished nearly completely the increased toxicity to endotoxin by zymosan or BCG (Benacerraf *et al.*, 1959).

The reported corticosteroid-induced depression of the global phagocytic RES activity has been confirmed by findings *in vitro* that hydrocortisone significantly inhibited erythrophagocytosis and phagocytosis of yeast cells by peritoneal macrophages from rats (Gemsa *et al.*, 1974) and from mice (Raz and Goldman, 1976).

Supplementally, it must be mentioned that, following small doses of corticosteroids (0.5–50 mg/kg cortisone), no depression but a significant stimulation of phagocytosis occurred (Crabbé, 1956; Heller *et al.*, 1957; Snell, 1960a; Nicol *et al.*, 1965; Benveniste *et al.*, 1970). The assumption that large corticosteroid doses depress RES phagocytosis whereas small doses have no effect or even stimulate the RES, was also confirmed by studies on the effect of cortisone in mice pretreated with phagocytosis stimulants (Flemming, 1974). A large dose of cortisone (5 mg i.v. per mouse) abolished the phagocytosis stimulation by bacterial endotoxins and triolein and strongly reduced the stimulating effect of PVNO, whereas a low dose of cortisone (0.2 mg i.v.) did not interfere with the effectiveness of the stimulants. The different and sometimes reverse effects of large and small doses of corticosteroids can also explain the bimodal effect with time found by Heller *et al.* (1957): a large cortisone dose (250 mg/kg) led to a depression 1 hr after injection followed by an increase in phagocytosis 24 hr later.

3.2. ANDROGENS

Testosterone propionate and androstene 3β-17α-diol induced a cortisone-like depression in male guinea pigs during the first 2 weeks of treatment. If testosterone treatment was not stopped, RES activity recovered during the weeks 3 and 4 (Snell and Nicol, 1956). In testosterone-treated rats, the phagocytic activity of the alveolar macrophages was also reduced (Schorn and Walter, 1975).

3.3. FATS AND LIPIDS

3.3.1. Liver Oil

In nonpregnant and pregnant rats, the phagocytic activity of the RES was depressed by an admixture of oxidized cod liver oil to a diet low in vitamin A; an admixture of triglycerides derived from cod liver oil did not produce an alteration of RES phagocytosis (McKay *et al.*, 1964).

3.3.2. Alkyl Esters of Fatty Acids

Following observations that ethyl oleate, ethyl stearate, ethyl palmitate, butyl oleate (Stuart *et al.*, 1960; Stuart, 1960, 1970; Biozzi *et al.*, 1963), and methyl palmitate (DiLuzio and Wooles, 1964; Morrow and DiLuzio, 1965) depressed RES phagocytosis in mice, alkyl esters of fatty acids were investigated in greater detail (DiLuzio and Blickens, 1966). Certain further methyl, ethyl, and *n*-butyl esters of fatty acids containing 14 to 20 carbon atoms of various degrees of saturation were found to induce a significant depression of the intravascular removal of colloidal carbon in mice 24 hr after injection. The fatty acid derivatives (number of C atoms in parentheses) are as follows: saturated—ethyl caprate (10), ethyl laureate (12), methyl myristate (14), methyl pentadecanoate (15), methyl palmitate (16), ethyl palmitate (16), *n*-butyl palmitate (16), methyl stearate (18), ethyl stearate (18), unsaturated—methyl palmitoleate (16), methyl oleate (18), ethyl oleate (18), *n*-butyl oleate (18), methyl elaidate (18), methyl linoleate (18), methyl linolenate (18), methyl arachidonate (20).

The most efficient depressants are those substances with 15 to 17 carbon atoms in their fatty acid chains, i.e., butyl oleate, ethyl palmitate, and methyl palmitate (Stuart, 1970). No changes in body or organ weight were found except for methyl pentadecanoate, which produced an increase in lung and spleen weight, and methyl palmitoleate and methyl arachidonate, which induced significant increases in spleen weights.

Fatty acid methyl esters containing 6 to 13 carbon atoms as well as ethyl laureate and ethyl caprate were toxic; they induced immediate death upon i.v. administration and could not be employed (DiLuzio and Blickens, 1966; Stuart, 1970). Ethyl esters of short-chain acids, either fatty, aromatic, or discarboxylic, had no effect on RES function.

Methyl palmitate has been studied very carefully and was found to induce a selective and pronounced impairment in the intravascular clearance of colloidal carbon (DiLuzio and Wooles, 1964; Morrow and DiLuzio, 1965; Blickens and DiLuzio, 1965; DiLuzio and Blickens, 1966). The most severe depression was induced in the mice by a dose of 35 mg/20 g. Following a single injection, a depression was induced as early as 5 hr after administration. Phagocytic function was significantly depressed for up to 17 days, maximal depression being observed at day 2. The decreased phagocytosis was due to a reduced hepatic and splenic macrophage activity. The administration of methyl palmitate to splenectomized mice produced a greater degree of phagocytic depression than that observed in intact mice. In view of the ease of preparation of methyl palmitate emulsions and the relatively long duration of the resultant depression, methyl palmitate is an ideal compound for inducing RE hypofunction (DiLuzio and Blickens, 1966). It is also remarkable that RE depression induced by methyl palmitate was not followed by a phase of hyperactivity, as observed by Kelly *et al.* (1960) after RES "blockade" by injection of inert colloids such as saccharated iron oxide and colloidal carbon.

As to ethyl palmitate, Stuart (1960) found not only suppression of phagocytosis but also widespread necrosis of the spleen designated as "chemical splenectomy" following i.v. injection of ethyl palmitate emulsions into mice (25 mg/20 g); bone marrow, thymus, and liver showed no significant lesions. Splenic necrosis has never been observed after treatment with ethyl stearate, ethyl oleate, or methyl palmitate. Thus, it is remarkable that the profound phagocytic depression found in ethyl palmitate-treated mice was confirmed in rats whereas the destructive necrotizing effect on the spleen could not be observed in this species (Kroma and Flemming, 1965).

As to the mechanism of action of the alkyl esters of fatty acids, it has been shown that certain lipid emulsions are removed from the vascular system by phagocytosis (DiLuzio and Riggi, 1964). In this case, impairment in the vascular clearance of the emulsified depressing esters in the presence of colloidal carbon particles would be manifested because of an increase in the number of circulating particles, which might lead to a functional "blockade" of the RES (Stuart and Davidson, 1963, 1964). Toxic damage of macrophage function also has to be taken in account as histological observations of RE organs of mice, with an ethyl stearate-induced depression of the RES, have indicated a marked depression of RE cells of the liver and spleen (Stuart and Cooper, 1962).

Based on these assumptions, the mechanism of ethyl palmitate-induced splenic destruction has been clarified (Kawasaki and Finch, 1972). Following i.v. injection of ^{14}C-labeled ethyl palmitate in mice, about 7% of the injected ethyl palmitate was present in the spleen 24 hr later with little remaining in other organs. There was only a slight change at 1 week. Marked localization of labeled ethyl palmitate was seen in the red pulp areas where there was extensive splenic necrosis, which seemed to be secondary to vascular trapping of the lipid emulsion particles in the red pulp of the spleen. An increase in either lipid emulsion particle size or splenic blood flow will result in reduced vascular trapping of ethyl palmitate by the spleen and less splenic necrosis. However, explanations such as functional "blockade" of the RES or structural cell damage cannot be accepted for methyl palmitate. Studies designed to evaluate radioactive clearance and tissue distribution showed that depression of phagocytic and immunological activity induced by methyl palmitate or other lipids cannot be explained by the retention of methyl palmitate or other lipids in macrophages (DiLuzio and Wooles, 1964; Blickens and DiLuzio, 1965). Therefore, it is generally assumed that the depression of phagocytosis by alkyl esters of fatty acids is the consequence of a direct cytotoxic effect of the ingested particles on the phagocytic cell either before or during their catabolism.

3.3.3. Oleic Acid

In the context of the preceding considerations, it is of interest that emulsions of oleic acid are potent inhibitors of RE phagocytic activity *in vivo* as well as *in vitro*. Spratt and Kratzing (1971) found that a single i.v. injection of an emulsion of oleic acid doubled the carbon clearance half-time in mice and depressed phagocytic activity for 24 hr. Carbon clearance half-time was increased fourfold in rats and phagocytic activity was still depressed after 72 hr. The inhibitory effect was also apparent in perfused livers of rats 5–7 hr after injection. The authors believe that the evidence from these results does suggest the possibility that the depression of phagocytic activity caused by methyl esters could be due to release of fatty acid following hydrolysis.

3.3.4. Cholesterol Oleate

Cholesterol esters, given i.v., are taken up by the RES. Emulsions of cholesterol oleate have been used in mice to modify the global phagocytic activity of the RES. For this reason, the phagocytic index K and the corrected phagocytic index α were determined using the carbon clearance method (Stuart, 1962, 1970; Flemming, 1963b, 1967). Stuart has found that the effects of cholesterol oleate depend on the dose given and range, with increasing doses, from mild stimulation through depression followed by temporary hyperfunction to a severe and relatively prolonged depression. The dose–response curve for K measured 24 hr after injection of this lipid showed a mild stimulation with a small dose (2.5–5 mg/20 g), and a profound depression after a large dose (10–30 mg).

The moderate stimulation produced by small doses lasted no more than 48 hr (Stuart, 1962, 1970). The time of onset of the stimulation depended on the amount of ester given, occurring promptly with small doses and being delayed with larger doses. The maximum dose of 30 mg was well tolerated but induced a marked depression of RES phagocytic function lasting for 2–3 days. By day 5, K values had returned to normal although α values remained low because, although there was a slight enlargement of the liver and spleen, the total body weight did not increase. After treatment with cholesterol oleate the spleen showed numerous vacuolated cells throughout the red pulp and at the periphery of the Malpighian bodies.

Cholesterol has been used as a "blockading agent." It affects RE phagocytic function in the same way as does inert material such as carbon or saccharated iron oxide (Stiffel, 1959) but possesses the advantage that it is eventually metabolized and thus eliminated from the tissues. The degree of "blockade" that follows a single dose of cholesterol oleate is significant and the duration is as long, if not longer than that obtained by colloids such as trypan blue or thorothrast. Apparently, the RE cells are capable of ingesting surprisingly large quantities of cholesterol oleate.

3.3.5. Phospholipids

To determine whether another class of lipids, phospholipids, would exert an effect on the phagocytic function of the RES, mice were injected with emulsions of either egg lecithin, sphingomyelin, or cephalin, which were prepared in the same manner as the fatty acid ester and triglyceride emulsions mentioned above (DiLuzio and Blickens, 1966; Blickens and DiLuzio, 1965). Lecithin and cephalin preparations induced phagocytic depression, although no significant alterations were observed in body weight or in liver, lung, or spleen weight. Sphingomyelin emulsions did not alter phagocytic function.

3.4. IMMUNODEPRESSANTS

3.4.1. Polyanions: Carrageenan, Dextran Sulfate, Polyanethole Sulfonate, Suramin

Between 2 and 6 days after the last i.v. injection of pyran (10–50 mg/kg for 2 days), a depression of phagocytosis occurred that was associated with a depression in the hepatic and splenic uptake of lipid emulsion and SRBC (Munson *et al.*, 1968, 1970). The high-moleculear-weight species (> 30,000) of pyran copolymer were found to be responsible for this depression (Drummond and Munson, 1975).

In vitro studies on the phagocytosis of yeast cells by peritoneal macrophages showed that, contrary to the stimulation induced by small doses (Section 2.7.4), higher doses of carrageenan (100 and 300 μg) as well as polyanethole sulfonate (400 μg) produced phagocytic inhibition. Parallel to *in vivo* experiments with mice, polyanethole sulfonate, suramin, and carrageenan suppressed RES phagocytosis 4 and 24 hr after administration; dextran sulfate caused an inhibition only after 4 hr, and at 72 hr only polyanethole sulfonate showed a depression (Bloksma *et al.*, 1980). Carrageenan injected i.v. with SRBC induced marked reduction in liver uptake and blood clearance of antigen, resulting in diversion of increased amounts of antigen to the spleen (Turner and Higginbothan, 1979).

3.4.2. Concanavalin A, Cytochalasin B, Azathioprine, Frentizole, Cycloleucine, 6-Mercaptopurine

Concanavalin A-treated neutrophils showed a decreased ability to phagocytize polyvinyltoluene beads (Berlin, 1972). The phagocytosis of polystyrene latex particles by monolayers of mouse peritoneal macrophages was inhibited by concanavalin A (Friend *et al.*, 1975).

Cytochalasin B inhibited the phagocytosis of various kinds of ingestible particles, immune complexes, and bacteria by human polymorphonuclear leukocytes (Davis *et al.*, 1971; Malawista *et al.*, 1971; Cannarozzi and Malawista, 1973; Zeigler and Schugar, 1979), peritoneal macrophages (Klaus, 1973; Axline and Reaven, 1974; Pesanti and Nugent, 1981), and rabbit alveolar macrophages (Malawista *et al.*, 1971; Sannes and Spicer, 1979). Due to cytochalasin B, the phagocytosis of live bacteria by human blood leukocytes was somewhat diminished but the phagocytosis of starch particles was almost completely inhibited (Cannarozzi and Malawista, 1973).

Azathioprine (Imurek) had no effect on clearance of gelatinized RE test lipid emulsion or colloidal carbon in rats (Pisano *et al.*, 1972) or on colloidal gold clearance in chronically treated rabbits (Kaufmann and McIntosh, 1971). Moreover, it did not inhibit the hepatic clearance of IgM-sensitized erythrocytes or the splenic clearance of IgG-coated erythrocytes (Atkinson and Frank, 1974). For man, however, reduced phagocytosis of *E. coli* and latex particles by blood monocytes has been reported (Bennedsen *et al.*, 1979). Similar results were found in murine macrophages, in which azathioprine depressed erythrophagocytosis *in vitro* as well as *in vivo* (Scheetz *et al.*, 1976).

Frentizole [1-(methoxy-2-benzothiazolyl)-3-phenyl urea] inhibited erythrophagocytosis by murine peritoneal macrophages *in vitro* (Scheetz *et al.*, 1976). Cycloleucine had no effect on clearance of gelatinized RE test lipid emulsion, but profoundly depressed clearance of colloidal carbon (Pisano *et al.*, 1972). 6-Mercaptopurine was ineffective in both tests.

3.4.3. Alkylating Agents

The effect of cyclophosphamide on the phagocytic activity of the RES was investigated in mice, rats, and guinea pigs using chromphosphate and carbon clearance. Friedberg *et al.* (1971) reported an initial phagocytic increase in mice 12 hr after an i.v. injection of 300 mg/kg, which was followed by a long-lasting suppression and a marked reduction in spleen weight. The depression but not the initial increase was confirmed by Flemming *et al.* (1983). Other studies in mice (Zschiesche and Augsten, 1968; Buhles and Shifrine, 1977), rats (Sharbaugh and Grogan, 1969; Lockhard *et al.*, 1971), and guinea pigs (Atkinson and Frank, 1974) failed to show any influence of cyclophosphamide on the phagocytic activity of the RES. This is apparently due to the fact that these authors used lower cyclophosphamide doses and i.p. and s.c. injections.

Other alkylating agents that depress RES phagocytosis are chlorambucil (administered orally) and thioTEPA (parenterally); busulfan had no effect (Megirian *et al.*, 1959; Megirian, 1965). The effects on the RES of a congeneric series of immunosuppressive nitrogen mustard benzimidazoles [1,2-substituted 5-bis(β-chloroethyl)-amino-benzimidazoles] and related compounds were studied in mice (Zschiesche, 1972). Several derivatives were found that more or less depressed the carbon clearance rate of the blood. In these detailed studies, distinct structure–function relationships were found. The biological effectiveness of the compounds is due to both the nitrogen mustard group substituted in position 5 and an alkyl group, alkanoic or amino acid-substituted in position 2 of the benzimidazole ring; furthermore, the efficacy of the substances was affected by either alkyl or aryl substitutions in position 1 or the dissociability of the substituent in position 2.

Regardless of their different effects on carbon clearance, all the compounds diminished the absolute number of both Kupffer cells of the liver and peritoneal macrophages but had no effect on the number of RE spleen cells. In contrast to these results, the benzimidazole derivatives that did decrease phagocytosis also caused a reduction of lysosomal and ATP-splitting enzyme activities, both being involved in the cellular uptake of particles. From these and other findings it was concluded that the phagocytosis-depressing effect of alkylating agents is based on alterations at the subcellular level rather than on the reduction of RE cell numbers. Further results indicated that both the inhibition of phagocytosis and the reduction in spleen weight can be explained by the hydrophobic and electronic properties of the R_1 substituent and the steric properties of the R_2 substituent (Franke *et al.*, 1974).

3.4.4. Antimetabolites

Methotrexate and pyrimidine analogs caused a significant reduction in the rate of $CrPO_4$ clearance in rats when administered i.p. or orally (Megirian *et al.*, 1959); 6-mercaptopurine failed to show any influence on the carbon clearance rate in mice (Zschiesche and Augsten, 1968). Triethylenemelamine induced a phagocytic depression in mice between 6 and 10 days following i.v. injection (Raake and Tempel, 1977).

In connection with antimetabolites, it may also be mentioned that the protein synthesis inhibitors cycloheximide and emetine were found to exert a dose-dependent, temporary preventive effect against autophagocytosis in chicken pancreatic acinar cells that had been induced by neutral red (Kiss *et al.*, 1980). Phlorizin, which acts as a metabolic inhibitor for the phosphorylating enzymes, has been shown to inhibit the phagocytosis activity of rats (Ludany *et al.*, 1957) and man (Enomato, 1959). Moreover, phagocytic inhibition occurred in fixed macrophages of the chick embryo liver if the eggs had been pretreated with phlorizin (Mizejewski and Ramm, 1972).

3.4.5. Alkaloids

Colchicine was found to depress the global RES phagocytic activity as indicated by the blood clearance of carbon in hamsters, mice, and rabbits (Galton, 1967). The most pronounced effects were seen in states of heightened phagocytic activity, as in the pregnant hamster and in hamsters treated with female sex hormones. Male hamsters, which displayed lower initial levels of phagocytic activity than females, were not significantly susceptible to the depressing action of colchicine. Male mice, however, which also possessed lower initial levels of phagocytic activity than females, exhibited a definite phagocytosis depression in response to colchicine. In the rabbit, colchicine produced a similar degree of phagocytosis inhibition in both sexes.

3.5. HEAVY METALS AND RARE EARTH METALS

Lead acetate [$Pb(CH_3COO)_2$] administered to rats (Trejo and DiLuzio, 1971; Trejo *et al.*, 1972b) and mice (Flemming and Schwörer 1982) induced a remarkable reduction of the carbon clearance rate. In rats, the depression of phagocytosis occurred after lead doses between 2.5 and 10 mg/rat and lasted from 6 hr to more than 72 hr; 10 mg was less effective than 2.5 and 5.0 mg and caused significant mortality. Further experiments using RE test lipid emulsion confirmed the impairment of hepatic macrophage phagocytic activity and showed its association with a reduced hepatic uptake; splenic and lung uptake were increased. The relatively greater participation of extrahepatic phagocytosis during the lead-induced hepatic phagocytic depression emphasized that the potential phagocytosis capacity of the spleen and lungs is unchallenged during normal conditions (Trejo *et al.*, 1972b).

Cadmium is known to be rapidly localized in the liver (Decker *et al.*, 1957; Perry *et al.*, 1970). Following i.v. injection, cadmium acetate increased blood clearance and enhanced Kupffer cell localization of the RE test lipid emulsion in rats (Cook *et al.*, 1974) and of colloidal carbon in mice (Flemming and Schwörer, 1982). In mice, the cadmium acetate-induced phagocytic increase was dose-dependent and lasted from 3 hr to more than 48 hr. Combined application with RES modulators led either to a reduction (trioein, endotoxin) or even to an abolition (cyclophosphamide) of the stimulating effect of cadmium acetate. Increases of plasma enzyme activities (GOT, GPT, GLDH) due to cadmium acetate were influenced by the RES modulators in a complex way. It was concluded that cadmium acetate would exert a toxic effect on the parenchymal liver cells which appears to be causally connected with the stimulation of phagocytosis (Flemming *et al.*, 1983, 1984). Stimulation of SRBC phagocytosis was also observed with peritoneal macrophages from mice that had been given cadmium chloride orally for 10 weeks; phagocytosis increased with increasing cadmium doses (Koller and Roan, 1977). It remains questionable, however, to what extent these results are comparable to those obtained with cadmium acetate. Moreover, prolonged exposures to cadmium and lead may produce different results than do single doses (Koller *et al.*, 1976).

Although the mechanism of the increasing effect of cadmium acetate on RES phagocytosis has not yet been clarified in full detail, there are strong indications that it is an indirect consequence of the initial acute cadmium intoxication (Hoffmann *et al.*, 1975; Flemming *et al.*, 1983). This assumption is supported by findings that the combined administration of cadmium acetate and stimulants like triolein or bacterial endotoxin did not result in an additional increase but converted the original increase into a phagocytic decrease (Flemming *et al.*, 1983).

Recently, a new effect of cadmium on the RES was discovered (Knutson *et al.*, 1980). Following chronic administration to mice by dissolving $CdCl_2$ in their drinking water for 8 months, cadmium caused an impaired liver uptake of A-IgG that was correlated with increased liver cadmium. This effect was specific in that clearance of aggregated human serum albumin and colloidal carbon was normal in cadmium-treated mice, suggesting that cadmium may affect either Fc or complement receptors of Kupffer cells in the liver. In this connection, long-term exposure of man to cadmium induces pathological alterations of the phagocytic system (Legoza *et al.*, 1983). In monocytes separated from the blood of workers who had been exposed to air pollution containing cadmium exceeding the MAC values for 9 years, Fcγ-receptor-mediated relative phagocytosis as well as intracellular killing capability were diminished.

Following i.v. injection of beryllium sulfate ($BeSO_4$) in rats and mice, most of it was converted to a nondiffusible colloidal beryllium phosphate–α-globulin complex that was removed from the blood by the RES and induced a pronounced depression of RES phagocytosis that was attributed to the physicochemical properties of beryllium (Vacher and Stoner, 1968; Vacher *et al.*, 1973).

Nontoxic colloidal gallium hydroxide [$Ga(OH)_3$] is accumulated by the RES cells of the liver, spleen, and bone marrow of mice, thus inducing a decreased hepatic uptake of subsequently administered toxic colloidal indium hydroxide [$In(OH)_3$]. The increasing depression of the phagocytic uptake of $In(OH)_3$ by the liver observed following increasing doses of $Ga(OH)_3$ was correlated with a decreased toxicity of $In(OH)_3$. It was concluded that hepatic phagocytosis of $In(OH)_3$ enhances the toxicity of indium. This conclusion was supported by the finding that both gelatin and thorotrast "blockade" of the RES also decreased the liver uptake of $In(OH)_3$ and decreased again its toxicity (Evdokimoff and Wagner, 1972a,b).

In vitro studies on peritoneal macrophages from mice showed that the rate of phagocytosis of bacteria was also inhibited by low as well as high doses of zinc

(Karl *et al.*, 1973). Other experiments performed on alveolar macrophages showed that nickelous chloride (Ni^{2+}) selectively depressed the phagocytic activity at concentrations lower than those causing cell death. This effect was increased with increasing nickelous concentration ranging from 5.1×10^{-4} to 1.1×10^{-3} M (Graham *et al.*, 1975).

Rare earth metal salts, among them gadolinium chloride, depress RE activity and significantly inhibit or abolish the RES-stimulating affect of zymosan, triolein, and BCG (Lázár, 1973b). Gadolinium chloride also inhibits the hormonally induced RE stimulation by estradiol in mice (Husztik *et al.*, 1977).

Investigations with heterologous erythrocytes labeled with ^{51}Cr show that gadolinium chloride-induced RE blockade is due to the depressed phagocytic activity of the Kupffer cells. Light and electron microscopic studies suggest that the failure of the Kupffer cells to incorporate carbon during the RE "blockade" induced by rare earth metal chloride is due to defects in the surface attachment and in the engulfment phase of phagocytosis (Husztik *et al.*, 1980).

REFERENCES

Altura, B. M., Hershey, S. G., and Mazzia, V. D. B., 1965, Influence of choline pretreatment on phagocytosis and survival after experimental shock, 2nd National Scientific Meeting, Salt Lake City, Utah, Abstr. No. 9.

Altura, B. M., Hershey, S. G., and Hyman, C., 1966, Influence of choline on the reticuloendothelial system and on survival after experimental shock, *J. Reticuloendothel. Soc.* **3**:57.

Ashworth, C. T., DiLuzio, N. R., and Riggi, S. J., 1963, A morphologic study of the effect of reticuloendothelial stimulation upon hepatic removal of minute particles from the blood of rats, *Exp. Mol. Pathol.* **1**:83.

Atkinson, J., and Frank, M., 1974, Failure of cytotoxic agents to inhibit the clearance of sensitized erythrocytes, *J. Reticuloendothel. Soc.* **16**:122.

Axline, S. C., and Reaven, E. P., 1974, Inhibition of phagocytosis and plasma membrane mobility of the cultivated macrophage by cytochalasin B, *J. Cell Biol.* **62**:647.

Altura, B. M., and Hershey, S. G., 1971, Acute intestinal ischemia shock and reticuloendothelial system function, *J. Reticuloendothel. Soc.* **10**:361.

Benacerraf, B., Biozzi, G., Halpern, B. N., and Stiffel, C., 1957, Physiology cof phagocytosis of particles by the RES, in: *Physiopathology of the Reticulo-Endothelial System* (B. N. Halpern, C. Benacerraf, and J. F. Delafresnaye, eds.), pp. 52–79, Charles C. Thomas, Springfield, Illinois.

Benacerraf, B., Thorbecke, G. J., and Jacoby, D. B., 1959, Effect of zymosan on endotoxin toxicity in mice, *Proc. Soc. Exp. Biol. Med.* **100**:796.

Benacerraf, B., and Sebestyén, M., 1957, The effect of bacterial endotoxins on the RES, *Fed. Proc.* **16**:860.

Bennedsen, J., Rhodes, J. M., Larsen, S. C., and Halberg, P. H., 1979, A profile of monocyte functions in patients with rheumatoid arthritis, 16th Annu. Natl. Meet. RE Soc., Abstr. 109, p. 57.

Benveniste, J., Higounet, F., and Salomon, J.-C., 1970, Effects of various doses of prednisolone on the phagocytic activity in axenic and holoxenic mice, *J. Reticuloendothel. Soc.* **8**:499.

Berlin, R. D., 1972, Effect of concanavalin A on phagocytosis, *Nature New Biol.* **235**:44.

Bilbey, D. L. J., and Nicol, T., 1958, Effect of various natural steroids on the phagocytic activity of the reticuloendothelial system, *Nature (London)* **182**:674.

Biozzi, G., Benacerraf, B., Grumbach, F., Halpern, B. N., Levaditi, J., and Rist, N., 1954, Étude de l'activité granulopexique du système LRE au cours de l'infection tuberculeuse expérimentale de la souris, *Ann. Inst. Pasteur (Paris)* **87**:291.

Biozzi, G., Benacerraf, B., and Halpern, B. N., 1955, The effect of Salm. typhi and its endotoxin on the phagocytic activity of the reticuloendothelial system in mice, *Br. J. Exp. Pathol.* **36**:226.

Biozzi, G., Halpern, B. N., Bilbey, D., Stiffel, C., Benacerraf, B., and Mouton, D., 1957a, Oestrogènes et fonction phagocytaire du systéme réticuloendothelial, (S.R.E.), *C.R. Soc. Biol.* **151**:1326.

Biozzi, G., Halpern, B. N., Benacerraf, B., and Stiffel, C., 1957b, Phagocytic activity of the reticuloendothelial system in experimental infections, in: *Physiopathology of the ReticuloEndothelial System* (B. N. Halpern, B. Benacerraf, and J. F. Delafresnaye, eds.) pp. 204–225, Charles C. Thomas, Springfield, Illinois.

Biozzi, G., Stiffel, C., and Mouton, D., 1963, Stimulation et dépression de la function phagocytaire du système réticuloendothélial par des emulsions de lipids: Relation avec quelques phénomènes immunologiques, *Rev. Fr. Etud. Clin. Biol.* **8**:341.

Bird, D. C., and Sheagren, J. N., 1970, Evaluation of reticuloendothelial system phagocytic activity during systemic *Candida albicans* infection in mice, *Proc. Soc. Exp. Biol. Med.* **133**:34.

Blickens, D. A., and DiLuzio, N. R., 1964, The effect of methyl cellulose on the reticuloendothelial system, *J. Reticuloendothel. Soc.* **1**:68.

Blickens, D. A., and DiLuzio, N. R., 1965, Metabolism of methyl palmitate, a phagocytic and immunologic depressant, and its influence of tissue lipids, *J. Reticuloendothel. Soc.* **2**:60.

Bliznakov, E., Casey, A., and Premuzie, E., 1970, Coenzymes Q: Stimulants of the phagocytic activity in rats and immune response in mice, *Experientia* **26**:953.

Bloksma, N., de Reuver, M. J., and Willers, J. M. N., 1980, Influence on macrophage functions as a possible basis of immunomodification by polyanions, *Ann. Immunol. (Paris)* **131D**:255.

Bloksma, N., de Reuver, M. J., and Willers, J. M. N., 1983, Impaired macrophage functions as a possible basis of immunomodification by microbial agents, tilorone and dimethyldioctadecylammoniumbromide, *Antonie van Leeuwenhoek J. Microbiol. Serol.* **49**:1.

Blumenstock, F., Saba, T. M., Weber, P., and Cho, E., 1976, Purification and biochemical characterization of a macrophage stimulating alpha-2-globulin opsonic protein, *J. Reticuloendothel. Soc.* **19**:157.

Blumenstock, F., Saba, T. M., Weber, P., and Laffin, R., 1978, Biochemical and immunological characterization of human opsonic α2SB glycoprotein: Its identity with cold-insoluble globulin, *J. Biol. Chem.* **253**:4287.

Boehme, D., and Dubos, R., 1958, The effect of bacterial constituents on resistance of mice to heterologous infection and on the activity of their reticuloendothelial system, *J. Exp. Med.* **107**:523.

Bragdon, J. H., and Gordon, R. S., 1958, Tissue distribution of ^{14}C after the intravenous injection of labelled chylomicrons and unesterified fatty acids in the rat, *J. Clin. Invest.* **37**:574.

Brauns, F. E., and Brauns, D. A., 1960, *The Chemistry of Lignin*, pp. 630–633, Academic Press, New York.

Brown, J. B., 1955, Urinary excretion of oestrogens during menstrual cycle, *Lancet.* **1**:320.

Brown, J. B., 1956, Urinary excretion of oestrogens during pregnancy, lactation and the reestablishment of menstruation, *Lancet* **1**:704.

Buhles, W. C., and Shifrine, M., 1977, Effects of cyclophosphamide on macrophage numbers, functions and progenitor cells, *J. Reticuloendothel. Soc.* **21**:285.

Burdzy, K., Munder, P. G., Fischer, H., and Westphal, O., 1964, Steigerung der Phagocytose von Peritonealmakrophagen durch Lysolecithin, *Z. Naturforsch.* **19**:1118.

Burgaleta, C., Territo, M. C., Quan, S. G., and Golde, D. W., 1978, Glucan-activated macrophages: Functional characteristics and surface morphology, *J. Reticuloendothel. Soc.* **23**:195.

Burger, H., and Leonhardt, K., 1952, Über die Beeinflussung der Leukocytenphagocytose durch die weiblichen Sexualhormone in vitro, *Arch. Gynaekol.* **181**:300.

Cannarozzi, N. A., and Malawista, S. E., 1973, Phagocytosis by human blood leukocytes measured by the uptake of 131 I-labelled human serum albumin: Inhibitory and stimulatory effects of cytochalasin B1, *Yale J. Biol. Med.* **46**:117.

Carr, I., and Williams, M. A., 1966, The cellular basis of reticuloendothelial stimulation, *Int. Symp. Atheroscler. RES Como, Italy, Summaries* p. 18.

Cook, J. A., Marconi, E. A., and DiLuzio, N. R., 1974, Lead and cadmium, endotoxin interaction: Effect on mortality and hepatic function, *Toxicol. Appl. Pharmacol.* **28**:292.

Cooper, G. N., 1964, Functional modification of reticuloendothelial cells by simple triglycerides, *J. Reticuloendothel. Soc.* **1**:50.

Cooper, G. N., and Stuart, A. E., 1961, Sensitivity of mice to bacterial lipopolysaccharide following alteration of activity of the reticuloendothelial system, *Nature (London)* **191**:294.

Cooper, G. N., and West, D., 1962, Effects of simple lipids on the phagocytic properties of peritoneal macrophages: Stimulatory effects of glyceryl trioleate, *Aust. J. Exp. Biol. Med. Sci.* **40**:485.

Crabbé, J., 1956, Enhancing action of small doses of cortisone on macrophage phagocytosis of staphylococci on rabbits, *Acta Endocrinol. (Copenhagen)* **21**:41.

Cutler, J. L., 1960, The enhancement of hemolysin production in the rat by zymosan, *J. Immunol.* **84**:416.

Cutler, J. L., 1961, The effect of zymosan on the phagocytosis of foreign erythrocytes, *J. Immunol.* **86**:73.

Davis, A. T., Estensen, R., and Quie, P. G., 1971, Cytochalasin B. III. Inhibition of human polymorphonuclear leukocyte phagocytosis, *Proc. Soc. Exp. Biol. Med.* **137**:161.

Decker, C. F., Byerrum, R. U., and Hoppert, C. A., 1957, A study of distribution and retention of cadmium-115 in the albino rat, *Arch. Biochem. Biophys.* **66**:140.

Degré, M., and Rollag, H., 1979, Influence of interferon on the in vivo phagocytic activity of reticuloendothelial system cells, *J. Reticuloendothel. Soc.* **25**:489.

DiCarlo, F. J., and Fiore, J. V., 1958, On the composition of zymosan, *Science* **127**:756.

DiCarlo, F. J., Beach, V. L., Haynes, L. J., Silver, N. J., and Steinetz, B. G., 1963a, Effect of hypophysectomy upon phagocytosis in the mouse, *Endocrinology* **73**:170.

DiCarlo, F. J., Haynes, L. J., and Phillips, G. E., 1963b, Effect of *Mycobacterium phlei* upon the reticuloendothelial system of mice of different ages, *Proc. Soc. Exp. Biol. Med.* **112**:651.

DiCarlo, F. J., Haynes, L. J., Silver, N. J., and Phillips, G. E., 1964a, Reticuloendothelial system stimulants of botanical origin, *J. Reticuloendothel. Soc.* **1**:224.

DiCarlo, F. J., Haynes, L. J., Silver, N. J., and Phillips, G. E., 1964b, Protection of mice against gram-positive bacteria with *Maytenus laevis* and other RES stimulants, *Proc. Soc. Exp. Biol. Med.* **116**:195.

DiLuzio, N. R., 1955, Effect of X-irradiation and choline on the reticuloendothelial system of the rat, *Am. J. Physiol.* **181**:595.

DiLuzio, N. R., 1960, Reticuloendothelial involvement in lipid metabolism, *Ann. N.Y. Acad. Sci.* **88**:244.

DiLuzio, N. R., 1976, Pharmacology of the reticuloendothelial system-accent on glucan, *Adv. Exp. Med. Biol.* **73a**:412.

DiLuzio, N. R., and Blickens, D. A., 1966, Influence of intravenously administered lipids on reticuloendothelial function, *J. Reticuloendothel. Soc.* **3**:250.

DiLuzio, N. R., and Riggi, S. J., 1964, The relative participation of hepatic parenchymal and Kupffer cells in the metabolism of chylomicrons, *J. Reticuloendothel. Soc.* **1**:248.

DiLuzio, N. R., and Riggi, S. J., 1970, The effects of laminarin, sulfated glucan and oligosaccharides of glucan on reticuloendothelial activity, *J. Reticuloendothel. Soc.* **8**:465.

DiLuzio, N. R., and Wooles, W. R., 1964, Depression of phagocytic activity and immune response by methylpalmitate, *Am. J. Physiol.* **206**:939.

DiLuzio, N. R., Pisano, J. C., and Saba, T. M., 1970, Evaluation of the mechanism of glucan-induced stimulation of the reticuloendothelial system, *J. Reticuloendothel. Soc.* **7**:731.

Dobson, E. L., 1957, Factors controlling phagocytosis, in: *Physiopathology of the Reticuloendothelial System* (B. N. Halpern, B. Benacerraf, and J. F. Delafresnaye, eds.), pp. 80–114, Blackwell, Oxford.

Dobson, E., and Kelly, L. S., 1973, The combined stimulation of the reticuloendothelial system by estradiol and endotoxin, *J. Reticuloendothel. Soc.* **13**:61.

Donahoe, R. M., and Huang, J. Y., 1976, Interferon preparations enhance phagocytosis in vivo, *Infect. Immun.* **13**:1250.

Doran, J. E., Mansberger, A. R., and Reese, A. C., 1980, Cold insoluble globulin enhanced phagocytosis of gelatinized targets by macrophage monolayers: A model system, *J. Reticuloendothel. Soc.* **27**:471.

Doran, J. E., Mansberger, A. R., Edmondson, H. T., and Reese, A. C., 1981a, Cold insoluble globulin and heparin interactions in phagocytosis by macrophage monolayers: Lack of heparin requirement, *J. Reticuloendothel. Soc.* **29**:275.

Doran, J. E., Mansberger, A. R., Edmondson, H. T., and Reese, A. C., 1981b, Cold insoluble globulin and heparin interactions in phagocytosis by macrophage monolayers: Mechanism of heparin enhancement, *J. Reticuloendothel. Soc.* **29**:285.

Drummond, D., and Munson, A., 1974, Effect of molecular weight of pyran copolymer on vascular clearance of colloidal carbon, *Abstr. 10th Annu. Natl. Meet. RE Soc.* **15**:2.

Enomato, T., 1959, Movement and phagocytosis of leucocytes with respect to their energy metabolism. I. Relation between the maintenance of movement and phagocytosis and the energy metabolism of leucocytes, *Asaka Igaku Zasshi* **11**:1199.

Eufinger, H., 1932, Das retikuloendotheliale System in der Gestationsperiode und im mensuellen Zyklus, *Monatsschr. Geburtshilfe Gynaekol.* **91**:312.

Evdokimoff, V., and Wagner, H. N., 1972a, Hepatic phagocytosis as a mechanism for increasing heavy-metal toxicity, *J. Reticuloendothel. Soc.* **11**:148.

Evdokimoff, V., and Wagner, H. N., 1972b, Reduction of indium toxicity by blockade of the reticuloendothelial system, *J. Reticuloendothel. Soc.* **11**:599.

Fauve, R. M., 1974, Immunostimulation with phospholipids, in: *Activation of Macrophages* (W.-H. Wagner and H. Hahn, eds.), pp. 157–161, Excerpta Medica, Amsterdam.

Filkins, J. P., and DiLuzio, N. R., 1967, Comparative effects of endotoxin and gelatin on reticuloendothelial activity, *Proc. Soc. Exp. Biol. Med.* **125**:908.

Flemming, K., 1963a, Strahlenschutzwirkung von Äthylstearat, *Naturwissenschaften* **50**:332.

Flemming, K., 1963b, Radiation protection effect and pharmacologically changed activity of the reticuloendothelial system, *Nature (London)* **200**:1117.

Flemming, K., 1965a, Radiation protection effect of chlorotrianisene (TACE), *Prog. Biochem. Pharmacol.* **1**:564.

Flemming, K., 1965b, Steigerung der Phagocytoseaktivität durch Maytenus laevis-Blätter und Scholler-Tornesch-Lignin (Porlisan), *Naturwissenschaften* **52**:346.

Flemming, K., 1966a, Langdauernde Stimulation des reticuloendothelialen Systems durch Chlortrianisen, *Naturwissenschaften* **53**:555.

Flemming, K., 1966b, Phagocytosesteigerung des RES durch das Pro-Östrogen Chlortrianisen, *Naunyn-Schmiedebergs Arch. Exp. Pathol. Pharmakol.* **255**:14.

Flemming, K., 1967, Pharmacological stimulation and depression of the phagocytic function of the RES, *Adv. Exp. Med. Biol.* **1**:188.

Flemming, K., 1974, Stimulation by various drugs of RES phagocytosis in mice, *Excerpta Med. Int. Congr. Ser.* **325**(2):280.

Flemming, K., 1977, Experimental animals and in vitro systems for testing substances enhancing the phagocytosis rate, in: *International Symposium on Experimental Animals and "in Vitro Systems*, Med. Microbiol. WHO Collab. Center, Veterinary Faculty, University of Munich, 1976.

Flemming, K. B. P., 1984, Effects of RES phagocytosis of physiological and pharmacological agents, in: *Tissue Culture and RES* (P. Röhlich and E. Bácsy, eds.), pp. 127–140, Akadémiai Kiadó, Budapest.

Flemming, K., and Graack, B., 1967, Zur Steigerung der Phagocytoseaktivität des reticuloendothelialen Systems durch Stoffe pflanzlicher Herkunft, *Arzneim. Forsch.* **17**:1541.

Flemming, K., and Langendorff, M., 1965, Das Pro-Östrogen Chlortrianisen, (TACE) als Strahlenschutzsubstanz, *Strahlentherapie* **128**:109.

Flemming, K., and Nothdurft, W., 1968, Phagocytoseanstieg im reticuloendothelialen System durch Polyvinylpyridin-N-oxide, *Klin. Wochenschr.* **46**:904.

Flemming, K., and Nothdurft, W., 1982, Investigations on the biphasic response of the reticuloendothelial system induced by the lipopolysaccharide of Salmonella abortus equi (Pyrexal), *Acta Biol. Acad. Sci. Hung.* **33**:353.

Flemming, K. B. P., and Schwörer, H., 1982, Decrease of RES phagocytosis following whole body X-irradiation and its interaction with responses to RES affecting drugs, 9th International RES Congress, Davos, Book of Abstracts, No. 94, p. 19.

Flemming, K., Flemming, C., and Graack, B., 1967, Strahlenresistenz bei pharmakologisch veränderter Phagocytoseaktivität des RES, *Strahlentherapie* **133**:280.

Flemming, K., Elias, S., and Schwörer, H., 1983, The RES phagocytosis in acute cadmium loading without and with RES modulators, *J. Congr. ETCS and EURES*, Budapest, Abstracts, p. 18.

Franke, R., Zschiesche, W., Augsten, K., Güttner, J., and Hesse, G., 1974, Quantitative structure–activity relationships in immunosuppressive nitrogen mustard benzimidazoles, *J. Reticuloendothel. Soc.* **16**:87.

Freudenberg, K., 1933, *Tannin-Celluslose-Lignin*, Springer-Verlag, Berlin.

Friedberg, K. D., Garbe, G., and Westermann, M., 1971, Beeinflussung des reticuloendothelialen Systems durch Cyclophosphamid, Endotoxin und Polyvinylpyridin-N-oxid, *Naunyn-Schmiedebergs Arch. Exp. Pathol. Pharmakol.* **269**:57.

Friend, K., Ekstedt, R. D., and Duncan, J. L., 1975, Effect of concanavalin A on phagocytosis by mouse peritoneal macrophages, *J. Reticuloendothel. Soc.* **17**:10.

Fukushima, K., Teller, M. N., Mountain, J. M., Tarnowski, G. S., and Stock, C. C., 1979, Predictive relationship of phagocytic activity to tumor regression in indoloquinolinone derivative-treated mice, *J. Reticuloendothel. Soc.* **26**:187.

Gaillard, D., Pipy, B., and Derache, R., 1974, Influence de la composition en acides gras d'huiles végétales alimentaires sur les activitès des enzymes de détoxication des microsomes hépatiques du rat, *Ann. Nutr. Aliment.* **28**:17.

Galanos, C., Lüderitz, O., Rietschel, E. T., and Westphal, O., 1977, Newer aspects of the chemistry and biology of bacterial lipopolysaccharides with special reference to their lipid A component, *Int. Rev. Biochem.* **14**:239.

Galton, M., 1967, Effect of colchicine on RES phagocytic activity, *J. Reticuloendothel. Soc.* **4**:476.

Gemsa, D., Fudenberg, H., and Schmid, R., 1974, Erythrophagocytosis: Regulation of the heme-degrading enzyme system, in: *Activation of Macrophages* (W.-H. Wagner and H. Hahn, eds.), Excerpta Medica, Amsterdam.

Ghys, R., 1961, Action radiomodificatrice des hormones sexuelles chez le rat, *J. Belge Radiol.* **44**:641.

Ghys, R., 1963, L'influence des facteurs métaboliques sur la radiosensibilité, *Laval Med.* **34**:69.

Gotjamanos, T., 1970, Alterations in reticuloendothelial organ structure and function following cortisone administration to mice, *J. Reticuloendothel. Soc.* **8**:421.

Graack, B., and Flemming, K., 1966, Untersuchungen zur Steigerung der Phagocytoseaktivität des RES durch Stoffe pflanzlicher Herkunft, *Naunyn-Schmiedebergs Arch. Exp. Pathol. Pharmakol.* **253**:37.

Graham, J. A., Gardner, D. E., Waters, M. D., and Coffin, D. L., 1975, Effect of trace metals on phagocytosis by alveolar macrophages, *Infect. Immun.* **11**:1278.

Gudewicz, P. W., 1979, The effects of cortisone acetate therapy on alveolar macrophage function and glucose metabolism, 16th Annu. Natl. Meet. RE Soc. Abstr. 28a.

Halpern, B. N., Prévot, A. R., Biozzi, G., Stiffel, C., Mouton, D., Morard, J. C., Bouthiller, Y., and Decreusefond, C., 1964, Stimulation de l'activité phagocytaire du systém réticuloendothélial provoquée par Corynebacterium parvum, *J. Reticuloendothel. Soc.* **1**:77.

Harborne, J. B., 1964, *Biochemistry of Phenolic Compounds*, Academic Press, New York.

Heller, J. H., 1953, Stimulation of the reticuloendothelial system with choline, *Science* **118**:353.

Heller, J. H., 1955, Cortisone and phagocytosis, *Endocrinology* **56**:80.

Heller, J. H., 1960, Nontoxic RES stimulatory lipids, *Ann. N.Y. Acad. Sci.* **88**:116.

Heller, J. H., Meier, R. M., Zucker, R., and Mast, G. W., 1957, The effect of natural and synthetic estrogens on reticuloendothelial system function, *Endocrinology* **61**:235.

Heller, J. H., Pasternak, V. Z., Ransom, J. P., and Heller, M. S., 1963, A new reticuloendothelial system stimulating agent (restim) from shark livers, *Nature (London)* **199**:4896.

Heller, J. H., Bliznakow, E. G., Ransom, J. P., Wilkins, D. J., and Pasternak, V. Z., 1965, The effect of a new RES stimulant on neoplasia, in: *The Reticuloendothelial System*, Nisha, Kyoto.

Hoebeke, J., 1976, Levamisole, an anti-anergic chemotherapeutic agent: Experimental and clinical findings, in: *The Reticuloendothelial System in Health and Disease: Functions and Characteristics* (S. M. Reichard, M. R. Escobar, and H. Friedman, eds.), p. 422, Plenum Press, New York.

Hoebeke, J., and Franchi, G., 1973, Influence of tetramisole and its optical isomers on the mononuclear phagocytic system, *J. Reticuloendothel. Soc.* **14**:317.

Hoffmann, E. O., Cook, J. A., DiLuzio, N. R., and Coover, J. A., 1975, The effects of acute cadmium administration on the liver and kidney of the rat, *Lab. Invest.* **32**:655.

Hofhuis, F. M. A., van der Meer, C., Kersten, M. C. M., Rutten, V. P. M. G., and Willers, J. M. N.,

1981, Effects of dimethyldioctadecylammonium bromide on phagocytosis and digestion of *Listeria monocytogenes* by mouse peritoneal macrophages, *Immunology* 43:425.

Hornnes, N., and Rygaard, J., 1960, Determination of inhibited blood clearance in cortisone treated mice by the intravenous injection of Au[198], *Acta Radiol.* 53:42.

Huang, K. Y., Donahoe, R. M., Gordon, F. B., and Dressler, H. R., 1971, Enhancement of phagocytosis by interferon containing preparations, *Infect. Immun.* 4:581.

Husztik, E., Lázár, G., and Szilágyi, S., 1977, Study on the mechanism of Kupffer-cell phagocytosis blockade induced by gadolinium chloride, in: *Kupffer Cells and Other Liver Sinusoidal Cells* (E. Wisse and D. L. Knook, eds.), pp. 387–395, Elsevier, Amsterdam.

Husztik, E., Lázár, G., and Párducz, A., 1980, Electron microscopic study of Kupffer-cell phagocytosis blockade induced by gadolinium chloride, *Br. J. Exp. Pathol.* 61:624.

Janssen, P. A. J., 1976, The levamisole story, *Prog. Drug Res.* 20:347.

Kampine, J. P., Banaszak, E. F., and Smith, J. J., 1965, Alteration of RES activity and circulatory responsiveness in the dog, *J. Reticuloendothel. Soc.* 2:172.

Kapila, D., Smith, C., and Rubin, A. A., 1971, Effect of pyran copolymer on phagocytosis and tumor growth, *J. Reticuloendothel. Soc.* 9:447.

Karl, L., Chvapil, M., and Zukoski, C. F., 1973, Effect of zinc on the viability and phagocytic capacity of peritoneal macrophages, *Proc. Soc. Exp. Biol. Med.* 142:1123.

Kaufmann, D. B., and McIntosh, R. M., 1971, The effects of azathioprine on reticuloendothelial clearance, *Clin. Res.* 19:221.

Kawasaki, D., and Finch, S. C., 1972, Study of the mechanism of ethyl-palmitate-induced splenic destruction, *J. Reticuloendothel. Soc.* 11:555.

Kelly, L. S., Dobson, E. L., Finney, C. R., and Hirsch, J. D., 1960, Proliferation of the reticuloendothelial system in the liver, *Am. J. Physiol.* 198:1134.

Kelly, L. S., Brown, B. A., and Dobson, E. L., 1962, Cell division and phagocytic activity in liver reticuloendothelial cells, *Proc. Soc. Exp. Biol. Med.* 110:555.

Kiss, A. L., Réz, G., and Kovács, J., 1980, Influence of protein synthesis inhibitors on neutral red-induced autophagocytosis in chicken pancreatic acinar cells, *Acta Biol. Acad. Sci. Hung.* 31:165.

Klaus, G. G., 1973, Cytochalasin B., Dissociation of pinocytosis and phagocytosis by peritoneal macrophages, *Exp. Cell Res.* 79:73.

Knutson, D. W., Vredevoe, D. L., Aoki, K. R., Hays, E. J., and Levy, L., 1980, Cadmium and the reticuloendothelial system (RES): A specific defect in blood clearance of soluble aggregates of IgG by the liver in mice given cadmium, *Immunology* 40:17.

Kojima, M., 1960, Morphological changes accompanying RES stimulation, *Ann. N.Y. Acad. Sci.* 88:196.

Kojima, M., Shishido, K., Kobayashi, S., and Dobashi, M., 1973a, A *Chlorella* polysaccharide as a factor stimulating RES activity, *J. Reticuloendothel. Soc.* 14:192.

Kojima, M., Kasajima, T., Imai, Y., Kobayashi, S., Dobashi, M., and Uemura, T., 1973b, A new *Chlorella* polysaccharide and its accelerating effect on the phagocytic activity of the reticuloendothelial system, *Recent Adv. RES Res.* 13:101.

Koller, L. D., and Roan, J. G., 1977, Effects of lead and cadmium on mouse peritoneal macrophages, *J. Reticuloendothel. Soc.* 21:7.

Koller, L. D., Exon, J. H., and Roan, J. G., 1976, Humoral antibody response in mice after single dose exposure to lead or cadmium, *Proc. Soc. Exp. Biol. Med.* 151:339.

Kroma, E., and Flemming, K., 1965, Äthylpalmitatwirkung auf die Milz und das reticuloendotheliale System der Ratte, Inaugural-Dissertation, Faculty of Medicine, Albert Ludwig University, Freiburg.

Lanser, M. E., and Saba, T. M., 1981, Fibronectin as a co-factor necessary for optimal granulocyte phagocytosis of *Staphylococcus aureus*, *J. Reticuloendothel. Soc.* 30:415.

Lázár, G., 1973a, Observations on the activity of the reticuloendothelial system in estradiol- and diethylstilbestrol-treated rats, *Endokrinologie* 61:152.

Lázár, G., 1973b, The reticuloendothelial-blocking effect of rare earth metals in rats, *J. Reticuloendothel. Soc.* 13:231.

Legoza, S., Gyimesi, E., and Biró, Z., 1983, Alterations of phagocytic functions in cadmium exposed workers, Jt. Congr. ECTS and EURES, Abstr. p. 32.

Lockhard, V. G., Sharbaugh, R. J., Arhelger, R. E., and Grogan, J. B., 1971, Ultrastructural altera-tions in phagocytic functions of alveolar macrophages after cyclophosphamide administration, *J. Reticuloendothel. Soc.* **9**:97.

Loose, L. D., and DiLuzio, N. R., 1976, Dose-related reticuloendothelial system stimulation by diethylstilbestrol, *J. Reticuloendothel. Soc.* **20**:457.

Ludany, G., Koklen, A., and Toth, E., 1957, Die Beeinflussung der Leukocytenphagocytose mit Phlorrhizin, *Experientia* **13**:409.

Lurie, M. B., 1960, The reticuloendothelial system, cortisone, and thyroid function: Their relation to native resistance to infection, *Ann. N.Y. Acad. Sci.* **88**:83.

Mackaness, G. B., and Blanden, R. Y., 1967, Cellular immunity, *Prog. Allergy* **11**:89.

McKay, D. G., Margaretten, W., and Rothenberg, J., 1964, Blockade of the reticuloendothelial system induced by dietary lipids, *Lab. Invest.* **13**:54.

Malawista, S. E., Gee, J. B. L., and Bensch, K. G., 1971, Cytochalasin B reversibly inhibits phagocy-tosis: Functional, metabolic, and ultrastructural effects in human blood leukocytes and rabbit alveolar macrophages, *Yale J. Biol. Med.* **44**:286.

Marcus, S., Esplin, D. W., and Hill, G. A., 1953, Effects of cortisone, ascorbic acid and piromen on phagocytosis in mice, *Proc. Soc. Exp. Biol. Med.* **84**:565.

Megirian, R., 1965, Effect of chlorambucil on the blood clearance of injected particulate matter, *J. Reticuloendothel. Soc.* **2**:238.

Megirian, R., Walton, M. S., and Laug, E. P., 1959, The effect of eight anticancer agents on the phagocytic properties of the reticuloendothelial system, *J. Pharmacol. Exp. Ther.* **127**:81.

Metchnikoff, E., 1901, *L'immunité dans les maladies infectieuses*, Paris.

Miake, S., Taleya, K., Matsumotot, T., Yoshikai, Y., and Nomoto, K., 1980, Relation between bactericidal and phagocytic activities of peritoneal macrophages induced by irritants, *J. Re-ticuloendothel. Soc.* **27**:421.

Mizejewski, G. J., and Ramm, G. M., 1972, Effect of phloridzin on phagocytosis in the chick embryo, *J. Reticuloendothel. Soc.* **11**:11.

Molnar, J., McLain, S., Allen, C., Laga, H., Gara, A., and Gelder, F., 1977, The role of an α 2-macroglobulin of rat serum in the phagocytosis of colloidal particles, *Biochim. Biophys. Acta* **493**:37.

Morrow, S. H., and DiLuzio, N. R., 1965, The fate of foreign red cells in mice with altered reticuloen-dothelial function, *Proc. Soc. Exp. Biol. Med.* **119**:647.

Möse, J. R., 1963, Versuche über die Wirksamkeit von Aristolochiasäure, *Planta Med.* **11**:72.

Möse, J. R., and Lukas, G., 1961, Versuche über die Wirkungsweise von Aristolochia clematitis, *Arzneim. Forsch.* **11**:33.

Munder, P. G., Modolell, M., Ferber, E., and Fischer, H., 1966, Phospholipide in quarzgeschädigten Makrophagen, *Biochem. Z.* **344**:310.

Munson, A. E., Regelson, W., Lawrence, W., and Wooles, W. R., 1968, Biphasic response of the reticuloendothelial system induced by pyran copolymer, *J. Reticuloendothel. Soc.* **5**:590.

Munson, A. E., Regelson, W., Lawrence, W., Jr., and Wooles, W. R., 1970, Biphasic response of the reticuloendothelial system (RES) induced by pyran copolymer, *J. Reticuloendothel. Soc.* **7**:375.

Munson, A. E., Munson, J. A., and Regelson, W., 1972a, Tilorone and congeners: Effect on host defense mechnisms, 8th Annu. Nat. Meet. RE Soc., Abstr. No. 27.

Munson, A. E., Munson, J. A., Regelson, W., and Wampler, G. L., 1972b, Effect of tilorone hydro-chloride and congeners on reticuloendothelial system, tumors, and the immune response, *Cancer Res.* **32**:1397.

Najjar, V. A., 1980, Biochemistry and physiology of tuftsin Thr-Lys-Pro-Arg, in: *The Reticuloen-dothelial System: A Comprehensive Treatise*, Volume 2 (A. J. Sbarra and R. R. Strauss, eds.), pp. 45–71, Plenum Press, New York.

Najjar, V. A., and Constantopoulos, A., 1972, A new phagocytosis-stimulating tetrapeptide hor-mone, tuftsin and its role in disease, *J. Reticuloendothel. Soc.* **12**:197.

Nicol, T., 1935, The female reproductive system of the guinea pig: Intravitam staining: fat produc-tion: influence of hormones, *Trans. R. Soc. Edinburgh* **58**:449.

Nicol, T., and Abou-Zirky, A, 1953, Influence of oestradiol benzoate and orchidectomy on the reticuloendothelial system, *Br. J. Med.* **1**:133.

Nicol, T., and Bilbey, D. L. J., 1957, Reversal by diethyl-stilbestrol of the depressant effect of cortisone on the phagocytic activity of the reticuloendothelial system, *Nature (London)* **179**:1137.

Nicol, T., and Bilbey, D. L. J., 1958, Substances depressing the phagocytic activity of the reticuloendothelial system, *Nature (London)* **182**:606.

Nicol, T., and Bilbey, D. L. J., 1960, The effect of various steroids on the phagocytic activity of the reticuloendothelial system, in: *Reticuloendothelial Structure and Function* (J. H. Heller, ed.), pp. 301–320, Ronald Press, New York.

Nicol, T., and Druce, C., 1961, Effect of dexamethasone on the phagocytic activity of the reticuloendothelial system, *Nature (London)* **190**:91.

Nicol, T., and Helmy, I. D., 1951, Influence of oestrogenic hormones on the reticuloendothelial system in the guinea pig, *Nature (London)* **167**:199.

Nicol, T., and Snell, R. S., 1955, Effect of deoxycorticosterone on the reticuloendothelial system, *Nature (London)* **175**:995.

Nicol, T., and Vernon-Roberts, B., 1965, The influence of the oestrous cycle, pregnancy, and ovariectomy on RES activity, *J. Reticuloendothel. Soc.* **2**:15.

Nicol, T., and Ware, C. C., 1960, Minimum dose of diethylstilbestrol required to stimulate the phagocytic activity of reticuloendothelial system, *Nature (London)* **185**:42.

Nicol, T., Snell, R. S., and Bilbey, D. L. J., 1956, Effect of cortisone on the defense mechanisms of the body, *Br. Med. J.* **2**:1.

Nicol, T., Bilbey, D. L. J., and Ware, C. C., 1958, Effect of various stilbene compounds on the phagocytic activity of the reticuloendothelial system, *Nature (London)* **181**:1538.

Nicol, T., Bilbey, D. L. J., and Druce, C. G., 1961, Effect of tri-*p*-anisylchloroethylene, dienoestrol and stilboestrol diphosphate, *Nature (London)* **190**:418.

Nicol, T., Bilbey, D. L. J., Charles, L. M., Cordingley, J. L., and Vernon-Roberts, B., 1964, Oestrogen: The natural stimulant of body defense, *J. Endocrinol.* **30**:277.

Nicol, T., Vernon-Roberts, B., and Quantock, D. C., 1965, The influence of various hormones on the reticuloendothelial system: Endocrine control of body defence, *J. Endocrinol.* **33**:365.

Nicol, T., Vernon-Roberts, B., and Quantock, D. C., 1966a, The effects of oestrogen: Androgen interaction on the reticuloendothelial system and reproductive tract, *J. Endocrinol.* **34**:163.

Nicol, T., Vernon-Roberts, B., and Quantock, D. C., 1966b, The effect of various anti-oestrogenic compounds on the reticuloendothelial system and reproductive tract in the ovariectomized mouse, *J. Endocrinol.* **34**:377.

Nicol, T., Quantock, D. C., and Vernon-Roberts, B., 1966c, Stimulation of phagocytosis in relation to the mechanism of action of adjuvants, *Nature (London)* **209**:1142.

Nothdurft, W., and Flemming, K., 1970, Die Wirkung von Polyvinylpyridin-N-oxid auf die Phagocytoseaktivität des reticuloendothelial Systems, *Naunyn-Schmiedebergs Arch. Pharmacol.* **267**:341.

Nothdurft, W., and Flemming, K., 1971, Quantitative study of sex difference in RE phagocytosis, in: *The Reticuloendothelial System and Immune Phenomena* (N. R. DiLuzio and K. Flemming, eds.), pp. 95–110, Plenum Press, New York.

Perry, H. M., Erlanger, M., Yunics, M., Schoepple, E., and Perry, E. F., 1970, Hypertension and tissue metal levels following intravenous cadmium, mercury and zinc, *Am. J. Physiol.* **219**:755.

Pesanti, E. L., and Nugent, K. M., 1981, Inhibition of macrophage phagocytosis after contact with ingestible particles, *J. Reticuloendothel. Soc.* **30**:157.

Pipy, B., Gaillard, D., and Derache, R., 1975, Influence de la qualité de diverses émulsions d'huiles végétales sur l'activité phagocytaire du système réticuloendothélial du rat, *Ann. Nutr. Aliment.* **29**:271.

Pisano, J. C., Patterson, J. T., and DiLuzio, N. R., 1972, Reticuloendothelial function in immune suppressed animals, *J. Reticuloendothel. Soc.* **12**:361.

Raake, W., and Tempel, K., 1977, Zur Wirkung von 6-Methyluracil auf die Phagozytoseaktivität von Mäusen nach Einwirkung von Ganzkörperröntgenbestrahlung oder 2,4,6-Triäthylenimino-s-triazin, *Strahlentherapie* **153**:843.

Rabinovitch, M., Hamburg, S. I., and Fleit, H. B., 1980, Interferon-induced enhancement of Fc receptor-mediated macrophage phagocytosis, *J. Reticuloendothel. Soc.* **28**(Suppl.):27.

Ransom, J. P., Pasternak, V. Z., and Heller, J. H., 1962, Effect of reticuloendothelial stimulating agent (restim) on resistance of mice, *J. Bacteriol.* **84**:466.

Raz, A., and Goldman, R., 1976, The in vitro effect of hydrocortisone on endocytosis in cultured mouse peritoneal macrophages, *J. Reticuloendothel. Soc.* **20**:177.

Regelson, W., and Munson, A. E., 1970, The reticuloendothelial effects of interferon inducers: Polyanionic and non-polyanionic prophylaxis against microorganisms, *Ann. N.Y. Acad. Sci.* **173**:831.

Reichard, S. M., Edelmann, A., and Gordon, A. S., 1956, Adrenal and hypophyseal influence upon the uptake of radioactive gold (Au^{198}) by the reticuloendothelial system, *Endocrinology* **59**:55.

Riggi, S. J., and DiLuzio, N. R., 1961a, Identification of a reticuloendothelial stimulating agent in zymosan, *Am. J. Physiol.* **200**:297.

Riggi, S. J., and DiLuzio, N. R., 1961b, Characterization of a reticuloendothelial stimulating agent in zymosan, *Fed. Proc.* **20**:265.

Ringle, D. A., Herndon, B. L., and Bullis, H. R., Jr., 1966, Effects of RES-stimulating lipids and zymosan on shock, *Am. J. Physiol.* **210**:1041.

Rooks, W. H., and Dorfman, R. I., 1961, Estrogen radioprotection in mice, *Endocrinology* **68**:838.

Rotta, J., Masek, K., Zeman, K., Vanecek, J., and Roskova, H., 1966, Palmitoylethanolamid and the RES, *Int. Symp. Atheroscler. RES, Como Summaries* p. 59.

Russo, V., and Travaglini, P. A., 1978, Possible active mechanisms of leucotrofina; thymic extract, Symposium on Cancer Modality Treatment and Cell Proliferation, Budapest.

Saba, T. M., and DiLuzio, N. R., 1969, Reticuloendothelial blockade recovery as a function of opsonic activity, *Amer. J. Physiol.* **216**:197.

Sannes, P. L., and Spicer, S. S., 1979, Inhibitory effects of cytochalasin B and the ionophores A23187 and X537A on binding and uptake of immune complexes by alveolar macrophages, *J. Reticuloendothel. Soc.* **26**:317.

Scheetz, M. E., Thomas, L. J., Harrington, J., and Schinitzky, M. R., 1976, Frentizole, a novel immunosuppressive, and azathioprine; their comparative in vivo and in vitro effect on murine peritoneal macrophages as measured in a novel assay for macrophage phagocytosis, *J. Reticuloendothel. Soc.* **20**(Suppl.):49a.

Schildt, B. E., and Löw, H., 1971, Relationship between trauma, plasma corticosterone and reticuloendothelial function in anaesthetized mice, *Endocrinologia (Bucharest)* **67**:141.

Schlipköter, H.-W., Dolgner, R., and Brockhaus, A., 1963, Ein Beitrag zur experimentellen Therapie der Silikose, *Dtsch. Med. Wochenschr.* **88**:1895.

Schmähl, D., 1957, Untersuchungen über die Beziehungen zwischen Konstituenten und Wirkung bei Östrogenen, *Arzneim. Forsch.* **7**:211.

Schorn, H., and Walter, C., 1975, Some hormonal effects on alveolar phagocytosis in the rat, *J. Reticuloendothel. Soc.* **18**(Suppl.):35a.

Sharbaugh, R. J., and Grogan, J. B., 1969, Suppression of reticuloendothelial function in the rat with cyclophosphamide, *J. Bacteriol.* **100**:117.

Sikl, D., Masler, L., and Bauer, S., 1969, Relationship between extracellular and cell wall polysaccharides of selected yeasts and yeast-like microorganisms, *Antonie van Leeuwenhoek J. Microbiol. Serol.* **35**(Suppl.):A9.

Snell, J. F., 1960a, The reticuloendothelial system. I. Chemical methods of stimulation of the reticuloendothelial system, *Ann. N.Y. Acad. Sci.* **88**:56.

Snell, J. F., 1960b, Relationship of chromium phosphate clearance rates to resistance. I. The effects of some corticosteroids on blood clearance rates in mice, in: *Reticuloendothelial Structure and Function* (J. H. Heller, ed.), Ronald Press, New York.

Snell, R. S., and Nicol, T., 1956, Effect of testosterone and androstene 3β-17d-diol on the activity of the reticuloendothelial system, *Nature (London)* **178**:1405.

Spratt, M. G., and Kratzing, C. C., 1971. The effect of dietary lipids and α-tocopherol on RES activity in choline deficiency, *J. Reticuloendothel. Soc.* **10**:319.

Stiffel, C., 1959, Etude de la fonction phagocytaire des cellule du système réticuloéndothelial au contact du sang, D.Sc. Thesis, University of Paris.

Stiteler, R. D., Proctor, J. W., Yamamura, Y., and Mansell, P. W. A., 1978, The effect of glucan on the clearance of intravenously injected tumor cells from the lung, *J. Reticuloendothel. Soc.* **24**:687.

Stuart, A. E., 1960, Chemical splenectomy, *Lancet* **2**:896.

Stuart, A. E., 1962, Effect of cholesterol oleate on the reticuloendothelial system, *Nature (London)* **196**:78.

Stuart, A. E., 1970, *The Reticuloendothelial System*, Livingstone, Edinburgh.

Stuart, A. E., and Cooper, G. N., 1962, Susceptibility of mice to bacterial endotoxin after modification of reticuloendothelial function by simple lipids, *J. Pathol. Bacteriol.* **83**:245.

Stuart, A. E., and Cooper, G. N., 1963, Stimulation of the reticuloendothelial phagocytosis function by glyceryl tricaprate and 2-oleodistearin, *Exp. Mol. Pathol.* **2**:215.

Stuart, A. E., and Davidson, A. E., 1963, The effect of intravenous cholesterol oleate on the function of the reticuloendothelial system, *Br. J. Pathol.* **64**:24.

Stuart, A. E., and Davidson, A. E., 1964, Effect of simple lipids on antibody formation after injection of foreign red cells, *J. Pathol. Bacteriol.* **87**:305.

Stuart, A. E., Biozzi, G., Stiffel, C., Halpern, B. N., and Mouton, D., 1960, The stimulation and depression of reticuloendothelial phagocytic function by simple lipids, *Br. J. Exp. Pathol.* **41**:599.

Symoens, J., and Rosenthal, M., 1977, Levamisole in the modulation of the immune response: The current experimental and clinical state. A review, *J. Reticuloendothel. Soc.* **21**:175.

Tanaka, A., Nagao, S., Nagao, R., Kotani, S., Shiba, S., and Kusumotot, S., 1979, Stimulation of the reticuloendothelial system of mice by muramyl dipeptide, *J. Reticuloendothel. Soc.* **24**:302.

Tennant, R. J., and Donald, K. J., 1976, The ultrastructure of platelets and macrophages in particle clearance stimulated by zymosan, *J. Reticuloendothel. Soc.* **19**:269.

Thomas, H. C., Slameron, J., and Tsitsikas, K., 1980, Immunostimulants in the therapy of chronic liver disease, in: *The Reticuloendothelial System and the Pathogenesis of Liver Disease* (H. Liehr and M. Grün, eds.), pp. 385–393, Elsevier/North-Holland, Amsterdam.

Thomas, R. G., and Chiffelle, T. L., 1974, Experimental alteration of rat lung clearance patterns by zymosan injection, *J. Reticuloendothel. Soc.* **15**:48.

Thompson, C. R., and Werner, H. W., 1953, Fat storage of an estrogen in women following orally administered Tace, *Proc. Soc. Exp. Biol. Med.* **84**:491.

Thorbecke, G. J., and Benacerraf, B., 1962, The reticuloendothelial system and immunological phenomena, *Prog. Allergy* **6**:559.

Timar, M., 1982, *Rolul splinei in hepatoprotectie* [The Role of the Spleen in Liver Protection], Centrala Industr. de Medicam., Cosmet. Color, si Lacuri, Bucharest.

Trejo, R. A., and DiLuzio, N. R., 1971, Impaired detoxification as a mechanism of lead acetate-induced hypersensitivity to endotoxin, *Proc. Soc. Exp. Biol. Med.* **136**:889.

Trejo, R. A., Loose, L. D., and DiLuzio, N. R., 1972a, Influence of diethylstilbestrol (DES) on reticuloendothelial function, tissue distribution and detoxication of *S. enteritidis* endotoxin, *J. Reticuloendothel. Soc.* **11**:88.

Trejo, R. A., DiLuzio, N. R., Loose, L. D., and Hoffmann, E., 1972b, Reticuloendothelial and hepatic functional alterations following lead acetate administration, *Exp. Mol. Pathol.* **17**:145.

Trnovec, T., Gajdosik, A., Bezek, S., Sikl, D., Koprda, V., Zemanek, M., and Faberova, V., 1977, The effect of fractions isolated from *Candida albicans* on phagocytic activity of the reticuloendothelial system in mice, *J. Reticuloendothel. Soc.* **22**:111.

Turner, E. V., and Higginbotham, R. D., 1979, Effect of intravenous carrageenan on immune responses and on the reticuloendothelial system, *J. Reticuloendothel. Soc.* **26**:763.

Vacher, J., and Stoner, H. B., 1968, The removal of injected beryllium from the blood of the rat: The role of the reticuloendothelial system, *Br. J. Exp. Pathol.* **49**:317.

Vacher, J., Deraedt, R., and Benzoni, J., 1973, Compared effects of two beryllium salts (soluble and insoluble): Toxicity and blockade of the reticuloendothelial system, *Toxicol. Appl. Pharmacol.* **24**:497.

van Ginckel, R. F., and de Brabander, M., 1979, The influence of a levamisole metabolite (DL-2-oxo-3-2-mercaptoethyl-5-phenyl-imidazolidine) on carbon clearance in mice, *J. Reticuloendothel. Soc.* **14**:317.

van Ginckel, R. F., and Hoebeke, J., 1974, Reversal of corticoid-depressed carbon clearance by levamisole in mice, Janssen Pharmaceutica, Biological Research Report on Levamisole, No. 4, April 1974.

van Ginckel, R. F., and Hoebeke, J., 1975, Carbon clearance enhancing factor in serum from levamisole treated mice, *J. Reticuloendothel. Soc.* **17**:65.

Verhaegen, H., DeCree, J., De Cock, W., and Verbruggen, F., 1973, Levamisole and the immune response, *N. Engl. J. Med.* **289**:1148.

Warr, G. W., and Sljivić, V. S., 1974, Studies on the organ uptake of ^{51}Cr-labelled sheep erythrocytes in the evaluation of stimulation of RES phagocytic function in the mouse, *J. Reticuloendothel. Soc.* **16**:193.

Waters, R. V., and Ferraresi, R. W., 1980, Muramyl dipeptide stimulation of particle clearance in several animal species, *J. Reticuloendothel. Soc.* **28**:457.

Watnick, A. S., and Gordon, A. S., 1964, Endotoxin influences on carbon clearance and resistance to bacterial infection, *J. Reticuloendothel. Soc.* **1**:170.

Westphal, O., 1975, Bacterial endotoxins, *Int. Arch. Allergy Appl. Immunol.* **49**:1.

Westphal, O., Nowotny, A., Lüderitz, O., Hurni, D., Eichenberger, E., and Schönholzer, G., 1958, Die Bedeutung der Lipoid-Komponente (Lipoid-A) für die biologischen Wirkungen bakterieller Endotoxine (Lipopolysaccharide), *Pharm. Acta Helv.* **33**:401.

Wierner, J., Cottrell, T. S., Mararetten, W., and Spiro, D., 1967, An electron microscopic study of steroid induced reticuloendothelial blockade, *Am. J. Pathol.* **50**:187.

Willers, J. M. N., Bloksma, N., van der Meer, C., Snippe, H., van Dijk, H, de Reuver, M. J., and Hofhuis, F. M. A., 1979, Regulation of the immune response by macrophages, *Antonie van Leeuwenhoek J. Microbiol. Serol.* **45**:41.

Wooles, W. R., and DiLuzio, N. R., 1964, The phagocytic and proliferative response of the reticuloendothelial system following glucan administration, *J. Reticuloendothel. Soc.* **1**:160.

Zeigler, Z., and Schugar, S., 1979, The effect of cytochalasin B and alkaloid compounds on human monocyte functions, *J. Reticuloendothel. Soc.* **25**:235.

Zschiesche, W., 1972, Alkylating anticancer agents and phagocytosis. II. Effects of alkylating agents on numerical distribution and histochemistry of reticuloendothelial cells, *J. Reticuloendothel. Soc.* **12**:16.

Zschiesche, W., and Augsten, K., 1968, Experimental studies on the effect of antibiotics and anticancer compounds on the phagocytic activity of the reticuloendothelial system (RES), *Chemotherapy (Basel)* **13**:257.

Zschiesche, W., Augsten, K., Ozegowski, W., and Krebs, D., 1970, Alkylating anticancer agents and phagocytosis. I. Effects of a homologous series of 1,2-substituted 5-bis (β-chloroethyl)-amino-benzimidazole derivatives on carbon clearance, *J. Reticuloendothel. Soc.* **8**:538.

11

Immunopotentiation by the Antitumor Polysaccharide Lentinan
Its Immunopharmacology and Physiology

JUNJI HAMURO and GORO CHIHARA

1. INTRODUCTION

Despite the enormous efforts of researchers around the world, promising cancer chemotherapeutics do not as yet exist, excluding some agents acting against certain cancer types with special characteristics and against certain leukemias. Chemotherapeutic agents possessing direct cytocidal activities on target cancer cells intend to kill the total mass of cancer, but they clearly also have accompanying detrimental toxic side effects on various lymphoid cells and bone marrow cells which have recently been considered to have relevant roles in host defense–surveillance mechanisms against cancer and they, therefore, limit the effectiveness of immunotherapy.

On the other hand, there is reliable clinical evidence of the presence of intrinsic resistance in the human body against cancer, and experimental evidence indicates that the host possesses the capability to attack even autologous cancer through cell-mediated immune reactions. To clarify the mechanisms of this resistance and to find a substance that will increase this resistance seems to be the most important means to opening a new way for immunotherapy in the treatment of cancer.

From this viewpoint we have investigated many folk remedies said to be

JUNJI HAMURO • Department of Basic Immunological Research, Central Research Laboratories, Ajinomoto Company, Yokohama, Japan.   GORO CHIHARA • National Cancer Center Research Institute, Tsukiji, Chuo-ku, Tokyo, Japan.

effective against cancer in Japan and Asian countries, and have found that lentinan, a polysaccharide extracted and isolated from *Lentinus edodes* (Berk.) Sing., a most popular edible mushroom in Japan, exerted a strong growth inhibitory action on sarcoma 180 transplanted in ICR or Swiss mice, resulting in almost complete regression of this tumor (Chihara *et al.*, 1969, 1970a).

Lentinan interestingly exerts its inhibitory action not only on allogeneic tumors, but also on syngeneic and autologous tumors; in addition, it prevents chemical and viral carcinogenesis. At the same time, lentinan is effective against bacterial, viral, and parasitic infections. In this review, we summarize chemical, biological, immunopharmacological, and physiological aspects of lentinan including its effects on tumors and infectious diseases.

2. CHEMICAL CHARACTERISTICS

In contrast to BCG, *Corynebacterium parvum*, and many other immunostimulants of polyanionic nature, lentinan is distinct in that it is a strictly chemically defined polysaccharide sufficiently purified after extraction and in that its physical and chemical characteristics have been completely clarified (Chihara *et al.*, 1970a). Therefore, biological activities of lentinan are reproducible and no differences are observed from lot to lot.

Lentinan is a $\beta(1 \rightarrow 3)$glucan with an average molecular weight of 500,000; its repeating unit is composed of five $\beta(1 \rightarrow 3)$glucopyranoside linkages with two $\beta(1 \rightarrow 6)$glucopyranoside-linked branches (Chihara *et al.*, 1970a; Sasaki and Takasuka, 1976). Thus, lentinan is composed solely of glucose with no other sugar components. Elementary analysis verified the molecular formula as $(C_6H_{10}O_5)n$ consistent with structural elucidation, and no nitrogen, phosphorus, or sulfur was detected. According to X-ray analysis, lentinan has a triple-helical structure (Bluhm and Sarko, 1977). The higher-order structure or micelle formation in solution of polysaccharides seems to have an important role in their biological activities. Pachyman and laminaran, possessing the same skeletal structure as lentinan, $\beta(1 \rightarrow 3)$glucans with $\beta(1 \rightarrow 6)$ branches, are devoid of antitumor activity; however, pachymaran, a $\beta(1 \rightarrow 3)$ linear glucan obtained by chemical scission of $\beta(1 \rightarrow 6)$ branchings in pachyman, has strong antitumor activity (Chihara *et al.*, 1970b). In addition, pachyman has been modified to U-pachyman, which has strong antitumor activity, by merely heating pachyman in 4 M aqueous urea at 45°C for 4 hr (Maeda *et al.*, 1973).

It is also interesting that a class of polysaccharides with antitumor activity such as lentinan only increase the content of α-helical structure in serum albumin or β structure in serum globulin, while antitumor-inactive polysaccharides are completely devoid of this effect (Hamuro and Chihara, 1973). The importance of the higher-order structure of polysaccharides for the appearance of this activity suggests the capacity, in biological systems of the host, to recognize conformational adaptability of polysaccharides. We also found that "linear $\beta(1 \rightarrow 3)$lentinan," obtained by chemical scission of $\beta(1 \rightarrow 6)$ branches (Smith degradation) (Hamuro *et al.*, 1971), and "small lentinan" (M_r 6000–10,000), obtained by degradation of parent lentinan in formic acid, are also effective in inhibiting tumor growth (Sasaki *et al.*, 1976).

3. ANTITUMOR EFFECTS

Lentinan exerts prominent antitumor effects on various allogeneic tumors in animal models and is devoid of direct cytocidal effects on these tumors when tested in cell culture systems (Maeda and Chihara, 1973). Specifically, lentinan does not possess any direct effects on tumor cells in terms of their growth rate and DNA synthesis (Akiyama and Hamuro, 1981). In this context, lentinan is surely a potentiator of host defense mechanisms since it shows growth inhibitory action on various syngeneic tumors *in vivo*. Lentinan also exerts no direct cytocidal action on normal cells, whereas most chemotherapeutic agents show such detrimental effects.

To date there have been almost no systematic experimental results reported on antitumor effects of the polysaccharides on syngeneic hosts, except the work using syngeneic A/PH,MC.S1 fibrosarcoma (Zákány *et al.*, 1980a). Thus, it is unclear whether these polysaccharides show similar antitumor activities in syngeneic systems as in allogeneic murine tumor system such sarcoma 180–SWM/Ms. As already mentioned, lentinan causes strong growth inhibition of sarcoma 180 at the optimal dose range, while higher dosages show considerably decreased activity (Maeda *et al.*, 1973). Thus, one of the characteristic features of the antitumor activity of lentinan is that of optimal dosage. The other relevant feature is that, depending on the responding character of the host to lentinan action, optimal doses, frequency and timing of administration showing optimal activity differ greatly.

In order to understand the antitumor action of lentinan on syngeneic tumors in more detail, we investigated the effects of lentinan using administration protocols in animals similar to those undertaken in clinical applications, namely lentinan was injected intravenously several days or weeks after tumor transplantation. As shown in Fig. 1, lentinan exerted growth inhibitory activity when administered 10–14 days after sarcoma 180 transplantation to the same extent as was observed when lentinan was injected just 1 day after sarcoma 180 transplantation. This fact suggests that injection of lentinan at the time when transplanted tumors are recognized by the host after established growth also has considerable effects.

The growth inhibitory effects of lentinan on syngeneic P815, L5178Y, MM46, and MM102 tumors are illustrated in Fig. 2 and Table 1, respectively. As can be seen from the results shown in Table 1, the time of injection of lentinan seems to be critical for significant antitumor activity in the MM102–C3H/He system. The results suggest that lentinan, as an immunological adjuvant, demonstrates its action depending on the state of the host–tumor immunological relationship. In contrast, the activity of lentinan on the P815–DBA/2 system is remarkable regardless of the timing of administration. Interestingly, the later the injection of lentinan at the same dose and frequency, the stronger is the growth

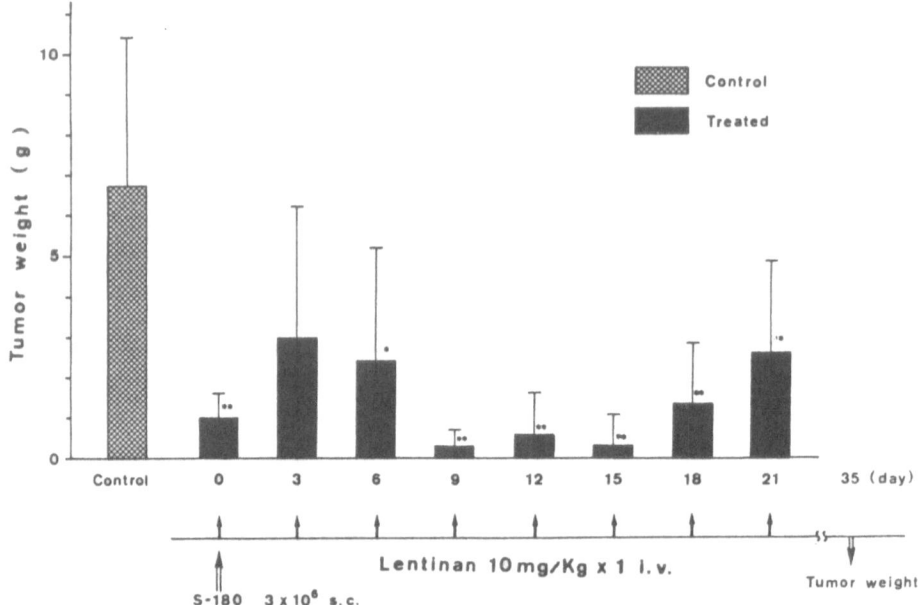

FIGURE 1.   Effect of lentinan on the growth of sarcoma 180.

inhibition. Optimal timing of administration appears to be 2 or 3 weeks after P815 transplantation. Results showing the same tendency were also obtained in the L5178Y–DBA/2 and MM46–C3H/He syngeneic systems. The reason why administration of lentinan at this period causes strong growth inhibition is at present unclear.

It can be safely said that lentinan shows antitumor effects also on syngeneic murine tumors even when administered without any other chemotherapeutic agents such as cyclophosphamide or 5-fluorouracil. Depending on the host–tumor relationship, however, the antitumor effects of lentinan can be far less, as exemplified in the EL4–C57BL/6 system. The results demonstrate that combined administration of lentinan and indomethacin causes synergistic growth inhibition of EL4 even when injection of lentinan alone did not cause any effect. The augmented growth inhibition observed may be attributed to the diminished suppression of immune responses mediated by prostaglandins, which may be released by tumor cells or by suppressor macrophages.

Lentinan also showed growth inhibitory action against other tumors such as Lewis lung cancer, B16 melanoma (Shiio and Yugari, 1980), SR–C3H/He sarcoma, and colon 26 in syngeneic murine systems as well as A/Ph,MC.S1 fibrosarcoma produced by methylcholanthrene in A/Ph(A/J) mice (Zákány et al., 1980a).

These results have prompted us to claim that lentinan is a "true antitumor substance" capable of potentiating host defense mechanisms against syngeneic tumors and is not merely a substance promoting the rejection of a foreign graft.

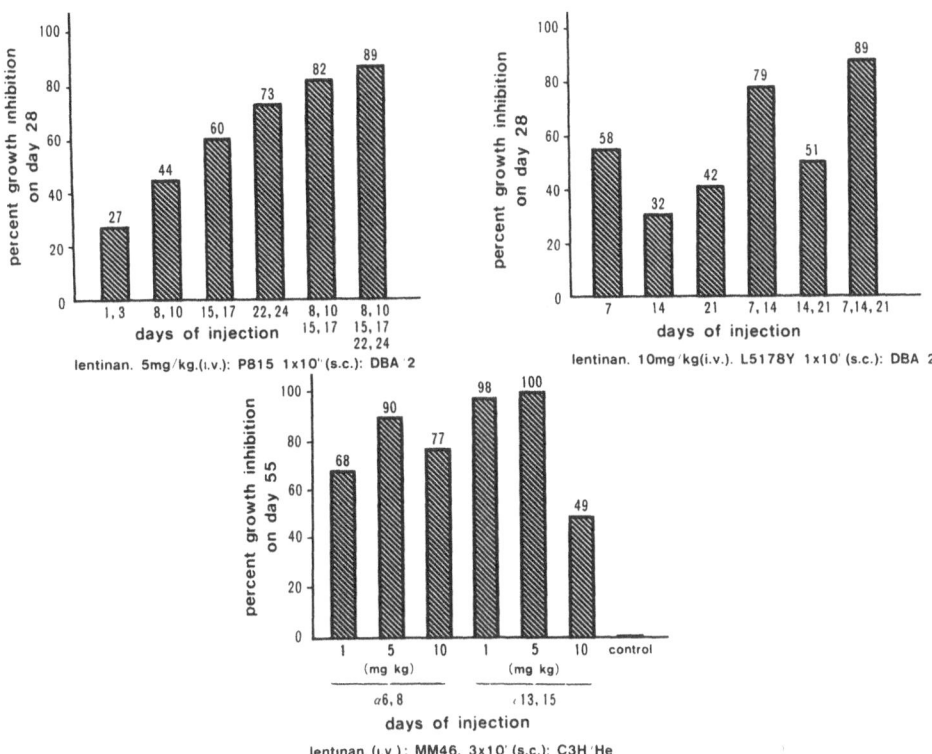

FIGURE 2.   Effect of lentinan on the growth of P815, L5178Y, and MM46 tumors in syngeneic hosts.

TABLE 1. Growth Inhibitory and Survival Effect of Lentinan on Mammary Carcinoma MM102 in C3HH/HeN Mice

Treatment[a]	Day of lentinan injection[b]	Tumor size (mm²)[c]	Survival[d]
Lentinan	Day 0	458 ± 215	1/7
	Day 7	529 ± 180	4/6
	Day 14	198 ± 125	7/7
	Day 21	637 ± 256	2/6
	Day 28	477 ± 241	5/7
Control		425 ± 253	3/6

[a]Lentinan (10 mg/kg) was injected i.v.
[b]The day of lentinan injection after the transplantation of 3×10^6 MM102 mammary carcinoma cells s.c. into C3H/HeN mice.
[c]Means ± S.D. on day 35.
[d]Proportion alive on day 70.

TABLE 2. THE ANTITUMOR EFFECTS OF LENTINAN IN ALLOGENEIC, SYNGENEIC, AND AUTOCHTHONOUS HOSTS AND THE PREVENTION OF CARCINOGENESIS

Tumors[a]	Hosts	Dose of lentinan (mg/kg)	Days of lentinan injection[b]	Tumor inhibition ratio (%)	References
Allogeneic					
Sarcoma 180	ICR	1 × 10	1 to 11	100	Chihara et al. (1970)
CCM adenocarcinoma	SWM/Ms	1 × 10	1 to 11	65.3	Maeda et al. (1973)
MM102 carcinoma	C3H/Arima	1 × 10	1 to 11	40.3	Maeda et al. (1973)
NTF reticulum cell sarcoma	SWM/Ms	1 × 10	1 to 11	27.3	Maeda et al. (1973)
Syngeneic					
A/Ph,MC.S1 sarcoma	A/Ph(A/J)	1 × 10	1 to 11	100	Zákány et al. (1980)
Lewis lung cancer	C57BL/6	1 × 6	1 to 7	59.3	Shiio and Yugari (1980)
EL4 lymphoma	C57BL/6	10 × 1	1	72.	This chapter
B16 melanoma	BDF$_1$	1 × 5	1 to 6	50.7	Shiio and Yugari (1980)
MM46 carcinoma	C3H/HeN	5 × 2	13, 15	100	This chapter
MM102 carcinoma	C3H/HeN	10 × 1	7	60	This chapter
SR-C3H/He sarcoma	C3H/He	1 × 10	1 to 11	47.5	Maeda et al. (1973)
P815 mastocytoma	DBA/2	5 × 4	8, 10, 15, 17	82	This chapter
L5178Y lymphoma	DBA/2	10 × 3	7, 14, 21	89	This chapter
Autochthonous					
MC-induced primary tumor	C3H/HeN	1 × 20	21 to 41[c]	Over 200% survival	Shiio and Yugari (1980)
Prevention of carcinogenesis	C3H/HeN	1 × 10	21 to 31	83 → 33%[d]	Shiio and Yugari (1980)

[a]All tumors were solid forms implanted s.c.
[b]Tumors were implanted on day 0.
[c]8-mm tumor diameter was day 0, when 100 mg/kg cyclophosphamide was injected.
[d]Determination at 30 weeks after methylcholanthrene treatment.

Thus, immunogenetic analysis of the hosts will become an important issue in the future as well as analysis of the common basis of host response to transplantation antigens and tumor antigens.

It was also demonstrated that lentinan when administered together with cyclophosphamide could prolong more than twofold the survival of C3H/HeN mice bearing primary autologous tumors induced by methylcholanthrene.

In this context, it might be worthwhile to mention that lentinan prevents methylcholanthrene-induced carcinogenesis when it is administered before or within 3 weeks after methylcholanthrene inoculation (83% → 30%). Antitumor effects and preventive effects of carcinogenesis by lentinan are summarized in Table 2.

4. ANTIBACTERIAL, ANTIVIRAL, AND ANTIPARASITIC EFFECTS

Lentinan not only exerts inhibitory effects on syngeneic and autologous tumors, but also has been demonstrated to possess strong inhibitory action against various bacteria, viruses, and parasites as summarized in Table 3.

When lentinan was administered to normal mice by i.p. injection, conspicuously enlarged lung granulomas were formed in response to either *Schistosoma mansoni* or *S. japonicum* eggs or to antigen-coated polyacrylamide beads (Byrum *et al.*, 1979). Liver granulomas in cercariae of *S. mansoni* infection were augmented up to eightfold in volume. In contrast, athymic nude mice showed a complete absence of hypersensitivity granulomas. Lentinan-potentiated granulomas show a distinct histopathological picture characterized by frequent, extensive central necrosis, uncommon in unpotentiated schistosome foci.

Recent studies have indicated that lentinan reduced the frequency of postchemotherapy relapse in experimental tuberculosis. (Kanai *et al.*, 1980). After termination of 5 months of intensive chemotherapy (streptomycin, isoniazid, rifampicin), one group of the mice received lentinan for 4 weeks and again for 4 weeks after a 1-month interval. The results indicate that the later multiplication of the latent bacilli was strongly reduced by lentinan treatment during the postchemotherapy period.

TABLE 3. INCREASE OF HOST RESISTANCE TO INFECTIONS BY
LENTINAN

Bacteria	
Mycobacterium tuberculosis	Kanai *et al.* (1980)
Mycobacterium leprae	Delville and Jacques (1980)
Listeria monocytogenes	Kawamura and Numazaki (1980)
Viruses	
VSV encephalitis virus	Chang (1981)
Abelson virus	Chang (1981)
Adenovirus type 12	Hamada (1981)
Parasites	
Schistosoma mansoni	Byrum *et al.* (1979)
Schistosoma japonicum	Byrum *et al.* (1979)

These results clearly suggest the effectiveness of lentinan against chronic infectious diseases and various infections frequently observed among patients with neoplastic diseases.

Prophylactic effects of lentinan to prolong survival in VSV encephalitis and Abelson virus infection have been reported (Chang, 1981). Preventive effects on viral tumorigenesis by adenovirus type 12 were also reported (Hamada, 1981).

5. IMMUNOLOGICAL CHARACTERISTICS

Several immunopotentiators such as the BCG strain of *Mycobacterium bovis* and *C. parvum* have been studied for their potency as antitumor immunotherapeutic agents. Among the well-known immunopotentiators, lentinan appears to represent a unique class of immunological adjuvants. Lentinan has little toxic side effects on *in vivo* application.

One of the distinct characteristics of its immunological reactivity is its capacity to act as a T-cell immunoadjuvant. In particular, lentinan appears to augment T-helper cell function to produce humoral antibody responses in normal and tumor-bearing murine systems. Here we describe the major immunological characteristics of lentinan relevant to its biological activities as an antitumor immunotherapeutic agent and the mechanism of that action.

5.1. ACTION ON T CELLS

Since the antitumor activity of lentinan against sarcoma 180 was markedly decreased by the administration of antilymphocyte serum (Maeda *et al.*, 1971), it seems likely that recirculating T lymphocytes have some role in the antitumor activity. Furthermore, the antitumor activity of lentinan against sarcoma 180 was not observed in neonatally thymectomized mice (Maeda and Chihara, 1971, 1973) and growth inhibition against syngeneic KKN-1 tumor was observed in *nu/+*BALB/c but not in *nu/nu* BALB/c mice (Yamada *et al.*, 1981). These experimental results clearly support the concept that the antitumor activity of lentinan requires an intact immunocompetent T-cell compartment and the activity is mediated through a thymus-dependent immune mechanism.

In vivo application of lentinan causes increases in the levels of certain types of serum proteins both acutely and subacutely (Maeda *et al.*, 1974). One of the increased serum proteins was functionally designated colony-stimulating factor (CSF) (Hamuro *et al.*, 1982). Upon *in vitro* incubation of nylon column-purified splenic T cells with lentinan, CSF is released into the supernatant in amounts five times greater than control. This CSF produced may then act on immunoregulatory Ia$^+$ macrophages resulting in augmented production of interleukin-1 (IL-1) [lymphocyte-activating factor (LAF)] by a positive feedback mechanism. On the other hand, lentinan directly induces peritoneal macrophages to produce increased amounts of IL-1. The augmented production of

IL-1 was also observed when peritoneal macrophages were incubated *in vitro* with lentinan, as assessed by the increased production of a factor mitogenic for thymocytes.

Recent studies clearly indicate that lentinan augments generation of anti-gen-specific cytotoxic T lymphocytes (CTL) against alloantigen and haptenated syngeneic cells *in vivo* and *in vitro* (Hamuro *et al.*, 1978a,b). Namely, lentinan is an effective immunoadjuvant for both alloreactive CTL responses and H-2-re-stricted CTL response specific to foreign antigens. In analyzing the mechanism of this adjuvant effect, it was noted that on *in vitro* incubation of splenic ad-herent cells or peritoneal exudate cells with a critical concentration of lentinan, a soluble product is generated, which in turn is able to augment the differentiation of antigenically triggered, clonally distinct CTL precursors into highly reactive CTL (Hamuro *et al.*, 1980). The complete failure to generate anti-H-2^d allokiller cells was confirmed in the absence of adherent splenic accessory cells, even in the presence of lentinan, and the successful transfer of the augmenting effect on anti-H-2^d allokiller cell generation by soluble factors from the 24-hr culture su-pernatant of spleen cells or splenic adherent cells in the presence of lentinan was observed.

As is well known, IL-1 is capable of differentiating premature T cells into immunocompetent mature T cells (IL-2-producing and -responding T cells). From these results, it is suggested that lentinan augments the production of IL-1 by Ia$^+$ immunoregulatory macrophages directly and/or indirectly via CSF pro-duction from T cells.

Recently, we have found that lentinan also exerts an augmentation of IL-1 production by macrophages even in syngeneic tumor-bearing murine systems.

It has also been found that lentinan is able to generate augmented CTL against LSTRA tumor cells in mixed syngeneic tumor–lymphocyte culture, and the effect was found by the method of limiting dilution to be due to an increase of CTL precursor cells (Levy *et al.*, 1981). All the findings presented here are consistent with the speculation that lentinan promotes differentiation of pre-mature (PNA$^+$) thymocytes into immunocompetent mature T cells (PNA$^-$) that circulate in the periphery. This interpretation may explain the requirement for an intact thymus for the appearance of the antitutmor activity of lentinan.

To evaluate the validity of the hypothesized reaction scheme presented, the generation of allokiller cells from thymocytes was tested. As shown in Fig. 3, thymocytes harvested from responder BALB/c mice treated with lentinan, in-duce augmented generation of allokiller cells in the presence of IL-2. This result indicates that thymocytes of lentinan-treated mice are more reactive to IL-2. In a syngeneic tumor-bearing system such as P815–DBA/2, allokiller cell generation from thymocytes is considerably suppressed even in the presence of IL-2. The generation, however, was restored to the level of non-tumor-bearing mice by the injection of lentinan. The generation of allokiller cells from splenocytes was also restored from 0 to around 40% in the absence of IL-2. These results may be explained by the augmented induction of mature T cells reactive to IL-2 as a second signal. Furthermore, spleen cells harvested from syngeneic tumor-bear-ing mice (P815/DBA/2) that received a triple i.p. injection of lentinan 2 weeks

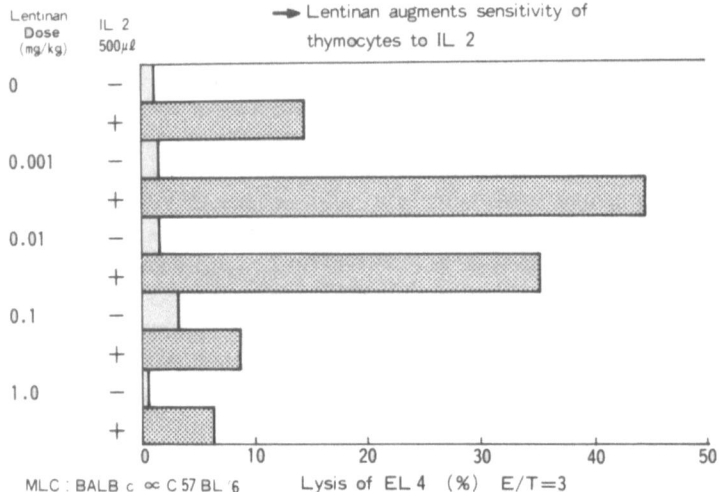

FIGURE 3. Augmented allokiller T induction by lentinan from thymocytes in the presence of interleukin-2 (IL-2).

after P815 transplantation were able to generate significant levels of antisyngeneic P815 tumor killer cells in the presence of IL-2.

Concerning an important nonspecific effector, NK cells, it was found that lentinan could augment NK activity in spleen cells and peritoneal exudate cells when administered i.p. or i.v. into NK high-responder C3H/He mice, but could not when administered into BALB/c mice. Lentinan did not activate NK cells when incubated *in vitro*, but a more marked augmentation of NK cell generation was observed when spleen cells obtained from lentinan-treated mice were cultured with the interferon inducer poly(I:C) or mixed lymphocyte culture supernatants. Recent unpublished data show that IL-2 produced in mixed lymphocyte culture supernatants can activate NK cells as well as IL-2 generated in supernatants of rat spleen cell cultures stimulated by Con A. At present, it is not clear whether the augmented NK activation observed by lentinan injection is due to the augmented reactivity of NK cells to interferon or to IL-2. Because we know that lentinan does not induce interferon different from other polyanionic immunoadjuvants and that lentinan does not activate NK cells *in vitro*, it seems possible that *in vivo* application of lentinan results in the augmented induction of IL-2-producing mature T cells and/or in the augmentation of NK cell reactivity to IL-2. Thus, lentinan may stimulate nonspecific antitumor effector NK cells via a T-cell-dependent pathway. In relation to the above hypothesis, the fact that serum obtained from lentinan-treated mice possesses IL-2 activity might draw our attention in the future to a detailed analysis of NK cell activation by lentinan.

The doses required to activate NK cells were found to be relatively higher than the doses required for antitumor activity and for other immunological activities of lentinan. Thus, it is at present difficult to ascertain the role of NK cells in the antitumor activity of lentinan.

Lentinan not only augments antigen-specific cellular immune responses, but can also trigger antigen-nonspecific immune responses against neoplastic cells. It was observed that lentinan and related substances with antitumor activity can induce cytotoxic peritoneal macrophages after i.p. injection. In contrast, inactive polysaccharides showed only a slight activity to induce (Hamuro *et al.*, 1980). In spite of many experiments, all attempts to render normal or thioglycollate-induced peritoneal exudate cells cytotoxic by the *in vitro* addition of lentinan have failed. Thus, lentinan is capable of rendering peritoneal exudate cells cytotoxic only under *in vivo* conditions in contrast to most other immunoadjuvants, which can render peritoneal exudate cells cytotoxic upon *in vitro* incubation. Lentinan did not cause elevated release of lysosomal enzymes from cultured macrophages, whereas most immunopotentiators do. The functions of lentinan-induced macrophages are distinct in many aspects from macrophages induced by other means.

Interestingly, lentinan augmented the reactivity of macrophages to macrophage-activating factor(s) (MAF), generated from activated T cells, resulting in the augmented generation of cytostatic and cytotoxic macrophages against tumor cells. Cell-free supernatants containing MAF were harvested from cultures of normal ICR mouse spleen cells incubated *in vitro* for 72 hr with Con A (5 μg/ml). As shown in Fig. 4, macrophages elicited by lentinan administered i.v. showed an augmented response to MAF.

To determine whether this augmentation of responsiveness would occur after direct action of lentinan on macrophages, peritoneal adherent cells were cocultured with lentinan *in vitro* for 24 hr and thus-treated macrophages were cultured in the presence of a suboptimal dose of MAF for another 24 hr. As shown in Fig. 5, lentinan augmented the responsiveness of macrophages to

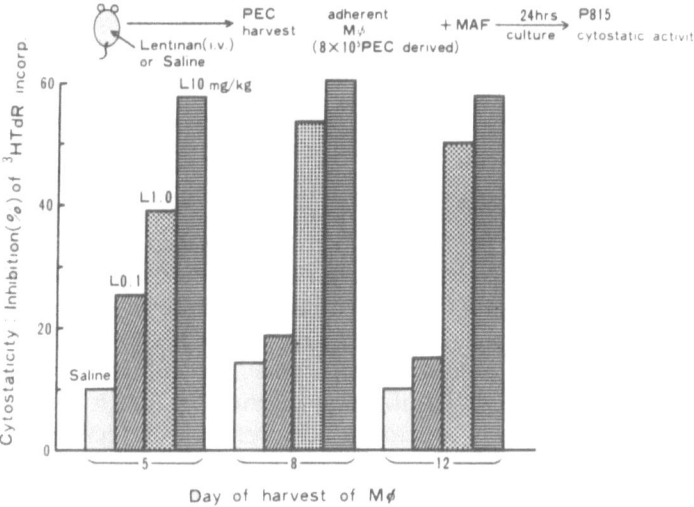

FIGURE 4. Augmentation by lentinan of macrophage-activating factor (MAF)-induced cytostatic macrophage generation.

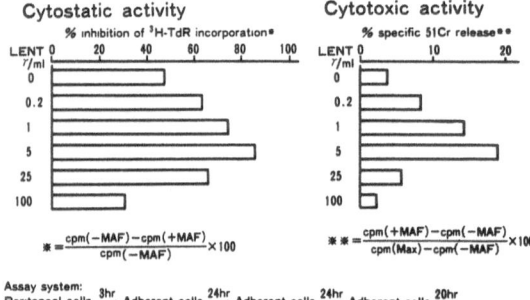

FIGURE 5. Augmented response of macrophages to MAF in the presence of lentinan *in vitro.*

MAF *in vitro,* although lentinan alone was not capable of rendering resident macrophages cytotoxic under this condition.

In this context, macrophages stimulated by lentinan *in vitro* are neither cytototxic nor cytostatic, but they possess elevated reactivity to MAF, one of the T-cell-derived lymphokines relevant in the induction of effector macrophages. Recently, we have also found that in mice bearing syngeneic tumors, lentinan augmented the responsiveness of peritoneal macrophages to MAF. The response of macrophages to MAF in mice bearing the syngeneic tumor L5178Y was significantly suppressed as compared with that in normal mice on day 25, but lentinan treatment of these L5178Y-bearing mice restored the response above control level (Table 4).

As already mentioned, lentinan is not capable of rendering resident or stimulated macrophages cytotoxic under *in vitro* conditions, so we suggest that the capacity of lentinan to induce *in vivo* cytotoxic macrophages is related to the ability of lentinan to activate the alternative pathway of complement to produce C3b, which may then be the essential component required to render macrophages cytotoxic, or to the ability of lentinan to augment the reactivity of macrophages to activated T-cell-derived MAF.

Masuko *et al.* (1979) and Zákány *et al.* (1980b, 1983) found that in MM46 and A/Ph,MC.S1 syngeneic tumor-bearing mice, lentinan augmented the antitumor delayed hypersensitivity reaction (DHR) measured by the footpad test or picryl chloride method and concluded that antibody-dependent macrophage-mediated cellular cytotoxicity (ADMC) was the effector mechanism in this case.

In order to elucidate the mechanism of action of lentinan to augment antitumor DHR, we examined whether antitumor DHR was adoptively transferred into normal syngeneic C3H/He mice by i.d. injection of tumor antigen with sensitized lymphoid cells from donor mice. As shown in Fig. 6, lentinan-treated recipient mice alone showed a significantly positive DHR. Also, the results are consistent with the previously described interpretation that lentinan stimulates effector macrophages to show augmented reactivity to activated T-cell-derived lymphokines (MAF).

Lentinan not only augments antitumor effector cell generation via T-cell-dependent pathways as described, but also is well known as an immunoadju-

TABLE 4. AUGMENTATION BY LENTINAN OF MAF-INDUCED CYTOSTATIC MACROPHAGE GENERATION IN L5178Y-TUMOR BEARING MICE

	Cytostatic activity Inhibition of [^{3}H]-TdR incorp. (%)[a]
Normal	30.1
Tumor (day 20)	34.3
Tumor + lentinan	72.4
Tumor (day 25)	8.1
Tumor + lentinan	74.6

DBA/2 mice:
L5178Y (1 × 10^6 cells s.c.) Lentinan (5 mg/kg) Peritoneal cells

0   7   14   20 21   25

Lentinan (5 mg/kg i.v.)

Peritoneal cells

Peritoneal cells ——— 3 hr ———→ Adherent cells ± MAF ——— 24 hr ———→ Cytostatic activity (target cell: P815)

[a] $\% = \dfrac{\text{cpm}(-\text{MAF}) - \text{cpm}(+\text{MAF})}{\text{cpm}(-\text{MAF})} \times 100.$

vant in humoral and cellular immune responses. As shown in Fig. 7, lentinan augments plaque-forming cell (PFC) induction against SRBC. Antigen SRBC was injected on day 0 and lentinan was injected i.p. three times on days 0, 1, and 2 in a wide dose range from 0.02 to 100 mg/kg. Depending on the number of inoculated SRBC, the augmenting and inhibiting effect of lentinan on PFC induction varied. In general, the smaller the dose of SRBC, the larger the dose of lentinan showing optimal augmentation.

Yoshikai *et al.* (1979) reported that macrophage activators such as *C. parvum* usually depressed anti-SRBC PFC induction and DHR. In this context, the impact of lentinan on macrophages may be distinct from that of *C. parvum* and other macrophage activators, which usually enhance the phagocytic activity of macrophages. It should be kept in mind that lentinan does not enhance phagocytic activity of macrophages as measured by carbon clearance. Augmentation of antibody production against SRBC was also observed in an *in vitro* culture system in the presence of 0.1 to 1 µg/ml lentinan and the augmenting effect may also be explained by the augmented production of IL-1, which in turn acts on helper T cells and/or B cells to augment antibody responses against T-cell-dependent antigens.

As described, lentinan strongly augments the *in vivo* generation of alloreactive CTL. The augmenting effect of i.p. administered lentinan on CTL exhibited

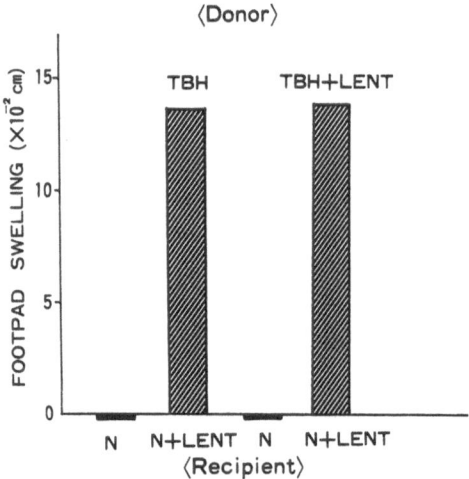

Female C 3H /He mice (Each group consisted of 5 animals)

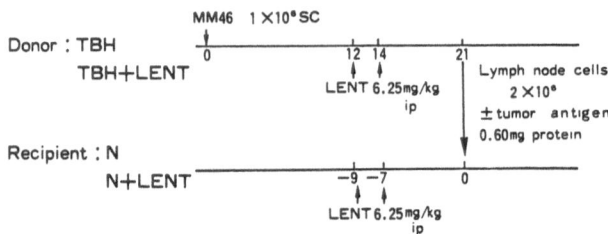

FIGURE 6.   Effect of lentinan on adoptive transfer of delayed hypersensitivity response.

a clear dose–response relationship and was strictly dependent on the injection schedule used. Injection of a high dose of lentinan (e.g., 100 mg/kg) as well as injection during the late phase of the immune response (7 or 8 days after antigen) markedly suppressed the lytic CTL activity. When the optimal conditions for augmented CTL responses are chosen, the augmented CTL activity within spleen cells and mesenteric lymph node cells persists for more than 25 days.

Lentinan increased the magnitude of the *in vitro* CTL response up to 28-fold when added into CTL culture at a concentration of 25 μg/ml. Lentinan appeared to enhance the responsiveness of alloreactive prekiller T cells rather than the immunogenicity of the stimulator cells and to influence the differentiation of antigenically triggered CTL precursors into cytotoxic effector cells.

Lentinan also augmented DHR to SRBC measured by foodpad swelling 1 day after SRBC rechallenge. Lentinan was injected i.v. according to protocols corresponding to those of standard antitumor assay on syngeneic tumors. In all strains of mice tested, 5 mg/kg lentinan significantly augmented DHR to SRBC consistent with the above-mentioned effect on PFC response to SRBC (Fig. 8).

There are several preliminary papers describing the specific impact of lentinan on T-cell compartments. One describes the augentation of antibody-de-

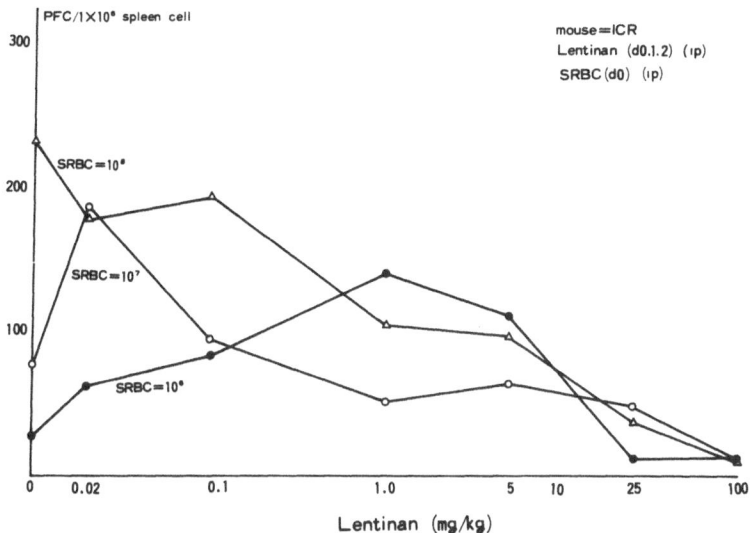

FIGURE 7.   Effect of lentinan on plaque-forming cell production to SRBC in mice.

pendent cellular cytotoxicity (ADCC) in spleen cells as assessed by cytotoxicity against CRBC as target cells (Dennert and Tucker, 1973). However, the augmenting effect was observed only at a critical dose of CRBC as an immunogen (10^7 cells). In the course of the analysis of the augmenting effects on antibody generation by lentinan in hapten–carrier conjugate systems, Dennert and Tucker (1973) reported that lentinan seemed to be a stimulator of helper T cells in normal murine systems. The same conclusion that lentinan stimulates helper T

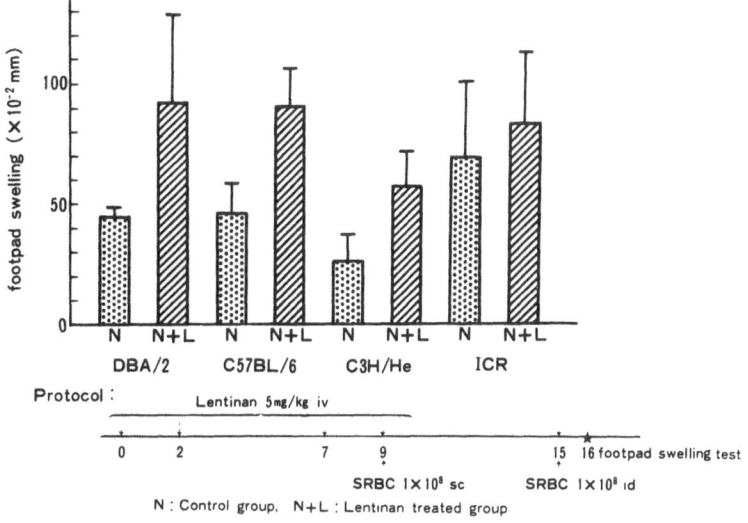

FIGURE 8.   Effect of lentinan on the delayed footpad reaction to SRBC in mice.

cells was made by Dresser and Phillips (1974) who analyzed the details of lentinan's effect on various classes of antibody against SRBC.

5.2. ACTION ON MACROPHAGES

Lentinan acts on macrophages to produce increased amounts of IL-1 and to augment the reactivity to MAF. The former macrophages are thought to be Ia$^+$ immune response regulators and the latter Ia$^-$ effectors. The different effects of lentinan on IL-1-producing macrophages and effector macrophages need clarification to determine more exactly the roles of different macrophage populations in various immune surveillance mechanisms against cancer.

Lentinan exerts various other complicated effects on macrophage functions. Host defense mechanisms of macrophages against cancer include phagocytosis, antigen presentation, various secretory functions, and cytotoxicity.

Lentinan-induced peritoneal macrophages showed no elevation of phagocytic activity compared to resident macrophages as assessed by carbon clearance tests. Macrophages harvested 7 days after injection of 0.1 mg/kg lentinan i.v. showed only a slight increase of phagocytic index expressed by K value. In contrast, the injection of zymosan or LPS markedly increased phagocytosis by macrophages within 2 days after injection.

Thus, lentinan seems to be distinct from zymosan, LPS, and most other immunoadjuvants, which act as RES stimulants. Intravenous injection of lentinan at a dose of 10 mg/kg, at which lentinan exerted strong growth inhibitory action against syngeneic murine tumors, did not increase carbon clearance of macrophages harvested from 2 to 7 days after injection in inbred mice such as C3H/HeN, BALB/c, DBA/2, and C57BL/6. These results indicate the absence of direct participation of phagocytic function of macrophages in the appearance of the antitumor activity of lentinan.

It is well known that LPS, zymosan, poly(I:C), pyran copolymer, C. parvum, BCG, and most known immunoadjuvants cause elevated release of lysosomal enzymes from macrophages when cocultured in vitro. However, again lentinan is completely devoid of this effect on cultured macrophages.

When peritoneal macrophages were harvested from mice that had received i.p. lentinan 4 days before, the spontaneous release of prostaglandin E and F (PGE, PGF) was strikingly reduced in resident macrophages (Hamuro et al., 1979). The diminished spontaneous release of both PGE and PGF was still apparent when macrophages were examined from mice that had received lentinan 8 days before. This effect is in contrast to that of C. parvum and BCG, which have been shown to induce a high spontaneous release of prostaglandins from spleen cells and peritoneal macrophages. This finding indicates a possible inverse correlation between the depression of prostaglandin release by lentinan-induced macrophages and augmentation by lentinan of T-cell functions. Thus, it is possible that a decrease in inhibitory activities of prostaglandins may facilitate the cytotoxic action of T cells and/or macrophages in cell-mediated immune responses.

5.3. SERUM PROTEIN COMPONENTS

A number of serum proteins are increased transiently after lentinan application. We have found that three major serum proteins in the α- and β-globulin regions are markedly increased in serum of ICR, DBA/2, or SWM/Ms mice 4 to 7 days after lentinan injection and these three major components were tentatively named LA, LB, and LC (Fig. 9) (Maeda *et al.*, 1974).

There is a clear parallelism between the antitumor activity of polysaccharides and the unique increase in these three serum protein components, except

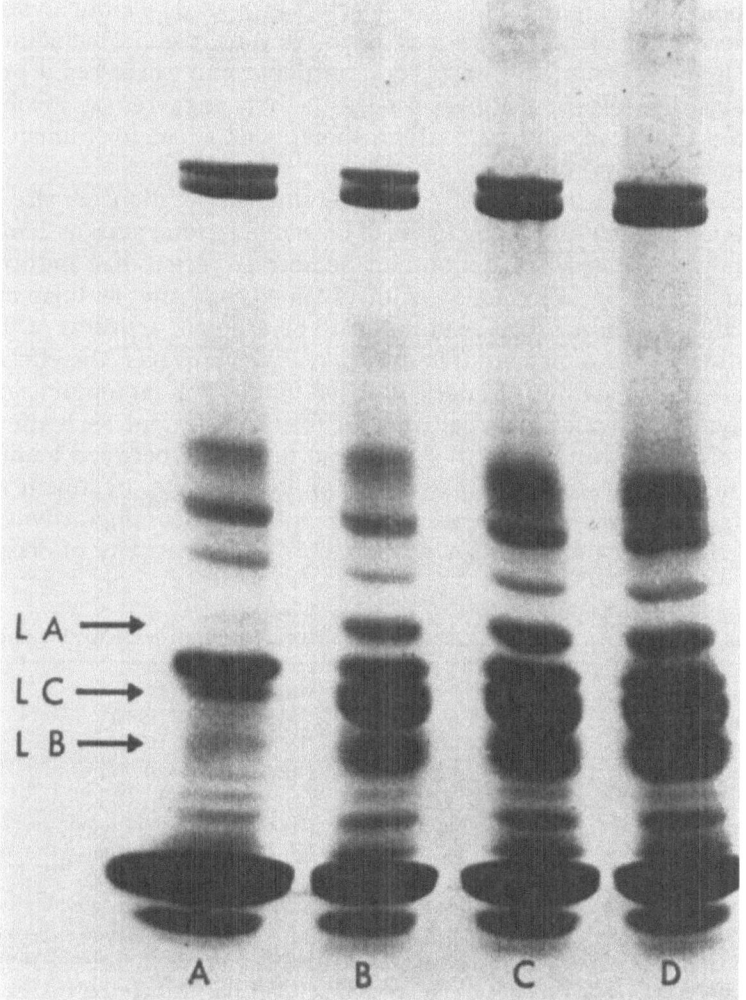

FIGURE 9.   The acrylamide gel pattern of serum from lentinan-treated ICR mice. A, control; B, 4 days; C, 7 days; D, 10 days after the last lentinan injection.

those in A/J mice. These increases in LA, LB, and LC were also detected after administration of zymosan, picibanil (a preparation of *Streptococcus hemolyticus*), C. *parvum*, and other immunostimulants, although the increase exhibited different kinetics from that of lentinan.

Recently, LA, LB, and LC have been identified by the micro two-dimensional polyacrylamide gel electrophoretic technique as haptoglobin–hemoglobin complex, hemopexin, and haptoglobin plus ceruloplasmin, respectively (Manabe *et al.*, 1983). These proteins are acute-phase proteins. In addition, marked increased in the amount of acute-phase proteins such as serum amyloid P and complement component C3 are also observed (A. J. S. Davies, personal communication).

It should be kept in mind that these factors increased by lentinan are probably synthesized in the liver and may have relevant roles in maintaining biochemical homeostasis of the host; e.g., ceruloplasmin possesses a protective effect against the lowering of liver catalase activity triggered by toxohormone (Itoh *et al.*, 1980) and may be a useful therapeutic agent for human aplastic anemia, cachexia, and others.

Various serum factors, increased after lentinan application, are also listed in Table 5. We have detected many kinds of bioactive factors, such as acute-phase protein inducer, vascular dilatation and hemorrage factor, IL-1 inducer, CSF, and antitutmor factor, from mouse serum obtained early after lentinan injection.

In addition, lentinan has been found to be a potent activator of the alternative pathway of complement (Okuda *et al.*, 1972); however, the effect to activate the alternative pathway is not correlated with action on tumors since inactive pachyman activates this pathway to the same extent as lentinan. The turnover of C3, C5, and factor B showed no difference between lentinan and pachyman. The polysaccharide particles (PX), isolated after treatment with C4-deficient guinea pig serum, showed prominent C3-consuming activity, which disappeared during prolonged incubation at 37°C. The activity of decayed en-

TABLE 5. VARIOUS SERUM FACTORS INCREASED AFTER LENTINAN APPLICATION

Acute-phase proteins (LA, LB, LC)	Increase	Maeda *et al.* (1974)
Haptoglobin	Increase	Manabe *et al.* (1983)
Hemopexin	Increase	Manabe *et al.* (1983)
Ceruloplasmin	Increase	Itoh *et al.* 81980)
Antitrypsin	No effect	Chihara (1980)
Transferrin	No effect	Manabe (personal communication)
Serum amyloid P	Increase	A. J. S. Davies (personal communication)
Complement system		
Classical pathway	Activation	Nishioka (personal communication)
Alternative pathway	Activation	Okuda *et al.* (1972)
C3 absolute value	Increase	A. J. S. Davies (personal communication)
Lysozyme activity	Activation	Chihara (1980)
Acute-phase protein inducer	Appearance	Chihara *et al.* (in press)
IL-1 inducer	Appearance	Hamuro *et al.* (1982)
Colony-stimulating factor	Increase	Hamuro *et al.* (1982)
Tumor necrosis factor	No effect	Chihara (1980)
Antitumor factor	Appearance	Chihara *et al.* (in preparation)

zyme could be regenerated by treatment with purified factor B (Hamuro *et al.*, 1978c). Thus, lentinan may activate or increase certain serum components in a nonspecific manner and these may play a yet to be defined role in the antitumor action of lentinan.

5.4. IMMUNE EFFECTOR CELL AGAINST TUMORS

Recently, we have analyzed in a more direct manner the role of lymphoid cells in the antitumor activity of lentinan and shown that the passive transfer of antitutmor activity can be achieved with the spleen cells and peritoneal exudate cells in syngeneic tumor–host systems. After establishment of P815 or L5178Y tumors in DBA/2 mice, lentinan was injected i.v., and peritoneal cells and spleen cells were harvested when the ratios of tumor growth inhibition reached 51 and 70%, respectively. These cells were transplanted to recipient DBA/2 mice together with 1×10^6 tumor cells s.c. to test for neutralizing effects on tumor target cells (cell ratio 1:8 for peritoneal cells, and 1:50 for spleen cells). In both P815 and L5178Y systems, spleen cells and peritoneal exudate cells obtained from tumor-regressing mice treated with lentinan exhibited more than 70% growth-inhibiting effects, whereas cells from control tumor-bearing mice elicited only marginal effects.

In the MM102–C3H/HeN system, a similar neutralizing effect was observed only when lentinan-treated spleen cells were transferred with serum from MM102-bearing mice, and in the MM46–C3H/HeN system only when lentinan-treated peritoneal exudate cells were transferred with serum from MM46-bearing mice. In these systems, antitumor effector mechanisms may involve an ADCC reaction.

We next examined the localization of cytotoxic effector cells *in situ* in the regressing tumor site. We tried to isolate cytotoxic effector cells from the tumor mass. In the L5178Y and P815–DBA/2 systems, regressing solid tumors were extirpated at the same time and single-cell suspensions were prepared by collagenase–trypsin–DNase treatment. After cell fractionation by sedimentation on a gradient of Ficoll, each cell fraction was tested for its cytotoxicity against the corresponding target tumor cells. Cell fractions obtained from tumors undergoing regression with lentinan treatment showed considerable cytotoxicity. The isolated cells were negative in neutral red staining and presumed to be lymphoid cells on the basis of morphology. The presence of effector cells in regressing tumors was also confirmed by the observation of augmented infiltration of lymphoid cells into P815 tumors of lentinan-treated syngeneic DBA/2 mice.

5.5. POSSIBLE MODE OF ACTION

The distinctive characteristics of lentinan include:

1. Chemically defined nature with reliable, reproducible activity
2. Effectiveness by systematic administration comparable to actual protocols used in clinical studies

3. No activation of macrophages or NK cells during *in vitro* cocultivation, but efficient activation of these cells upon *in vivo* application
4. No increase of interferon and lysosomal enzymes released from macrophages upon *in vitro* cultivation
5. Depression of prostaglandin release from macrophages induced by lentinan
6. Characteristic dependency on T cells as an immunoadjuvant such as to augment reactivity of precursor/effector cells to T-cell-derived lymphokines
7. No mitogenicity and absence of action as a polyclonal activator

As a tentative mechanism of action, we propose that lentinan triggers increased production of IL-1 by direct impact on macrophages or indirectly via augmented CSF production from lentinan-stimulated T cells. Thus, increased production of IL-1 results in the augmented maturation of premature lymphoid cells into mature cells capable of responding to IL-2; in turn, mature cells are differentiated into effector CTL and NK cells in the presence of IL-2. In addition, lentinan-induced augmentation of macrophage reactivity to MAF results in augmented generation of effector macrophages. Furthermore, increased or activated serum factors may complement these actions.

Lentinan is capable of positively influencing the immunologically specific limb of T-cell-mediated cytotoxic immune responses as well as the nonspecific limb of macrophage- and NK cell-mediated responses.

The postulated mode of action explains several observed characteristics of the antitumor action of lentinan, such as the absence of antitumor activity in neonatally thymectomized mice, the lack of activity in *nu/nu* mice, the decrease of activity by carrageenan treatment, the loss of activity by 400-R irradiation at an early phase after transplantation, and the loss of activity with the administration of immunosuppressive agents.

6. OTHER PHYSIOLOGICAL ASPECTS

Lentinan has several physiological and endocrinological effects. It increases histamine or serotonin sensitivity in mice in the same way as pertussis vaccine, but, by contrast, lentinan can also suppress the histamine shock of pertussis-treated mice (Homma and Kuratsuka, 1973). Lentinan also prevents toxic death due to the administration of cyclocytidine or vincristine (Tokuzen *et al.*, 1976); e.g., toxic death resulting from the administration of 500 mg/kg cyclocytidine for 20 days occurred in 7 out of 17 mice, but this toxic action is apparently suppressed when lentinan is used in combination with cyclocytidine, and there were no deaths during the corresponding period.

A marked difference between 25% and 75% in the tumor inhibitory effect of lentinan against the syngeneic LOU immunocytoma in rats was observed depending on the chronobiological best timing or worst timing and may relate the action of lentinan to other yet unsuspected systems (Levi *et al.*, 1982).

The antitumor activity of lentinan is strongly inhibited by thyroxine, the growth inhibitory activity lowering from 98% to 22% upon administration of thyroxine. Since thyroxine tends to enhance the growth of tumors, there remains a possibility that this inhibition may be the result of antagonism between the action of lentinan and thyroxine.

The antitutmor effect of lentinan is also inhibited by hydrocortisone. As the action of cortisol is synergistic with the action of antilymphocyte serum and this hormone is known to specifically attack the thymus-derived lymphocyte, it is natural that the antitumor effect of lentinan is inhibited by hydrocortisone acetate.

7. CONCLUSION

Lentinan exhibits potent antitumor, antibacterial, antiviral, and antiparasitic effects. As a chemically well-defined neutral polysaccharide, it is characterized by immunological and biological activities distinct from those of other immunostimulants, such as BCG, *C. parvum*, LPS, levamisole, pyran copolymer, poly(I:C), interferons, etc. Low toxicity (LD_{50} = 1500 mg/kg in mice) is also an important characteristic of lentinan when compared with other chemotherapeutic agents possessing detrimental toxic side effects. These characteristic features make lentinan a good candidate for application in clinical studies of cancer patients.

Human cancers should be considered as diseases with great diversities comparable to many infectious diseases. Host–tumor relationships may differ depending on the growth state of the cancer and on the course of curative treatments. Therefore, the study of lentinan with regard to human cancer should be based on strict injection time and dose schedules that successfully adapt the immunological and biological characteristics observed in animals administered lentinan.

A most important and urgent task for clinical immunologists is to determine parameters of host–tumor relationship useful in indicating which protocols best apply to immunopotentiators such as lentinan.

REFERENCES

Akiyama, Y., and Hamuro, J., 1981, Effect of antitumor polysaccharides on specific and non-specific immune responses and their immunological characteristics, *Tampakushitsu Kakusan Koso* **26**:208.

Bluhm, T. H., and Sarko, A., 1977, The triple helix structure of lentinan, a linear β-(1-3)-D-glucan, *Can. J. Chem.* **55**:293.

Byrum, J. E., Sher, A., DiPietro, J., and Von Lichtenberg, F., 1979, Potentiation of schistosome granuloma by lentinan, a T-cell adjuvant, *Am. J. Pathol.* **94**:201.

Chang, K. S. S., 1981, Lentinan-mediated resistance against VSV-encephalitis, Abelson virus induced tumor, and trophoblastic tumor in mice, in: *Manipulation of Host Defense Mechanisms* (T. Aoki, I. Urushizaki, and E. Tsubura, eds.), Excerpta Medica, Amsterdam.

Chihara, G., 1980, Lentinan and serum factors, in: *The Mechanisms of Host Defense* (D. Mizuno, K. Takeya, and N. Ishida, eds.), University of Tokyo Press, Tokyo.

Chihara, G., Maeda, Y. Y., Hamuro, J., Sasaki, T., and Fukuoka, F., 1969, Inhibition of mouse sarcoma 180 by the polysaccharides from *Lentinus edodes* (Berk.) Sing., *Nature (London)* **222**:687.

Chihara, G. Hamuro, J., Maeda, Y. Y., Arai, Y., and Fukuoka, F., 1970a, Fractionation and purification of the polysaccharides with marked antitumor activity, especially lentinan, from *Lentinus edodes* (Berk.) Sing. (an edible mushroom), *Cancer Res.* **30**:2776.

Chihara, G., Hamuro, J., Maeda, Y. Y., Arai, Y., and Fukuoka, F., 1970b, Antitumor polysaccharide derived chemically from natural glucan (pachyman), *Nature (London)* **225**:943.

Delville, J., and Jacques, P. J., 1980, Therapeutic and prophylactic effects of yeast glucan and related polysaccharidic immunomodulators in experimental leprosy, *Int. J. Immunopharmacol.* **2**:183.

Dennert, G., and Tucker, D., 1973, Antitumor polysaccharide lentinan, a T-cell adjuvant, *J. Natl. Cancer Inst.* **51**:1729.

Dresser, D. W., and Phillips, J. M., 1974, The orientation of the adjuvant activities of *Salmonella typhosa* lipopolysaccharide and lentinan, *Immunology* **27**:895.

Hamada, C., 1981, Inhibitory effect of lentinan on the tumorigenesis of adenovirus type 12 in mice, in: *Manipulation of Host Defense Mechanisms* (T. Aoki, I. Urushizaki, and E. Tsubura, eds.), Excerpta Medica, Amsterdam.

Hamuro, J., and Chihara, G., 1973, Effect of antitumor polysaccharides on the higher structure of serum protein, *Nature (London)* **245**:40.

Hamuro, J., Maeda, Y. Y., Fukuoka, F., and Chihara, G., 1971, The significance of higher structure of the polysaccharides lentinan and pachymaran with regard to their antitumor activity, *Chem. Biol. Interact.* **3**:69.

Hamuro, J., Röllinghoff, M., and Wagner, H., 1978a, β-1,3-glucan mediated augmentation of alloreactive murine cytotoxic T-lymphocytes *in vivo*, *Cancer Res.* **38**:3080.

Hamuro, J., Wagner, H., and Röllinghoff, M., 1978b, β-1,3-glucans as a probe for T-cell specific immune adjuvants: Enhanced *in vitro* generation of cytotoxic T-lymphocytes, *Cell. Immunol.* **38**:328.

Hamuro, J., Hadding, U., and Bitter-Seuermann, D., 1978c, Solid phase activation of alternative pathway of complement by β-1,3-glucans and its possible role for tumor regression, *Immunology* **34**:695.

Hamuro, J., Röllinghoff, M., Wagner, H., Seitz, M., Grimm, W., and Gemsa, D., 1979, Depressed prostaglandin release from peritoneal cells induced by a T-cell adjuvant, lentinan, *Z. Immunitaetsforsch.* **155**:28.

Hamuro, J., Röllinghoff, M., and Wagner, H., 1980, Induction of cytotoxic peritoneal exudate cells by T-cell immune adjuvants of the β-1,3-glucan type lentinan and its analogues, *Immunology* **39**:551.

Hamuro, J., Akiyama, Y., Iguchi, Y., Izawa, N., and Matsuo, T., 1982, Distinct roles of serum factor induced by a T cell specific immune adjuvant lentinan in cellular immune responses, *Int. J. Immunopharmacol.* **4**:268.

Homma, R., and Kuratsuka, K., 1973. The histamine sensitizing activity of lentinan, an antitumor polysaccharide, *Experientia* **29**:290.

Itoh, O., Torikai, T., Satoh, M., and Osawa, T., 1980, Purification and characterization of a mouse serum glycoprotein increased in level by administration of antitumor polysaccharide lentinan, *Gann* **71**:644.

Kanai, K., Kondo, E., Jacques, P. J., and Chihara, G., 1980, Immunopotentiating effect of fungal glucans as related by frequency limitation of post chemotherapy relapse in experimental mouse tuberculosis, *Jpn. J. Med. Sci. Biol.* **33**:283.

Kawamura, T., and Numasaki, Y., 1980. Effect of lentinan on host resistance against Listeria infections, *Proc. Jpn. Cancer Assoc.* **39**:134.

Levi, F., Halberg, F., Chihara, G., and Byrum, J. E., 1982, Chronoimmunomodulation: Circadian, circaseptan and circannual aspects of immunopotentiation or suppression with lentinan, in: *Toward Chrono-pharmacology*, Pergamon Press, (R. Takahashi, F. Halberg, and C. A. Walker, eds.), Elmsford, New York.

Levy, J.-P., Gomard, E., and Wibier-Franqui, J., 1981, Cellular interactions in vitro in a primary antitumor response, in: *Manipulation of Host Defense Mechanisms* (T. Aoki, I. Urushizaki, and E. Tsubura, eds.), Excerpta Medica, Amsterdam.

Maeda, Y. Y., and Chihara, G., 1971, Lentinan, a new immuno-accelerator of cell-mediated immune responses, *Nature (London)* **229**:634.

Maeda, Y. Y., and Chihara, G., 1973, The effects of neonatal thymectomy on the antitumor activity of lentinan, carboxymethylpachymaran and zymosan, and their effects on various immune responses, *Int. J. Cancer* **11**:153.

Maeda, Y. Y., Hamuro, J., and Chihara, G., 1971, The mechanism of action of antitumor polysaccharides: The effect of antilymphocyte serum on the antitumor activity of lentinan, *Int. J. Cancer* **8**:41.

Maeda, Y. Y., Hamuro, J., Yamada, Y. O., Ishimura, K., and Chihara, G., 1973, The nature of immunopotentiation by the antitumor polysaccharide lentinan and the significance of biogeneic amines in its action, in: *Immunopotentiation* (G. E. W. Wolstenholme and J. Knight, eds.), Elsevier, Excerpta Medica, North-Holland, Amsterdam.

Maeda, Y. Y., Chihara, G., and Ishimura, K., 1974, Unique increase of serum protein components and action of antitumor polysaccharides, *Nature (London)* **252**:250.

Manabe, T., Takahashi, Y., Okuyama, T., Maeda, Y. Y., and Chihara, G., 1983, Identification of mouse serum proteins increased by the administration of antitumor polysaccharide lentinan, by micro two-dimensional electrophoresis. *Electrophoresis* **4**:242.

Masuko, Y., Abe, S., and Mizuno, D., 1979, The time of antitumor action of immunopotentiators depend on immune reaction: Antitumor delayed hypersensitivity reaction, antibody and serum factor LB, *Proc. Jpn. Cancer Assoc.* **38**:92.

Okuda, T., Yoshioka, Y., Ikekawa, T., Chihara, G., and Nishioka, K., 1972, Anticomplementary activity of antitumor polysaccharides, *Nature New Biol.* **238**:59.

Sasaki, T., and Takasuka, N., 1976, Further study of the structure of lentinan, an antitumor polysaccharide from *Lentinus edodes*, *Carbohydr. Res.* **47**:99.

Sasaki, T., Takasuka, N., Chihara, G., and Maeda, Y. Y., 1976, Antitumor activity of degraded products of lentinan: Its correlation with molecular weight, *Gann* **67**:191.

Shiio, T., and Yugari, Y., 1980, Antitumor effect of lentinan on syngeneic and autologous tumor–host systems, and suppression of chemical carcinogenesis, *Int. J. Immunopharmacol.* **2**:172.

Tokuzen, R., Okabe, M., and Nakahara, W., 1976, Combined effect of cyclocytidine and lentinan on spontaneous mammary tumors in mice, *Gann* **67**:327.

Yamada, Y., Kubota, T., Hanatani, Y., Matsumoto, S., Kumai, K., Ishibiki, K., and Abe, O., 1981, Antitumor effect of lentinan in the mouse system, in: *Manipulation of Host Defense Mechanisms*, (T. Aoki, I. Urushizaki, and E. Tsubura, eds.), Excerpta Medica, Amsterdam.

Yoshikai, Y., Miake, S., Matsumoto, T., Nomoto, K., and Takeya, K., 1979, Effect of stimulation and blockage of mononuclear phagocyte system on the delayed footpad reaction to SRBC in mice, *Proc. Jpn. Soc. Immunol.* **9**:171.

Zákány, J., Chihara, G., and Fachet, J., 1980a, Effect of lentinan on tumor growth in murine allogeneic and syngeneic hosts, *Int. J. Cancer* **25**:31.

Zákány, J., Chihara, G., and Fachet, J., 1980b, Effect of lentinan on the production of migration inhibitory factor induced by syngeneic tumor in mice, *Int. J. Cancer* **26**:783.

Zákány, J., Jánossy, T., Németh, T., Chihara, G., Fachet, J., and Petri, G., 1983, Mechanism of the A/Ph.MC.S1 tumor graft rejection in syngeneic mice, *Gann* **74**:712.

12

Immunoregulation by Cancer Chemotherapeutic Agents

M. JANE EHRKE and ENRICO MIHICH

1. INTRODUCTION

Considerable progress in cancer therapeutics has been achieved since the inception, in the mid 1940s, of the initial trials of antifolates, steroids, and alkylating agents, which marked the beginning of the current phase of cancer chemotherapy. Notwithstanding the demonstrated value of chemotherapy in the treatment of certain types of neoplastic disease, ways must still be identified to circumvent basic limitations before drugs can be used broadly in the effective treatment of cancer. Consequently, as discussed elsewhere (Mihich, 1978), among the main approaches in cancer chemotherapy, has been the study of the mechanisms of selective toxicity of drugs; included in these studies have been those of the interactions of drugs with host defense mechanisms. As a result of these investigations, it became apparent quite early that most anticancer drugs are potentially capable of suppressing host defense mechanisms and that in many cases this effect is a consequence of the very antiproliferative action that is the basis of the agent's antitumor activity. In fact, despite a number of remarkably insightful experiments conducted between the mid 1950s and the mid 1960s, which indicated the unique immunomodulating potential of certain anticancer agents, the preponderance of the information obtained until the late 1970s has been restricted to their immunosuppressive properties (see Hersh, 1973; Mihich, 1975; Spreafico and Anaclerio, 1977; Bast, 1982). In light of the availability of these and other excellent reviews on the immunosuppression caused by anticancer agents (Mihich, 1979; Hersh, 1974; Bach, 1975) it is the intent of this presentation to concentrate on examples of the immunomodulating characteristics of these drugs.

M. JANE EHRKE and ENRICO MIHICH • Department of Experimental Therapeutics and Grace Cancer Drug Center, Roswell Park Memorial Institute, New York State Department of Health, Buffalo, New York 14263.

The interactions of drugs with immune reactions have, in general, been considered nonspecific in nature, in the sense that in many cases they appear to be the consequence of pharmacological perturbations, such as inhibition of cell proliferation, which would not affect the immunological system uniquely. Yet, as demonstrated by the results of early experiments, a drug may inhibit one type of response against one antigen without affecting (or conversely even augmenting) a different type of response against the same antigen or the same type of response against a different antigen (see Schwartz, 1968). Thus, selectivity in chemical immunomodulation might depend not only on the multifactorial biochemical and pharmacological parameters of drug–host interaction (see Rustum et al., 1976) but also on intrinsic characteristics of the immunological systems.

The host immunological response to antigen is the culmination of a multiplicity of cellular phenomena including specific metabolic activation, differentiation, and proliferation; complex and not fully elucidated interactions between different cells and cell products, and various mechanisms of interaction of effector with target leading to antigen neutralization, lysis, and/or phagocytic disposition. Specific cell functions are under strict genetic control and gene products are the determinants of the regulation of immune response, regardless of whether this response ultimately involves a specific effector cell or a nonspecific cell activated by a specific cell product.

With the rapidly increasing knowledge about both the complex network of circuits involved in immune responses and the biochemical and pharmacological events that follow drug administration, acquisition of basic information on selective drug effects on immune systems had become possible. In fact, there are now many well-documented examples of chemotherapeutic agents selectively affecting one type of immune response and not another as well as inducing immunomodulation (i.e., one agent under different conditions causing inhibition, no change, or augmentation of the same immune response). In at least one case where investigations have progressed to the point of identifying the primary site of selective activity at the cell level, it has become clear that the agent may be more discriminating than the monoclonal antibodies yet available (Ferguson and Simmons, 1978; Smith et al., 1982). Thus, these agents may have potential applications as exquisitely selective probes in basic investigations into the complex circuits of immunoregulation, as well as theoretical potential in remission maintenance protocols designed to optimize their immunomodulating characteristics without unduly compromising their antitumor toxicity. This chapter is devoted to a brief review of the salient information available on the immunomodulating properties of certain antineoplastic agents.

2. 6-MERCAPTOPURINE

The example of 6-mercaptopurine (6-MP) is cited first in deference to its historical significance as the first well-documented example of augmented immune responsiveness induced by an anticancer agent. The mechanism of the selective immunoregulatory activity of this agent has not been determined.

Schwartz and co-workers described the effects of 6-MP on the humoral and cellular responses against bovine γ-globulin (BGG) in rabbits (see Schwartz, 1968). They found that a dose of antigen (20 μg, i.v.) too small to evoke a primary response in control animals stimulated a rapid rise in both IgM and IgG anti-BGG antibodies when given after the last dose of a 1-week course of 6-MP, 10 mg/kg per day (Chanmougan and Schwartz, 1966). A somewhat shorter course of 6-MP (10 mg/kg per day for 4 days) begun simultaneously with the administration of BGG had no effect on the synthesis of circulating antibody but prevented the acquisition of delayed hypersensitivity (Borel and Schwartz, 1964). Finally, a slightly lower dose of 6-MP was shown to selectively eliminate IgG production and, under these conditions, IgM synthesis continued for many weeks (Borel *et al.*, 1965). This classical set of experiments clearly demonstrated that the results one obtains in these types of studies are dependent on the following parameters: (1) the timing of drug administration with respect to antigenic stimulus, (2) the dose of drug used, (3) the dose of antigen given, (4) the nature of antigenic challenge (e.g. the route of administration, use of adjuvants, type of antigen), and (5) the nature of the immune response assayed. These principles still apply and one must be cognizant of them when comparing experimental results from various studies.

Subsequent to these early studies, the investigations of 6-MP and its methylnitroimidazole derivative, azathioprine (AZ), have been concerned almost exclusively with their immunosuppressive properties. This emphasis has been the consequence, primarily, of the early recognition of the utility of these agents (particularly AZ) as chemical immunosuppressants in organ transplants. For a description of the immunosuppressive properties of thiopurines, see the reviews by Bach (1975), Spreafico and Anaclerio (1977), and Winkelstein (1979). The ability of AZ, at low concentrations, to selectively bind to T lymphocytes and inhibit their capacity to form rosettes with SRBC is the basis of a widely applied assay for functional T lymphocytes (see Bach, 1975). AZ, *in vitro*, also inhibits the proliferative and cytolytic responses of mixed lymphocyte cultures, whereas the mitogenic and T-independent response of B cells in culture are, in general, less sensitive to the thiopurines.

In contrast to the rather extensive literature on the immunosuppressive effects of the thiopurines, their ability to augment selected immune responses has received relatively little attention. Recently, however, Drossler *et al.* (1981) investigated the effects of 6-MP on antibody production in guinea pigs. They found that the drug augmented the production of hapten-specific IgG1 and prolonged the production of hapten-specific IgG2 without affecting the production of either set of carrier-specific antibodies. Thus, these workers were able to confirm and extend the observations concerning augmentation of antibody production that Schwartz and co-workers had made in the rabbit. Two other recent reports that dealt solely with the inhibitory effects of 6-MP may, nevertheless, have implications toward the understanding of the immunoaugmenting activity of the drug. Phillips *et al.* (1979) demonstrated that marked alterations in monocyte-macrophage generation and distribution occur following 6-MP treatment of guinea pigs. Since functional macrophages or their products have been shown to play pivotal roles in most immune responses, alteration in their distribution or maturation could have modulating effects. Another function that regulates the level of response is suppression. Medzihradsky *et al.* (1981), using a cell transfer model, demonstrated that the generation of carrier-specific suppressor cells is sensitive to 6-MP treatment. Thus, suppressor cells, under specific conditions, may be a target of selective 6-MP cytotoxic effects and under those conditions a modulation of the immune response could occur. Extensive experimentation is still required before the immunoregulatory potential of 6-MP is fully characterized.

3. CYCLOPHOSPHAMIDE

Cyclophosphamide (CY) is a second example of a putative immunosuppressive agent that, in early studies, appeared to increase immune responsiveness under certain conditions. In contrast to 6-MP, the immunoregulatory potential of CY has been investigated extensively.

Turk and co-workers suggested that the augmentation of delayed hypersensitivity reactions observed when CY was administered prior to sensitization was the result of the elimination of a regulatory cell (for reviews of the early studies, see Bach, 1975; Turk and Parker, 1979a,b). On the basis of their findings, they concluded that the regulatory cell belonged to the B-cell lineage (Polak and Turk, 1974), although they did not rule out the possibility that regulatory cells of the T or macrophage lineages could also be affected. It was subsequently demonstrated that doses of CY too low to affect antibody production were immunoaugmenting for delayed-type hypersensitivity (DTH). This suggested that a B-cell-linked function was not the sole regulator of delayed reactions and that suppressor T cells might also be involved (Askenase *et al.*, 1975).

That cell types, which regulate cell-mediated immune responses, might be selectively sensitive to CY was inferred at a time when interest in such cell subsets was rapidly expanding. This combination of circumstances resulted in the extensive use of CY, at low doses, as a probe in studies designed to elucidate the properties of suppressor cells. On the other hand, a large number of studies were also designed to further evaluate the mechanism of CY immunoaugmenting action in tumor models and to define conditions under which it would be possible to use the knowledge gained to potential advantage in experimental chemoimmunotherapy. Recent developments in these two areas are discussed below. For discussions of the studies reported up to the mid 1970s, the reader is referred to a number of excellent reviews (e.g., Bach, 1975; Spreafico and Anaclerio, 1977; Turk and Parker, 1979a).

3.1. CHARACTERIZATION OF THE REGULATORY CELL SUBSET(S) SELECTIVELY SENSITIVE TO CY

The studies that have been directed toward the identification of the subset(s) of cells selectively sensitive to CY can be grouped under three general headings, namely studies involving: (1) low-dose CY *in vivo*, (2) *in vitro* active analogs of CY, and (3) high-dose CY *in vivo*.

The selective sensitivity of T regulatory (suppressor) cells to CY was established as a result of a large number of experiments in animals in which primarily low *in vivo* doses of CY were used. These findings have more recently been confirmed and extended to cells of human origin in *in vitro* studies made possible by the availability of *in vitro* active CY metabolites or synthetic precursors of *in vitro* active CY metabolites. Conversely, the immunomodulation seen in the studies utilizing high-dose CY has, in general, been interpreted as being the consequence of inhibition of CY-sensitive B-cell regulation.

3.1.1. Studies with Low-Dose CY

Askenase *et al.* (1975) were the first to report that modulations in DTH can be produced by CY pretreatment (low dose, 1–2 days before antigen) without comcomitant detectable alterations in antibody responses. Based on their data, these authors suggested that suppressor T cells may be affected by the drug. Similar conclusions have been reported by a number of different groups and the information concerning this mode of CY action has been extended to other model systems. Mitsuoka *et al.* (1976) evaluated the effect of CY on the DTH to methylated human serum albumin (MHSA) and also concluded that the augmentation following CY pretreatment was due to damage of suppressor T cells and not of B cells. In studies of the *in vitro* IgM response against trinitrophenylated polyacrylamide, Duclos *et al.* (1977) found that CY pretreatment decreased antibody production by spleen cells from nude mice and increased it by cells from conventional mice. They concluded that CY (low dose, day −4) affects B cells in the spleens of both mice but that in the conventional mice its effect on a pre-T-suppressor cell predominates. Burrows *et al.* (1976) demonstrated that CY induced augmentation of DTH to SRBC in mice that had been rendered incapable of an antibody response by treatment with anti-μ serum. Thus, the independence of the CY-induced effects on cell-mediated responses from the possible modulation of B-cell responses by the drug has been established in a variety of experimental models.

In a similar manner, the differential sensitivity of T subsets to CY-induced modulation has also been examined. Bash *et al.* (1976) found that the T-cell-dependent suppressive effect on *in vitro* PHA-stimulated spleen cell proliferation, which is elicited by large i.v. doses of antigen, was present if CY was administered at the same time as antigen. Rollinghoff *et al.* (1977) demonstrated that CY-sensitive T cells suppress the *in vivo* differentiation of antigen-specific CTL following immunization with either allogeneic lymphocytes or syngeneic hapten-conjugated lymphocytes and in their absence higher levels of lytic activity develop. Consistent with this observation, findings by a number of workers have also indicated the relative CY insensitivity of cytotoxic T-cell precursors. In fact, Glaser (1979) demonstrated that CY treatment converts mice from a state of low to high CTL responsiveness against SV40-induced tumor-associated antigens by depletion of suppressor T cells. Ferguson and Simmons (1978), using spleen cells from CY-treated mice as responder cells in cell-mediated cytoxicity (CMC) cultures, demonstrated that precursors of T-suppressor cells are sensitive to a dose of CY that does not appear to affect the lymphoid cells' ability to develop CTL. They suggested, therefore, that this differential sensitivity to CY could separate two subpopulations, both bearing the Ly-23$^+$ phenotype. Cantor *et al.* (1978) showed that another T-cell subset, the Ly-123$^+$ Qa-1$^+$, T_H-inducible, "feedback" suppressor cell, is also CY sensitive. Debre *et al.* (1976) used CY (a relatively high dose, 2 days before antigen) to show that following injection of GT (Copolymer of L-glutamic acid and L-tyrosine), the inability of BALB/c mice to respond to immunization with GT-MBSA was due to specific T-suppressor cell development and not to a T-helper deficiency. Information obtained utilizing the differential sensitivity of T subsets to CY provided part of the basis for the unifying hypothesis, proposed by Benacerraf and co-workers, which involves at least three distinct T-suppressor cell subsets, two of which are CY sensitive, in the pathway of cellular interaction leading to immunosuppression after antigen exposure (Sunday *et al.*, 1981). The generation of Ts_1, the induction-phase suppressor cell, and that of Ts_3, one of the two effector-phase suppressor cell populations, are sensitive to CY. These cells also are I-J positive and may bear the same or similar idiotype determinants, whereas the other effector-phase suppressor cell (Ts_2) is CY insensitive and bears antiidiotype. More recently, they defined an I-J-restricted event in the activation of Ts_3 effector cells and have shown that it appears to be dependent on a CY-sensitive I-J$^+$, I-A$^-$ adherent antigen-presenting cell (Lowy *et al.*, 1983). They suggest that the deficiency of these cells in CY-treated mice may explain how the drug inhibits T_s function *in vivo*. The implications of this proposal are obvious and testing of this premise in various experimental systems is needed.

3.1.2. Studies *in Vitro* with Active CY Metabolites

Since CY is not active *in vitro*, all the studies reviewed above involved treatment of mice. The direct proof for differential sensitivity to CY of lymphocyte subsets was dependent on experimental approaches in which cells could be exposed to *in vitro* active compounds derived from CY. Shand (1978) activated CY *in vitro* with rat liver microsomes plus cofactors and showed that treatment of mouse spleen cells with the activated drug did not affect the graft-versus-host reactivity of the cells but abolished their capacity to develop a primary antibody response following their transfer to irradiated syngeneic mice. The effect on antibody production appeared to be reversible as immunocompetence was recovered in 7–10 days. Following this demonstration that the treatment of murine spleen cells *in vitro* with microsomally activated CY could reproduce the activity displayed by high-dose CY *in vivo*, this technique was utilized to show that suppressor T cells for anti-SRBC DTH responses are sensitive to much lower concentrations of activated CY than are helper T cells for anti-SRBC antibody responses (Shand and Liew, 1980).

A number of the chemical intermediates produced by the microsomal activation of CY have been defined and following their chemical synthesis (Colvin *et al.*, 1973; Conners *et al.*, 1974), Shand and Howard (1979) tested their effects on B-cell function *in vitro*. They found that only those compounds that have alkylating activity [4-hydroperoxycyclophosphamide (4-OOHCY), 4-hydroxycyclophosphamide (4-OHCY), phosphoramide mustard] inhibited B-cell responses but that the inhibition was reversible and not dependent on cell death. Diamantstein and co-workers (Diamantstein *et al.*, 1979, 1981; Kaufmann *et al.*, 1980) have used 4-OOHCY in a series of investigations and have found that: (1) the effects of 4-OOHCY *in vitro* on spleen cells parallel those of CY *in vivo* in terms of ability to augment or inhibit lymphocyte functions; (2) T-cell subsets involved in DTH are sensitive to 4-OOHCY as follows: precursors of suppressor T cells > antigen-activated suppressor T cells > T cells mediating DTH; (3) T-cell subsets involved in humoral responses also differ in their sensitivities to CY (helper T cells of humoral response = suppressor T cells of DTH > suppressor T cells of humoral response = T cells mediating DTH).

Recently, Cowens *et al.* (1981) have reported that the use of 4-OOHCY allows the separation of 4-OOHCY-sensitive precursor T-suppressor cells from 4-OOHCY-resistant precursor cytotoxic T cells as defined functionally in a model involving T-cell-mediated responses to alloantigen. Since both populations are reported to be Lyt-23$^+$, this was a direct demonstration that differential CY sensitivity can separate two populations bearing the same Lyt phenotype as had been suggested earlier by Ferguson and Simmons (1978). The same group (Ozer *et al.*, 1982) has extended the studies to human peripheral blood lymphocytes and has shown a differential sensitivity to 4-OOHCY between human presuppressor cells for B-effector functions and inducer T cells, although both T subsets express the OKT4$^+$8$^-$ phenotype. The precursor suppressor cells are 4-OOHCY sensitive before Con A induction but the mature suppressor and the inducer functions are relatively insensitive. Finally, they (Smith *et al.*, 1982) have shown differential sensitivity to 4-OOHCY of subsets of cells involved in the regulation of the development of human allospecific cytotoxic T lymphocytes in culture. While CTL effectors are resistant to 4-OOHCY, precursors of suppressor cells and precursors of CTL may be separated on the basis of their 4-OOHCY sensitivity, precursors of suppressor cells being the most sensitive. The treatment of the OKT4$^+$8$^-$ subset with very-low-dose 4-OOHCY appeared to selectively block suppressor cell development and substantial cytotoxic activity was detected. These findings again indicate that subset separation on the basis of sensitivity to CY may be more discriminating than the separation obtained on the basis of the reactivity of the monoclonal antibodies that are available at this time.

3.1.3. Studies with High-Dose CY

It may be helpful to state at the outset that the results obtained with high-dose CY are perhaps more ambiguous than those obtained with low-dose CY. This may reflect a more general (pan) cytotoxic effect at high dose as opposed to a more selective effect at low dose or in fact, at the high dose, quite selective effects may occur involving opposing functions, which could lead to confusion.

Nevertheless, a good deal of research has been done with high-dose CY as the following summary indicates.

In 1967, Magiure and Ettore noted that guinea pigs treated with CY (10 mg, i.p.) for 5 days prior to sensitization with DNCB showed enhanced responsiveness to challenge with DNCB. Following this initial observation, Turk and co-workers demonstrated that pretreatment with CY at 30 mg/kg, a dose that depletes B-cell but not T-cell-dependent areas of peripheral lymphoid tissues (Turk and Poulter, 1972), augments both contact sensitivity and DTH to simple antigens (Polak and Turk, 1974). On the basis of their findings, they concluded that a regulatory cell, belonging to the B-cell lineage, had been eliminated.

Other reports have also linked augmentation of cellular responses to the release of T cells from the influence of CY-sensitive B-cell regulation. Lagrange *et al.* (1974) suggested that CY freed the mediators of DTH to SRBC from the influence of blocking factors that were formed as a consequence of the interaction of antigen with antibody. They found that the augmentation of DTH was dependent on temporal factors related to drug and antigen administration and suggested that, in general, T cells are resting cells that are insensitive to CY until induced to proliferate by exposure to specific antigen, whereas B cells are from a rapidly replicating precursor pool and are susceptible to CY at all times. Turk and co-workers have advanced a similar hypothesis, namely that CY is cyotoxic to any short-lived, rapidly turning over cell and that long-lived, slowly turning over cells are insensitive to the drug. From this it follows that any cell under appropriate conditions might be CY sensitive, but that augmentation of an immune response would only occur when the precursor suppressor cell was short-lived and the precursor effector cell was long-lived (Turk and Parker, 1979a,b); however, as the authors state, this may be an oversimplification. Recently, Turk and co-workers (B. Noble *et al.*, 1977), using a panel of four antigens, have also shown the dissociation, in terms of CY sensitivity, of cells regulating DTH and precursors of plasma cells making three different types of antibodies. Further, these studies demonstrated a difference in the CY sensitivity of precursors of the various antibody-producing cells, which was interpreted in terms of long-lived and short-lived B-cell populations.

Other studies with high-dose CY have included those of Otterness and Chang (1976) who described conditions of immunization and CY administration (relatively low dose, orally) under which lymphocyte-mediated lysis of EL4 target cells was augmented while antibody-mediated lysis was suppressed. They suggested that the stimulation of the cellular response was consequent to the elimination of either antigen–antibody complex or B-cell feedback inhibition. Wood and Monaco (1977) demonstrated time-dependent effects of CY on the specific unresponsiveness to skin allografts induced in ALS-treated mice infused with bone marrow from untreated donor mice. CY before bone marrow infusion decreased graft survival. This result was interpreted as being due to decreased blocking antibody production. CY after bone marrow infusion increased graft survival, which was interpreted as being the result of selective effects on proliferating cytotoxic T cells. While studying the inability of high antigen doses to induce DTH, Marchal and co-workers (Marchal *et al.*, 1978; Milon and Marchal,

1978) found that DTH developed when spleen cells from mice rendered non-responsive by priming with high doses of antigen were transferred with antigen to footpads of nonsensitized mice. Limiting dilution studies in this model indicated that spleen cells from the nonresponsive mice contained greater numbers of DTH-mediating cells than spleen cells from mice undergoing DTH. Furthermore, CY pretreatment restored DTH responsiveness in the mice primed with large doses of antigen and CY pretreatment of spleen cell-recipient mice increased the infiltration at the DTH site. From these results they concluded that the defect in the high-dose antigen-primed mice resulted from a decrease in the number of circulating DTH cells. Since CY pretreatment inhibited antibody production and increased circulating DTH cells, they postulated that there was a CY-sensitive, B-cell-dependent retention of DTH cells in the spleens of high-dose antigen-primed mice. Based on their observations, they also postulated that in the CY-pretreated recipient mice, there may be a CY-dependent increase in the number of monocytes recruited to the DTH site.

Not all studies with high-dose CY have led to the conclusion that the elimination of CY-sensitive B cells was the best interpretation of the results. Based on the effects of varying a number of factors on the CY-induced modulation of DTH and anti-SRBC antibody formation, Kerckhaert et al. (1977) concluded that CY interferes with more than one regulatory mechanism. Thus, while under some conditions inhibition of antibody formation correlated with increased DTH, under other conditions it did not and they concluded that T-suppressor cells were also CY sensitive.

Merluzzi and co-workers have shown that Thy-1.2$^+$, Ly-1$^+$2$^-$, helper cells are CY sensitive (Merluzzi et al., 1979, 1980) and that the CY-inhibited generation of CTL against allogeneic tumor cells can be restored by the addition of T-helper cells (thymocytes) or MLC supernatants containing T-cell-derived helper factor (Merluzzi et al., 1981b). They extended these studies to show that a low in vivo CTL response, induced by CY administration, can be restored by injection of the MLC supernatant containing T-cell-derived helper factor (Merluzzi et al., 1981a). Thus, these findings are consistent with those of Sy et al. (1977), Ferguson and Simmons (1978), Hurme (1979), and Taswell et al. (1979) indicating that cytotoxic T-cell precursors are relatively CY insensitive and may explain the inhibition of T-cell-mediated responses under certain conditions (e.g., high dose or CY administration after antigen) reported by others (Gerber et al., 1978; Giampietri et al., 1978–79; Mitsuoka et al., 1979; Goto et al., 1981). Hancock and Kilburn (1982) have recently confirmed the findings of Merluzzi and co-workers and extended them to a syngeneic tumor system in which they find an apparently similar lesion at the level of T help, but also suggest a reduction in cytotoxic T-cell precursors.

The findings of Schwartz and co-workers make a somewhat different, albeit cautionary point that may have implications toward understanding apparent paradoxes. They found that under the same conditions of CY pretreatment: (1) with different antigens it was possible to observe augmented DTH and inhibited GVH (Schwartz et al., 1976); (2) with the same antigen, when DTH response was high, CY pretreatment inhibited it, and when the response was low, CY augmented it (Schwartz *et al.*, 1978). From these findings they ruled out that the CY-sensitive regulatory T cells were obligatory suppressors. In contrast, they suggest that the regulatory T cells affected by CY belong to two functional subsets: (1) DTH amplifier (helper) and (2) suppressor amplifier (helper). Thus, under conditions where the summation of the signals from the underlying immune response would result in a high cellular response, pretreatment with low doses of CY may eliminate the positive feedback regulatory function and result in inhibition of the response.

Other findings that can lead to conflicting conclusions have been described by several groups. Hurme *et al.* (1982), Yu *et al.* (1980), and Mitsuoka *et al.* (1979) all found that initially more than one functional subset was sensitive to CY but that the rapid recovery of functional activity of some subsets together with the markedly delayed recovery of others made it appear as if only the latter were sensitive. It may also be pertinent that Sy *et al.* (1977) have shown that the suppressor cells can be regenerated within 7–14 days following CY treatment. The fact that the low immunoresponsiveness of aged animals is not potentiated by CY treatment (Bach, 1979; Mitsuoka, 1979) indicates the dependence of drug action on the age of the mice used in the studies. Finally, the enzymatic activation of CY appears to vary between the mouse strains (probably under genetic control) and to vary within a strain depending on enzyme induction above the baseline level (Goto *et al.*, 1981; Hurme *et al.*, 1980).

3.2. CY AND HOST ANTITUMOR DEFENSES

Before discussing the deliberate use of CY in conjunction with host antitumor defenses, a few considerations should be added to those just mentioned above. For instance, despite the demonstrated sensitivity to the drug of the precursor regulatory (suppressor) cells, there is considerable evidence that mature T-suppressor cells are resistant to CY. These include splenic MLC suppressor cells (Bonavida, 1977), thymic cells that inhibit both antigen- and mitogen-induced proliferation in culture (Neta *et al.*, 1977), and the T-repressor cells that are involved in the induction of specific antibody unresponsiveness under defined conditions (Debre *et al.*, 1976; Ramshaw *et al.*, 1977; for a review on drug-induced B-cell tolerance, see Howard and Shand, 1979). Similar questions as to the relevance of CY-induced B-cell modulation were raised by the recent report of Gagnon and MacLennan (1981) who found little evidence to suggest that CY given on a daily basis causes suppression of established antibody responses. On the other hand, McIntosh *et al.* (1979) and Braciale and Parish (1980) have described the appearance of a cell, in spleens of mice 5 to 14 days after CY treatment, that inhibits antibody responses, either directly or indirectly, through the action of a T-regulatory cell. Furthermore, the Ly-123$^+$, Qa-1$^+$, T_H-inducible, CY-sensitive suppressor cell described by Cantor *et al.* (1978) is part of a negative-feedback circuit and the elimination of this CY-sensitive subset during chemotherapy could lead to disruption of homeostatic

regulation, while its activation during immunotherapy could also be counterproductive.

Another example of a potentially negative consequence of CY-induced disruption of immune regulation is provided by L'age-Stehr and Diamantstein (1978). They found autoreactive T cells following the injection of normal mice with CY. They postulated that this was because CY induced both the appearance of "new" or altered-self antigenic sites and the transient depletion of the negative regulatory T-suppressor cells. In contrast, Hurme (1979) found that cells from CY-treated mice responded normally to alloantigen but failed to develop H-2-restricted (TNP-coupled syngeneic cells or H-Y antigen) responses in culture; this would indicate that precursors of H-2-restricted (altered-self) responses were CY sensitive.

Despite the multiplicity of factors having the potential to give rise to conflicting results, a considerable amount of evidence has been accumulated over the past 15 years suggesting that host immunoreactivity contributes to the therapeutic effect of CY in neoplastic disease. The data have been obtained in a variety of experiments involving either allogeneic or syngeneic tumor–host models and single-agent or combination (immunotherapeutic–chemotherapeutic) treatments (for a review of the early studies, see Fefer, 1974).

3.2.1. Single-Agent Treatments

Among the first to examine the possibility of cooperative relationships between CY and antitumor host defenses were Moore and Williams (1973) who stressed that the ability of CY to inhibit the growth of a methylcholanthrene-induced sarcoma was dependent on the size of the tumor, the timing of drug administration, and host immune factors. Radov et al. (1976), using a highly immunogenic mouse mammary adenocarcinoma, confirmed Moore and Williams' findings and established the critical dependence of the outcome on the development of a T-cell-dependent antitumor immune response by the host and not on the size of the tumor only. The significance of host immune responses in determining tumor cures following CY therapy has subsequently been described also with other mouse-tumor models (Chassouex et al., 1978; Lubet and Carlson, 1978). In a recent series of papers, Hengst, Mokyr, and Dray (Hengst et al., 1980, 1981; Mokyr et al., 1982) have reconfirmed the importance of the variables mentioned above to the outcome of CY therapy. They used the MOPC-315 plasmacytoma–syngeneic BALB/c mouse model and showed: (1) the importance of timing of drug administration relative to tumor inoculation (day 4 does not cure, day 8–14 cures); (2) that tumor cures depend on the development of T-cell-dependent immune responses; and (3) that the failure of early treatment (day 4) to produce cures correlates with low levels of host antitumor immunity. Recently, Vidovic et al. (1982) reported similar results in an adult WVM rat–Yoshida ascites sarcoma model.

These findings appear to be consistent with the proposals discussed in the previous sections. Lagrange et al. (1974) suggested that shortly after antigen

presentation, the T cells that had been induced to proliferate would be sensitive to CY. Thus, CY early (day 4) would be ineffective since it would eliminate the cells mediating the host response. In fact, Balow et al. (1975, 1977) reported that replicating T cells that mediate cellular immunity are CY sensitive. Turk and Parker (1979a,b) suggested that for CY to induce immunopotentiation, there would have to be a rapidly turning over suppressor cell population regulating a slowly turning over effector cell population. Radov et al. (1976) have shown that mature cytotoxic T cells (Tc) are CY insensitive, and thus CY late (day 8–14) would eliminate suppressor cell regulation without decreasing host antitumor activity if the suppressor cell population was turning over rapidly. Consistent with this, Yu et al. (1980), using a tumor neutralization assay, found that CY administration early, before initiation of T-cell proliferation, or later, after the development of Tc, apparently inhibited suppressor cell activity without affecting tumor-neutralizing activity, whereas CY administration near the time Tc were first detected inhibited both activities. North (1982) has also suggested that delayed CY treatment of tumor-bearing animals eliminates T-suppression. In the face of the considerable evidence that the mature T-suppressor cell is CY resistant, this would also suggest that the mature suppressor cell is a short-lived cell that is constantly being renewed from the CY-sensitive precursor suppressor cell pool.

The possibility that macrophages are induced by CY has also been suggested. Milon and Marchal (1978) observed increased numbers of macrophages recruited to the site of DTH response. Evans et al. (1980) studied the leukocytes associated with regressing and recurring tumors following CY treatment and found increases in macrophages and granulocytes at the tumor site. Dye and North (1980), on the basis of similar observations, postulated that it might be therapeutically advantageous to activate these macrophages. They found that appropriately timed intratumor endotoxin injections resulted, after a long delay, in tumor cures. The long delay suggested that the endotoxin-induced effects involved the stimulation of host antitumor immunity and not just activation of the macrophages to become tumoricidal. The possible involvement of the macrophage product, tumor necrosis factor (Carswell et al., 1975), should also be considered. Mantovani et al. (1980) have shown that CY treatment did not affect spontaneous or BCG-stimulated macrophage cytotoxic activity, while Lespinats et al. (1979) found increased cytostatic activity associated with adherent cells following CY treatment. In considering the effects of CY on macrophages, it is important to mention the results reported by Bennett and Mitchell (1979) indicating that appropriately timed administration of CY potentiates the activation by BCG of immature monocyte suppressor cells, which may function as negative regulators of host defenses.

Finally, there are a few examples of the effective use of CY prophylactically. The report by Hellstrom and Hellstrom (1978) provides an example where the elimination of CY-sensitive cells prior to administration of 3-methylcholanthrene (3-MC) was beneficial to the host in terms of a delay in the appearance of chemically induced primary tumors. Similarly, Ray and Raychaudhuri (1981)

reported that pretreatment of mice with low-dose CY delayed or inhibited tumor appearance following the inoculation of 3-MC-induced transplantable fibrosarcomas.

3.2.2. Combination Treatments

Various combination modalities involving CY have been examined. Fefer and co-workers studied a number of models for adoptive immunochemotherapy (for reviews of early findings, see Fefer, 1974; Fefer *et al.*, 1976a,b). Recently, they have published a series of reports evaluating, in depth, one of these models involving C57BL/6 mice and a Friend virus-induced tumor (FBL-3). Using this sytem, they have shown that for adoptive chemoimmunotherapy of established syngeneic tumors to be effective, the transferred immune cells must have been sensitized against the same tumor (Cheever *et al.*, 1980). The effect of the combined therapy on the established tumor is biphasic in that there is a rapid chemoimmuno-reduction of the number of tumor cells followed by a transient increase over several weeks in the number of tumor cells before final rejection. The late phase of tumor reduction is sensitive to ALS (Greenberg *et al.*, 1980) and may be similar to the delayed rejection observed by Dye and North (1980) following LPS (see above). Fefer and co-workers have recently shown that the success of the combined treatment was dependent on the transfer of Lyt-1^{+}2^{-} T cells, while cells that were cytotoxic for the FBL tumor *in vitro* were shown to develop from the Lyt-1^{+}2^{+} and Lyt-1^{-}2^{+} subsets (Greenberg *et al.*, 1981). This suggested that the critical cells in the adoptive immunotherapy may function *in vivo* predominantly as amplifier cells. As mentioned above, Merluzzi *et al.* (1979, 1980) had shown that Lyt-1^{+}2^{-} cells are CY sensitive and therefore could be limiting in the CY-treated tumor-bearing mice.

By repeatedly supplementing cultures with IL-2, a T-cell growth factor produced by Lyt-1^{+}2^{-} cells, lymphocytes that are cytotoxic to tumors can be grown and nonspecifically expanded to large numbers (Gillis and Smith, 1977). With the advent of this methodology for the maintenance of specific CTL in long-term culture, it was possible for the first time to determine if, after their adoptive transfer, these effector cells also functioned *in vivo*. Using this technique, Cheever *et al.* (1981) were able to show that cells sequentially immunized *in vivo*, rechallenged with the same tumor *in vitro*, and then grown in culture with IL-2 prolonged the median survival time of tumor-bearing mice to a greater extent than did cells that were tested after *in vivo* immunization only; however, no mice were cured. They subsequently found that multiple injections of purified IL-2 greatly increased the efficacy of the cultured cells but had no effect on the noncultured cells (Cheever *et al.*, 1981) in the standard combination therapy model. Hardt *et al.* (1981) reported that a Lyt-23^{+}, CY-sensitive T cell regulates the activity of an IL-2 inhibitor *in vivo*. Thus, as suggested by Cheever *et al.* (1982), if the noncultured, but not the long-term-cultured, immune spleen cells reconstituted the CY-treated mice with IL-2-inhibitor-producing cells, this could explain the lack of potentiation when IL-2 plus noncultured cells were used.

Other groups have also studied models of CY-facilitated, adoptive immunotherapy. As mentioned in the preceding section, Dray and co-workers had shown that CY treatment of early nonpalpable tumors failed to induce cures and this failure was shown to correlate with low levels of antitumor immunity. They found that cures were inducible, however, by the adoptive transfer of immune spleen cells 1 day following day 4 CY treatment or delayed (day 10) CY treatment (Mokyr et al., 1982). In contrast to their findings, using a different tumor–host model, North (1982) found that CY treatment alone had only a temporary effect on the progression to death whether CY treatment was initiated early or late. Adoptive immunotherapy alone was ineffective. Combined chemo-immunotherapy was, however, effective in this model also, in that the i.v. infusion of CY followed in 1 hr by the i.v. infusion of tumor-immune spleen cells caused small as well as large tumors to completely regress. Since tumor regression, however, could be inhibited by injection of spleen cells from tumor-bearing but not normal donor mice, it was suggested that the presence of a tumor-induced population of CY-sensitive suppressor T cells was responsible for the failure of adoptive immunotherapy alone. This would seem to be in opposition to the findings of others that the mature T-suppressor cell is relatively CY insensitive but could be explained if this population was rapidly turning over and the precursors were CY sensitive (see Section 3.2.1). Nevertheless, it is clear that CY treatment of tumor-bearing mice eliminates antigen-exposed subsets of cells and that following their elimination, existing or adoptively transferred appropriate immune cell populations can successfully eradicate even large tumor masses. The studies of Kataoka et al. (1978) utilizing Con A-bound L1210 cells as a vaccine and CY administration 1 to 3 days before the second of two vaccinations led to a similar conclusion.

Several investigations of combined modalities involving CY and non-specifically immunostimulating agents have also been reported. Kobayashi and co-workers (Akiyama et al., 1977) found, in a syngeneic tumor–rat model, that appropriate timing of administration of tumor, CY, and PS-K, a nonspecifically immunostimulating protein-bound polysaccharide, resulted in 78% long-term survivors as compared to no long-term survivors when either agent was used singly. Fisher and co-workers have published a series of reports evaluating a variety of parameters involved in the inhibition of tumor growth by *Corynebacterium parvum* in combination with CY (see Fisher and Gunduz, 1979). As Dye and North (1980) found with CY plus LPS treatment, alterations in macrophage functions did not seem to play a direct role in the increased efficacy of the combined treatment. They have, in fact, suggested that the greater inhibition of tumor growth by the chemoimmunotherapy correlates with cytokinetic changes in the tumor during such treatment, but it is not known if this is a direct or an indirect effect.

In conclusion, while there is still much to be learned relative to the appropriate therapeutic application of CY, a great deal has been elucidated concerning its immunomodulating properties. On the basis of this knowledge, the drug has been successfully employed as a selective probe in basic research on the regulation of the immune responses and in chemoimmunotherapy model systems.

4. ADRIAMYCIN

The anthracycline aminoglycosidic antibiotic, Adriamycin (doxorubicin, ADM), was first described in 1969 (DiMarco *et al.*, 1969) about 6 years after the isolation of its structurally close analog, daunorubicin, was reported (Grein *et al.*, 1963). Both agents were rapidly introduced into clinical trials and perhaps no other family of chemotherapeutic agents has been as quickly accepted, as important agents in the treatment of human malignancies. Although ADM differs from the parent compound, daunorubicin, only by the substitution of a hydroxyl group for a hydrogen on C-14, it has been shown to have a broader spectrum of activity and a superior therapeutic index than daunorubicin both in experimental animal models (Sandberg *et al.*, 1970; Schwartz and Grindey, 1973) and in man (Carter, 1980). The coincidence of the remarkably wide range of antitumor applications for ADM together with the apparent stringency of the structure–activity relationship between it and daunorubicin gave impetus to a profusion of investigations to determine which drug-induced-effects were the determinants of antitumor selectivity. The reader is referred to a number of recent reviews (Schwartz, 1983; Arcamone, 1981; Young *et al.*, 1981) and proceedings of recent symposia (Crooke and Reich, 1980; Muggia, 1983) for detailed information on the biochemical and pharmacological studies. Despite this considerable effort a consensus has not yet been reached as to the determinants of antitumor selectivity of the anthracyclines.

4.1. CONTRIBUTION OF DRUG-INDUCED EFFECTS ON HOST–TUMOR INTERACTIONS

The early realization of the apparent lack of correlation between effects on either drug–tumor or host–drug interactions and the differences in the antitumor efficacies of the two drugs led two groups, independently, to examine the effects of the drugs on the third arm of this trigonal relationship, namely host–tumor interaction. Schwartz and Grindey (1973) compared the effects of ADM and daunorubicin in immunosuppressed and nonsuppressed DBA/2 mice bearing the ascitic lymphocytic leukemia P-288. They found that ADM had a significantly greater antitumor efficacy than did daunorubicin in the nonsuppressed mice; however, the therapeutic response to the two drugs was similar after immunosuppression induced by either X-irradiation or chemicals. Since they also found that ADM was concentrated less in the spleen, they concluded that a relative sparing from inhibition of host antitumor defense mechanisms might contribute to the therapeutic advantage of ADM, as compared to daunorubicin. Subsequently, Schwartz and Kanter (1975) demonstrated a similar reduction of the therapeutic response of ADM in splenectomized mice. Giuliani *et al.* (1974) compared the activity of ADM and daunorubicin on two transplanted murine sarcoma virus-Moloney-induced tumor lines. One line had been adapted to growth in culture and was shown to be relatively nonantigenic; the other was highly antigenic. The activity of ADM was greater than that of daunorubicin on the highly antigenic tumor whereas the two had almost equal effects on the nonantigenic one, again suggesting the possible involvement of host defense mechanisms in ADM antitumor efficacy.

In order to substantiate this possibility, Mantovani and co-workers under-took a comparative analysis of the effects of ADM and daunorubicin in various types of immune responses (Mantovani et al., 1976a,b; Vecchi et al., 1976). They found, under the conditions examined, that ADM, when compared to daunoru-bicin, was more suppressive to primary humoral responses against SRBC and was less suppressive to primary humoral responses against a T-independent antigen or a tumor allograft, as well as secondary responses against SRBC. Similarly, they found that ADM-treated tumor-allografted mice had higher lev-els of cell-mediated cytotoxicity (CMC) in cells from the peritoneal cavity but not in those from the spleen. The ADCC activity of spleen cells from mice treated with ADM or daunorubicin was, in general, similar to controls. Finally, they examined the effects of these agents on total spleen cellularity and on spleen cell subpopulations. Daunorubicin induced a faster and longer-lasting cell depletion than ADM. The depletion appeared to be the consequence of a relatively general cytotoxic effect since the percentage of T cells and Fc receptor-positive cells was similar in the treated and untreated mice; however, they did observe an appar-ent sparing of macrophages from this cytotoxic effect.

Thus, the possibility, originally suggested by Schwartz and Grindey (1973), that differences in the immunodepressive activity between the two analogs could contribute to the increased efficacy of ADM appeared to be supported by the demonstrated quantitative and qualitative differences in the effects of the two agents on various immune response test systems. Following the establish-ment of this correlation, there have been, over the last 6 years, a large variety of in-depth studies investigating ADM–host defense interactions. As a conse-quence of these studies, it has become apparent that ADM is not only immu-nosuppressive but, in fact, has selective immunoaugmenting properties.

4.2. MODULATION OF HUMORAL RESPONSES

As mentioned above, the early studies indicated that ADM inhibited or had little effect on humoral responses against either SRBC or tumor allograft (Orsini and Mihich, 1975; Mantovani et al., 1976a,b; Vecchi et al., 1976). Dimitrov et al. (1978, 1979) demonstrated that both non-tumor-bearing mice and tumor-bearing mice that had been treated with ADM 3 days before challenge with SRBC devel-oped augmented direct and indirect plaque-forming cell (PFC) responses. Mihich and co-workers (Tomazic et al., 1981; Ehrke et al., 1983) reevaluated ADM-induced effects on the humoral response in a tumor allograft system and confirmed that under conditions of near-optimal response, ADM treatment of the mice either before (day −3, −1, or 0) or after (day +1, +2, or +4) tumor challenge inhibited the response. When the dose of antigen used for challenge was varied, however, they found that under conditions where the level of the control response was low, an ADM-induced augmentation of the humoral re-

sponse could be seen if the animals had been treated with drug on day -9, -7, or -5 (Tomazic et al., 1981; Ehrke et al., 1983). Similarly, Cohen et al. (1980) demonstrated that the addition of low concentrations (10^{-9} to 10^{-8} M) of ADM to primary anti-SRBC/PFC cultures augments the number of direct PFC that develop. They also evaluated the effect of varying the time of ADM treatment of mice on the level of PFC that would develop in culture (Ehrke et al., 1983). It was found that following day -3 treatment, augmented numbers of PFC developed; following day -9 or -1 treatment, reduced numbers of PFC developed; and following day -7 or -5, essentially control levels were observed. The importance of antigen dose was also demonstrated in these studies in that, under conditions that produced a high control response, day -5 treatment resulted in reduced response, while under conditions that produced a lower control response, day -5 treatment had little effect. Thus, ADM-induced immunomodulation of humoral response was demonstrable under defined conditions.

4.3. MODULATION OF CELL-MEDIATED LYTIC RESPONSES

The term cell-mediated lytic activity is considered by some to encompass the classically immunospecific activity of the CTL that develop in response to antigenic challenge, as well as NK and tumoricidal macrophage activities for which specificity in the classical sense cannot be ascribed at this time. Studies have been carried out to investigate ADM-induced effects on each of these cellular host defense systems.

4.3.1. Augmented CTL Development

As noted above, Mantovani et al. (1976a,b) reported that animals treated with ADM (15 mg/kg) 24 hr before tumor allograft implantation developed higher levels of CMC activity in the peritoneal cavity (but not in the spleen) than did mice treated with daunorubicin. While on a per cell basis the level of CMC activity attained at either site in the ADM-treated mice was similar to control levels, the marked decrease in cellularity at both sites induced by the dose of drug used resulted in a considerably lower total cytotoxic activity in terms of lytic units per mouse.

Mihich and co-workers (Orsini et al., 1977) found that spleen cells from mice treated with a somewhat lower dose (5 mg/kg) of ADM, 5 or 3 days before but not 1 day before challenge in culture with alloantigen, developed augmented CTL activity. This finding was the first suggestion that ADM may interact in a selective manner with cell functions involved in the immune response and lead to its modulation. On the basis of histological and cell separation studies, it was suggested that the cells selectively affected by ADM might be progenitors of cytotoxic T cells and/or macrophage (accessory) cells (Orsini et al., 1977).

Tomazic et al. (1980) reported that increased CTL activity was also demonstrable if ADM (0.1 μM) was added directly to the primary allogeneic response culture 24 hr before, at the same time as, or as late as 48 hr after antigen. The effect seen, however, was dependent on culture conditions; when the response was low, ADM augmented the response, but when the response was near optimal, ADM inhibited it. The ADM-induced effects were found to be associated with a silica-resistant or plastic-nonadherent population of cells. Since these populations, in the presence of ADM, could develop normal levels of CTL activity, it was suggested that ADM effects led to the replacement of the accessory cell function of the silica-sensitive, plastic-adherent, mature macrophage (Ehrke *et al.*, 1982).

Utilizing the accumulated information concerning the experimental conditions that affected the observed ADM-induced immunomodulations, Mihich and co-workers (Tomazic *et al.*, 1981; Ehrke *et al.*, 1982, 1983) examined its effects on the host defense mechanisms in a tumor allograft system. As mentioned above, augmentation or inhibition of the humoral response was seen in this model dependent on antigen dose and time between drug treatment and antigen challenge. Similarly, when alloantigen challenge was varied so that a less than optimal response occurred, mice pretreated with ADM (5 mg/kg) 5 days before allograft implantation developed augmented levels of CTL activity in both spleen and PEC populations. When the response was near optimal, ADM treatment did not affect CTL development. Evaluation of the dependence of effects on CTL development upon time of ADM (5 mg/kg) administration relative to tumor allografting on day 0, indicated that treatment on day -13, -11, -7, or -5 resulted in augmented response, treatment on day -15, -9, or -3 did not significantly affect the response, and only treatment on day -1 inhibited the response (Ehrke *et al.*, 1983). In addition, if mice that had received ADM on the various days were killed on day 0 and their spleen cells challenged in culture with alloantigen, a very similar kinetics of dependence on time of drug administration was seen.

Thus, ADM-induced modulation of both humoral and cellular immune responses was demonstrated under three experimental designs, namely (1) both drug addition and sensitization in culture; (2) drug administration to spleen donor mice and sensitization in culture; and (3) both drug administration and sensitization in mice. Consistent with the principles recognized in the early studies with 6-MP, the results seen were dependent on: (1) drug dose, (2) antigen dose, and (3) time between drug administration and antigen challenge. Finally, it should be noted that in general when the combination of conditions resulted in an augmented humoral response, little or no effect was seen on the cellular response, and when the cellular response was augmented, the humoral response was usually inhibited.

4.3.2. Cellular Basis of CTL Augmentation

Having established that, depending on conditions, ADM could selectively induce augmented CTL responses, investigations were initiated to determine the cellular basis of this selectivity. The model system selected was day -5 administration of the drug to the spleen donor mouse and challenge of the spleen cells in culture. This model allows all the usual pharmacokinetics of drug-host interaction to occur before the cells are removed and challenged in culture but also, since the cells are removed before stimulation, it permits the performance of experiments impossible in the animal.

It was found (Ehrke *et al.*, 1982) that, following ADM treatment, a spleen cell subset, which was nonadherent, silica insensitive, and nonphagocytic, appeared to have been modified so that there was associated with it an accessory cell function, which is usually only detected with the adherent, silica-sensitive, phagocytic cell subset from nontreated controls. This subset of cells was shown to develop, during 5 days of culture, detectable phagocytic activity (see Section 4.3.6). Thus, under conditions where mature macrophages were limited (adherent or silica-sensitive cells removed) at the time of alloantigen challenge, the cells from ADM-treated mice developed levels of CMC activity much higher than the low levels that were developed by similar subsets of cells from nontreated control mice. The levels of activity attained, however, were not greater than those attained by the unseparated spleen cells from nontreated mice. In contrast, when mature macrophages were not limited, the capability to develop an augmented level of CMC was shown to be associated with a subset of cells from ADM-treated mice that was adherent to either plastic or nylon wool. In cell separation/recombination experiments, it was found that the removal of Thy-1.2$^+$ cells from the adherent subset from ADM-treated mice had little effect on the response, whereas their removal from the adherent subset from nontreated mice resulted in elevated levels of response. This suggested that a Thy-1.2$^+$ cell, involved in the regulation of the response, was missing from or failed to develop in the ADM-treated population. Thus, ADM induced modifications in two subsets: (1) immature cells of the monocyte-macrophage lineage, which can provide accessory function, and (2) adherent, Thy-1.2-bearing cells, which cooperate in maintaining CMC activity at normal levels. It is tempting to speculate that in the latter case the cell selectively affected may be similar to the CY-sensitive, I-J$^+$ antigen-presenting cell required for Ts$_3$ activation recently described by Lowy *et al.* (1983).

4.3.3. ADM-Induced Effects on Suppressor Functions

In direct studies of ADM-induced effects on suppressor cells, Anaclerio *et al.* (1980) found that ADM significantly reduced the suppressive activity in a cell transfer system involving the humoral response of CDF$_1$ mice to SRBC challenge. In contrast, Cohen *et al.* (1980) showed that ADM addition to culture did not affect the suppression of anti-SRBC/PFC cultures by MLR- or Con A-induced supressor cells; however, it did inhibit macrophage-dependent SIRS (soluble immune response suppressor) activity. Similarly, Mihich and co-workers (Ehrke *et al.*, 1980; Ryoyama *et al.*, 1980, 1981) investigated the development during culture of cells that suppress primary CTL response cultures. They found that when cells from ADM-treated mice were used, there was a relatively small increase in the development of suppressor cell activity in two culture systems. When the activity of the culture-induced suppressor cells was compared in primary CTL cultures utilizing spleen cells from ADM-treated or nontreated mice as responding cells, however, it was found that the ADM-treated cells were relatively insensitive to suppression. Thus, these findings suggest that ADM may have little or no direct effect on suppressor cells but may modulate the sensitivity of the other subsets to suppressor cell or suppressor factor activity.

4.3.4. ADM Modulation of Soluble Mediators

Other evidence, gained primarily in studies of conditioned medium (CM) from cultures of cells from ADM-treated and nontreated mice, has also indicated that soluble mediators may be affected as a consequence of ADM treatment (Ehrke *et al.*, 1980, 1982). CM from cultures of spleen cells from mice treated with ADM 5 days (ADM-CM) but not 1 day before sacrifice has nearly twice the concentration of PGE_2 as does CM from nontreated spleen cells (N-CM) (S. A. Cohen, personal communication). Studies utilizing indomethacin indicate that the difference in the levels of PGE_2 produced, however, does not seem to correlate with effects on developing CTL activity but may be relevant in NK activity studies (see Section 4.3.5). The responsiveness of primary CTL cultures whose ability to respond had been abrogated by either silica treatment or use of heat-treated (45°C, 60 min) alloantigen could be restored by the addition of ADM-CM but not N-CM (Ehrke *et al.*, 1982). Further, ADM-CM, but not N-CM, was shown to be able to maintain long-term CTL cultures. Thus, these findings are consistent with increased IL-2 production by spleen cells from ADM-treated mice. This is further supported by the fact that spleen cells from ADM-treated mice can develop CTL in response to heat-treated alloantigen whereas nontreated spleen cells require an exogenous source of IL-2 in order to respond (Ehrke *et al.*, 1980, 1982). Also, the relative insensitivity to suppression of cells from ADM-treated mice and their suggested increased IL-2 production are consistent with the proposal of Smith *et al.* (1979) that the level of suppression observed in culture may be the result of a competition for endogenous IL-2 between responding and suppressing cells. Despite these apparent correlations, it is not clear at this time whether the increased IL-2 production is a primary ADM-induced effect or secondary to ADM-induced modulations of cells of the macrophage lineage that may result in increased IL-1 production. In fact, when CM from cultures of PEC from ADM-treated mice was examined, significant levels of IL-1-"like" but no IL-2 activity was found (Salazar and Cohen, 1983). Thus, again, the effects seen may be the consequence of selective effects on the monocyte-macrophage cell type.

4.3.5. Modulation of NK Activity

Initial reports indicated that ADM did not affect NK activity (Mantovani *et al.*, 1978; Djeu *et al.*, 1979). Subsequent detailed studies by two groups have indicated, however, that ADM can, depending on conditions, inhibit or augment NK activity (Santoni *et al.*, 1980; Ehrke *et al.*, 1982). A single i.p. injection of ADM results in a rapid increase of NK cytolytic activity by PEC. In contrast to the stimulatory effect on PEC, ADM administration (either i.p. or i.v.) can result in reduced NK activity in the spleen. Santoni et al. (1980) found that the reduction peaked 3 days after drug treatment with rapid recovery thereafter. The depressed NK activity could be reversed by removal of adherent cells, and in cell-mixing experiments, plastic-adherent spleen cells from ADM-treated mice, but not from nontreated mice, inhibited the NK activity of normal spleen cells. In contrast, little difference was found in the NK activity of spleen cells from nontreated mice or from mice treated with ADM on day −5 when assayed on day 0 (Ehrke et al., 1982); however, if the cells were cultured for 5 days, those from the ADM-treated mice had a reduced NK activity. If indomethacin was added at the initiation of culture, the NK activity of both populations was increased and the levels attained were essentially equal. Additionally, CM from cultures of spleen cells from ADM-treated mice also suppressed the NK activity of spleen cells from nontreated mice and these CM have been shown to have increased levels of PGE_2 (see above). The suggestion, therefore, that the reduced NK activity is the consequence of this PGE_2 production was made and is consistent with the observation that the activity of NK cells appears to be subjected to considerable regulation by macrophages (Cudkowicz and Hochman, 1979; Santoni et al., 1980) and their soluble factors (Santoni et al., 1980; Brunda et al., 1980).

4.3.6. Modulation of Macrophage Functions

As noted above, Orsini et al. (1977) reported histological findings indicating a relative increase in cells of the monocyte-macrophage lineage in the spleens of mice 3 to 5 days following ADM (5 mg/kg) treatment. At nearly the same time, Mantovani and co-workers reported the relative sparing of macrophages from the cytotoxic effects of ADM in the mouse (Mantovani et al., 1976a) and in culture (Mantovani, 1977).

In subsequent studies (Ehrke et al., 1980; Cohen et al., 1982), the ADM-induced modulations of cells of the macrophage lineage have been evaluated by assessing drug effects on the mature macrophage function of phagocytizing opsonized SRBC (Fc-dependent phagocytosis). When spleen cells were exposed to 4–10 μM concentrations of ADM for short periods of time (4–6 hr), inhibition of phagocytosis was seen (Ehrke et al., 1978; Facchinetti et al., 1978; Cohen et al., 1980). In contrast, cells exposed to a lower concentration (0.1 μM ADM) for 4 days in culture have increased levels of phagocytic activity compared to those of cells from control cultures (Ehrke et al., 1982). No difference in phagocytic activity was observed with spleen cells from nontreated mice or mice treated with ADM (5 mg/kg) on day −5 when assayed on day 0; however, after 5 days in culture, increased activity was seen with the spleen cells from ADM-treated mice (Ehrke et al., 1980; Cohen et al., 1982). When mature macrophages were removed before the 5-day culture period either by 24-hr silica treatment (followed by its removal) or by plastic-adherence separation, the remaining spleen cell population from nontreated mice had no detectable phagocytic activity before or after culture. In contrast, while the corresponding populations from ADM-treated mice had no detectable phagocytic activity before culture, after culture they had a phagocytic activity essentially equivalent to that obtained with unseparated spleen cell populations from nontreated mice (Cohen *et al.*, 1982; Ehrke *et al.*, 1982). Thus, ADM treatment of mice appears to result in an increase in the number of nonphagocytic, nonadherent, immature macrophages in the spleen 5 days later and these cells can mature during subsequent culture.

The following points can be added in support of this interpretation: (1) when silica was added to the cultures on day 4 (24 hr before assay), the phagocytic activities of spleen cells from both ADM-treated and nontreated mice were completely abrogated; (2) when cells from ADM-treated and nontreated mice were separated on the basis of plastic adherence after culture the phagocytic activity was found to be associated with plastic-adherent cells and while on a per cell basis their phagocytic activities were equivalent to those of control cells, there were twice as many adherent cells in the cultures from ADM-treated mice (Cohen *et al.*, 1982); and (3) as indicated above (Section 4.3.2), these silica-insensitive, plastic-nonadherent cells were capable of supplying accessory cell function (a function thought to be associated with mature macrophages) during primary CTL response cultures (Ehrke *et al.*, 1982).

The possible *in vivo* relevance of these observations is suggested by the fact that the phagocytic activity of spleen cells from mice treated with ADM on day -9, -11, or -13 is augmented compared to that of spleen cells from nontreated mice when assayed on day 0 (Cohen *et al.*, 1982). Thus, the time-dependent maturation of a subset of cells that was shown to occur during 4 or 5 days in culture may have an *in vivo* counterpart.

ADM-induced effects on macrophage tumoricidal activity have also been evaluated. Stoychkov *et al.* (1979) found that peritoneal macrophages from mice treated with ADM (10 mg/kg, i.p. or s.c.) 1 day earlier were as cytotoxic for MBL-2 lymphoblastoid leukemia cells as were cells from mice treated with 10^4 U of purified mouse fibroblast interferon. The effect was ADM-dose dependent (10 mg/kg > 5 mg/kg > 2.5 mg/kg) and time dependent, in that cells obtained 4 days or later after treatment were not tumoricidal. Facchinetti *et al.* (1978) had reported assessing, by fluorescence microscopy, the accumulation of ADM within the nucleus of macrophages exposed to drug *in vitro*. Haskill (1981) combined these two approaches and found that macrophages displaying ADM-induced tumor-cytostatic activity in the peritoneal exudate paralleled the presence of macrophages exhibiting red fluorescent cytoplasmic particles. He found the same time dependence that Stoychkov *et al.* (1979) had reported. He also observed that the ADM-stimulated macrophages caused HeLa cell growth inhibition in a manner similar to free ADM and not like C. *parvum*-stimulated macrophages. Finally, whereas four freeze–thaw cycles destroy the activity of C. *parvum*-activated macrophages, they did not affect the activity of the ADM-stimulated macrophage preparation. He concluded, therefore, that drug retention may be the predominant effector mechanism involved in the ADM-activated tumoricidal macrophage phenomeonon.

Martin *et al.* (1982) found that peritoneal macrophages from rats collected 24 hr after an i.p. injection of ADM (10 mg/kg) were cytotoxic to syngeneic cancer cells; such an activity was not elicited by incubation of peritoneal macrophages with ADM over a large range of concentrations for 1–24 hr. They observed, as had been reported by Facchinetti *et al.* (1978) for mice, that rat macrophages exposed to ADM *in vitro* accumulated the drug in their nuclei, whereas the macrophages exposed to ADM in the rat accumulated it in cytoplasmic vacuoles, as Haskill (1981) had reported for mice. Examination of peritoneal cells at time points early after ADM administration to the rat indicated that while all cells had nuclear fluorescence, ADM appeared to accumulate in mast cell granules and that macrophages phagocytized AM-containing granules from degranulating mast cells. Based on these observations, they exposed mast cells to ADM *in vitro* and found that subsequently these ADM mast cells induced macrophages *in vitro* to become cytotoxic. Finally, they observed that ADM fluorescence appeares in the nuclei of tumor cells following their incubation with *in vivo* ADM-exposed macrophages that contained fluorescent cytoplasmic particles.

These findings, taken together, are consistent with the hypothesis that the role of ADM-induced tumoricidal macrophages may be a relatively passive one of concentrating drug (with the help of mast cells) and transferring it into the tumor cell. While this seems possible during the first few days after drug administration within the further restrictions of i.p. drug, i.p. effector cells, and i.p. tumor, there are certain lines of evidence that suggest that ADM may induce macrophages to play a more active tumoricidal role. Stoychkov *et al.* (1979) reported that s.c. administration of ADM was as effective as i.p. administration in inducing tumoricidal activity in peritoneal macrophages 1 day later and the dose dependency seen was similar for both inoculation sites. It is difficult to reconcile these findings with the suggestion that the transfer, to the target tumor cells, of drug concentrated within the peritoneal macrophages is the sole mechanism involved. Since the s.c. route of administration was not tested in any of the subsequent studies, this, however, is a moot point. Kleinerman *et al.* (1982), using a culture system to study the generation of spontaneous monocyte-mediated cytotoxicity in human cells, found a time-dependent augmented development of cytolytic activity in cells that had been exposed to ADM (1 μM) for 15 min prior to culture (free drug was washed away before culture). Neither control nor drug-exposed cells had cytolytic activity after 2 days of culture and while both had activity on days 3, 4, and 7, the cells exposed to ADM had greater activity than controls at each time point. The target cells in these studies were ^{51}Cr-labeled chicken RBC and despite the authors' statement that the monocyte effector cell capable of lysing tumor targets develops under these same culture conditions, no information concerning ADM-induced effects with tumor targets was given. Nevertheless, since following the 15-min exposure to drug the cells did not become cytotoxic until 3 days later, these results would suggest that the ADM-induced regulation of this spontaneous monocyte-mediated cytotoxicity probably occurs by a mechanism other than drug transfer. This possibility is further supported by the fact that the lysis of the targets was not affected by their prior exposure to free drug and the fact that cultures that received ADM-treated cells did not have decreased viability, which might have been expected if a phenomenon similar to the mast cell degranulation and disappearance reported by Martin *et al.* (1982) had occurred. Further, Salazar and Cohen (1983) have recently demonstrated, by quantitative spectrofluorometry, that, while peritoneal cells from mice 1 day after i.p. ADM administration do contain concentrations of drug sufficient to be cytotoxic for P815 tumor cells in an 18-hr assay, cells from mice 5 and 7 days after ADM administration do not, but all three populations are equally cytolytic for the P815 targets. They also found that, in response to PMA, peritoneal cells from mice 1, 3, or 5 days after ADM administration produced 6–10 times the concentration of superoxide anion as was produced by cells from control mice and suggest the possibility of the involvement of active oxygen species with ADM-induced tumoricidal macrophage activity (see Volume 2 of this series for reviews of oxidative metabolism and macrophage function). Finally, Hisano and Fidler (1982) found that 14 days but not 7 days after i.v. administration of ADM (15 mg/kg), alveolar macrophages had tumoricidal activity, again a time dependency suggesting a cytocidal mechanism other than drug transfer. They also found that, as had been reported earlier by Mantovani et al. (1980) with BCG, ADM did not affect the ability of the macrophage to be activated to a tumoricidal state in situ by a derivative of MDP, which again indicates the relative ADM-insensitivity of mature macrophages.

Thus, ADM has been shown to induce modulations in populations of cells of the monocyte-macrophage lineage localized in spleen, lungs, or the peritoneal cavity. The question of macrophages being activated to tumoricidal activity by ADM as opposed to serving as a drug depot and transfer vehicle remains to be clarified. As will be indicated in the following section, however, there is evidence that macrophages may play a pivotal role in determining the final outcome of ADM administration in various syngeneic tumor–host models.

4.4. ADM AND HOST ANTITUMOR DEFENSES

Mantovani et al. (1979a,b,c) utilized three tumors having different immunogenic characteristics to evaluate ADM effects in vivo on host antitumor defenses. The tumor lines used were the poorly immunogenic L1210Cr leukemia, the immunogenic SL2 lymphoma, and the strongly immunogenic L1210Ha leukemia. In confirmation of earlier studies (Schwartz and Grindey, 1973; Giuliani et al., 1974), ADM antitumor efficacy was greater in the model with the greatest potential for host antitumor response. Thus, in the strongly immunogenic L1210Ha leukemia system, ADM (10 mg/kg, day 1) treatment produced 45% cures with a mean percent ILS of 150, whereas in the SL2 and L1210Cr tumor systems the mean percent ILS was 85 and 42, respectively, with cures of only 10% in the former and none in the latter. These differences were abolished if 5 days prior to tumor implantation the mice had received an immunodepressive dose of DTIC [5-(3,3-dimethyl-1-triazeno) imidazole-4-carboxamide]. Similarly, ADM treatment of L1210Ha leukemia in thymus-deprived mice was markedly less effective than in thymus-intact mice. Using the DTIC-resistant L1210Ha leukemia, they also were able to show that administration of an immunodepressive dose of DTIC as late as 10 days, but not 20 days, after tumor inoculation (day 0) significantly reduced the number of cures induced by ADM treatment (10 or 8 mg/kg, day 1). This suggests the persistence of viable L1210Ha cells for at least 9 days after ADM treatment and that these cells were capable of growing and killing the host if the host immune responses were inhibited. Finally, the animals cured of L1210Ha leukemia by ADM treatment were reported to be resistant to a second challenge with 10^5 L1210Ha cells. These findings, therefore, further support the importance of host antitumor defenses to the antineoplastic effectiveness of ADM and suggest a requirement for thymus-dependent cells.

Mantovani *et al.* (1979a,b,c) also evaluated the possible role macrophages play in the antitumor effectiveness of ADM by utilizing the macrophage toxins silica and carrageenan. Silica administration to the mice on days −2 and 0 or on days 0 and 2, but not at earlier or later times, markedly reduced ADM therapeutic effectiveness in the L1210Ha leukemia and SL2 lymphoma systems but did not alter the effects of ADM against the nonimmunogenic L1210Cr leukemia. Similar findings were obtained with carrageenan. Further, macrophages obtained from L1210Ha leukemia-inoculated ADM-cured mice were, by morphological criteria, activated and were able to inhibit the growth and the DNA synthesis of unrelated tumors *in vitro*.

Riccardi *et al.* (1979) reported that mice lethally irradiated 5–6 hr before tumor inoculation and assayed 3 days later displayed significant tumor growth inhibitory activity in syngeneic as well as allogeneic tumor–host combinations if they had been pretreated with ADM. This ADM-induced antitumor response was dependent on drug dose and independent of its route of administration. The fact that it was detectable 5, 15, or 30 days after drug administration indicated that it was not due to direct antitumor action by the drug. In fact, a crucial role for phagocytic cells in this ADM-induced response was suggested when antimacrophage agents (silica or carrageenan) were shown to abrogate the antitumor activity, and consequently the involvement of ADM-activated tumoricidal macrophages was postulated.

In another series of studies also involving ADM pretreatment of mice followed by inoculation (s.c.) of syngeneic lymphoma, Ehrke *et al.* (1981, 1982) found significant inhibition of tumor growth, both in terms of wet weights of tumor and increased survival time. A correlation was demonstrated between these findings and the antitumor activity of spleen cells from similarly treated mice in that the spleen cells from the ADM-treated EL4 lymphoma-bearing mice developed augmented levels of CTL activity in response to rechallenge with the lymphoma in culture and caused significant tumor neutralization in a Winn assay. Finally, the migration of EL4 cells to the spleen from the site of the s.c. inoculation was inhibited in the mice that had been treated with ADM. The probable involvement of cells of the monocyte-macrophage lineage was implied when these findings were considered together with the demonstrated ADM-induced modulations of the immature macrophage population (see Section 4.3.6) and the reported role macrophages can play in control of metastatic disease (Eccles, 1978; Fidler, 1980).

The results of a series of studies evaluating combination chemo-immunotherapy with ADM and a number of nonspecific immunostimulants in various experimental tumor systems are also consistent with the hypothesis that mono-cyte-macrophage cells play a key role in ADM-induced effects. Houchens *et al.* (1976) showed that the combination of ADM and the macrophage-activating agent *C. parvum* was better than either alone in increasing the life span of mice with P388 leukemia or Lewis lung carcinoma but was ineffective in nude mice, suggesting a possible T-cell requirement. Tagliabue *et al.* (1977) evaluated ADM, CY, and 5-fluorouracil in combination with *C. parvum*, BCG, and levamisole against L1210Ha leukemia and found ADM–*C. parvum* the most active combina-tion. They found that the antitumor activity was dependent on dose of ADM and on time between ADM and *C. parvum* administration, a 5-day interval resulting in maximal activation. These findings were confirmed and extended by similar observations in the SL2 lymphoma systems (Mantovani *et al.*, 1979b). The strict time dependency of the effects seen was confirmed and it was found that when assessed 6 days after *C. parvum* administration, splenic macrophages from mice that had received ADM 5 days before *C. parvum* had greater tumoricidal activity than those that had not. The correlations between the time dependency of these events and those described by Cohen *et al.* (1982; see Section 4.3.6) for the appearance of immature macrophages and their maturation in the spleen following ADM treatment of mice are apparent.

In conclusion, while it is clear that a great deal concerning ADM immu-noregulatory potential remains to be understood, considerable progress has been made. The relatively tenuous nature of any single line of evidence present-ed as to a probable primary role of cells of the monocyte-macrophage lineage in ADM-induced effects is offset by the preponderance of evidence from the many experimental designs suggesting the same conclusion. The T cell dependency of certain observations has been suggested but it is not clear at this time whether modulations of T-cell functions are a primary ADM-induced effect or are second-ary to ADM-induced modulation of immature macrophages. Further confusing this issue is the fact that T cells and/or their products may provide obligatory signals involved in macrophage regulation.

Finally, as indicated at the beginning, a consensus has not been reached as to the determinants of antitumor selectivity of the anthracyclines; nevertheless, the areas being currently evaluated, namely membrane interactions, oxidation–reduction properties (free radical formation), and DNA damage, all are potential determinants of immunoregulation.

5. VINCA ALKALOIDS

5.1. BACKGROUND

The vinca alkaloids [vincristine (VCR) and vinblastine (vincaleukoblastin, VLB)] provide a slightly different example than those cited heretofore, in that the study of immunoregulation by these two chemically similar agents may not only provide information of an immunopharmacological nature but also infor-mation critical to the understanding of a basis for the considerable differences in their biological activities. Although VLB and VCR differ structurally only at a single carbon moiety (methyl versus formyl), they appear to differ broadly in many of their activities. For instance, whereas both drugs have been reported to induce useful responses in broad spectrums of human cancers, they differ markedly in their clinical application. In fact, in combination with other agents, VCR is the first-line therapy for induction of remission in childhood and adult acute lymphoblastic leukemia and for non-Hodgkin's lymphomas, whereas VLB is the indicated treatment of Hodgkin's disease and some solid tumors such as non-seminomatous cancer of the testes. The vinca alkaloids also vary in the frequency and severity of the toxic side effects they produce. The dose-limiting toxicities with VCR are neurological and neuromuscular, whereas with VLB they are hematological, primarily leukopenia (Creasey, 1975).

It has proven impossible, as of yet, to reconcile the structural similarity of the two vinca alkaloids with their quite different biological actions. This problem has been further complicated by the realization that the differential actions of the vinca alkaloids must be based on some biological process other than their reaction with tubulin or the microtubules *per se* (Himes *et al.*, 1976). In fact, their actions on brain microtubules *in vivo* and tubulin *in vitro* are quite similar. Their rate of binding to tubulin (equilibrium attained in less than 5 min) and the affinity of this binding (VCR, $K_a = 8 \times 10^6$; VLB, $K_a = 6 \times 10^6$ liters/mole) are examples of this similarity (Owellen *et al.*, 1972). Consistent with this is also the suggestion that their antitumor (cytotoxic) effect cannot be directly linked to their antimitotic activity (Schreck, 1974). This was based, in part, on the fact that inhibition of formation of the mitotic spindle and arrest of the cell division in metaphase occurs *in vivo* at dose levels that do not affect tumors. Further, there are the reports that VCR preferentially destroys stationary populations of human lymphoid cells (Rosner *et al.*, 1973) or Chinese hamster cells (Olah *et al.*, 1978) growing in long-term or plateau-phase cultures. The studies of the effects of vinca alkaloids on hemopoietic precursor cells have also indicated, where data are available for comparison, that their effects, at least in rodents, are entirely similar (Marsh, 1976).

Beer and co-workers (Gout *et al.*, 1978) have shown that in rats, following i.p. administration of tritium-labeled agents, the level of VLB in the blood rose much more rapidly than that of VCR but it also fell much more rapidly and these distribution patterns correlated with the binding of the agents to platelets. In parallel experiments, in culture, they showed similar differences in the uptake and retention of the two vinca alkaloids by platelets, by cells isolated from a sensitive rat lymphoma, or by L5178Y cells. Of particular interest is the fact that while *in vitro* cells isolated from the rat lymphoma release VLB rapidly, in the animal the lymphoma retains the alkaloid long after the level of VLB in the circulation has fallen (R. L. Noble *et al.*, 1977). Thus, in a sensitive target tissue in the animal, the pharmacokinetics of VLB resembles that of VCR.

While the pharmacokinetic distributions of VLB and VCR in the blood and their binding by cells are surely important variables mediating their toxic and oncolytic effects, it is difficult to reconcile the differences in the latter with information available on the former. For instance, VLB, when compared to VCR, attains a significantly higher blood level that is maintained over the first 6 hr and this would be consistent with the induction of leukopenia by VLB but not necessarily with the advantage VCR is shown to have in remission induction in acute leukemia.

5.2. IMMUNOMODULATION

Recently, differences in the effects of VCR and VLB on immune responses have been described and it can be suggested that information obtained in this area about some of their unique selective effects may contribute to the elucidation of the basis of their different biological actions.

The immunosuppressive effects of the vinca alkaloids were reported by Aisenberg and Wilkes (1964). They found in rats, using BSA as antigen, that the vinca alkaloids not only inhibit antibody formation, delayed hypersensitivity development, and homograft rejection but also suppress established delayed hypersensitivity. Since that time, there have been reports of vinca alkaloid effects in other immune systems, but unfortunately few of these studies directly compared the two vinca alkaloids.

In studies in which VLB was administered to mice before, at the same time as (Syeklocha et al., 1966), or after (Romanycheva et al., 1978) SRBC, a time-dependent inhibition of PFC formation was observed. It was suggested (Romanycheva et al., 1978) that VLB did not prevent the recruitment of precursor cells into PFC but that the utlimate decrease in PFC numbers was due to "unbalanced growth" induced by the cytostatic agent. Under the conditions of their studies, however, these investigators did not observe any increase in PFC. In contrast, Shek and Coons (1978) found that the administration of VLB at the same time as antigen resulted in augmented hapten-specific PFC response and suggested the inhibition of suppressor cell development as the mechanism.

Bartocci et al. (1980) have reported that the in vitro generation of B10-A cytotoxic lymphocytes against irradiated B10 spleen cells is augmented or inhibited depending on: (1) dose of VCR administered to responder spleen donor mice or (2) concentrations of VCR added to the sensitization culture. Further, they reported (Riccardi et al., 1980) a large percentage of long-term survivors among mice, which had received a single dose of VCR 3 days after being inoculated with tumor cells incompatible at multiple minor histocompatibility loci. VCR did not have the same effect in F_1 (histocompatible) hosts although there was some increase in MST. They found that the antitumor efficacy of VCR was markedly reduced in preirradiated (immunodepressed) hosts, suggesting that VCR increased the antilymphoma graft response, rather than producing direct cytotoxic effects on the tumor. Kataoka et al. (1981) identified a tumor vaccine-induced macrophage suppressor cell and showed that VLB may preferentially inhibit its production. When mice received VLB together with the second of two tumor vaccine injections, significant numbers survived subsequent inoculation of live tumor cells, whereas those receiving either VLB or vaccine alone did not survive.

Orsini *et al.* (1980) found that VCR and VLB inhibited the development of primary cell-mediated immunity of C57BL/6 spleen cells against X-irradiated allogeneic P815 tumor cells (P815x) in culture. A clear concentration and time of addition dependency was shown. A positive correlation was found between results obtained in culture and those obtained in a comparable CMC response in a primary immunization system in C57BL/6 mice. In the *in vivo* system, the vinca alkaloids were given on day 0 or +2 with respect to antigen inoculation. Their effects on the CMC response and on the antibody-mediated complement-dependent cellular cytotoxic (CDCC) responses were determined. The data suggested that there is a difference in the sensitivity of the humoral and cellular responses to the two alkaloids, VLB being more suppressive to the CMC and VCR to the CDCC. Of equal interest was an early (day 7) augmentation of the CMC by VCR administration on day 0 and an augmentation (day 6 and 7) of the CDCC by VLB administration on day 0.

In order to obtain further insight into the possible differences between the effects of VLB and VCR on humoral and cellular immune responses of spleen cells from C57BL/6 mice, Mihich and co-workers (Ryoyama *et al.*, 1982) examined, in parallel, the effects of these agents on three parameters in culture, namely (1) suppressor T-cell development, (2) CMC response against P815x, and (3) anti-SRBC/PFC responses. When the alkaloids were given to the spleen donor mice 24 hr before sacrifice, 3 or 1 mg/kg VLB (1/2 or 1/6 LD_{10} dose) caused inhibition of development of suppressor T-cell activity in culture and the LD_{10} or 1/2 LD_{10} dose of VLB also reduced the level of CMC activity that developed in culture at all R:S ratios tested except 5:1. In contrast, VCR, at doses lower than 3 mg/kg (LD_{10}), had no effect on suppressor cell development or CMC development in culture. Furthermore, when the alkaloids were added at equimolar concentrations directly to the culture, even though they appeared equally toxic in terms of viable cell recoveries, VLB inhibited suppressor T-cell development whereas VCR did not and VLB was also more inhibitory to CMC development. VCR was, however, significantly more inhibitory to PFC development than VLB at equimolar concentrations. These findings are consistent with those obtained *in vivo* and suggest that VCR selectively affects B-cell functions and that VLB selectively affects T-cell functions. While under the conditions of these studies no augmentation of CMC was seen when the alkaloids were added directly to the cultures, augmentation was seen when spleen cells from pretreated mice were cultured at R:S ratios of 5:1. The augmentation was greater following pretreatment with VLB than with VCR.

Thus, immunoregulation is another biologically relevant area in which these two vinca alkaloids appear to differ in their activities. The investigation of the possible relevance of the divergence of their selective immunoregulatory properties to their respective applications in different neoplastic diseases may be an area in which future investigation will yield fruitful insights. Furthermore, the fact that two such structurally similar analogs that have apparently very similar reactions with tubulin (thought to be their mechanism of biological activity) affect immune responses so differently suggests their possible utility as probes in immunoregulatory studies.

6. CONCLUDING REMARKS

The examples of drug-induced effects on immunoregulation that have been discussed provide evidence for the potential utility of using antineoplastic agents as probes in basic studies of immunoregulation and suggest opportunities for the improved utilization of such drugs in chemoimmunotherapy.

In general, antineoplastic agents are considered to be cytotoxic in their antitumor and toxic effects. Questions should be asked, therefore, as to whether the immunomodulating effects of some of these agents are also due to their cytotoxicity. This possibility would be consistent with the majority of the experimental data indicating the dependence of CY-induced immunoregulation on the elimination of cells involved in the development of suppression. This possibility would not necessarily be compatible, however, with findings such as those indicating a probable correlation between ADM-induced immunoregulation and the appearance of a population of immature cells differentiating into macrophages. Indeed, it may be suggested that the cellular events that are responsible for a drug-induced immunoregulatory response are, in general, more selective in their occurrence than the events usually associated with the drug's lethal toxicity. It may be reasonable to postulate that certain anticancer agents exert effects on immunoregulation not only through the selective inhibition or elimination of critical cell types and/or functions but also through mechanisms similar to those involved in the effects on cell differentiation and maturation recently demonstrated for some of these agents (Lotem and Sachs, 1980; Takeda et al., 1982). Indeed, differentiation of cells and functions is pivotal in the regulation and development of the immune response.

The differences in immunomodulation between two such closely related active agents as the vinca alkaloids may depend on determinants of selectivity expressed in the target cell. A multiplicity of cellular phenomena, either pharmacological or immunological in nature, are operative within the many intra- and interregulatory circuits that form the complex network of the immune response and are likely to affect selectivity of drug action. Following antigen challenge, a cascade of positive and negative signals involving both direct cell-to-cell interactions and interactions between cells and cellular products must occur in a defined sequence within rather stringent time restraints. Even a seemingly small perturbation in this cascade of effects could result in a manyfold alteration at the effector level of the response. The constraints related to the timing of drug administration with respect to antigenic stimulus, the dose of drug used, the dose of antigen given, and the nature of the immune response assayed, which were demonstrated in the early studies and which have been repeatedly confirmed, are consistent with the suggestion that the determinants of selectivity in immunomodulation reside primarily within target cells.

Future investigations into the selective sensitivity of target cells to drugs should contribute further to the understanding of the intricate patterns of the regulation of the immune response. Moreover, the application of the information thus acquired to the design of experimental therapy would aid in the ultimate development of optimal remission maintenance treatments that may provide distinctive therapeutic advantages in the clinic.

REFERENCES

Aisenberg, A. C., and Wilkes, B., 1964, Studies on the suppression of immune responses by the periwinkle alkaloids vincristine and vinblastine, *J. Clin. Invest.* **43**:2394.

Akiyama, J., Kawamura, T., Gotohda, E., Yamada, Y., Hosokawa, M., Kodama, T., and Kobayashi, H., 1977, Immunochemotherapy of transplanted KMT-17 tumor in WKA rats by combination of cyclophosphamide and immunostimulatory protein-bound polysaccharide isolated from Basidiomycetes, *Cancer Res.* **37**:3042.

Anaclerio, A., Conti, G., Goggi, G., Honorati, M. C., Ruggeri, A., Moras, M. L., and Spreafico, F., 1980, Effect of cytotoxic agents on suppressor cells in mice, *Eur. J. Cancer* **16**:53.

Arcamone, F., 1981, *Doxorubicin Anticancer Antibiotics*, Academic Press, New York.

Askenase, P. W., Hayden, B. J., and Gershon, R. K., 1975, Augmentation of delayed-type hypersensitivity by doses of cyclophosphamide which do not affect antibody responses, *J. Exp. Med.* **141**:697.

Bach, J.-F., 1975, *The Mode of Action of Immunosuppressive Agents*, pp. 93–225, American Elsevier, New York.

Bach, M.-A., 1979, Influence of aging on T-cell subpopulations involved in the *in vitro* generation of allogeneic cytotoxicity, *Clin. Immunol. Immunopathol.* **13**:222.

Balow, J. E., Hurley, D. L., and Fauci, A. S., 1975, Cyclophosphamide suppression of established cell-mediated immunity: Quantitative vs. qualitative changes in lymphocyte populations, *J. Clin. Invest.* **56**:65.

Balow, J. E., Parrillo, J. E., and Fauci, A. S., 1977, Characterization of the direct effects of cyclophosphamide on cell-mediated immunological responses, *Immunology* **32**:899.

Bartocci, A., Riccardi, C., and Bonmassar, E., 1980, *In vivo* or *in vitro* modulating effects of vincristine on the generation of allogeneic cytotoxic lymphocytes *in vitro*, *J. Immunopharmacol.* **2**:61.

Bash, J. A., Singer, A. M., and Waksman, B. H., 1976, The suppressive effect of immunization on the proliferative responses of rat T cells *in vitro*. II. Abrogation of antigen-induced suppression by selective cytotoxic agents, *J. Immunol.* **116**:1350.

Bast, R. C., 1982, Effects of cancers and their treatment on host immunity, in: *Cancer Medicine*, (J. F. Holland and E. Frei, III, eds.), pp. 1134–1173, Lea & Febiger, Philadelphia.

Bennett, J. A., and Mitchell, M. S., 1979, Induction of suppressor cells by intravenous administration of bacillus Calmette-Guerin and its modulation by cyclophosphamide, *Biochem. Pharmacol.* **28**:1947.

Bonavida, B., 1977, Antigen-induced cyclophosphamide-resistant suppressor T cells inhibit the *in vitro* generation of cytotoxic cells from one-way mixed leukocyte reactions, *J. Immunol.* **119**:1530.

Borel, Y., and Schwartz, R. S., 1964, Inhibition of immediate and delayed hypersensitivity by 6-mercaptopurine, *J. Immunol.* **92**:754.

Borel, Y., Fauconnet, M., and Miescher, P. A., 1965, Effect of 6-mercaptopurine on different classes of antibody, *J. Exp. Med.* **122**:263.

Braciale, V. L., and Parish, C. R., 1980, Inhibition of *in vivo* antibody synthesis by cyclophosphamide-induced suppressor cells, *Cell. Immunol.* **51**:1.

Brunda, M. J., Herberman, R. B., and Holden, H. T., 1980, Inhibition of murine natural killer cell activity by prostaglandins, *J. Immunol.* **124**:2682.

Burrows, P. D., Gershon, R. K., Lawton, A. R., and Mowry, R. W., 1976, Regulation of delayed hypersensitivity (DTH) in B-cell deprived mice, *Fed. Proc.* **35**:861.

Cantor, H., McVay-Boudreau, L., Hugenberger, J., Naidorf, K., Shen, F. W., and Gershon, R. K., 1978, Immunoregulatory circuits among T-cell sets. II. Physiologic role of feedback inhibition *in vivo*: Absence in NZB mice, *J. Exp. Med.* **147**:1116.

Carswell, E. A., Old, L. J., Kassel, R. L., Green, S., Fiore, N., and Williamson, B., 1975, An endotoxin-induced serum factor that causes necrosis of tumors, *Proc. Natl. Acad. Sci. USA* **72**:3666.

Carter, S. K., 1980, The clinical evaluation of analogs. III. Anthracyclines, *Cancer Chemother. Pharmacol.* **4**:5.

Chanmougan, D., and Schwartz, R. S., 1966, Enhancement of antibody synthesis by 6-mercaptopurine, *J. Exp. Med.* **124**:363.

Chassouex, D. M., Gotch, F. M., and MacLennan, I. C. M., 1978, Analysis of synergy between cyclophosphamide therapy and immunity against a mouse tumor, *Br. J. Cancer* **38**:211.

Cheever, M. A., Greenberg, P. D., and Fefer, A., 1980, Specificity of adoptive chemoimmunotherapy of established syngeneic tumors, *J. Immunol.* **125**:711.

Cheever, M. A., Greenberg, P. D., and Fefer, A., 1981, Specific adoptive therapy of established leukemia with syngeneic lymphocytes sequentially immunized *in vivo* and *in vitro* and nonspecifically expanded by culture with interleukin 2, *J. Immunol.* **126**:1318.

Cheever, M. A., Greenberg, P. D., Fefer, A., and Gillis, S., 1982, Augmentation of the antitumor therapeutic efficacy of long-term cultured T lymphocytes by *in vivo* administration of purified interleukin 2, *J. Exp. Med.* **155**:968.

Cohen, S. A., Ehrke, M. J., and Mihich, E., 1980, Selective imbalances of cellular immune responses by Adriamycin, in: *Advances in Enzyme Regulation* (G. Weber, ed.), pp. 335–346, Pergamon Press, Elmsford, N.Y.

Cohen, S. A., Ehrke, M. J., Ryoyama, K., and Mihich, E., 1982, Augmentation of the phagocytic activity of murine spleen cell populations induced by Adriamycin, *Immunopharmacology* **5**:75.

Colvin, M., Padgett, C. A., and Fenselou, C., 1973, A biologically active metabolite of cyclophosphamide, *Cancer Res.* **33**:915.

Conners, T. A., Cox, P. J., Farmer, P. B., Foster, A. B., and Jarman, M., 1974, Some studies of the active intermediates formed in the microsomal metabolism of cyclophosphamide and isophosphamide, *Biochem. Pharmacol.* **23**:115.

Cowens, J. W., Ozer, H., Ehrke, M. J., Colvin, M., and Mihich, E., 1981, Inhibition of the development of suppressor cells in culture by 4-hydroperoxycyclophosphamide (400H-CYP), *Fed. Proc.* **40**:1096.

Creasey, W. A., 1975, Vinca alkaloids and colchicine, in: *Antineoplastic and Immunosuppressive Agents II* (A. C. Sartorelli and D. G. Johns, eds.), pp. 670–694, Springer-Verlag, Berlin.

Crooke, S. T., and Reich, S. D., 1980, *Anthracyclines: Current Status and New Developments*, Academic Press, New York.

Cudkowicz, G., and Hochman, P. S., 1979, Do natural killer cells engage in regulated reaction against self to ensure homeostasis?, *Immunol. Rev.* **44**:13.

Debre, P., Waltenbaugh, C., Dorf, M. E., and Benacerraf, B., 1976, Genetic control of specific immune suppression. IV. Responsiveness to random copolymer L-glutamic acid^{50}-L-tyrosine^{50} induced in BALB/c mice by cyclophosphamide, *J. Exp. Med.* **144**:277.

Diamantstein, T., Willinger, E., and Reiman, J., 1979, T-suppressor cells sensitive to cyclophosphamide and to its *in vitro* active derivative 4-hydroperoxycyclophosphamide control the mitogenic response of murine splenic B cells to dextran sulfate: A direct proof for different sensitivities of lymphocyte subsets to cyclophosphamide, *J. Exp. Med.* **150**:1571.

Diamantstein, T., Klos, M., Hahn, H., and Kaufmann, S. H. E., 1981, Direct *in vitro* evidence for different susceptibilities to 4-hydroperoxycyclophosphamide of antigen-primed T cells regulating humoral and cell-mediated immune responses to sheep erythrocytes: A possible explanation for the inverse action of cyclophosphamide on humoral and cell-mediated immune responses, *J. Immunol.* **126**:1717.

DiMarco, A., Gaetani, M., and Scarpinato, B., 1969, Adriamycin (NSC-123,127): A new antibiotic with antitumor activity, *Cancer Chemother. Rep.* **53**:33.

Dimitrov, N. V., Denny, T. N., and LaVigne, R., 1978, Immune responses during administration of Adriamycin and *Corynebacterium parvum*, *Clin. Immunol. Immunopathol.* **9**:177.

Dimitrov, N. V., Denny, T. N., Weisman, M. F., and Cameron, D. G., 1979, Effect of Adriamycin and *Corynebacterium parvum* in tumor-bearing mice: Modulation of response to sheep red blood cells, *J. Natl. Cancer Inst.* **63**:423.

Djeu, J. Y., Heinbaugh, J. A., Vieira, W. D., Holden, H. T., and Herberman, R. B., 1979, The effect of immunopharmacological agents on mouse natural cell-mediated cytotoxicity and on its augmentation by poly I:C, *Immunopharmacol.* **1**:231.

Drossler, K., Klima, F., and Ambrosius, H., 1981, The influence of cyclophosphamide and 6-mercaptopurine on the IgG1 and IgG2 immune response in guinea pigs, *Immunology* **44**:61.

Duclos, H., Galanaud, P., Devinsky, O., Maillot, M.-C., and Dormont, J., 1977, Enhancing effect of low dose cyclophosphamide treatment on the *in vitro* antibody response, *Eur. J. Immunol.* **7**:679.

Dye, E. S., and North, R. J., 1980, Macrophage accumulation in murine ascites tumors. I. Cytoxan-induced dominance of macrophages over tumor cells and the antitumor effect of endotoxin, *J. Immunol.* **125**:1650.

Eccles, S. A., 1978, Macrophages and cancer, in: *Immunological Aspects of Cancer* (J. E. Castro, ed.), pp. 123–145, University Park Press, Baltimore.

Ehrke, M. J., Cohen, S. A., and Mihich, E., 1978, Selectivity of inhibition by anticancer agents of mouse spleen immune effector functions involved in responses to sheep erythrocytes, *Cancer Res.* **38**:521.

Ehrke, M. J., Ryoyama, K., Tomazic, V., Cohen, S. A., and Mihich, E., 1980, Selective imbalances of cellular immune responses by Adriamycin, *Recent Results Cancer Res.* **75**:204.

Ehrke, M. J., Ryoyama, K., and Mihich, E., 1981, Generation of cytotoxic lymphocytes in cultures of spleen cells from tumor bearing mice: Modification by Adriamycin and cyclophosphamide treatment of the mice, *Proc. Am. Assoc. Cancer Res.* **22**:273.

Ehrke, M. J., Cohen, S. A., and Mihich, E., 1982, Selective effects of Adriamycin on murine host defense systems, *Immunol. Rev.* **65**:594.

Ehrke, M. J., Tomazic, V., Ryoyama, K., Cohen, S. A., and Mihich, E., 1983, Adriamycin induced immunomodulation: Dependence upon time of administration, *Int. J. Immunopharmacol.* **5**:43.

Evans, R., Madison, L. D., and Eidlen, D., 1980, Cyclophosphamide-induced changes in the cellular composition of a methylcholanthrene-induced tumor and their relation to bone marrow and blood leukocyte levels, *Cancer Res.* **40**:395.

Facchinetti, T., Raz, A., and Goldman, R., 1978, A differential interaction of daunomycin, Adriamycin and N-trifluoroacetyl Adriamycin 14-valerate with mouse peritoneal macrophages, *Cancer Res.* **38**:3944.

Fefer, A., 1974, Tumor immunotherapy, In: *Antineoplastic and Immunosuppressive Agents I*, (A. C. Sartorelli and D. G. Johns, eds.), pp. 528–554, Springer-Verlag, Berlin.

Fefer, A., Einstein, A. B., Jr., and Cheever, M. A., 1976a, Adoptive chemoimmunotherapy of chancer in animals: A review of results, principles and problems, *Ann. N.Y. Acad. Sci.* **277**:492.

Fefer, A., Einstein, A. B., Jr., Cheever, M. A., and Berenson, J. R., 1976b, Models for syngeneic adoptive chemoimmunotherapy of murine leukemias, *Ann. N.Y. Acad. Sci.* **276**:573.

Ferguson, R. M., and Simmons, R. L., 1978, Differential cyclophosphamide sensitivity of suppressor and cytotoxic cell precursors, *Transplantation* **25**:36.

Fidler, I. J., 1980, Therapy of spontaneous metastases by intravenous injection of liposomes containing lymphokines, *Science* **208**:1469.

Fisher, B., and Gunduz, N., 1979, Further observations on the inhibition of tumor growth by *Corynebacterium parvum* with cyclophosphamide. X. Effect of treatment on tumor cell kinetics in mice, *J. Natl. Cancer Inst.* **62**:1545.

Gagnon, R. F., and MacLennan, I. C. M., 1981, The effect of chronic daily cyclophosphamide administration on established antibody responses, *Clin. Exp. Immunol.* **46**:178.

Gerber, M., Andress, D., Pioch, Y., Radal, M., and Serrou, B., 1978, Effect of cyclophosphamide and methyl prednisolone on *in vitro* cellular immune response to allogeneic tumor cells, *Transplantation* **26**:142.

Giampietri, A., Bonmassar, E., and Goldin, A., 1978–79, Drug induced modulation of immune responses in mice: Effects of 5-(3,3-dimethyl-1-triazeno)-imidazole-4-carboxamide (DTIC) and cyclophosphamide (CY), *J. Immunopharmacol.* **1**:61.

Gillis, S., and Smith, K. A., 1977, Long-term culture of tumor-specific cytotoxic T-cells, *Nature (London)* **268**:154.

Giuliani, F., Casazza, A. M., and DiMarco, A., 1974, Virologic and immunologic properties and response to daunomycin and Adriamycin of a non-regressing mouse tumor derived from MSV-induced sarcoma, *Biomedicine* **21**:435.

Glaser, M., 1979, Regulation of specific cell-mediated cytotoxic response against SV40-induced tumor associated antigens by depletion of suppressor T cells with cyclophosphamide in mice, *J. Exp. Med.* **149**:774.

Goto, M., Mitsuoka, A., Sugiyama, M., and Kitano, M., 1981, Enhancement of delayed hypersensitivity reaction with varieties of anti-cancer drugs: A common biological phenomenon, *J. Exp. Med.* **154**:204.

Gout, P. W., Wijcik, L. L., and Beer, C. T., 1978, Differences between vinblastine and vincristine in distribution in the blood of rats and binding by platelets and malignant cells, *Eur. J. Cancer* **14**:1167.

Greenberg, P. D., Cheever, M. A., and Fefer, A., 1980, Detection of early and delayed antitumor effects following curative adoptive chemoimmunotherapy of established leukemia, *Cancer Res.* **40**:4428.

Greenberg, P. D., Cheever, M. A., and Fefer, A., 1981, Eradication of disseminated murine leukemia by chemoimmunotherapy with cyclophosphamide and adoptively transfered immune syngeneic Lyt-1⁺2⁻ lymphocytes, *J. Exp. Med.* **154**:952.

Grein, A., Spalla, C., and DiMarco, A., 1963, Descrizione e classificazione di un attinomicete (*Streptomyces peucetius* sp. nova) produttore di un sostanza ad attivita antitumorale: La Daunomicina, *G. Microbiol.* **11**:109.

Hancock, E. J., and Kilburn, D. G., 1982, The effects of cyclophosphamide on *in vitro* cytotoxic responses to a syngeneic tumor, *Cancer Immunol. Immunother.* **14**:54.

Hardt, C., Rollinghoff, M., Pfizenmaier, K., Mosmann, H., and Wagner, H., 1981, Lyt-23⁺ cyclophosphamide-sensitive T cells regulate the activity of an Interleukin 2 inhibitor *in vivo*, *J. Exp. Med.* **154**:262.

Haskill, J. S., 1981, Adriamycin-activated macrophages as tumor growth inhibitors, *Cancer Res.* **41**:3852.

Hellstrom, I., and Hellstrom, K. E., 1978, Cyclophosphamide delays 3-methylcholanthrene sarcoma induction in mice, *Nature (London)* **275**:129.

Hengst, J. C. D., Mokyr, M. B., and Dray, S., 1980, Importance of timing in cyclophosphamide therapy of MOPC-315 tumor-bearing mice, *Cancer Res.* **40**:2135.

Hengst, J. C. D., Mokyr, M. B., and Dray, S., 1981, Cooperation between cyclophosphamide tumoricidal activity and host antitumor immunity in the cure of mice bearing large MOPC-315 tumors, *Cancer Res.* **41**:2163.

Hersh, E. M., 1973, Modification of host defense mechanism, in: *Cancer Medicine* (J. F. Holland and E. Frei, III, eds.), p. 681, Lea & Febiger, Philadelphia.

Hersh, E. M., 1974, Immunosuppressive agents, in: *Antineoplastic and Immunosuppressive Agents I* (A. C. Sartorelli and D. G. Johns, eds.), pp. 577–617, Springer-Verlag, Berlin.

Himes, R. H., Kersey, R. N., Heller-Bettinger, I., and Samson, F. E., 1976, Action of the vinca alkaloids vincristine, vinblastine, and desacetyl vinblastine amide on microtubules *in vitro*, *Cancer Res.* **36**:3798.

Hisano, G., and Fidler, I. J., 1982, Systemic activation of macrophages by liposome-entrapped muramyl tripeptide in mice pretreated with the chemotherapeutic agent Adriamycin, *Cancer Immunol. Immunother.* **14**:61.

Houchens, D. P., Johnson, R. K., Ovejera, A., Gaston, M. R., and Goldin, A., 1976, Effects of *Corynebacterium parvum* alone and in combination with Adriamycin in experimental tumor systems, *Cancer Treat. Rep.* **60**:823.

Howard, J. G., and Shand, F. L., 1979, The nature of drug-induced B cell tolerance, *Immunolog. Rev.* **43**:43.

Hurme, M., 1979, Differential cyclophosphamide sensitivity of precursor cells in allogeneic and H-2 restricted cytotoxic responses, *J. Exp. Med.* **149**:290.

Hurme, M., Bang, B. E., and Sihvola, M., 1980, Genetic differences in the cyclophosphamide-induced immune suppression: Weaker suppression of T-cell cytotoxicity by cyclophosphamide activated by CBA mice, *Clin. Immunol. Immunolpathol.* **17**:38.

Hurme, M., Sihvola, M., and Bang, B., 1982, During lymphatic regeneration, precursors for major histocompatibility complex-restricted cytotoxic T cells appear before alloreactive precursors, *J. Exp. Med.* **155**:327.

Kataoka, T., Kobayashi, H., and Sakurai, Y., 1978, Potentiation of concanavalin A-bound L1210 vaccine *in vivo* by chemotherapeutic agents, *Cancer Res.* **38**:1202.

Kataoka, T., Oh-Hashi, F., Sakurai, Y., and Ogihara, K., 1981, Effect of antineoplastic agents on the induction of suppressor macrophages by concanavalin A-bound tumor vaccine, *Cancer Res.* **41**:5151.

Kaufmann, S. H. E., Hahn, H., and Diamantstein, T., 1980, Relative susceptibilities of T cell subsets involved in delayed-type hypersensitivity to sheep red blood cells to the *in vitro* action of 4-hydroperoxycyclophosphamide, *J. Immunol.* **125**:1104.

Kerckhaert, J. A., Hofhuis, F. M., and Willers, J. M., 1977, Effects of variation in time and dose of cyclophosphamide injection on delayed hypersensitivity and antibody formation, *Cell Immunol.* **29**:232.

Kleinerman, E. S., Zwelling, L. A., Schwartz, R., and Muchmore, A. V., 1982, Effect of L-phenylalanine mustard, Adriamycin, actinomycin D, and 4'-(9-acridinylamino)methanesulfon-*m*-anisidide on naturally occurring human spontaneous monocyte-mediated cytotoxicity, *Cancer Res.* **42**:1692.

L'age-Stehr, J., and Diamantstein, T., 1978, Induction of autoreactive T lymphocytes and their suppressor cells by cyclophosphamide, *Nature (London)* **271**:663.

Lagrange, P. H., Mackaness, G. B., and Miller, T. E., 1974, Potentiation of T-cell-mediated immunity by selective suppression of antibody formation with cyclophosphamide, *J. Exp. Med.* **139**:1529.

Lespinats, G. M., Kolb, J. P. B., and Poupon, M., 1979, Cytostatic effect of spleen cells of cyclophosphamide-treated mice on tumor cells, *J. Immunopharmacol.* **1**:175.

Lotem, J., and Sachs, L., 1980, Potential pre-screening for therapeutic agents that induce differentiation in human myeloid leukemia cells, *Int. J. Cancer* **25**:561.

Lowy, A., Tominaga, A., Drebin, J. A., Takaoki, M., Benacerraf, B., and Greene, M. I., 1983, Identification of an I-J+ antigen-presenting cell required for third order suppressor cell activation, *J. Exp. Med.* **157**:353.

Lubet, R. A., and Carlson, D. E., 1978, Therapy of the murine plasmacytoma MOPC 104E: Role of the immune response, *J. Natl. Cancer Inst.* **61**:897.

McIntosh, K. R., Segre, M., and Segre, D., 1979, Inhibition of the humoral response by spleen cells from cyclophosphamide-treated mice, *Immunopharmacol.* **1**:165.

Magiure, H. C., and Ettore, V. L., 1967, Enhancement of dinitro-chlorobenzene (DNCB) contact sensitization by cyclophosphamide in guinea-pigs, *J. Invest. Dermatol.* **48**:39.

Mantovani, A., 1977, *In vitro* and *in vivo* cytotoxicity of Adriamycin and daunomycin for murine macrophages, *Cancer Res.* **37**:815.

Mantovani, A., Tagliabue, A., Vecchi, A., and Spreafico, F., 1976a, Effects of Adriamycin and daunomycin on spleen cell populations in normal and tumor allografted mice, *Eur. J. Cancer* **12**:381.

Mantovani, A., Vecchi, A., Tagliabue, A., and Spreafico, F., 1976b, The effects of Adriamycin and daunomycin on antitumoral immune effector mechanisms in an allogeneic system, *Eur. J. Cancer* **12**:371.

Mantovani, A., Luini, W., Peri, G., Vecchi, A., and Spreafico, F., 1978, Effect of chemotherapeutic agents on natural cell-mediated cytotoxicity in mice, *J. Natl. Cancer Inst.* **61**:1255.

Mantovani, A., Candiani, G. P., Luini, W., Salmona, M., Spreafico, F., and Garattini, S., 1979a, Effects of chemotherapeutic agents on host defense mechanisms: Its possible relevance for the antitumoral activity of these drugs, in: *Current Trends in Tumor Immunology* (S. Ferrone, S. Gorini, R. B. Herberman, and R. A. Reisfeld, eds.), pp. 139–154, Garland Press, New York.

Mantovani, A., Polentarutti, N., Luini, W., Peri, G., and Spreafico, F., 1979b, Role of host defense mechanisms in the antitumor activity of Adriamycin and daunomycin in mice, *J. Natl. Cancer Inst.* **63**:61.

Mantovani, A., Vecchi, A., Tagliabue, A., and Spreafico, F., 1979c, The effect of chemotherapeutic agents on host defense mechanisms: Its relevance for chemoimmunotherapy combinations, in: *Tumor-Associated Antigens and Their Specific Immune Responses* (F. Spreafico and R. Arnon, eds.), pp. 271–286, Academic Press, New York.

Mantovani, A., Luini, W., Candiani, G. P., and Spreafico, F., 1980, Effect of chemotherapeutic agents on natural and BCG-stimulated macrophage cytotoxicity in mice, *Int. J. Immunopharmacol.* **2**:333.

Marchal, G., Milon, G., Hurtrel, B., and Lagrange, P. H., 1978, Titration and circulation of cells mediating delayed type hypersensitivity in normal and cyclophosphamide treated mice during response to sheep red blood cells, *Immunology* **35**:981.

Marsh, J. C., 1976, The effects of cancer chemotherapeutic agents on normal hematopoietic precursor cells: A review, *Cancer Res.* **36**:1853.

Martin, F., Caignard, A., Olsson, O., Jeannin, J. F., and Leclerc, A., 1982, Tumoricidal effect of macrophages exposed to Adriamycin *in vivo* or *in vitro*, *Cancer Res.* **42**:3851.

Medzihradsky, J. L., Hollowell, R. P., and Elion, G. B., 1981, Differential inhibition by azathioprine and 6-mercaptopurine of specific suppressor T cell generation in mice, *J. Immunopharmacol.* **3**:1.

Merluzzi, V. J., Faanes, R. B., and Choi, Y. S., 1979, Restoration of cyclophosphamide-induced suppression of thymus-derived cytotoxic cell generation by normal thymocytes, *Cancer Res.* **39**:3647.

Merluzzi, V. J., Faanes, R. B., and Choi, Y. S., 1980, Recovery of the capacity for cytotoxic T cell generation in cyclophosphamide-treated mice by the addition of Lyt-1^{+}2^{-} helper cells, *Int. J. Immunopharmacol.* **2**:341.

Merluzzi, V. J., Kenney, R. E., Schmid, F. A., Choi, Y. S., and Faanes, R. B., 1981a, Recovery of the *in vivo* cytotoxic T-cell response in cyclophosphamide-treated mice by injection of mixed-lymphocyte-culture supernatants, *Cancer Res.* **41**:3663.

Merluzzi, V. J., Walker, M. M., and Faanes, R. B., 1981b, Inhibition of cytotoxic T-cell clonal expansion by cyclophosphamide and the recovery of cytotoxic T-lymphocyte precursors by supernatants from mixed-lymphocyte cultures, *Cancer Res.* **41**:850.

Mihich, E., 1975, Immunosuppression in cancer therapeutics: Proceedings of the First International Symposium on Cancer and Transplantation, *Transplant. Proc.* **7**:275.

Mihich, E., 1978, Chemotherapy and immunotherapy as a combined modality of cancer treatment, in: *Advances in Tumor Prevention, Detection and Characterization*, Volume 4, (W. Davis and K. R. Harrap, eds.), p. 113, Excerpta Medica, Amsterdam.

Mihich, E., 1979, Drug selectivity in the suppression of the immune response, in: *Drugs and Immune Responsiveness* (J. L. Turk and D. Parker, eds.), pp. 25–39, Macmillan & Co., London.

Milon, G., and Marchal, G., 1978, Increased infiltration by monocytes in delayed type hypersensitivity site following cyclophosphamide treatment, *Immunology* **35**:989.

Mitsuoka, A., Baba, M., and Morikawa, S., 1976, Enhancement of delayed hypersensitivity by depletion of suppressor T cells with cyclophosphamide in mice, *Nature (London)* **262**:77.

Mitsuoka, A., Morikawa, S., Baba, M., and Harada, T., 1979, Cyclophosphamide eliminates suppressor T cells in age-associated central regulation of delayed hypersensitivity in mice, *J. Exp. Med.* **149**:1018.

Mokyr, M. B., Hengst, J. C. D., and Dray, S., 1982, Role of antitumor immunity in cyclophosphamide-induced rejection of subcutaneous nonpalpable MOPC-315 tumors, *Cancer Res.* **42**:974.

Moore, M., and Williams, D. E., 1973, Contribution of host immunity to cyclophosphamide therapy of a chemically-induced murine sarcoma, *Int. J. Cancer* **11**:358.

Muggia, F. M., Young, C. W., and Carter, S. K. (eds.), 1983, *Anthracycline Antibiotics in Cancer Therapy*, Nijhoff, The Hague.

Neta, R., Winkelstein, A., Salvin, S. B., and Mendelow, H., 1977, The effect of cyclophosphamide on suppressor cells in guinea pigs, *Cell. Immunol.* **33**:402.

Noble, B., Parker, D., Scheper, R. J., and Turk, J. L., 1977, The relation between B-cell stimulation and delayed hypersensitivity: The effect of cyclophosphamide pretreatment on antibody production, *Immunology* **32**:885.

Noble, R. L., Gout, P. W., Wijcik, L. L., Hebden, F., and Beer, C. T., 1977, The distribution of [^{3}H]vinblastine in tumor and host tissues of Nb rats bearing a transplantable lymphoma which is highly sensitive to the alkaloid, *Cancer Res.* **37**:1455.

North, R. J., 1982, Cyclophosphamide-facilitated adoptive immunotherapy of an established tumor depends on elimination of tumor-induced suppressor T cells, *J. Exp. Med.* **55**:1063.

Olah, E., Palyi, I., and Sugar, J., 1978, Effects of cytostatics on proliferating and stationary cultures of mammalian cells, *Eur. J. Cancer* **14**:895.

Orsini, F., and Mihich, E., 1975, Immunosuppression by Adriamycin (AM) and daunorubicin (DM), *Proc. Am. Assoc. Cancer Res.* **16**:130.

Orsini, F., Pavelic, Z., and Mihich, E., 1977, Increased primary cell mediated immunity in culture subsequent to Adriamycin or daunorubicin treatment of spleen donor mice, *Cancer Res.* **37**:1719.

Orsini, F., Eppolito, C., Ehrke, M. J., and Mihich, E., 1980, Inhibition by selected anticancer agents of the development of primary cell-mediated immunity against allogeneic tumor cells in culture, *Cancer Treat. Rep.* **64**:211.

Otterness, I. G., and Chang, Y.-H., 1976, Comparative study of cyclophosphamide, 6-mercaptopurine, azathioprine and methotrexate: Relative effects on the humoral and the cellular immune response in the mouse, *Clin. Exp. Immunol.* **26**:346.

Owellen, R. J., Owens, A. H., Jr., and Donigian, D. W., 1972, The binding of vincristine, vinblastine and colchicine to tubulin, *Biochem. Biophys. Res. Commun.* **47**:685.

Ozer, H., Cowens, J. W., Colvin, M., Nussbaum-Blumenson, A., and Sheedy, D., 1982, In vitro effects of 4-hydroperoxycyclophosphamide on human immunoregulatory T subset function. I. Selective effects on lymphocyte function in T–B cell collaboration, *J. Exp. Med.* **155**:276.

Phillips, S. M., Catanzaro, P. J., Carpenter, C. B., and Zweiman, B., 1979, Mechanisms in the suppression of delayed hypersensitivity in the guinea pig by 6-mercaptopurine. II. Kinetic and morphologic studies on the monocyte-macrophage component, *Immunopharmacol.* **1**:277.

Polak, L., and Turk, J. L., 1974, Reversal of immunological tolerance by cyclophosphamide through inhibition of suppressor cell activity, *Nature (London)* **249**:654.

Radov, L. A., Haskill, J. S., and Korn, J. H., 1976, Host immune potentiation of drug responses to a murine mammary adenocarcinoma, *Intl. J. Cancer* **17**:773.

Ramshaw, I. A., Bretscher, P. A., and Parish, C. R., 1977, Regulation of the immune response. II. Repressor T cells in cyclophosphamide-induced tolerant mice, *Eur. J. Immunol.* **7**:180.

Ray, P. K., and Raychaudhuri, S., 1981, Low-dose cyclophosphamide inhibition of transplantable fibrosarcoma growth by augmentation of the host immune response, *J. Natl. Cancer Inst.* **67**:1341.

Riccardi, C., Puccetti, P., Santoni, A., Herberman, R. B., and Bonmassar, E., 1979, Adriamycin-induced antitumor response in lethally irradiated mice, *Immunopharmacol.* **1**:211.

Riccardi, C., Bartocci, A., Puccetti, P., Spreafico, F., Bonmassar, E., and Goldin, A., 1980, Combined effects of antineoplastic agents and antilymphoma allograft reactions, *Eur. J. Cancer* **16**:23.

Rollinghoff, M., Starzinski-Powitz, A., Pfizenmaier, K., and Wagner, H., 1977, Cyclophosphamide-sensitive T lymphocytes suppress the in vivo generation of antigen-specific cytotoxic T lymphocytes, *J. Exp. Med.* **145**:455.

Romanycheva, V., Babichev, V. A., Uteshev, B. S., and Kalinkovitch, A. G., 1978, The kinetics of inhibition with methotrexate and vinblastine of the primary immune response to sheep red blood cells in mice (plaque-forming cells), *Folia Biol. (Prague)* **24**:343.

Rosner, F., Grunwald, H., and Hirshaut, Y., 1973, Mechanism of action of vincristine: Selective killing of stationary cell populations, *Blood* **42**:1014.

Rustum, Y. M., Grindey, G. B., Hakala, M. T., and Mihich, E., 1976, Multifactorial cellular determinants of the action of antimetabolites, in: *Advances in Enzyme Regulation* (G. Weber, ed.), p. 281, Pergamon Press, Elmsford, N.Y.

Ryoyama, K., Ehrke, M. J., and Mihich, E., 1980, Reduced sensitivity to "antigen-specific" suppression caused by Adriamycin (AM), *Proc. Abstr. Int. Congr. Immunol.* **4**:17.

Ryoyama, K., Ehrke, M. J., and Mihich, E., 1981, Cell–cell interaction in the generation of "nonspecific" suppressor cells in culture and its modification by anti-cancer drugs, in: *Proceedings of the EORTC Symposium on Immunopharmacologic Effects of Radiotherapy* (J. Dubois, B. Serrou, and C. Rosenfeld, eds.), pp. 23–27, Raven Press, New York.

Ryoyama, K., Mace, K., Ehrke, M. J., and Mihich, E., 1982, The differential sensitivity of T-cell immune functions to vincristine and vinblastine, *Int. J. Immunopharmacol.* **4**:187.

Salazar, D., and Cohen, S. A., 1983, Multiple tumoricidal effector mechanisms induced by Adriamycin, *Cancer Res.* **44**:2561.

Sandberg, J. S., Howsden, F. L., DiMarco, A., and Goldin, A., 1970, Comparison of antileukemic effect in mice of Adriamycin (NSC-123,127) and daunomycin (NSC-82151), *Cancer Chemother. Rep.* **54**:1.

Santoni, A., Riccardi, C., Sorci, V., and Herberman, R., 1980, Effects of Adriamycin on the activity of mouse natural killer cells, *J. Immunol.* **124**:2329.

Schreck, R., 1974, Cytotoxicity of vincristine to normal and leukemic cells, *Am. J. Clin. Pathol.* **62**:1.

Schwartz, A., Orbach-Arbouys, S., and Gershon, R. K., 1976, Participation of cyclophosphamide-sensitive T cells in graft-vs-host reactions, *J. Immunol.* **117**:871.

Schwartz, A., Askenase, P. W., and Gershon, R. K., 1978, Regulation of delayed-type hypersensitivity reactions by cyclophosphamide-sensitive T cells, *J. Immunol.* **121**:1573.

Schwartz, H. S., 1983, Mechanisms of selective cytotoxicity of Adriamycin, danuorubicin and related anthracyclines, in: *Molecular Aspects of Anticancer Drug Action* (S. Neidle and M. J. Waring, eds.), pp. 93–125, Macmillan Co., New York.

Schwartz, H. S., and Grindey, G. B., 1973, Adriamycin and daunorubicin: A comparison of antitumor activities and tissue uptake in mice following immunosuppression, *Cancer Res.* **33**:1837.

Schwartz, H. S., and Kanter, P., 1975, Cell interactions: Determinants of selective toxicity of Adriamycin and daunorubicin, *Cancer Chemother. Rep.* **6**:107.

Schwartz, R. S., 1968, Immunosuppressive drug therapy, in: *Human Transplantation* (F. T. Rapaport and J. Dausset, eds.), pp. 440–471, Grune & Stratton, New York.

Shand, F. L., 1978, The capacity of microsomally-activated cyclophosphamide to induce immunosuppression *in vitro*, *Immunology* **35**:1017.

Shand, F. L., and Howard, J. G., 1979, Induction *in vitro* of reversible immunosuppression and inhibition of B cell receptor regeneration by defined metabolites of cyclophosphamide, *Eur. J. Immunol.* **9**:17.

Shand, F. L., and Liew, F. Y., 1980, Differential sensitivity to cyclophosphamide of helper T cells for humoral responses and suppressor T cells for delayed-type hypersensitivity, *Eur. J. Immunol.* **10**:480.

Shek, P. N., and Coons, A. H., 1978, Effect of colchicine on the antibody response. I. Enhancement of antibody formation in mice, *J. Exp. Med.* **147**:1213.

Smith, J., Cowens, W., Nussbaum-Blumenson, A., Sheedy, D., Mihich, E., and Ozer, H., 1982, Functional separation of human suppressor and cytotoxic T subsets defined *in vitro* by 4-hydroperoxycyclophosphamide (4-HC), *Fed. Proc.* **41**:797.

Smith, K. A., Gillis, S., Baker, P. E., and McKenzie, D., 1979, T-cell growth factor-mediated T-cell proliferation, *Ann. N.Y. Acad. Sci.* **332**:423.

Spreafico, F., and Anaclerio, A., 1977, Immunosuppressive agents, in: *Immunopharmacology* (J. W. Hadden, R. G. Coffey, and F. Spreafico, eds.), pp. 245–278, Plenum Press, New York.

Stoychkov, J. N., Schultz, R. M., Chirigos, M. A., Pavlidis, N. A., and Goldin, A., 1979, Effects of Adriamycin and cyclophosphamide treatment on induction of macrophage cytotoxic function in mice, *Cancer Res.* **39**:3014.

Sunday, M. E., Benacerraf, B., and Dorf, M. E., 1981, Hapten-specific T cell responses to 4-hydroxy-3-nitrophenyl acetyl. VIII. Suppressor cell pathways in cutaneous sensitivity responses, *J. Exp. Med.* **153**:811.

Sy, M.-S., Miller, S. D., and Claman, H. N., 1977, Immune suppression with supraoptimal doses of antigen in contact sensitivity. I. Demonstration of suppressor cells and their sensitivity to cyclophosphamide, *J. Immunol.* **119**:240.

Syeklocha, D., Siminovitch, L., Till, J. E., and McCulloch, E. A., 1966, The proliferative state of antigen-sensitive precursors of hemolysin-producing cells, determined by the use of the inhibitor, vinblastine, *J. Immunol.* **96**:472.

Tagliabue, A., Polentarutti, N., Vecchi, A., Mantovani, A., and Spreafico, F., 1977, Combination chemo-immunotherapy with Adriamycin in experimental tumor systems, *Eur. J. Cancer* **13**:657.

Takeda, K., Minowada, J., and Block, A., 1982, Kinetics of appearance of differentiation-associated characteristics in ML-1, a line of human myeloblastic leukemia cells, after treatment with 12-O-tetradecanoylphorbol-13-acetate, dimethyl sulfoxide, or 1-β-D-arabinofuranosylcytosine, *Cancer Res.* **42**:5152.

Taswell, C., MacDonald, H. R., and Cerottini, J.-C., 1979, Limiting dilution analysis of alloantigen-reactive T lymphocytes. II. Effect of cortisone and cyclophosphamide on cytotoxic T lymphocyte precursor frequencies in the thymus, *Thymus* **1**:119.

Tomazic, V., Ehrke, M. J., and Mihich, E., 1980, Modulation of the cytotoxic response against allogeneic tumor cells in culture by Adriamycin, *Cancer Res.* **40**:2748.

Tomazic, V., Ehrke, M. J., and Mihich, E., 1981, Augmentation of the development of immune responses of mice against allogeneic tumor cells after Adriamycin treatment, *Cancer Res.* **41**:3370.

Turk, J. L., and Parker, D., 1979a, The effect of cyclophosphamide on the immune response, *J. Immunopharmacol.* **1**:127.

Turk, J. L., and Parker, D., 1979b, The effect of drugs on immunological control mechanisms, in: *Drugs and Immune Responsiveness* (J. L. Turk and D. Parker, eds.), pp. 73–84, Macmillan & Co., London.

Turk, J. L., and Poulter, L. W., 1972, Selective depletion of lymphoid tissue by cyclophosphamide, *Clin. Exp. Immunol.* **10**:285.

Vecchi, A., Mantovani, A., Tagliabue, A., and Spreafico, F., 1976, A characterization of immunosuppressive activity of Adriamycin and daunomycin on humoral antibody production and tumor allograft rejection, *Cancer Res.* **36**:1222.

Vidovic, D., Marusic, M., and Culo, F., 1982, Interference of anti-tumor and immunosuppressive effects of cyclophosphamide in tumor-bearing rats: Analysis of factors determining resistance of susceptibility to a subsequent tumor challenge, *Cancer Immunol. Immunother.* **14**:36.

Winkelstein, A., 1979, The effects of azathioprine and 6MP on immunity, *J. Immunopharmacol.* **1**:429.

Wood, M. L., and Monaco, A. P., 1977, The effect of cyclophosphamide on the specific unresponsiveness to skin allografts induced in ALS-treated mice infused with donor bone marrow, *J. Immunol.* **118**:1456.

Young, R. C., Ozols, R. F., and Myers, C. E., 1981, The anthracycline antineoplastic drugs, *N. Engl. J. Med.* **305**:139.

Yu, S., Lannin, D. R., Tsui-Collins, A. L., and McKhann, C. F., 1980, Effect of cyclophosphamide on mice bearing methylcholanthrene-induced fibrosarcomas, *Cancer Res.* **40**:2756.

Chemistry and Biological Profile of Immunosuppressants

T. Y. SHEN

1. INTRODUCTION

Immunosuppressive agents is a term describing a wide group of immunoregulants whose principal biological effects are suppression of cellular and/or humoral immunity manifested in disorders such as organ transplantation and autoimmune diseases. The influence of lineage and cytokinetic aspects of immunocytes on their sensitivity to drug actions is well appreciated. As the immune system is a dynamic and balanced network of macrophages, T and B lymphocytes, interacting with other cells such as neutrophils, mast cells, platelets, etc., it is not surprising that the activity of an immunological agent may vary both qualitatively and quantitatively according to experimental conditions. Indeed, in animal assays many immunoregulants have bell-shaped or biphasic dose–response curves: an agent may be stimulatory at lower doses but inhibitory at excessive doses. With the gradual characterization of various subsets of T and B lymphocytes and immune mediators such as lymphokines, interleukins, mitogenic or inhibitory factors, it became clear that a T-helper antiproliferative agent and a T-suppressor inducer may achieve similar immunosuppressive effects. Furthermore, a suppression of humoral response by some agents may result in immune deviation with concomitant augmentation of the cellular response. In other words, depending on the mechanism of action and the sensitivity of immune cells at different stages, an immunoregulant may exert differential effects on the overall immune process in a concentration-dependent and protocol-dependent manner.

In the early stage of the development of immunosuppressants, emphasis was on lymphocytotoxic actions. Inhibition of antibody production, mitogenic response of lymphocytes, and delayed hypersensitivity *in vivo* were used as primary biological assays. As a consequence, antineoplastic cytotoxic agents and antimetabolites, e.g., cyclophosphamide and 6-mercaptopurine, and antiinflammatory corticosteroids were recognized as the first generation of immunosup-

T. Y. SHEN • Merck Sharp & Dohme Research Laboratories, Rahway, New Jersey 07065.

pressants (Hersh, 1974). In the past decade with the development of more sophisticated immunological systems, the functional aspects of cells and mediators became feasible therapeutic targets. Encouraged by an increasing clinical interest in organ transplantation and chronic immunological disorders such as rheumatoid arthritis and lupus erythematosus, a wide search of immunoregulants has uncovered a variety of agents, including many novel structures from natural products. Unfortunately, despite some genuine attempts to rationalize the immunoregulatory effect in terms of specific and quantitative biochemical actions, such as receptor blockage, mediator inhibition, or intracellular cAMP/cGMP levels, our understanding of the mechanism of action of most immunosuppressants is still very fragmentary (Sigel *et al.*, 1982).

In the following survey, a representative group of immunosuppressants are selected from the recent literature to illustrate their discovery, general chemical characteristics, and principal biological properties. In several cases, because of the duality of their immunological actions, certain overlap with previous discussions on immunostimulants is unavoidable. Not included in this chapter are a group of soluble immunosuppressive proteins and glycoproteins produced by T and B lymphocytes or macrophages. Most of them, such as α-globulins, α-fetoprotein, C-reactive protein, interferons, antigen-specific and nonspecific factors for T lymphocytes, factors for B cells and for macrophages, etc., are still being purified and characterized. Their properties and biological significance have been reviewed recently (Cathcart and Krakauer, 1982). The extensive studies on the immunoregulatory effects of prostaglandins and sex hormones are also beyond the scope of this discussion.

2. ALKYLATING AGENTS

The cytotoxic alkyalting agents, initially developed as potential antitumor agents, were investigated as immunosuppressants at an early stage (Brune and Whitehouse, 1979). This family of compounds is characterized by the presence of two chemically reactive groups such as aziridine or its precursor (e.g., β-chloroethylamine), sulfonate or ethylene oxide, in the molecule. The bifunctional structure forms a cross-link between nucleophiles present in biopolymers such as DNA. The remaining structure in the alkylating molecule may be considered as a "carrier moiety" that influences the pharmacodynamics of the agent, thus achieving varying degrees of potency and cellular or organ specificity. The cytotoxicity of alkylating agents is not specific to the phase of the cell cycle but is usually more lethal to cells in cycle than to resting cells. Most alkylating agents in use today were developed empirically. The possible clinical attributes observed with some of them are still being rationalized in newer testing systems according to current immunological understandings.

2.1. CYCLOPHOSPHAMIDE

The most widely used alkylating agent within the last two decades is cyclophosphamide (**1**) (Hersh, 1974). Cyclophosphamide is a prodrug. *In vivo* it

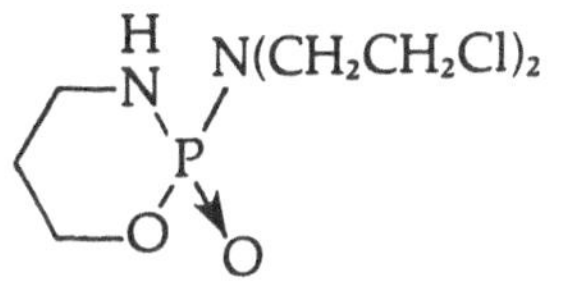

1

is converted by hepatic microsomal enzymes to a series of metabolites (Fig. 1), several of which, as their chemical structures would indicate, are chemically reactive (Jardine *et al.*, 1978). Its overall activity in an *in vivo* system depends on the pharmacokinetics of the drug, local tissue metabolic capacity, and the distribution of various intermediary metabolites. Cyclophosphamide is generally more toxic to B lymphocytes and inhibits antibody response *in vivo* effectively. It also has a suppressive effect on T-cell functions, especially precursor T cells, but it has no significant effect on delayed hypersensitivity. The effect of cyclophosphamide and other alkylating agents on the induction and expression of suppressor cells may depend on the relative timing of antigen and drug administration as well as the kinetics and susceptibility of different subsets of T-suppressor cells (i.e., inducer, precursor, and effector). Clinically, cyclophosphamide has been used in the treatment of a variety of diseases with direct or indirect immune etiology, such as systemic lupus erythematosus, graft rejection, rheumatoid arthritis, and even multiple sclerosis (Hauser *et al.*, 1983).

2.2. OTHER ALKYLATING AGENTS

Other antitumor alkylating agents useful in immunosuppression are chlorambucil (**2**), CCNU (**3**), and melphalan (**4**). In melphalan, phenylalanine is used

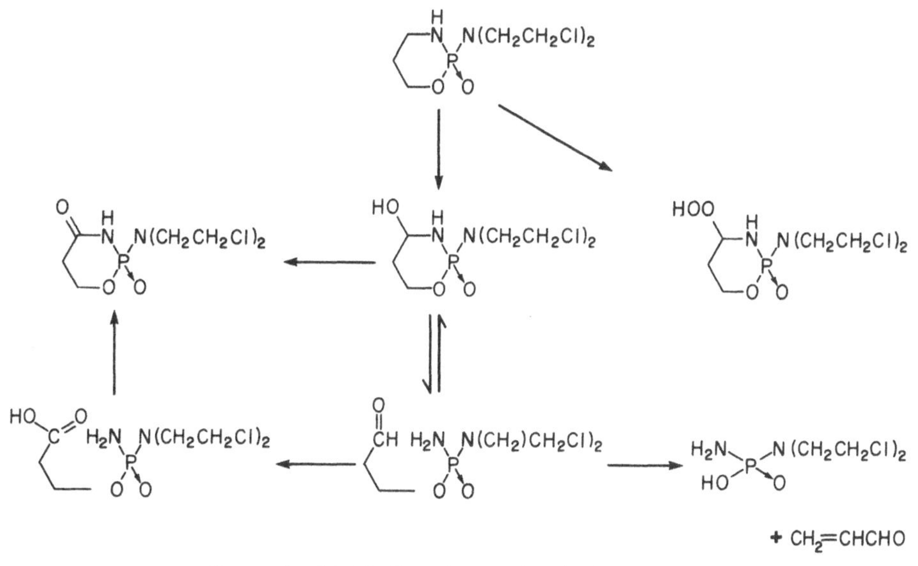

FIGURE 1. Metabolic pathway of cyclophosphamide.

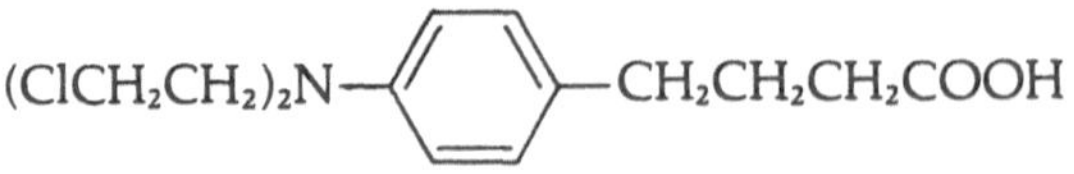

$$(ClCH_2CH_2)_2N--CH_2CH_2CH_2COOH$$

2

$$ClCH_2CH_2NCONH-$$
$$\underset{NO}{|}$$

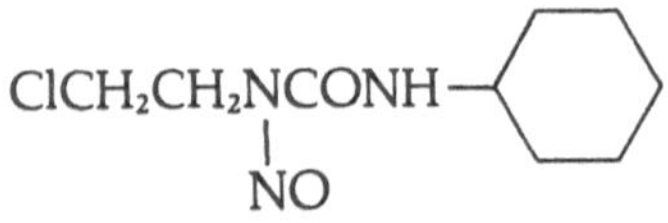

3

$$(ClCH_2CH_2)_2N--CH_2CH-COOH$$
$$\underset{NH_2}{|}$$

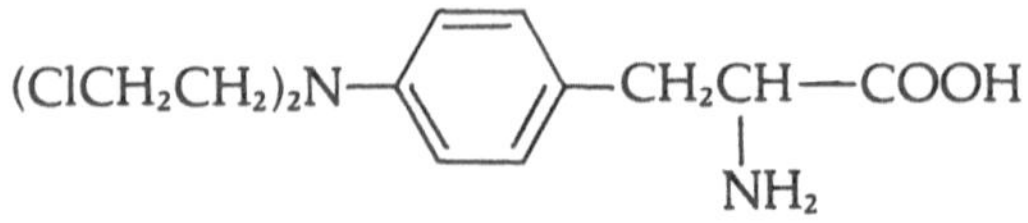

4

as a carrier moiety for the alkylating groups. Another immunomodulating bifunctional alkylating agent is busulfan (**5**), which enhances T-cell-mediated immune responses to tumor cells (Mizushima *et al.*, 1981).

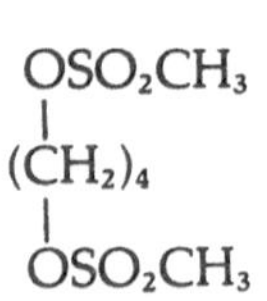

$$OSO_2CH_3$$
$$|$$
$$(CH_2)_4$$
$$|$$
$$OSO_2CH_3$$

5

Several alkylating agents, through their preferential elimination of suppressor T cells, have shown immunomodulating activities under various conditions. A good example is the cyano aziridine derivative azemexone (BM 12531) (**6**) (Luckenbach *et al.*, 1981). Administered before antigen, azemexone stimulates both humoral ir   · and delayed hypersensitivity, but it suppresses antibody formation v   nistered after antigen. It increases host resistance to experimental tumc   ial infection, and irradiation. A related derivative BM 41332 (**7**) was repo..... to inhibit the development of polyarthritic lesions induced by Freund's adjuvant in the rat (Bicker, 1982).

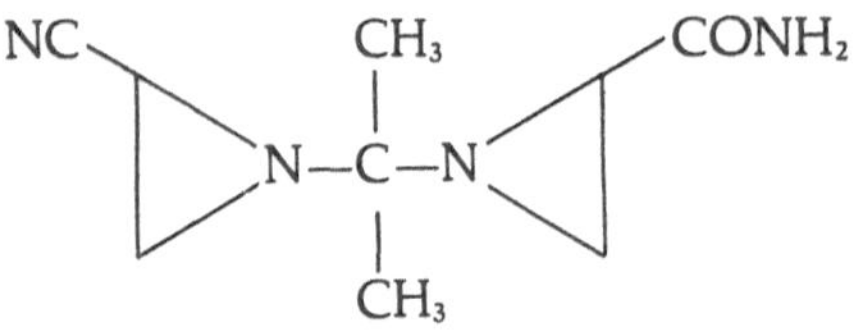

6

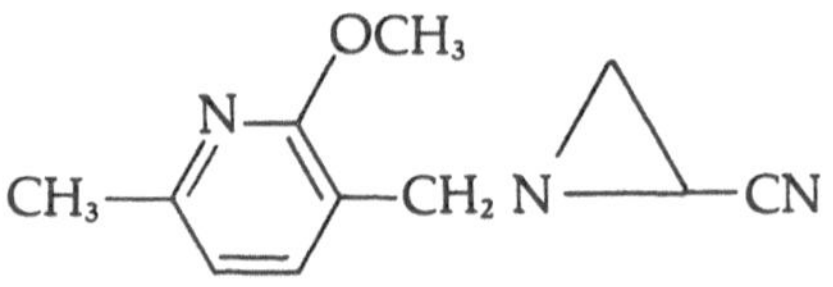

7

Obviously, experiments with isolated and well-characterized subpopulations of T cells are needed to resolve many apparently differential or conflicting effects of these alkylating agents.

3. ANTIMETABOLITES OF NUCLEOSIDE METABOLISM

Numerous cytotoxic antimetabolites and nucleoside analogs that interfere with nucleic acid biosynthesis have been investigated in many years of cancer research. Not unexpectedly, many of them can alter the proliferation and function of lymphocytes or other immunological responses. As inhibitors of DNA synthesis, they are mainly effective against cells in the S phase and not resting cells. A few well-known examples are described below.

3.1. METHOTREXATE

As a folic acid antagonist and an inhibitor of purine biosynthesis (Hitchings and Elion, 1963), methotrexate (**8**) depresses antibody response, delayed hypersensitivity, homograft rejection, and graft-versus-host reaction. Because of its severe hepatotoxicity, the long-term use of methotrexate in autoimmune diseases, psoriasis, and rheumatoid arthritis must proceed with caution (Brune and Whitehouse, 1979).

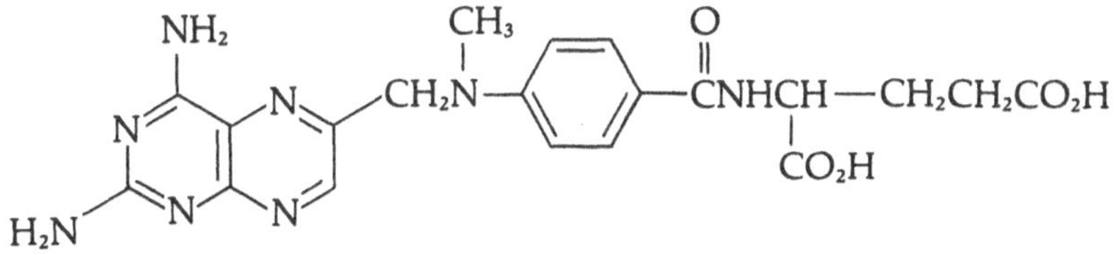

8

The inhibition of dihydrofolate reductase from different species and cell types by methotrexate is under extensive investigations. X-ray crystallography (Matthews *et al.*, 1977), resonance Raman spectroscopy, ^{13}C NMR, and computer modeling techniques are also used to define the precise mode of interaction at the molecular level and to guide the possible synthesis of more selective inhibitors. Prodrug derivatives and new analogs of methotrexate are also being studied in an attempt to improve its therapeutic index.

3.2. THIOPURINES

6-Mercaptopurine (6-MP) (**9**) and its prodrug, the methylnitroimidazole derivative azathioprine (Az) (**10**), have been extensively studied as immunosuppressive agents (Winkelstein, 1979). 6-MP is a competitive inhibitor of hypoxanthine phosphoribosyl transferase. It is also converted to thioinosinic acid and other metabolites. Together these metabolites inhibit various pathways of pu-

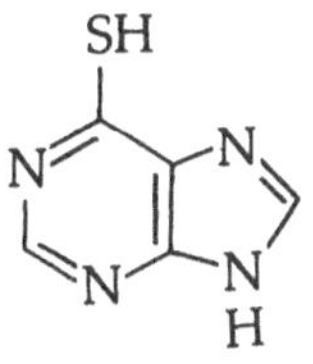

9 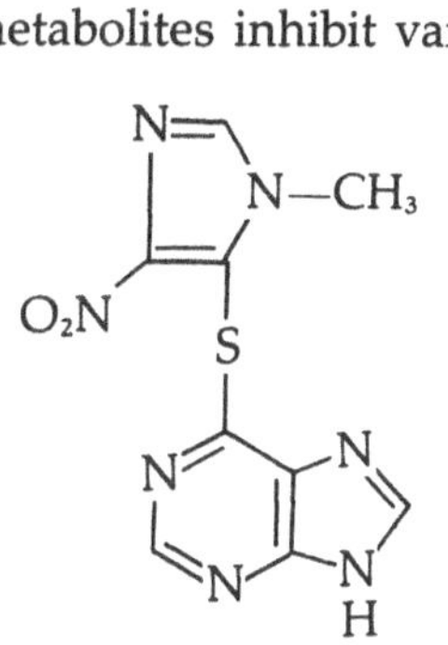   10

rine metabolism. Az was designed as a transport form of 6-MP and is metabolized almost quantitatively into 6-MP *in vivo*. Both 6-MP and Az have a direct action on cellular differentiation during immune induction, presumably associated with inhibition of DNA, RNA, and protein synthesis. However, some differential effects of the two drugs have also been noted (Medzihradsky *et al.*, 1981). 6-MP appears to be more effective than Az in blocking the production of specific suppressor T cells *in vivo* at equimolar doses. On the other hand, Az is more active in inhibiting various *in vitro* T-cell-dependent responses. The immunosuppression by thiopurines is reversible and time-dependent. A better recovery from the cytotoxic effect of Az was also observed. A more complete analysis of the biochemical properties of these two well-known immunosuppressants is still being pursued.

3.3. CYTOSINE ARABINOSIDE

Cytosine arabinoside (Ara-C) (**11**) a cytidine analog, is an inhibitor of DNA synthesis. The nucleoside is first phosphorylated to Ara-CTP by deoxycytidine

11

kinase; the nucleotide then inhibits mammalian DNA polymerase competitively with the natural substrate CTP. Ara-C has multiple effects on immune functions (Heppner and Calabresi, 1976). It suppresses B and/or T cells under different conditions. It can exert a profound inhibitory effect on Fc receptor cells without affecting NK cells (Zighelbolm and Shih, 1981). *In vivo*, it inhibits antibody response and antibody-dependent cytotoxicity. It does not affect delayed cutaneous hypersensitivity and graft-versus-host responses.

3.4. RIBAVIRIN

Ribavirin (**12**), initially developed as an antiviral agent, interferes with influenza virus RNA polymerase and prevents capping of *Vaccinia* mRNA (Sidwell *et al.*, 1972; Streeter *et al.*, 1973). It inhibits specifically inosine 5'-monophosphate dehydrogenase, a cellular enzyme required for guanosine 5'-monophosphate biosynthesis. Its suppression of the lymphoproliferative response is reversible by guanosine (Peavy *et al.*, 1980). At higher concentrations it exerts a cytotoxic

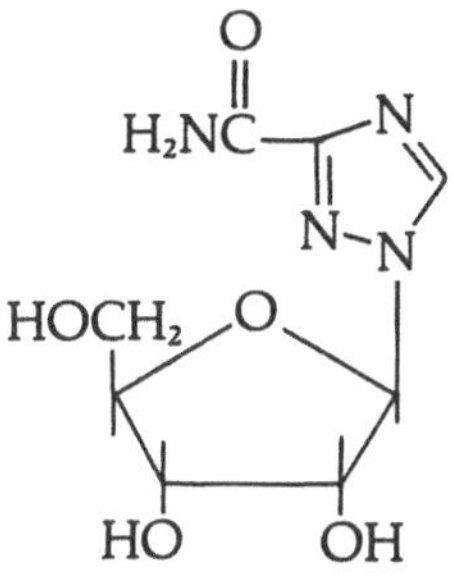

12

effect on B lymphocytes (Powers *et al.*, 1982). Ribavirin prolongs the survival of NZB/W F_1 mice and may have some potential in treating virus-induced autoimmune diseases.

3.5. ADENOSINE DEAMINASE INHIBITORS

Deficiencies in several enzymes related to purine catabolism, such as purine nucleoside phosphorylase (PNP) or adenosine deaminase, cause marked abnormalities in immunological functions (Fishman *et al.*, 1980). An inherited deficiency of PNP in man is associated with profound cellular immune dysfunction but with intact humoral immunity. Genetic absence of adenosine deaminase causes a severe combined immunodeficiency disease with suppression of both cellular and humoral responses (Trotta *et al.*, 1981; Sordillo *et al.*, 1981). Increased urinary excretion of purine metabolites has also been observed in some patients with cancer and/or acquired immune deficiency syndrome (AIDS). The cause-and-effect relationship between inhibition of adenosine deaminase, accumulation of adenine metabolites, and lymphocyte dysfunction has been well demonstrated by several investigations with purine nucleosides and specific adenosine deaminase inhibitors (Kazmers *et al.*, 1983).

Adenosine, cAMP, and agents that increase the intracellular levels of cAMP, at 10^{-4} M *in vitro*, selectively suppress lymphocyte blastogenesis induced by different lectins. ATP, presumably via its degradation to adenosine, is also suppressive. The metabolically more stable analog, 2-chloroadenosine (**13**), which binds to cell surface receptors and mimics the action of adenosine in

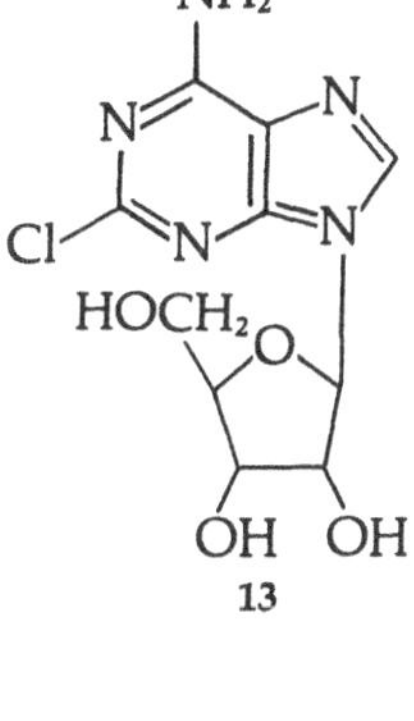

13

several tissues, is more potent at 10^{-5} M. The antilymphoproliferative effects of other adenosine derivatives, N^6-isopentenyl (**14**) and N^6, N^6-dimethyladenosine (**15**) at 1–5 µM *in vitro*, were observed earlier.

$R_1 = H$ $R_2 = CH_2 - CH = C \langle \substack{CH_3 \\ CH_3}$

14 $R_1 = R_2 = CH_3$

                                                                15

The lymphotoxicity of adenosine and 2'-deoxyadenosine (**16**) is potentiated by the presence of adenosine deaminase inhibitors, 2'-deoxycoformycin (DCF) (**17**) and *erythro*-9-(2-hydroxy-3-nonyl) adenine (**18**) (Ratech *et al.*, 1982; Lum *et al.*, 1979) in micromolar concentrations. Used alone, these adenosine deaminase inhibitors do not significantly interfere with lymphocyte function *in vitro*. *In vivo*, constant infusion of low doses of DCF produces a highly specific impairment of lymphocyte function and affects the differentiation of bone marrow stem cells.

16   **17**   **18**

Lymphoid degeneration, lymphopenia, and marked decrease in response to both B- and T-cell mitogens are observed. In this study, the continued presence of adenosine deaminase inhibitors is required for maximum efficacy. The potential application of adenosine deaminase inhibitors in leukemia and bone marrow transplantation is under investigation.

3.6. OTHER PURINE ANALOGS

9-Deazaadenosine (**19**), a cyclicnucleoside, inhibits lymphocyte-mediated cytolysis at 1–10 μM. It is metabolized rapidly to the 5′-triphosphate by adenosine kinase and causes a decrease of ATP within the cytolytic lymphocytes (Zimmerman *et al.*, 1983).

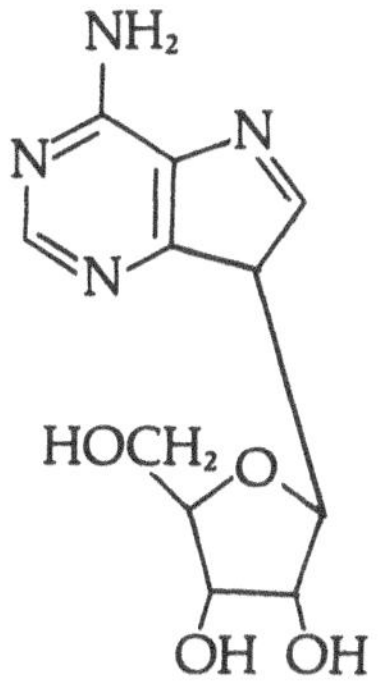

$$NH_2$$

HOCH$_2$

OH OH

19

An isomer, 3-deazaadenosine (**20**), inhibits antibody-dependent cellular cytotoxicity of mouse spleen cells at 3 μM and the antibody-dependent phagocytosis of mouse peritoneal cells (Medzihradsky *et al.*, 1982). It controls *S*-adenosylmethionine-mediated transmethylation by inhibiting *S*-adenosylhomocysteine hydrolase and intracellular accumulation of 3-deaza-*S*-adenosylhomocysteine.

$$NH_2$$

HOCH$_2$

OH OH

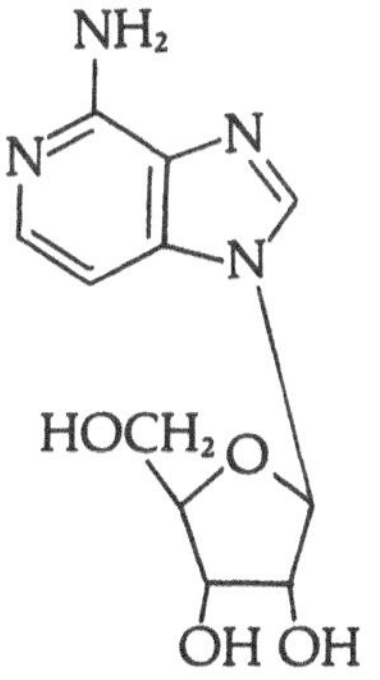

20

Two inosine derivatives, isoprinosine (**21**) and NPT 15392 (**22**), are modulators of lymphocyte and macrophage functions (Hadden and Wybran, 1981; Ikehara *et al.*, 1981). NPT 15392 is more potent than isoprinosine on suppressor functions. At 0.01–10 μg/ml, it induces suppressor cells that inhibit a mixed leukocyte culture reaction and an autologous response to Con A.

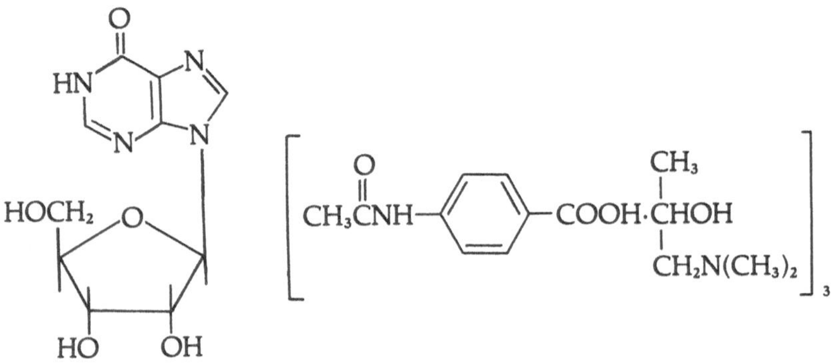

21

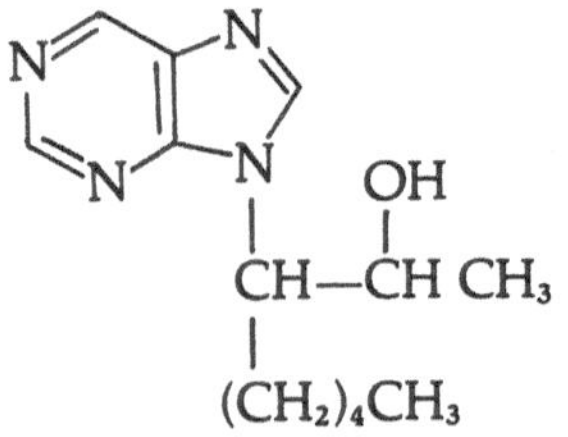

22

In the NZB murine model of autoimmune hemolytic anemia, NPT 15392 also retards the development of antierythrocyte antibody accompanied by some improvement of disease parameters (Jones *et al.*, 1983). As discussed in Chapter 8, *in vivo* NPT 15392 exerts an overall immunostimulating and immunorestorative effect in tumor-suppressed mice and cancer patients.

A resurgence of interest in nucleoside analogs as potential immunopharmacological agents is evident. With continued elucidation of the critical metabolic pathways involved in the proliferation and function of subsets of T and B lymphocytes and phagocytes, further development of specific immunosuppressive nucleosides is expected.

4. MEMBRANE REGULATORS

Membrane receptors, ligands, and transport systems are involved in cellular interactions and responses to external stimuli. Agents affecting the integrity and function of submembrane elements such as microtubules and microfilaments clearly would exert immunoregulatory activities. For example, the microtubule-disrupting agents colchicine (**23**) and vinblastine (**24**) decrease or abolish the effect of macrophage inhibitory factor (MIF) or macrophage-activating factor (MAF) on the macrophage (McCarthy *et al.*, 1979). They also inhibit lectin-induced lymphocyte mitogenesis and receptor mobility, as well as humoral antibody response to SRBC (Trottier and Fitzgerald, 1981). Vinblastine, but not the closely related vincristine (**25**), suppresses the generation of cytotoxic T-

23

lymphocyte response *in vitro* and *in vivo* (Ryoyama *et al.*, 1982). It was suggested that T-cell responses are more sensitive to vinblastine, whereas B-cell responses are more sensitive to vincristine. In the NZB/NZW lupus model, greater toxicity was seen with vinblastine. At carefully chosen doses, vincristine is erythrosuppressive without affecting primary antibody response. Vincristine and a new analog, vindesine (**26**), appear to have better safety margins in prolonging the survival time of these animals (Olsen and Gabrielsen, 1982).

R^1	R^2	R^3	
$CONH_2$	.OH	CH_3	26
$COOCH_3$	$OCOCH_3$	CHO	25
$COOCH_3$	$OCOCH_3$	CH_3	24

Lymphocyte activation by the mitogen phytohemagglutinin (PHA) requires an accumulation of intracellular Ca^{2+}, which induces turnover of monophosphoinositide and cGMP synthesis. The microfilament inhibitor cytochalasin B (**27**) exerts a biphasic effect on the uptake of Ca^{2+} in antibody- and complement-treated L cells (Shearer and Moore, 1981). It enhances uptake at lower concentrations (10^{-6} M) and inhibits the uptake only at higher concentrations (10^{-4} M).

5. METALS

5.1. GOLD DERIVATIVES

The potential of metal salts or organometallic compounds as cytotoxic or immunomodulatory agents has received increasing attention in recent years. The antirheumatic effect of injectable gold salts such as sodium aurothiomalate (28) and gold thioglucose (29) was recognized early. Various inhibitory actions on cellular and enzymatic functions were attributed to colloidal gold accumulated in the tissue, but the antirheumatic and possible immunological effects of gold are still poorly understood (Leibfarth and Persellin, 1981). A major action of gold may involve interference with macrophage functions essential in the activation of lymphocytes (Lipsky and Ziff, 1982).

$HO_2CCH(SAu)CH_2CO_2H$

28

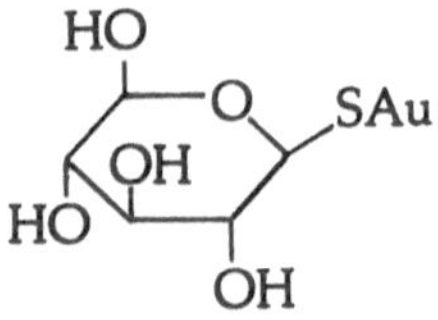

29

An orally active derivative, auranofin (**30**), has been developed (Sutton *et al.*, 1972). Auranofin is a coordination complex of acetylated gold thioglucose with a highly lipophilic phosphine group. *In vitro*, auranofin at 5 μM inhibits the

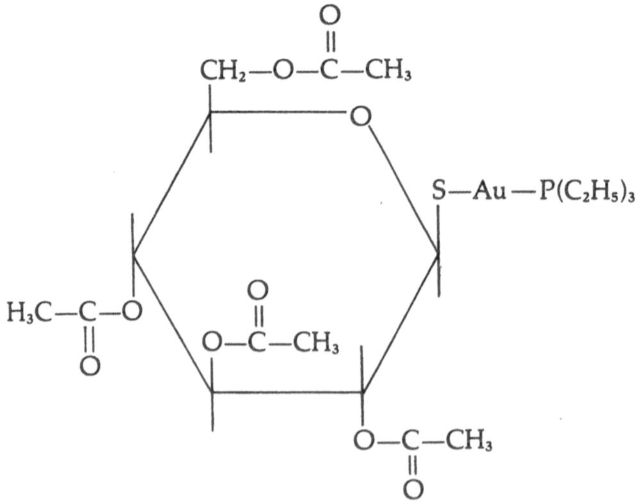

30

release of lysosomal enzymes from zymosan-stimulated rat leukocytes (DiMartino and Walz, 1977) and immune-complex-treated human leukocytes (Finkelstein *et al.*, 1977). It blocks PMN-mediated antibody-dependent lysis of L cells. It also interferes with the membrane transport of thymidine and 2-deoxy-D-glucose. These properties are not shared by sodium aurothiomalate. Apparently, the lipophilic and metabolic properties of this coordination compound not only change oral absorption and other pharmacodynamic properties of gold but also its membrane and intracellular actions. *In vivo*, auranofin at a dose equivalent to 10 mg gold/kg per day significantly decreases 7 S antibody production in adjuvant-arthritic rats and produces a 60% reduction in the number of hemolytic plaque-forming cells in normal rats. In rheumatoid arthritic patients at a daily dose of 6–9 mg, auranofin decreases IgG and rheumatoid factor titers and the abnormal erythrocyte sedimentation rate. The common side effects of auranofin are diarrhea, rashes, and renal and hematological disorders. The detailed cellular and *in vivo* metabolism of auranofin has not been described. Since there are multiple metabolizable groups and bonds in auranofin, it is conceivable that some of its biological properties may be attributable to various intermediary metabolites.

5.2. PLATINUM COMPLEXES

A family of platinum complexes have been investigated primarily for their antitumor activities (Plowman, 1983). Bioactive platinum complexes have a generic structure of *cis*-(Pt-A$_2$X$_2$). The *trans* stereoisomers are often inactive. The lability of the anionic leaving group X affects the *in vivo* stability, the tissue distribution, and, consequently, the toxicity and activity of the complex. The optimal groups are chloride, bromide, or oxalate anions. The N-donor group A (e.g., NH$_3$, RNH$_2$, R$_2$NH, etc.) are likely to remain in the coordination complex *in vivo*. As in the case of auranofin, their lipophilicity may alter the membrane permeability of the complex and exert a secondary effect on bioactivity. Platinum complexes interact with the N^7 guanine and N^3 cytosine in the DNA in an interstrand or intrastrand manner comparable to the cross-linking of DNA by bifunctional alkylating agents.

Bioactive platinum complexes, CDDP (**31**) and the diaminocyclohexane analog PHM (**32**), exert their immunosuppressive action at least partly by inhibition

31   **32**

of lymphocyte transformation. CDDP suppresses adjuvant-induced arthritis in rats at 1 mg/kg with marked lymphocytopenia. CDDP also suppresses antibody plaque-forming cells and various cellular immune responses such as skin graft rejection and graft-versus-host reactions in mice. The less nephrotoxic analog PHM has shown similar properties. It is also effective in experimental allergic encephalomyelitis. The immunosuppressive action of platinum complexes is short-lived and can be followed by a rebound immunostimulation. The severe toxicity of these complexes, i.e., renal tubular necrosis, myelosuppression, autoimmune hemolytic anemia, etc., has so far confined their therapeutic applications to cancer therapy and possibly intralesional injections, such as intraarticular injection in rheumatoid arthritis.

5.3. OTHER METALS

Results on the immunomodulatory effects of other metals are still preliminary (Rainsford *et al.*, 1983). The inhibition of helper T cells by D-penicillamine (**59**) and other thiol compounds appears to require copper (see below). Zinc deprivation is associated with an immunodeficiency syndrome (Bach, 1981). Zinc supplement enhances the mitogenic responses of human lymphocytes in an age-dependent fashion through action on the cytochalasin B-sensitive microfilaments. Other metal derivatives have shown immunostimulatory effects. Lithium carbonate at a serum level of 1 meq/liter enhances granulocyte production via stimulation of monocyte colony-stimulating factor production (Lee and Hopkins, 1980). It may also have a direct stimulatory effect on helper cells and it abrogates suppresses cells. Several organogermanium compounds, e.g., (Ge $CH_2CH_2CO_2H)_2O_3$, are orally active immunoadjuvants (Aso *et al.*, 1981). Further clarification of the immunochemical mechanisms of metals and their derivatives is needed to ascertain their immunosuppressive/modulatory activities under different conditions.

6. ANTIMICROBIAL AGENTS

With obvious clinical implications, the immunological activity of various types of antimicrobial agents has been surveyed broadly. The immunosuppressive activity of the cytostatic antitumor mitomycin C (**33**) has been demonstrated by its prolongation of skin graft survival and suppression of the graft-versus-host reaction (Lemmel and Good, 1969). Adriamycin (**34**) is immunosuppressive and antiinflammatory in many *in vitro* and *in vivo* systems (Ehrke *et al.*, 1983; Gieldanowski and Skowronska, 1980). Its cytostatic effect suppresses lymphocyte transformation and B-cell proliferation. *In vivo* at 1 mg/kg, it causes suppression of both primary and secondary antibody response, preferably given 2 days after immunization.

The antibiotic chloramphenicol (**35**) was reported to be immunosuppressive in homologous skin transplantation in rats and nerve transplantation in rabbits at 100 mg/kg per day (Parekh, 1981). Its *p*-methylsulfonyl analog, thiamphenicol (**36**), has shown immunosuppressive properties in several systems. It inhibits

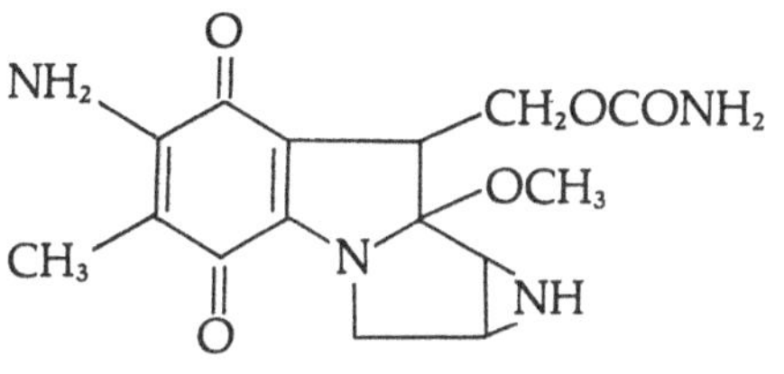

33

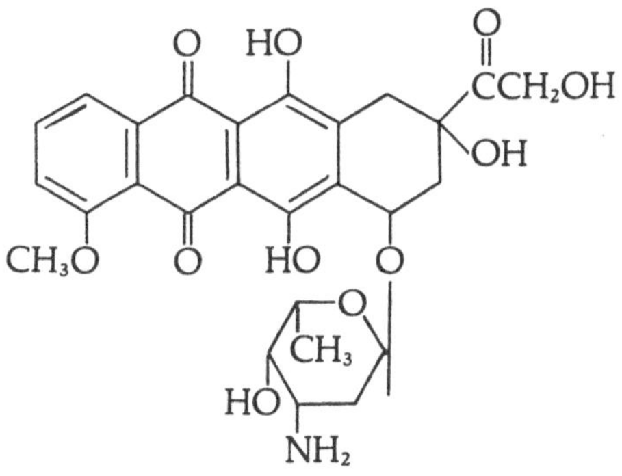

34

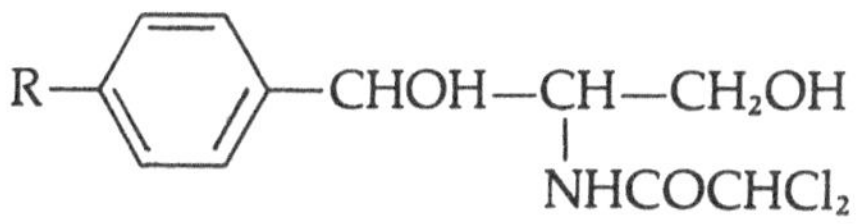

R=NO$_2$ 35
R=CH$_3$SO$_2$ 36

PHA-induced lymphocyte transformation and depresses primary antibody production but not secondary immune responses. Like cyclophosphamide, it prolongs the survival of renal allografts and life span of NZB/W mice. In preliminary clinical trials with lupus nephritis patients, thiamphenicol suppresses various laboratory indices of SLE such as antinuclear factor titers, LE cell numbers, elevated erythrocyte sedimentation rate and serum complement C3 levels. The main side effects are some reversible hematological disorders (Richmond, 1979).

A number of tetracyclines suppress PHA-induced blastogenesis and delayed hypersensitivity in mice (Thong and Ferrante, 1980). Tetracyclines also inhibit leukocyte migration and phagocytosis (Finch, 1980).

With aminoglycosides, a transient impairment of chemotaxis of PMN from healthy volunteers treated with gentamicin (37) or amikacin (38) was reported

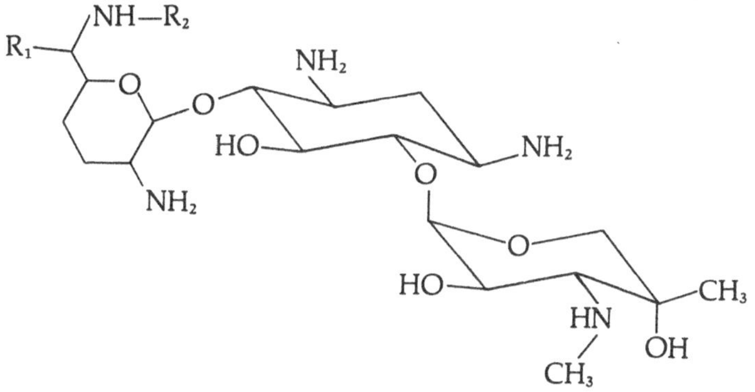

37

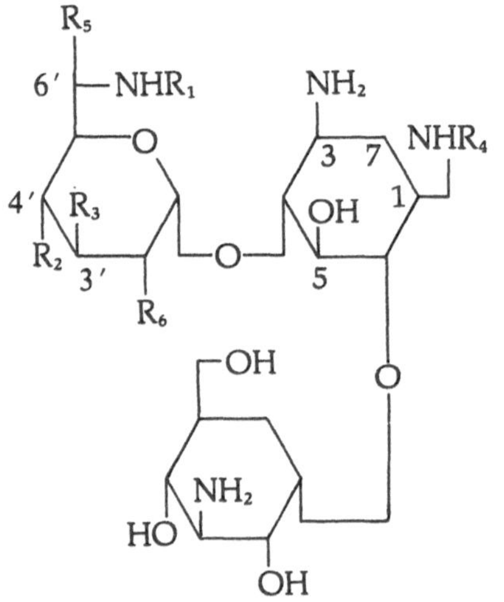

$$R_1 = R_5 = H, R_2 = R_3 = R_6 = OH, R_4 = COCH(OH)CH_2CH_2NH_2$$

38

(Khan *et al.*, 1979). However, a recent study using a different methodology found that neither gentimycin nor sisomicin (**39**) at therapeutic doses interferes with PMN chemotaxis and phagocytosis (LeMoli *et al.*, 1983). Further clarifications are needed.

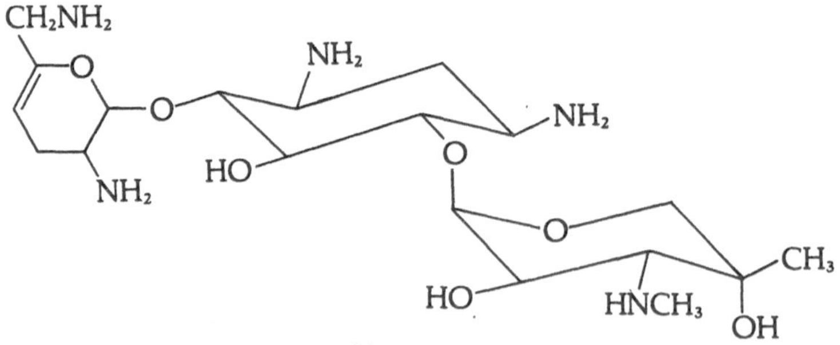

39

Rifampicin (**40**) also suppresses PHA-induced blastogenesis of human lymphocytes and delayed hypersensitivity in guinea pigs. It increases the survival time of skin allograft in rabbits (Finch, 1980) and heart allograft in rats (Schwartz and Charpentier, 1982).

The antimycotic amphotericin B (**41**) inhibits PHA blastogenesis of lymphocytes but enhances phagocytosis of macrophages and promotes selective toxicity for thymocytes and suppressor T cells (Stewart *et al.*, 1981).

40

41

7. CYCLOSPORIN A AND RELATED CYCLOPEPTIDES

One of the highlights in the current advances in transplant medicine is the discovery of cyclosporin A (Kolata, 1983).

Cyclosporin A (CyA) (**42**) is a fungal metabolite with profound immunosuppressive properties (Borel *et al.*, 1976). The discovery of CyA from screening of fermentation broths in a simple mouse assay of hemagglutinin formation and the demonstration of its selective immunosuppressive activities greatly heightened interest in the study of natural products as a source of novel immunotherapeutic agents. CyA is a hydrophobic cyclo-undecapeptide with a molecular weight of 1203. Early synthetic chemical studies showed that the presence of unnatural amino acids in the molecule is essential to maintain its high potency (Petcher *et al.*, 1976).

An extensive literature has been published on the immunological and clinical properties of CyA (Borel *et al.*, 1977; Burckhardt and Guggenheim, 1979; reviews by Borel, 1981; Britton and Palacios, 1982; White, 1982). CyA preferentially inhibits the generation of cytotoxic T lymphocytes but not that of suppressor T cells. Earlier investigations showed that CyA is a potent and reversible

```
                                              CH₃    H
                                                \   /
                                                 C
                                                 ‖
                                                 C
                                                / \
                                               H   CH₂
                                                    |
        CH₃    CH₃              CH₃    CH₃  HO      CH          CH₃
          \   /                   \   /      \      |            |
           CH              CH₃     CH   CH₃   CH   CH₃   CH₂    CH₃
           |                \     /      |     \   /      |      |
           CH₂              CH₃  CH    CH₃ CH  CH₃        CH₂   CH₃
           |                 |    |     |   |             |      |
  CH₃—N—CH—CO—N——CH—C—N——CH—CO—N—CH—C—N—CH₂
       |    L          L    ‖            |   L    ‖        |
       CO                   O            H        O        CO
 CH₃                                     ┊        ┊        |
   \                                     ┊        ┊        N—CH₃
    CH—CH₂—CH L                          ┊        ┊        |
   /                                     H        O        |
 CH₃                                              ‖        N—CH₃
   CH₃—N                                  H       |   H    |
       |    D            L    |       L   |    L  |   |  L |
      OC—CH——N—CO—CH—N—CO—CH—N—C—CH—N—CO—CH
           |       |        |        |      |        |
          CH₃      H       CH₃       CH₂   CH₃       CH₂
                                      |     CH        |
                                      CH   /  \       CH
                                     /  \ CH₃ CH₃    /  \
                                   CH₃  CH₃        CH₃  CH₃
                                          42
```

inhibitor of lymphocyte proliferation and primary mixed lymphocyte reaction probably by affecting an early event after stimulation. A recent analysis (Bunjes *et al.*, 1981) suggested that CyA impaired the release of IL-1 from activated macrophages. It also blocks the release of, or response to, IL-2 or T-cell growth factor from activated T-helper cells (Larsson, 1980), thus depriving the activation of cytotoxic T-lymphocyte precursors. In humans, both T and B lymphocytes seem to be affected. Numerous animal experiments have demonstrated the efficacy of CyA in skin, nerve, and renal allografts. In man, CyA is active orally or intravenously. A 92% survival rate with CyA, compared with 45% survival with Az, was observed in a 1981 study. As the antilymphocyte activity may require the constant presence of CyA in the treatment of human allotransplantation, e.g., kidney, liver, heart, lung, and pancreas, continuous therapy with CyA and concomitant therapy with adrenal corticoids has been suggested.

Impressed by the activity of CyA and at the same time concerned about its severe side effects, e.g., nephrotoxicity and an increased incidence of lymphoma, several laboratories have searched for safer agents. Herbicolin is a lipophilic cyclic heptapeptide produced by *Erwinia lerbicola*. Its chemical and biological properties are similar to CyA (Bockhorn *et al.*, 1983).

Cyclomunine is another hexacyclodepsipeptide of undefined structure extracted from *Fusarium equiseti* (Pompidou *et al.*, 1980; Navarro and Touraine, 1983). It has a moderate immunopotentiating effect at very low doses (10^{-3} μg/ml) and a potent inhibitory effect on mitogen-induced lymphocyte proliferation at > 1 μg/ml. *In vivo*, it suppresses graft-versus-host reaction and rejection of skin allograft in mice. These immunosuppressive properties have been attributed to its cytotoxic and cytostatic activities on lymphoblasts. A comparative study of cyclomunine and cyclosporin A showed some similar *in vitro* properties.

8. OTHER NATURAL PRODUCTS

8.1. L-ASPARAGINASE

An interesting development in immunosuppressive therapy is the use of an enzyme, L-asparaginase from *E. coli* cultures, that hydrolyzes asparagine to aspartic acid (Ohno and Hersh, 1970). Lymphoid tissue in man is deficient in asparagine synthetase and is consequently highly susceptible to the depletion of asparagine. Human T lymphocytes are more sensitive to this enzyme than B lymphocytes (Holland and Ohnuma, 1979). L-Asparaginase induces lymphopenia and reduces the size of lymph nodes, thymus, and spleen. It is a potent immunosuppressant of humoral and cell-mediated immunity. The enzyme preparation also has some glutaminase activity, which may contribute to the immunosuppressive action as well. Clinically, L-asparaginase induces remissions in acute lymphoblastic leukemia (Tallal *et al.*, 1970). Covalent attachment of this enzyme to polyethylene glycol reduces its antigenicity and prolongs its plasma half-life to 72 hr in man (Abuchowski *et al.*, 1981).

8.2. SERUM THYMIC FACTOR ANALOGS

Thymic factors (FTS) induce T-cell differentiation and maturation, and enhance T-cell functions (Bach *et al.*, 1975; Lau and Goldstein, 1980). Similar to other thymic factors and thymopoietin, FTS also increases the activity of T suppressors (Kaiserlian *et al.*, 1981). FTS and several metabolically more stable structural analogs, which possess similar biological activities and binding affinity to FTS-specific cellular receptors, were also found to suppress skin graft rejection. Thus, according to the immune status of the animal, FTS may act either as an immunostimulator or as an immunosuppressor.

8.3. VITAMIN D DERIVATIVES

A link between the immune system and bone metabolism was indicated by the action of a lymphokine, osteoclast-activating factor, that stimulates osteoclasts to resorb bone *in vitro*. The production of osteoclast-activating factor requires T lymphocytes and macrophages. Recently, an impairment of the mitogenic response of T cells from thymus and spleen and a decrease of thymus weight were found to be associated with defective bone resorption induced by clodronate, dichloromethylene diphosphonate (**43**), treatment (Milhaud *et al.*, 1983).

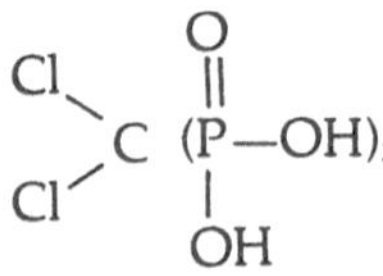

43

Addition of 0.01 µg/ml of 1α,25-dihydroxy, 1α,24(*R*), and 1α,24(*S*)-dihydroxy derivatives of cholecalciferol (vitamin D$_3$) to human peripheral blood lymphocytes significantly suppresses mitogen-induced lymphoproliferation (Miyakoshi *et al.*, 1981). However, the possible *in vivo* immunomodulatory effects of these and other vitamin D metabolites in normal and immunosuppressed patients remain to be clarified.

8.4. CHOLESTEROL DERIVATIVES

The roles of various types of lipids in the development, reactivity, and regulation of the immune systems and their possible effects on tumor development were reviewed at a workshop recently (Newberne and Thurman, 1981). Dietary fats, cholesterol, and other sterols appear to influence cancer induction either directly or indirectly. Lipemia is associated with aberrations of immune function in humans. Polyunsaturated fats have a regulatory effect on lymphocyte reactivity, possibly via the oxygenated metabolites of arachidonic acid and other fatty acids as well as an altered hormone metabolism. As a consequence, skin graft and renal transplant survivals are improved, and mitogenic responses and delayed hypersensitivity are suppressed. Hypercholesterolemia also diminishes lymphocyte response to antigens and decreases host resistance to infection and to transplantable tumors. Oxidized derivatives of cholesterol are potent immunosuppressives. 25-Hydroxycholesterol (**44**) inhibits *in vitro* humoral and cellular responses. These effects are not related to its inhibition of cellular 3-hydroxy-3-methylglutaryl cholesterol (HMG CoA) reductase, the enzyme controlling the rate of cholesterol formation. Compactin (**45**), a specific fungus-derived inhibitor of HMG CoA reductase, has no immunosuppressive activity (Humphries, 1981).

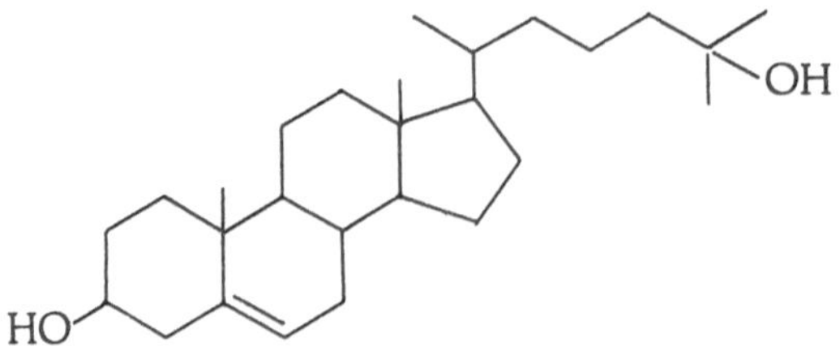

44

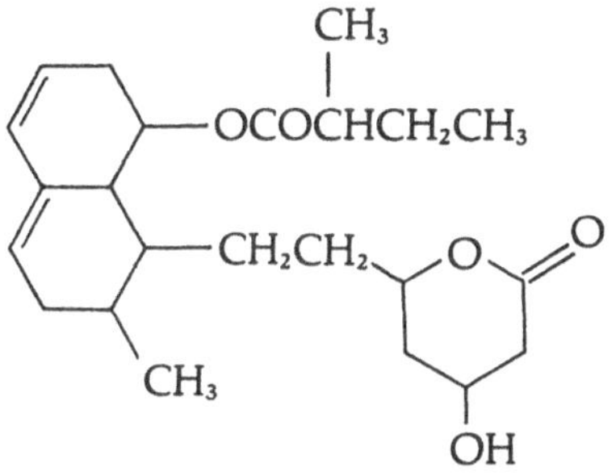

$$CH_3$$
$$\text{—OCOCHCH}_2\text{CH}_3$$
$$\text{—CH}_2\text{CH}_2$$
O   O

$$CH_3$$

OH

45

Plasma lipoproteins are also involved in some regulatory aspects of lymphocytes, inhibiting their *in vivo* and *in vitro* functions. Lymphocytes have surface receptors for different subsets of lipoproteins. Occupancy of LDL receptors suppresses PHA-enhanced accumulation of Ca^{2+} and the subsequent increase of cGMP and phosphatidylinositol turnover in human lymphocytes (Harmony and Hui, 1981). LDL also influences the activation of T lymphocytes into suppressor cells or into killer cells. The overall *in vivo* results may fluctuate according to the levels of lipoproteins and the immune status.

8.5. CARRAGEENAN

A variety of polysaccharides and their derivatives have been found to have immunomodulatory activity, enhancing host resistance to infection, etc. (see Chapters 10 and 12). Most of those are nonionic β(1→3)glucans.

Carrageenans are a group of sulfated polysaccharides isolated from marine algae that can markedly suppress immune responses both *in vivo* and *in vitro* (Thomson and Fowler, 1981). The primary structures of κ, ι, and λ carrageenans are shown in Fig. 2 (Rochas and Rinaudo, 1980). Carrageenan has been used in the past two decades as an inflammatory stimulus in the laboratory investigation of nonsteroidal antiinflammatory agents. The polyanionic carrageenan blocks the chemical pathway of complement activation. Recently, carrageenan was shown to be cytotoxic to macrophages due to its persistence within secondary lysosomes after ingestion, being resistant to degradation by lysosomal glycosidases. The ι form of carrageenan is also a mitogen for subpopulations of mouse B cells (Kolb *et al.*, 1981). *In vivo*, carrageenan is a potent immunosuppressant and prolongs graft survival. However, repeated systemic administration of carrageenan causes disseminated intravascular coagulation, hepatotoxicity, and nephrotoxicity. These toxicities obviously preclude any clinical applications.

8.6. CARBOHYDRATE DERIVATIVES

A novel glucoside of plant origin, sarmentosine (**46**), was shown to inhibit cell-mediated immune responses (Zhai *et al.*, 1982). It suppresses plaque-form-

κ - carrageenan

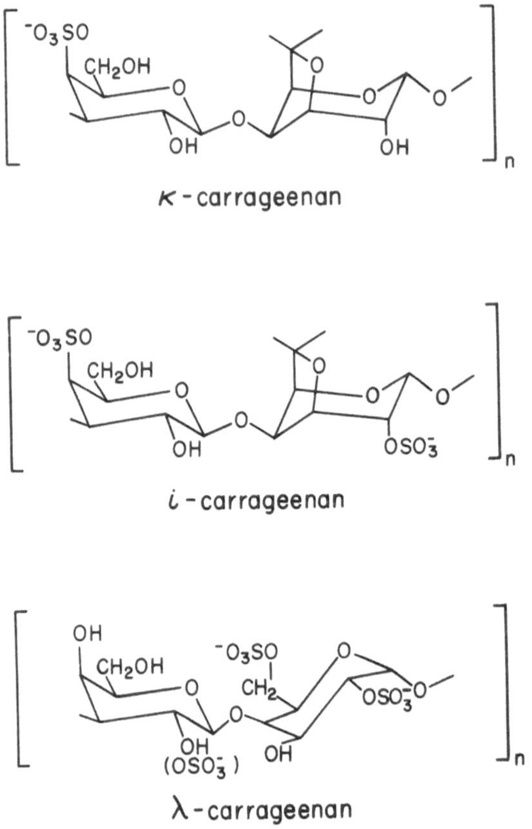

ι - carrageenan

λ - carrageenan

FIGURE 2.   Structural formulas of carra-geenans.

ing cell response and graft-versus-host response in rats. Very low toxicity was observed.

A simple carbohydrate derivative, n-pentyl-β-D-fructopyranoside (**47**), was found to inhibit IgE formation in passive cutaneous anaphylaxis in mice and rats (Haraguchi *et al.*, 1982).

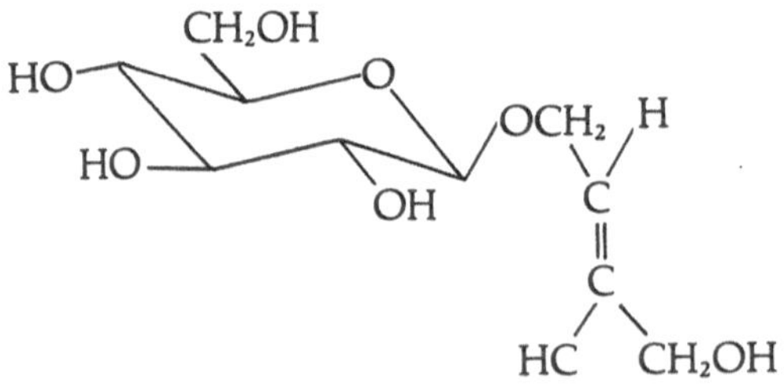

46

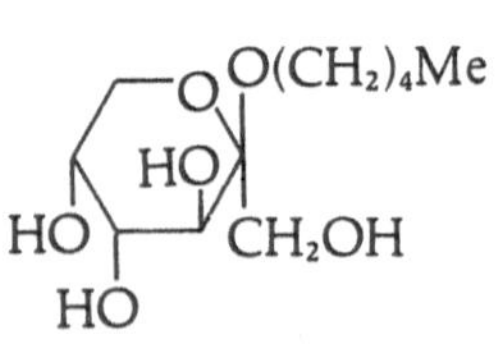

47

8.7. DIVERSIFIED STRUCTURES

The diversity of natural products and close analogs possessing immunosuppressive properties was further shown by many preliminary reports. Cytostipin and vermiculine (**48**) (Horakova *et al.*, 1980) inhibit the graft-versus-host reaction. Cimicifugocide (**49**) inhibits blastogenesis of mouse splenocytes at 50 ng/ml. It inhibits primary antibody response to SRBC at 0.1 mg i.p. and delayed hypersensitivity at 1 mg i.v. Its immunosuppressive action is preferentially directed toward B-cell function (Hemmi and Ishida, 1980).

The immunosuppressive effects of mycotoxins, e.g., trichothecenes T2 toxin, have also been observed (Ito *et al.*, 1982). These mycotoxins inhibit DNA synthesis, mitogenic responses of guinea pig spleen cells, and anti-DNP antibody response *in vivo*.

The development of hyporesponsiveness, or tolerance, to the immunosuppressive Δ^8-tetrahydrocannabinol (**50**) has been demonstrated (Loveless *et al.*, 1981). The ED_{50} for the inhibition of hemolytic plaque-forming cells (PFC)/spleen after immunization with SRBC was estimated to be 40 mg/kg. However, the ED_{50} was elevated significantly higher after daily treatment with 5–10 mg/kg Δ^8 THC for 5 days prior to SRBC immunization.

A unique sesquiterpene, qinghaosu (**51**), isolated from *Artemesia annua* L., is an antimalaria agent reported to have some modest effect on the immune system (Ge *et al.*, 1982). A water-soluble sodium hemisuccinate derivative of qinghaosu inhibits mitogenic responses of mouse spleen cells or human peripheral lymphocytes at 1 μg/ml, but shows only marginal effects *in vivo*.

9.   SYNTHETIC IMMUNOPHARMACOLOGICAL AGENTS

Interest in synthetic compounds as potential immunopharmacological agents has steadily grown in recent years in many pharmaceutical laboratories. There is also an increasing concern for the potential immunotoxicity of new drugs. As a result, a variety of pharmacological agents and many novel synthetic compounds have been investigated in newer immunological assays. In general, these compounds are first characterized by their effects on lymphocyte proliferation, macrophage and neutrophil functions, antibody production, and the development of plaque-forming cells, delayed hypersensitivity, graft-versus-host reaction, etc. Chronic inflammatory models such as adjuvant- or collagen II-induced polyarthritis in rats and disease models like NZB/W autoimmune mice are occasionally used as follow-up assays. *In vitro* assays measuring specific biochemical or cellular processes in immune response such as production or function of individual interleukins, receptor blockage of chemoattractants C5a, f-Met-Leu-Phe, LTB_4, platelet-activating factor, etc. and differential effects on subsets of B and T lymphocytes are being used with increasing frequency to elucidate their possible mechanism of actions. At the present time, the determination and prediction of potential immunotoxicity is still dependent on long-term safety assessment in animals. Nevertheless, with the rapid growth of "immunotoxicity" as a new descipline, further progress in developing cellular assays and more predictive toxicity models to eliminate potentially toxic structures as therapeutic agents will undoubtedly be made in the near future. Some current studies in the search for new immunosuppressive agents are illustrated by the following examples.

9.1.   PROCARBAZINE

Procarbazine (**52**) was originally synthesized as a monoamine oxidase inhibitor and was found to possess antitumor and immunosuppressive activities (Zeller *et al.*, 1963). It is used clinically in the treatment of Hodgkin's disease. The cytotoxicity of procarbazine is related to its *in vivo* metabolism, liberating the methyl hydrazine moiety, which is a precursor of reactive methyl radicals. Procarbazine suppresses the circulatory antibody response and prolongs the survival of skin allografts. With an appropriate dosage schedule, procarbazine, like cyclophosphamide and methotrexate, strongly inhibits antibody response to SRBC in mice without affecting delayed hypersensitivity (Doherty, 1981) . Procarbazine also potentiates the immunosuppressive effect of antilymphocyte serum (Floersheim, 1973).

$$\begin{array}{c} CH_3 \\ CH_3 \end{array} CH-NHCO-\!\!\!\!\bigcirc\!\!\!\!-CH_2-NH-NH-CH_3$$

52

9.2.   NIRIDAZOLE

Niridazole is a nitrothiazole derivative (**53**). At the therapeutic doses used in the treatment of schistosomiasis in man, niridazole was found to suppress both *in vitro* and *in vivo* manifestations of cell-mediated immunity primarily by interfering with the afferent arm of T-cell sensitization (Vadas and Bernard, 1981). It markedly inhibits the development of experimental autoimmune encephalomyelitis (EAE), resulting from the attack of activated T lymphocytes on the myelin of the central nervous system, in mice and in rats. Niridazole also decreases the severity of thyroid infiltration in a laboratory model of autoimmune murine thyroiditis at 100 mg/kg (Vladutiu, 1982).

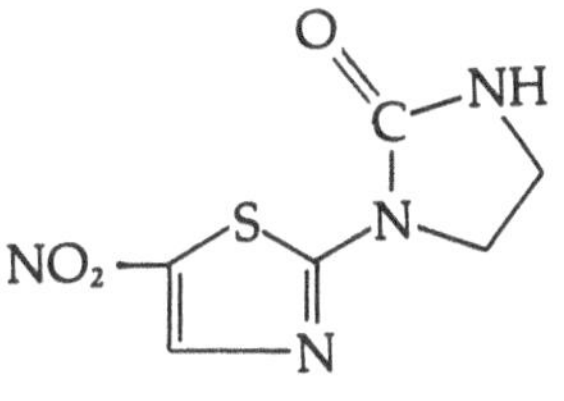

53

It may be noted that, analogous to levamisole (**55**), both niridazole and

$$S$$
$$|$$

TEI-3096 (see below) have the partial structure of thiourea (N—C—N) in their ring systems. The sulfhydryl derivative of levamisole (**56**) was recognized as an active metabolite. Similarly, the ring-opened metabolite of niridazole, 1-thiocarbamoyl-2-imidazolidinone (**54**), was shown to mimic its immunosuppressive effects (Tracy *et al.*, 1982; Gautman *et al.*, 1982).

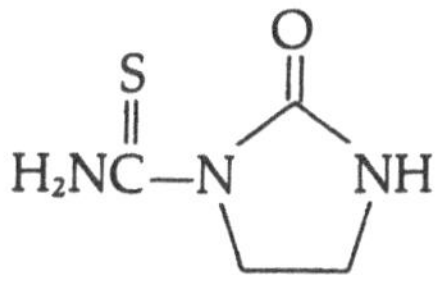

54

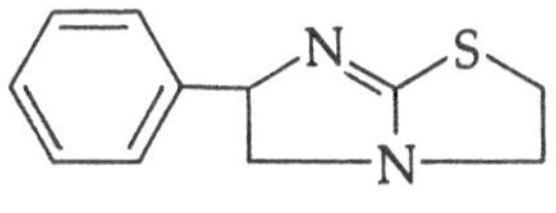

55

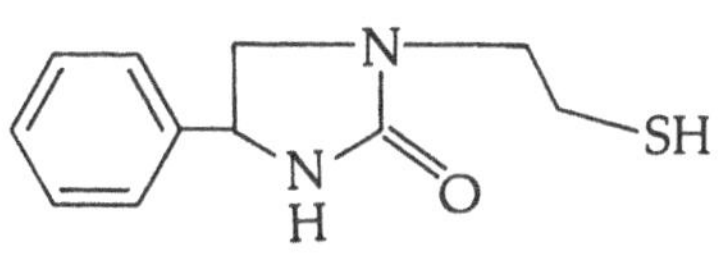

56

9.3.   TEI-3096

From the testing of a series of thiazolopyrimidine derivatives, TEI-3096 (**57**) was found to suppress adjuvant arthritis but not acute inflammation in rats at 10-50 mg/kg (Yamamoto *et al.*, 1980). It inhibits blast formation induced by Con

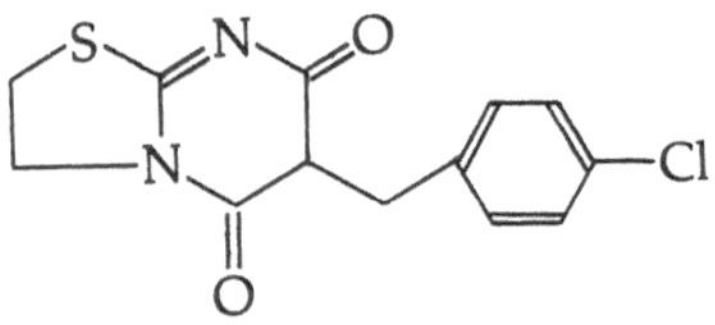

57

A or LPS at > 50 μM and suppresses elevated PFC response against a T-cell-dependent antigen. It also enhances delayed hypersensitivity in mice and rats (Komoriya *et al.*, 1981).

9.4. CP-17,193

In the development of piroxicam as a nonsteroidal antiinflammatory agent, several related structures were found to be immunosuppressive agents (Lombardino and Otterness, 1981). CP-17,193 (58) is not lymphocytotoxic but displays marked immunosuppressive activity in mice (Otterness, 1981). At low doses (1–3 mg/kg p.o.), CP-17,193, like cyclophosphamide, preferentially inhibits the humoral immune response to the antigen EL_4 tumor cells (Otterness and Chang, 1976), which possess major H-2 differences and are strongly linked with T-cell mitogenicity. The inhibition of humoral response to SRBC, as a weak polyclonal B-cell mitogen, requires higher doses of CP-17,193. Above 10 mg/kg p.o., both humoral and cellular responses are completely suppressed. For both antigens the order of suppressive potency on a weight basis is methotrexate > CP-17,193 > cyclophosphamide > 6-MP > Az.

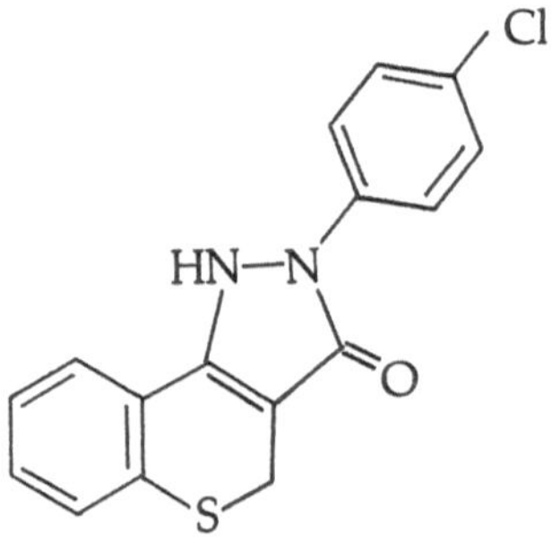

58

10. GLUCOCORTICOIDS

Following the dramatic demonstration of the potent antiarthritic effect of cortisone in 1948, a family of synthetic and more potent steroid derivatives have been used widely as antiinflammatory and immunosuppressive agents. The chemical structures of commonly used glucocorticoids are shown in Fig. 3. Among these, dexamethasone is often used as a standard reference in many

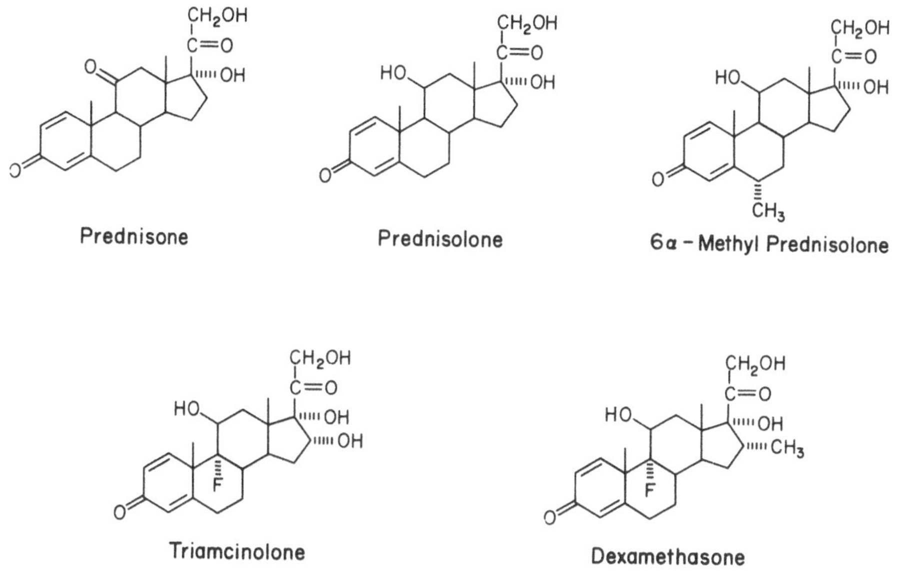

Prednisone   Prednisolone   6α – Methyl Prednisolone

Triamcinolone   Dexamethasone

FIGURE 3.   Commonly used glucocorticoids.

laboratory and clinical experiments. The biological actions of these compounds are very similar; they differ mainly in potency (on a weight basis), pharmacokinetics, and, to some extent, partial dissociation of various systemic side effects. The major metabolic, hormonal, cardiovascular, and sodium-retaining effects of these steroids have been extensively reviewed (Jasani, 1979; Nelson and Conn, 1980; Munck and Leung, 1977; Baxter and Harris, 1975; Bach, 1975).

The common mechanism of action of glucocorticoids at the molecular level involves a sequence of events starting from interaction with cellular membrane receptors as shown in Fig. 4.

The induction of protein synthesis by glucocorticoids in a diversity of tissues leads to the production of enzymes, e.g., tryptophan pyrrolase and tyrosine amino transferase in the liver, and enzyme inhibitors such as lipomodulin, which blocks the release of arachidonic acid by phospholipase A_2 in inflamed tissue and induces suppressor T cells as well (Hirata and Iwata, 1983).

At the cellular level, the immunosuppressive effects of glucocorticoids are manifested by lymphopenia, not due to lympholysis but through a redistribution of the circulating lymphocytes to extravascular compartments. The reduction of T lymphocytes is more pronounced than B lymphocytes. Glucocorticoids also inhibit the blastogenic response of lymphocytes to antigens, mitogens, and autologous mixed lymphocytes. These effects are transient, reversible, and require the presence of glucocorticoid receptors (Homo *et al.*, 1980). For example, 10–100 nM dexamethasone suppresses the production of the T-cell growth factor by stimulated human peripheral monocytes through a receptor-mediated process (Crabtree *et al.*, 1980). Dexamethasone (at > 10 nM), prednisolone, and hydrocortisone (at 1 μM) also reduce the number of Fc receptors, which are

Target Cell

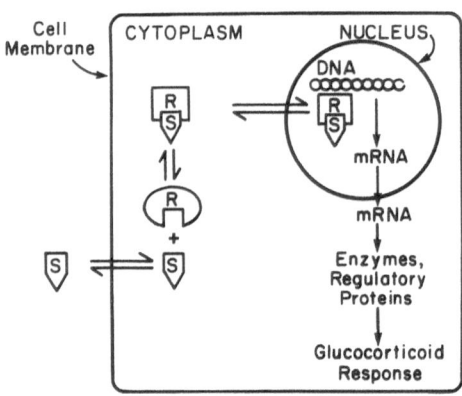

FIGURE 4.   Steps in glucocorticoid action. S, steroid; R, specific glucocorticoid receptor. (Adapted from Nelson *et al.*, 1980.)

important in initiating phagocytosis and antibody-dependent cell-mediated cytotoxicity, in a human progranulocyte cell line. At pharmacological or non-physiological concentrations (up to 10^{-5} M), steroids may exert an inhibitory effect on lymphoid tissue by a nonspecific process associated with an alteration of cell membranes.

Glucocorticoids induce monocytopenia and eosinopenia in a similar fashion. Monocyte functions such as chemotaxis, adherence, phagocytosis, granuloma formation, and responsiveness to lymphokines released from specifically sensitized lymphocytes are also impaired. Glucocorticoids further cause neutrophilic leukocytosis, via the release of mature neutrophils from the bone marrow. Granulocyte functions such as adherence, aggregation, release of pyrogen, mediators, and lysosomal hydrolases are inhibited by steroids under different conditions (Oseas *et al.*, 1982).

In addition, glucocorticoids have a protective effect on blood vessels and microcirculation. They reduce the vasodilatory effects of histamine, kinins, and prostaglandins, directly or indirectly.

Such profound physiological actions of glucocorticoids produce highly effective antiinflammatory and immunosuppressive effects in a wide range of immunological disorders such as autoimmune diseases, lupus erythematosus, rheumatoid arthritis, psoriasis, skin and organ transplantation, etc. Unfortunately, their long-term clinical applications are severely limited by many well-known side effects including adrenal suppression, electrolyte imbalance, osteoporosis, glucose intolerance, muscle catabolism, impaired wound healing and host resistance to infections. In the 1950s, extensive efforts in many research laboratories to improve the therapeutic safety margin of glucocorticoid analogs were largely unsuccessful. Nevertheless, those studies provided a biological foundation for the search of nonsteroidal structures, which may possess some of the immunoregulatory effects of glucocorticoids but without their hormonal or metabolic side effects.

11. ANTIARTHRITIC AGENTS

The involvement of immunological derangement in the pathogenesis of rheumatoid arthritis has long been recognized (McCarthy *et al.*, 1979; Ziff *et al.*, 1982). In chronic inflammation, the interaction of macrophages, T and B lymphocytes leads to the elaboration of lymphokines, the formation of antigen–antibody complexes, and the activation of PMNs, macrophages, and local cells to produce swelling, tissue proliferation, and cartilage destruction. A schematic representation is shown in Fig. 5. Not surprisingly, the possible immunomodulatory or immunosuppressive effects of antiarthritic agents, especially the "disease-modifying antirheumatic drugs" (DMARDs) such as gold (see above), D-penicillamine, and antimalarials, received much attention. In the search for nonsteroidal antiinflammatory agents (NSAIDs) during the past two decades, adjuvant-induced polyarthritis, and more recently collagen II-induced arthritis, in rats were also used extensively as secondary assays to determine their effects on immune-based chronic inflammatory processes. In the past few years, various *in vitro* assays, such as neutrophil and macrophage functions, lymphocyte responses, and chemotaxis, were employed to characterize their specific mechanisms of action. Although antiarthritic agents in general are not potent immunosuppressive agents, as shown by the following examples, some of their immunopharmacological properties may be contributory to their therapeutic effects clinically.

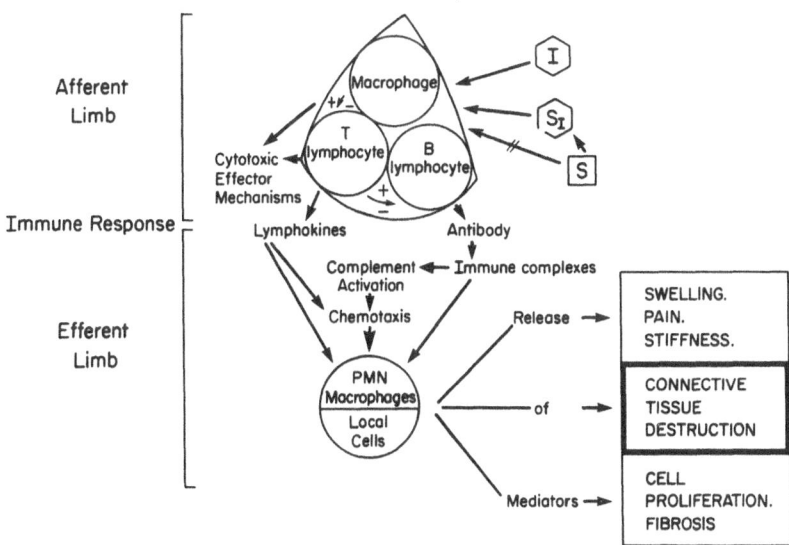

FIGURE 5. Schematic representation of the pathogenesis of chronic inflammatory diseases. (From Davies *et al.*, 1982.)

11.1.   D-PENICILLAMINE

D-Penicillamine (**59**), first obtained from the acid hydrolysates of penicillin, is a copper chelator developed originally to promote urinary copper excretion in Wilson's disease patients. As a sulfhydryl compound, it is capable of dissociating macroglobulins such as rheumatoid factor *in vitro*. This observation led to a prolonged clinical investigation that demonstrated its slow-acting antirheumatic effects accompanied by a reduction of the level of circulating immune complexes (Jaffe, 1975). The mechanism of action of D-penicillamine is still not fully understood. In animal models, it has no inhibitory effect on acute inflammation.

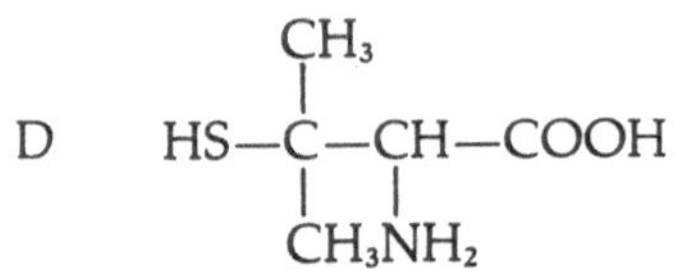

$$D \quad HS-\overset{\overset{\textstyle CH_3}{|}}{\underset{\underset{\textstyle CH_3NH_2}{|}}{C}}-CH-COOH$$

59

Depending on the dosing regimen, it can suppress or stimulate different versions of adjuvant arthritis. It also increases response to delayed hypersensitivity in rats and guinea pigs (Arrigoni-Martelli, 1982). *In vitro*, D-penicillamine in the presence of copper ions markedly decreases mitogen-induced T-cell proliferation and the generation of immunoglobulin-secreting cells. A selective action on T-cell functions was observed without concomitant alteration in the activity of either B cells or monocytes (Lipsky, 1982). In other systems, D-penicillamine acts as a polyclonal B-cell activator, significantly enhancing the primary humoral immune response (Goodman and Weigle, 1981).

11.2.   DAPSONE

Dapsone (**60**), the treatment of choice for leprosy (Modderman, 1980), was only recently demonstrated to possess moderate antirheumatic effect (McConkey *et al.*, 1976; Swinson *et al.*, 1981). After chronic therapy, dapsone significantly improves the erythrocyte sedimentation rate, reduces C-reactive proteins and other clinical parameters in rheumatic patients. Dapsone is also effective in treating the immune-based dermatitis herpetiformis. Unfortunately, its clinical applications are limited by its tendency to induce methemoglobinemia or hemo-

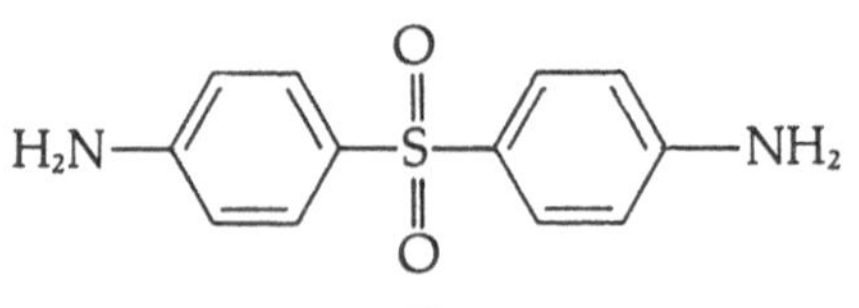

$$H_2N-\underset{\underset{O}{\overset{\overset{O}{\|}}{S}}}{}-NH_2$$

60

lysis in almost all patients (*Lancet*, 1981). In laboratory studies, dapsone and the close analog AUS (**61**), which has activity in treating avian leukosis (Shen *et al.*, 1971), are inhibitors of lecithin biosynthesis and the release of lysosomal en-

61

zymes in macrophages (Shigeura *et al.*, 1975; Bonney *et al.*, 1979; Davies *et al.*, 1982).

11.3. CCA

CCA is an anthranilic acid derivative (**62**) initially synthesized as an anti-rheumatic agent (Abe *et al.*, 1979). Its mode of action is not clear. As an immunomodulator, it potentiates antibody responses in animals with impaired immunity. On the other hand, it shows an immunosuppressive effect in animals with enhanced immune responses. For example, CCA suppresses the *in vitro* PFC response in spleen cells from NZB/W F_1 mice and reduces their kidney disease *in vivo* (Ohsugi *et al.*, 1978). It restores the T-suppressor activity in mice treated with colchicine (**23**), which inhibits the induction of T-suppressor cells. The action of CCA is believed to be mainly on T lymphocytes and not B lymphocytes (Yamamoto *et al.*, 1982). The effect of CCA on the production of rheumatoid factor and other immunological parameters in rheumatoid arthritic patients is still being ascertained (Warabi and Shiokawa, 1979).

62

12. INDUSTRIAL CHEMICALS

With the general concern regarding the potential environmental hazards of industrial chemicals and waste disposal, many publications on the immunotoxicity of various chemical intermediates or by-products have appeared. As non-specific metabolic poisons or cytotoxic agents, their detrimental effects on host immunity are not surprising. Benzene inhibits T- and B-lymphocyte mitogenesis and the production of PFC against SRBC in mice, probably via its oxidized metabolites, hydroquinone, catechol, etc., formed in the liver (Wierda *et al.*, 1981). A polychlorinated biphenyl mixture, Aroclor 1242, which stimulates hepatic mixed-function oxidases and conjugating enzymes, can decrease the amount of benzene metabolites in lymphoid tissues. However, Aroclor itself suppresses the *in vivo* primary splenic response to SRBC in mice. TCDD, 2,3,7,8-tetrachlorodibenzo-*p*-dioxin (**63**), is a persistent halogenated hydrocarbon with cumulative toxicity *in vivo*. At total doses of 40–100 µg/kg, TCDD causes cellular depletion in lymphoid tissues in mice and impairs antibody responses to SRBC and other antigens. It suppresses delayed hypersensitivity to oxazolone at 4

63

µg/kg. *In vitro*, it inhibits the generation of alloantigen-specific cytotoxic T cells at 0.004 µg/ml (Clark *et al.*, 1981). Similar immunotoxicities have been observed with other polyhalogenated biphenyls, naphthalenes, dibenzofurans and dibenzo-*p*-dioxins, and chlorinated phenols, including pentachlorophenol (PCP) (Exon and Koller, 1983).

13. OUTLOOK

In the past two decades, immunosuppressants have clearly evolved from cytotoxic alkylating agents and antimetabolites, as by-products of anticancer research, to a large group of immunoregulants of diverse chemical structures that can intervene in one or more pathways in the complex and dynamic immune system. With further progress in the characterization of humoral factors and subsets of immune cells, the current trend of developing more specific immunosuppressants with well-defined biochemical mechanism of action is certainly going to continue.

The principal clinical applications of available immunosuppressants are organ transplantation and severe autoimmune diseases. Because of their potential immunotoxicity such as an impairment of host resistance to infectious agents and possible tumorigenicity, applications to many other immunological disorders, which are less life-threatening, are still very limited. Hopefully, newer immunosuppressants will have more tolerale benefit/risk ratios to broaden their therapeutic utilities.

An increasing awareness of immunotoxicity has also prompted a widespread evaluation of the potential immunosuppressive effect of chemicals and drugs that were developed mainly for their pharmacological actions, such as captopril (Kallenberg *et al.*, 1981) and cephalosporins (Forsgren, 1981). In some cases the demonstrated immunosuppressive effects are relatively minor and probably not clinically significant. Nevertheless, such effort further bridged the traditional gap between two related disciplines, immunology and pharmacology.

The emergence of a unified immunopharmacological approach to drug development is clearly in evidence in the current research on antiarthritic agents. As indicated above, the pathogenesis of rheumatoid arthritis, lupus erythematosus, psoriasis, and other chronic inflammatory and degenerative diseases involves varying aspects of immunological disorders. Several classical inflammatory mediators have also been shown to have immunoregulatory properties. For example, prostaglandin E inhibits IL-2 production and exerts broad-range suppressive effects on B-cell and T-cell responses (Rogers *et al.*, 1982; Bonta and Parnham, 1982; Walker *et al.*, 1983) and alters the functional response of neutrophils to chemotactic peptides (Fantone *et al.*, 1983). On the other hand, LTB_4 and other oxygenated metabolites of arachidonic acid induce neutrophil chemotaxis and degranulation (Samuelsson, 1983; Bokoch and Reed, 1981). Several NSAIDs, in addition to their cyclooxygenase inhibitory activity, are also capable of blocking the receptor of the chemotactic peptide f-Met-Leu-Phe (Smith and Iden, 1980; Cost *et al.*, 1981) and/or suppressing the inflammatory responses of macrophages and neutrophils (Davies *et al.*, 1982). Undoubtedly, more potent leukocyte regulators with greater effects on cellular and humoral immunity than NSAIDs will be forthcoming. In the search for superior antiinflammatory and immunosuppressive agents, approaches aiming at receptor blockade, enzyme inhibition or suppression of mediator functions may provide an effective pharmacological intervention of an aggressive immune process, presumably with less long-term immunotoxicities.

REFERENCES

Abe, C., Warabi, H., and Shiokawa, Y., 1979, Immunopharmacological effects of CCA in human rheumatoid arthritis and in experimental animals, *The Ryumachi (Japan)* **19**:554.

Abuchowski, A., Davis, F. F., and Davis, S., 1981, Immunosuppressive properties and circulating life of achromobacter glutaminase-asparaginase covalently attached to polyethylene glycol in man, *Cancer Treat. Rep.* **65**:1077–1081.

Arrigoni-Martelli, E., 1982, Antirheumatic drugs, *Med. Actual.* **18**:461–508.

Aso, H., Yamaguchi, T., Ebina, T., and Ishida, N., 1981, *12th Int. Congr. Chemother., Florence* p. 129.

Bach, J. F., 1975, Corticosteroids, in: *The Mode of Action of Immunosuppressive Agents* (A. Neuberger and E. L. Tatum, eds.), pp. 21–91, Elswier, New York.

Bach, J. F., 1981, The multi-faceted zinc dependency of the immune system, *Immunol. Today* **2**:225.

Bach, J. F., Dardenne, M., Pleau, J. M., and Bach, M. A., 1975, Isolation, biochemical characterization and biological activity of a circulating thymic hormone in the mouse and in the human, *Ann. N.Y. Acad. Sci.* **249**:186.

Baxter, J. D., and Harris, A. W., 1975, Mechanisms of glucocorticoid action: General features with reference to steroid-mediated immunosuppression *Transplant. Proc.* **7**:55–65.

Bicker, U., 1982, Effect of the immunomodulant 2-cyanaziridine derivative BM 41.332 on adjuvant arthritis in the rat, *Arzneim. Forsch.* **32**:746–752.

Bockhorn, H., Baron, D. P., Hark, T., Degen, H., Hopt, U., Mueller, G. H., and Winkelmann, G., 1983, Herbicolin, another cyclic peptide with immunosuppressive activities, *Transplant. Proc.* **15**:560.

Bokoch, G. M., and Reed, P. W., 1981, Effect of various lipoxygenase metabolites of arachidonic acid on degranulation of polymorphonuclear leukocytes, *J. Biol. Chem.* **256**:5317–5320.

Bonney, R. J., Wightman, P. D., and Davies, P., 1979, Selective inhibitors of lecithin biosynthesis in mouse peritoneal macrophages, *Biochem. Pharmacol.* **28**:2471–2478.

Bonta, I. L., and Parnham, M. J., 1982, Immunomodulatory-antiinflammatory functions of E-type prostaglandins, *Int. J. Immunopharmacol.* **4**:103–110.

Borel, J. F., 1981, Cyclosporin-A: Present experimental status, *Transplant. Proc.* **13**:344.

Borel, J. F., Feurer, C., Gubler, H. U., and Stahelin, H., 1976, Biological effects of cyclosporin A: A new antilymphocytic agent, *Agents Actions* **6**:468–475.

Borel, J. F., Feurer, C., Magnee, C., and Stahelin, H., 1977, Effects of the new antilymphocytic peptide cyclosporin A in animals, *Immunology* **32**:1017–1025.

Britton, S., and Palacios, R., 1982, Cyclosporin A—usefulness, risks and mechanism of action, *Immunol. Rev.* **65**:5.

Brune, K., and Whitehouse, M. W., 1979, Cytostats with effects in chronic inflammation, in: *Handbook of Experimental Pharmacology*, Volume 50, Part 2 (J. R. Vane and S. H. Ferreira, eds.), pp. 531–578, Springer-Verlag, Berlin.

Bunjes, D., Hardt, C., Rollinghoff, M., and Wagner, H., 1981, Cyclosporin A mediates immunosuppression of primary cytotoxic T cell responses by impairing the release of interleukin 1 and interleukin 2, *Eur. J. Immunol.* **11**:657–661.

Burckhardt, J. J., and Guggenheim, B., 1979, Cyclosporin A: In vivo and in vitro suppression of rat T-lymphocyte function, *Immunology* **36**:753–757.

Cathcart, M. K., and Krakauer, R. S., 1982, Soluble factors in the suppression of the immune response, in: *Immune Regulation, Evolutionary and Biological Significance* (L. R. Ruben and M. E. Gershwin, eds.), pp. 167–199, Dekker, New York.

Clark, D. A., Gauldie, J., Szewczuk, M. R., and Sweeney, G., 1981, Enhanced suppressor cell activity as a mechanism of immunosuppression by 2,3,7,8-tetrachlorodibenzo-*p*-dioxin (41275), *Proc. Soc. Exp. Biol. Med.* **168**:290–299.

Cost, H., Gespach, C., and Abita, J.-P., 1981, Effect of indomethacin on the binding of the chemotactic peptide formyl-Met-Leu-Phe on human polymorphonuclear leukocytes, *FEBS Lett.* **132**:85–88.

Crabtree, G. R., Gillis, S., Smith, K. A., and Munck, A., 1980, Mechanisms of glucocorticoid-induced immunosuppression: Inhibitory effects on expression of Fc receptors and production of T-cell growth factor, *J. Steroid Biochem.* **12**:445–449.

Davies, P., Bonney, R. J., Humes, J. L., and Kuehl, F. A., Jr., 1982, The effect of anti-rheumatic agents on macrophage function, *Int. J. Immunopharmacol.* **4**:111–118.

DiMartino, M. J., and Walz, D. T., 1977, Inhibition of lysosomal enzyme release from rat leukocytes by auranofin: A new chrysotherapeutic agent, *Inflammation* **2**:131–142.

Doherty, N. S., 1981, Selective effects of immunosuppressive agents against the delayed hypersensitivity response and humoral response to sheep red blood cells in mice, *Agents Actions* **11**:237–242.

Ehrke, M. J., Tomazin, V., Ryoyama, K., Cohen, S. A., and Mihich, E., 1983, Adriamycin induced immunomodulation: Dependence upon time of administration, *Int. J. Immunopharmacol.* **5**:43–48.

Exon, J. H., and Koller, L. D., 1983, Effects of chlorinated phenols on immunity in rats, *Int. J. Immunopharmacol.* **5**:131–144.

Fantone, J. C., Marasco, W. A., Elgas, L. J., and Ward, P. A., 1983, Anti-inflammatory effects of prostaglandin E_1: In vivo modulation of the formyl peptide chemotactic receptor on the rat neurophil, *J. Immunol.* **130**:1495–1497.

Finch, R., 1980, Immunomodulating effects of antimicrobial agents, *J. Antimicrob. Chemother.* **6**:691–694.

Finkelstein, A. E., Roisman, F. R., and Walz, D. T., 1977, The effect of auranofin, a new antiarthritic agent, on immune complex-induced release of lysosomal enzymes from human leukocytes, *Inflammation* **2**:143–150.

Fishman, R. F., Rubin, A. L., Novogrodsky, A., and Stenzel, K. H., 1980, Selective suppression of blastogenesis induced by different mitogens: Effect of noncyclic adenosine-containing compounds, *Cell. Immunol.* **54**:129–139.

Floersheim, G. L., 1973, Induction of unresponsiveness to skin and heart allografts in mice by a synergistic treatment with procarbazine, anti-lymphocyte serum, and donor-type cells, *Transplantation* **15**:195.

Forsgren, A., 1981, The immunosuppressive effect of cephalosporins and cephalosporin–gentamicin combinations, *J. Antimicrob. Chemother.* **8**:183–186.

Gautman, S. C., Scissors, D. L., and Webster, L. T., Jr., 1982, Further observations on the effects of 1-thiocarbamoyl-2-imidazolidinone (TCI) on cell-mediated immunity, *Int. J. Immunopharmacol.* **4**:201–212.

Ge, H. L., Shen, M., He, Y. X., and Zhang, H. Z., 1982, Immunosuppressive action of qinghaosu, *Int. J. Immunopharmacol.* **4**:362.

Gieldanowski, J., and Skowronska, J., 1980, Studies on immunosuppressive and anti-inflammatory effect of adriamycin, *Arch. Immunol. Ther. Exp.* **28**:439–446.

Goodman, M. G., and Weigle, W. O., 1981, Nonspecific activation of murine lymphocytes, *Cell. Immunol.* **65**:337–351.

Hadden, J. W., and Wybran, J., 1981, Immunopotentiators. II. Isoprinosine, NPT 15392 and azimexone: Modulators of lymphocyte and macrophage development and function, in: *Advances in Immunopharmacology* (J. W. Hadden, L. Chedid, P. Mullen, and F. Spreafico, eds.), pp. 457–468, Pergamon Press, Elmsford, N.Y.

Haraguchi, Y., Yagi, A., Koda, A., Inagaki, N., Noda, K., and Nishioka, I., 1982, A specific inhibitor of IgE-antibody formation: *n*-Pentyl β-D-fructopyranoside, *J. Med. Chem.* **25**:1495–1499.

Harmony, J. A. K., and Hui, D. Y., 1981, Inhibition by membrane-bound low-density lipoproteins of the primary inductive events of mitogen-stimulated lymphocyte activation, *Cancer Res.* **41**:3799–3802.

Hauser, S. L., Dawson, D. M., Lehrich, J. R., Beal, M. F., Kevy, S. V., Propper, R. D., Mills, J. A., and Weiner, H. L., 1983, Intensive immunosuppression in progressive multiple sclerosis: A randomized 3-arm study of high-dose intravenous cyclophosphamide, plasma exchange, and ACTH, *N. Engl. J. Med.* **308**:173–180.

Hemmi, H., and Ishida, N., 1980, The immune response of splenic lymphocytes after cimicifugoside treatment in vitro and pretreatment in vivo, *J. Pharmacobio-Dyn.* **3**:643–648.

Heppner, G. H., and Calabresi, P., 1976, Selective suppression of humoral immunity by antineoplastic drugs, *Annu. Rev. Pharmacol.* **16**:367–379.

Hersh, E. M., 1974, Immunosuppressive agents, in: *Antineoplastic and Immunosuppressive Agents,* Volume 1 (A. C. Sartorelli and D. G. Johns, eds.), pp. 577–617, Springer-Verlag, Berlin.

Hirata, F., and Iwata, M., 1983, Role of lipomodulin, a phospholipase inhibitory protein, in immunoregulation by thymocytes, *J. Immunol.* **130**:1930–1936.

Hitchings, G. H., and Elion, G. B., 1963, Chemical suppression of the immune resonse, *Pharmacol. Rev.* **15**:365–405.

Holland, J. F., and Ohnuma, T., 1979, Lessons from the study of induced alterations in amino acids in patient with cancer, *Cancer Treat. Rep.* **63**:1013–1018.

Homo, F., Picard, F., Durant, S., Gagne, D., Simon, J., Dardenne, M., and Duval, D., 1980, Glucocorticoid receptors and their functions in lymphocytes, *J. Steroid Biochem.* **12**:433–443.

Horakova, L., Nousa, K., Pospisil, M., Konopaskova, E., Klapacova, J., and Fuska, J., 1980, Immunosuppressive properties of the antibiotics cytostipin and vermiculine, *Folia Biol. (Prague)* **26**:312–326.

Humphries, G. M. K., 1981, Difference in the ability of compactin and oxidized cholesterol, both known inhibitors of cholesterol biosynthesis, to suppress in vitro immune responses, *Cancer Res.* **41**:3789–3791.

Ikehara, S., Hadden, J. W., Good, R. A., Linzer, D. G., and Pahwa, R. N., 1981, In vitro effects of two immunopotentiators, isoprinosine and NPT 15392, on murine T-cell differentiation and function, *Thymus* **3**:87–95.

Ito, H., Watanabe, K., and Koyama, J., 1982, The immunosuppressive effects of trichothecenes and cyclochlorotine on the antibody responses in guinea pigs, *J. Pharmacobio-Dyn.* **5**:403–409.

Jaffe, I. A., 1975, Penicillamine treatment of rheumatoid arthritis: Effect on immune complexes, *Ann. N.Y. Acad. Sci.* **256**:330–337.

Jardine, I., Fenselau, C., Appler, M., Kan, M.-N., Brundrett, R. B., and Colvin, M., 1978, Quantitation by gas chromatography chemical ionization mass for nitrogen mustard in the plasma and urine of patients receiving cyclophosphamide therapy, *Cancer Res.* **38**:408–415.

Jasani, M. K., 1979, Anti-inflammatory steroids: Mode of action in rheumatoid arthritis and homograft reaction, in: *Handbook of Experimental Pharmacology,* Volume 50, Part 2 (J. R. Vane and S. H. Ferreira, eds.), pp. 598–660, Springer-Verlag, Berlin.

Jones, C., Lee, C., Hoehler, F., Koyama, P., Skinner, W., and Lamott, J. A., 1983, Observations on the immunomodulator NPT 15392 in New Zealand black mice, *Int. J. Immunopharmacol.* **5:**85–590.

Kaiserlian, D., Dujic, A., Dardenne, M., Bach, J. F., Blanot, D., and Bricas, E., 1981, Prolongation of murine skin grafts by FTS and its synthetic analogues, *Clin. Exp. Immunol.* **45:**338–343.

Kallenberg, C. G. M., Van Der Lann, S., and De Zeeuw, D., 1981, Captopril and the immune system, *Lancet* **2:**92.

Kazmers, I. S., Daddona, P. E., Dalke, A. P., and Kelley, W. N., 1983, Effect of immunesuppressive agents on human T and B lymphoblasts, *Biochem. Pharmacol.* **32:**805–810.

Khan, A., Hogan, S., and Hill, J. M., 1979, Immunosuppressive effects of sulfato-*trans*-(−)-1,2-diaminocyclohexane platinum (II), *Cancer Res.* **39:**3476–3478.

Kolata, G., 1983, Drugs transform, transplant medicine, *Science,* **221:**40–42.

Kolb, J.-P. B., Quan, P. C., Poupon, M.-F., and Desaymard, C., 1981, Carrageenan stimulates populations of mouse "B" cells mostly nonoverlapping with those stimulated with LPS or dextran sulfate, *Cell. Immunol.* **57:**348–360.

Komoriya, K., Tsuchimoto, M., Naruchi, T., Okimura, T., and Yamamoto, I., 1983, Immunopharmacological profile of TEI-3096: A new immunomodulator, *J. Immunopharmacol.* **4:**285–301.

Lancet, 1981, Adverse reactions to dapsone, **2:**184–185.

Lau, C., and Goldstein, G., 1980, Functional effects of thymopoietin 32–36 (TP$_5$) on cytotoxic lymphocyte precursor units (CLP-U), *J. Immunol.* **124:**186.

Lee, M., and Hopkins, L. E., 1980, Attenuation of chemotherapy-induced neutropenia with lithium carbonate, *Am. J. Hosp. Pharm.* **37:**1066–1071.

Leibfarth, J. H., and Persellin, R. H., 1981, Mechanism of action of gold, *Agents Actions* **11:**458–472.

Lemmel, E. M., and Good, R. A., 1969, Tolerance of cell-mediated immune responses after *in vitro* treatment of competent cells with mitomycin C, *Int. Arch. Allergy Appl. Immunol.* **36:**554.

LeMoli, S., Seminara, R., D'Amelio, R., and Aiuti, F., 1983, In vitro and in vivo effect of sisomicin and gentamycin on polymorphonuclear chemotaxis and phagocytosis, *Int. J. Immunopharmacol.* **5:**49–54.

Lipsky, P. E., 1982, Studies on the mechanism of action of D-penicillamine in rheumatoid arthritis, *Adv. Pharmacol. Ther. Proc. 8th Int. Congr.* **4:**181–191.

Lipsky, P. E., and Ziff, M., 1982, The mechanisms of action of gold and D-penicillamine in rheumatoid arthritis, *Adv. Inflammation Res.* **3:**219–235.

Lombardino, J. G., and Otterness, I. C., 1981, Novel immunosuppressive agents. Potent immunological activity of some benzothiopyrano (4,3-c) pyrazol-3-ones, *J. Med. Chem.* **24:**830.

Loveless, S. E., Harris, L. S., and Munson, A. E., 1981, Hyporesponsiveness to the immunosuppressant effects of delta-8-tetrahydrocannabinol, *Int. J. Immunopharmacol.* **3:**371–383.

Luckenbach, G. A., Cortez-Campeao, D., Modolell, M. D., Munder, P. G., and Bicker, U., 1981, Immunomodulation by the new synthetic compound BM 12,531 (azimexone), *Exp. Pathol.* **19:**37.

Lum, C. T., Sutherland, D. E. R., and Najarian, J. S., 1979, Inhibition of PHA and NaIO$_4$ mitogenesis by the adenosine deaminase inhibitors *erythro*-9-(2-hydroxy-3-nonyl) adenine (EHNA) and 2-deoxycoformycin (2-dCF), *Clin. Immunol. Immunopathol.* **12:**453–459.

McCarthy, P. L., Shaw, J. E., and Remold, H. G., 1979, The role of microtubules in the response of macrophages to MIF, *Cell. Immunol.* **46:**409–415.

McConkey, B., Davies, P., Crockson, R. A., Crockson, A. P., Butler, M., and Constable, J. J., 1976, Dapsone in rheumatoid arthritis, *Rheumatol. Rehabil.* **15:**230–234.

Matthews, D. A., Alden, R. A., Bolin, J. T., Freer, S. T., Hamlin, R., Young, N., Kraut, J., Poe, M., Williams, M., and Hoogsteen, K., 1977, Dihydrofolate reductase: X-ray structure of the binary complex with methotrexate, *Science* **197:**452.

Medzihradsky, J. L., Zimmerman, T. P., Wolberg, G., and Elion, G. B., 1982, Immunosuppressive effects of the S-adenosylhomocysteine hydrolase inhibitor, 3-deazaadenosine, *J. Immunopharmacol.* **4:**29–41.

Medzihradsky, R. P., Hollowell, R. P., and Elion, G. B., 1981, Differential inhibition by azathioprine and 6-mercaptopurine of specific suppressor T cell generation in mice, *Int. J. Immunopharmacol.* **3:**1–16.

Milhaud, G., Labat, M.-L., and Moricard, Y., 1983, (Dichloromethylene)diphosphonate-induced impairment of T-lymphocyte function, *Proc. Natl. Acad. Sci. USA* **80:**4469–4473.

Miyakoshi, H., Aoki, T., and Hirasawa, Y., 1981, Immunological effects of 1α-hydroxycholecalciferol (1α-OH-D$_3$) and its metabolites, *Clin. Nephrol.* **16:**119–125.

Mizushima, Y., Sendo, F., Takeichi, N., Hosohawa, M., and Kobayashi, H., 1981, Enhancement of antitumor transplantation resistance in rats by appropriately timed administration of busulfan, *Cancer Res.* **41:**2917–2921.

Modderman, E. S. M., 1980, Dapsone, still first choice in leprosy, *Pharm. Int.* October:198–202.

Munck, A., and Leung, K., 1977, Glucocorticoid receptors and mechanisms of action, in: *Receptors and Mechanism of Action of Steroid Hormones*, Part II (J. R. Pasqualini, ed.), pp. 311–397, Dekker, New York.

Navarro, J., and Touraine, J. L., 1983, Comparative study of cyclomunine and cyclosporin A on human lymphocyte proliferation in vitro: The lack of an immunosuppressive effect by specific clonal deletion, *Int. J. Immunopharmacol.* **5:**157–162.

Nelson, A. M., and Conn, D. L., 1980, Glucocorticoids in rheumatic disease, *Mayo Clin. Proc.* **55:**758–769.

Newberne, P. M., and Thurman, G. B., 1981, Working Group IV: Lipids and the immune system. Report and recommendations., *Cancer Res.* **41:**3803–3804.

Ohno, R., and Hersh, E. M., 1970, Immunosuppressive effects of L-asparaginase, *Cancer Res.* **30:**1605.

Ohsugi, Y., Nakano, T., Hata, S., Niki, R., Matsuno, T., Mishii, Y., and Takagaki, Y., 1978, N-(2-carboxyphenyl)-4-chloroanthranilic acid disodium salt: Prevention of autoimmune kidney disease in NZB/W F$_1$ hybrid mice, *J. Pharm. Pharmacol.* **30:**126.

Olsen, C. T., and Gabrielson, A. E., 1982, Vindesine and other vinca alkaloids in treatment of NZB/NZW mice, *Int. J. Immunopharmacol.* **4:**358.

Oseas, R. S., Allen, J., Yang, H.-H., Baehner, R. L., and Boxer, L. A., 1982, Mechanism of dexamethasone inhibition of chemotactic factor induced granulocyte aggregation, *Blood* **59:**265–269.

Otterness, I. G., 1981, Comparative activity of CP-17,193 and five established immunosuppressives toward the antigens SRBC and EL$_4$, *Clin. Exp. Immunol.* **46:**332–339.

Otterness, I. G., and Chang, Y.-H., 1976, Comparative study of cyclophosphamide, 6-mercaptopurine, azathioprine and methotrexate: Relative effects on the humoral and cellular immune response in the mouse, *Clin. Exp. Immunol.* **26:**346.

Parekh, P. K., 1981, Homologous nerve transplantation and immunosuppression in rabbits, *Res. Exp. Med.* **179:**121–131.

Peavy, D. L., Koff, W. C., Hyman, D. S., and Knight, V., 1980, Inhibition of lymphocyte proliferative responses by ribavirin, *Infect. Immun.* **29:**583–589.

Petcher, T. J., Weber, H.-P., and Ruegger, A., 1976, Crystal and molecular structure of an iododerivative of the cyclic undecapeptide cyclosporin A, *Helv. Chim. Acta* **59:**1480–1488.

Plowman, P. N., 1983, Clinical pharmacology of platinum complexes and their possible usefulness outside oncology, *Agents Actions* **13:**88–90.

Pompidou, A., Touraine, J. L., Simon-Lavoine, N., and Hadden, J. W., 1980, Immunomodulatory effects of cyclomunine in vitro, *Int. J. Immunopharmacol.* **2:**141–144.

Powers, C. N., Peavy, D. L., and Knight, V., 1982, Selective inhibition of functional lymphocyte subpopulations by ribavirin, *Antimicrob. Agents Chemother.* **22:**108–114.

Rainsford, K. D., Schweitzer, A., and Brune, K., 1983, Distribution of the acetyl compared with the salicyl moiety of acetylsalicylic acid, *Biochem. Pharmacol.* **32:**1301–1308.

Ratech, H., Kuritski, L., Thorbecke, G. J., and Hirschhorn, R., 1982, Suppression of human lymphocyte DNA and protein synthesis in vitro by adenosine and eight modified adenine nucleosides in the presence or in the absence of adenosine deaminase inhibitors, 2'-deoxycoformycin (DCF) and *erythro*-9-(2-hydroxy-3-nonyl) adenine (EHNA), *Cell. Immunol.* **68:**244–251.

Richmond, D. E., 1979, Thiamphenicol as an immunosuppressant in active systemic lupus erythematosus with nephritis, *Aust. N.Z. J. Med.* **9:**670–675.

Rochas, C., and Rinaudo, M., 1980, Structural and conformational investigation of carrageenans, *Biopolymers* **19:**2165–2175.

Rogers, T. J., Campbell, L., Calhoun, K., Nowowiejski, I., and Webb, D. R., 1982, Suppression of B-cell and T-cell responses by the prostaglandin-induced T-cell-derived suppressor (PITS), *Cell. Immunol.* **66**:269–276.

Ryoyama, K., Mace, K., Ehrke, M. J., and Mihich, E., 1982, The differential sensitivity of T cell immune functions to vincristine and vinblastine, *Int. J. Immunopharmacol.* **4**:187–194.

Samuelsson, B., 1983, Leukotrienes: Mediator of immediate hypersensitivity reactions and inflammation, *Science* **220**:568.

Schwartz, J., and Charpentier, B., 1982, Immunosuppressive property of rifampicin antagonizes the beneficial effect of blood transfusion in rat organ allografting, *Transplantation* **34**:155–156.

Shearer, W. T., and Moore, E. G., 1981, Humoral immunostimulation. X. Cytochalasin B stimulates complement-dependent calcium uptake in antibody-treated cells, *Cell. Immunol.* **61**:62–77.

Shen, T. Y., Johnston, D. B. R., Jensen, N. P., Ruyle, W. V., Friedman, J. J., Fordice, M. W., McPherson, J. F., Boswell, K. H., Maag, T. A., Burg, R. W., Pellegrino, R. M., Jewell, M. E., Morris, C. A., Easterbrooks, H. L., and Skelly, B. J., 1971, New chemoprophylactic agents for Marek's disease, *Abstr. Pap., 162nd Natl. Meet. Am. Chem. Soc.* MEDI-44.

Shen, M., Ge, H., Song, Q., and Zhang, H., 1984, Immunosuppressive action of qinghaosu, *Scientia Sinica* **27**:398–406.

Shigeura, H. T., Hen, A. C., Burg, R. W., Skelly, B. J., and Hoogsteen, K., 1975, Metabolic studies on diphenylsulfone derivatives in chick macrophages, *Biochem. Pharmacol.* **24**:687–691.

Sidwell, R. W., Huffman, J. H., Khare, G. P., Allen, L. B., Witkowski, J. T., and Robins, R. K., 1972, Broad-spectrum antiviral activity of virazole: 1-α-D-ribofuranosyl-1,2,4-triazole-3-carboxamide, *Science* **177**:705–706.

Sigel, M. M., Ghaffar, A., McCumber, L. J., and Huggins, E. M., Jr., 1982, Immunosuppressive agents: A conceptual overview of their action on inductive and regulatory pathways, in: *Clin. Cell. Immunol.: Mol. Ther. Rev.* (A. A. Luderer, and H. H. Weetall, ed.), pp. 67–144, Humana, Clifton, New Jersey.

Smith, R. J., and Iden, S. S., 1980, Pharmacological modulation of chemotactic factor-elicited release of granule-associated enzymes from human neutrophils, *Biochem. Pharmacol.* **29**:2389–2395.

Sordillo, E. M., Ikehara, S., Good, R. A., and Trotta, P. P., 1981, Immunosuppression by 2'-deoxycoformycin: Studies on the mode of administration, *Cell. Immunol.* **63**:259–271.

Stewart, S. J., Spagnuolo, P. J., and Ellner, J. J., 1981, Generation of suppressor T lymphocytes and monocytes by amphotericin B, *J. Immunol.* **127**:135.

Streeter, D. G., Witkowski, J. T., Khare, G. P., Sidwell, R. W., Bauer, R. J., Robins, R. K., and Simon, L. N., 1973, Mechanism of action of 1-α-D-ribofuranosyl-1,2,4-triazole-3-carboxamide (Virazole), a new broad-spectrum antiviral agent, *Proc. Natl. Acad. Sci. USA* **70**:1174–1178.

Sutton, B. M., McGusty, E., Walz, D. T., and DiMartino, M. J., 1972, Oral gold antiarthritic properties of alkylphosphine gold coordination complexes, *J. Med. Chem.* **15**:1095–1098.

Swinson, D. R., Zlosnick, J., and Jackson, L., 1981, Double-blind trial of dapsone against placebo in the treatment of rheumatoid arthritis, *Ann. Rheum. Dis.* **40**:235–239.

Tallal, L., Tan, C., Oettgen, H., Wollner, N., McCarthy, M., Helson, L., Burchenal, J., Karnofsky, D., and Murphy, M. L., 1970, *E. coli* L-asparaginase in the treatment of leukemia and solid tumors in 131 children, *Cancer* **25**:306–320.

Thomson, A. W., and Fowler, E. F., 1981, Carrageenan: A review of its effects on the immune system, *Agents Actions* **11**:265–273.

Tracy, J. W., Kazura, J. W., and Webster, L. T., Jr., 1982, Suppression of cell-mediated immune response in vivo and in vitro by 1-thiocarbamoyl-2-imidazolidinone, *Int. J. Immunopharmacol.* **4**:187–200.

Thong, Y. H., and Ferrante, A., 1980, Effect of tetracycline treatment of immunological response in mice, *Clin. Exp. Immunol.* **39**:728–732.

Trotta, P. P., Tedde, A., Ikehara, S., Pahwa, R., Good, R. A., and Balis, M. E., 1981, Specific immunosuppressive effects of constant infusion of 2'-deoxycoformycin, *Cancer Res.* **41**:2189–2196.

Trottier, R. W., and Fitzgerald, T. J., 1981, The effects of colchicine derivatives on humoral antibody response in mice, *Drug Dev. Res.* **1**:241–244.

Vadas, M. A., and Bernard, C. C. A., 1981, Selective inhibition of the induction phase of delayed type hypersensitivity in mice by niridazole, *Clin. Immunol. Immunopathol.* **20**:313–320.

Vladutiu, A. P., 1982, Influence of immunomodulators, niridazole and levamisole, on autoimmune murine thyroiditis, *Immunol. Lett.* **4**:243–247.

Walker, C., Kristensen, F., Bettens, F., and de Weck, A. L., 1983, Lymphokine regulation of activated (G₁) lymphocytes. I. Prostaglandin E₂-induced inhibition of interleukin 2 production, *J. Immunol.* **130**:1770–1773.

Warabi, A. C., and Shiokawa, Y., 1979, Immunopharmacological effects of CCA in human rheumatoid arthritis and in experimental animals, *The Ryumachi (Japan)* **19**:554.

White, D. J. G. (ed.), 1982, *Cyclosporin A*, Elsevier, Amsterdam.

Wierda, D., Irons, R. D., and Greenlee, W. F., 1981, Immunotoxicity in C57BL/6 mice exposed to benzene and aroclor 1254, *Toxicol. Appl. Pharmacol.* **60**:410–417.

Winkelstein, A., 1979, The effects of azathioprine and G-MP on immunity, *J. Immunopharmacol.* **1**:429.

Yamamoto, I., Okimura, T., Ohmori, H., Komoriya, K., Ohba, T., Kurozumi, S., Naruchi, T., and Hashimoto, Y., 1980, An immunopharmacological profile, *Jpn. J. Inflammation* **1**:139.

Yamamoto, I., Ohmori, H., and Sasano, M., 1982, CCA: An immunopharmacological profile *in vivo* and *in vitro*, *Drugs Exp. Clin. Res.* **8**:5–10.

Zeller, P., Gutmann, H., Hegeolus, B., Kaiser, A., Langemann, A., and Muller, M., 1963, Methylhydrazine derivatives. A class of cytoxic agents, *Experientia* **19**:129.

Zhai, S., Shen, M., Xong, Y., Li, J., Ding, Y., and Gao, Y., 1982, Study on the immunosuppressive activity of sarmentosine, *Zhonghua Weishengwuxue He Mianyixue Zazhi* **2**:145–149.

Ziff, M., Velo, G. P., and Gorini, S. (eds.), 1982, *Advances in Inflammation Research*, Volume 3, Raven Press, New York.

Zighelbolm, J., and Shih, W., 1981, Effect of cytosine arabinoside on K cells and Fc receptors, *Prog. Cancer Res. Ther.* **19**:245–259.

Zimmerman, T. P., Deeprose, R. D., Wolberg, G., Stopford, C. R., Duncan, G. S., Miller, W. H., and Miller, R. L., 1983, Inhibition of lymphocyte function by 9-deazaadenosine, *Biochem. Pharmacol.* **32**:1211–1217.

14

The Effect of Environmental Agents on Cells of the Mononuclear Phagocyte System

JACK H. DEAN and DOLPH O. ADAMS

1. INTRODUCTION

The term macrophage ("large eater") was introduced by Metchnikoff (1901) to describe cells that he believed played an important role in resistance to bacterial infections through engulfment and digestion of microorganisms. Endocytic cells were further studied by Aschoff (1924) who used the ability to take up vital dyes to classify reticular cells of the spleen and lymph nodes, endothelial cells of the lymph and blood sinuses, histiocytes of the tissues including the liver and spleen, and blood monocytes, collectively constituting the reticuloendothelial system (RES). On the basis of common morphology, function, and origin, the highly phagocytic mononuclear cells and their precursors are now grouped into one family of cells termed the mononuclear phagocyte system (MPS).

Certain common characteristics can be outlined for cells of the MPS. Most are fairly large cells with varying amounts of cytoplasm, a reniform or oval nucleus and cytoplasmic organelles specialized for secretory activities. Ruffling of the surface membrane, easily recognized in phase-contrast or electron microscopy, is a frequent morphological characteristic of the mononuclear phagocyte as compared to lymphocytes. Other functional properties shared by cells of the MPS are avid phagocytosis, pinocytosis, and the ability to adhere firmly to glass or plastic surfaces. In fact, adherence to glass or plastic surfaces is a major means of isolating these cells. The phagocytosis of particles by mononuclear phagocytes is enhanced by the presence of specific immunoglobulins with or without the addition of complement, because these cells have cell membrane recep-

JACK H. DEAN • Department of Cell Biology, Chemical Industry Institute of Toxicology, Research Triangle Park, North Carolina 27709.   DOLPH O. ADAMS • Department of Pathology, Duke University Medical Center, Durham, North Carolina 27706.

tors for the Fc portions of antibody molecules and for the third component of complement.

Mononuclear phagocytes originate from precursor cells (CFU-GM) in the bone marrow, where they mature into promonocytes and monocytes. Monocytes are transported via the blood to organs and tissues, where they develop into macrophages. The macrophages of the MPS include the histiocytes of connective tissue; Kupffer cells of the liver; alveolar macrophages of the lungs; free and fixed macrophages of the spleen, lymph nodes, and bone marrow; and macrophages associated with serous membranes, such as the pleural and peritoneal serosa. Osteoclasts of bone tissue and microglial cells of the nervous system are also included in the MPS. Bloodborne monocytes and local replication in some cases continuously replenish these macrophage compartments with new cells. In sites of inflammation, the recruitment of monocytes from the blood is greatly enhanced and local multiplication of macrophages is also increased (for review see Adams, 1976).

Cells of the MPS provide a major defense against mechanically produced injuries as well as those produced by chemicals or biological toxins, infectious agents, and neoplastically transformed cells. Dysfunction of the MPS can lead to indirect tissue damage through altered host resistance to infectious agents or neoplastically transformed cells, or through direct tissue injury by the mononuclear phagocytes themselves or their cellular products (e.g., autoimmune diseases). Environmental agents, especially fibers, particulates, and gases (see review by Gardner, 1984), are well known to alter macrophage function. Chemicals and drugs have also been found to alter the MPS (see reviews by Loose *et al.*, 1981; Dean *et al.*, 1982, 1984; Lewis and Adams, 1984). The effects of environmental agents on macrophage function have been difficult to characterize precisely. This difficulty may be attributable, in part, to the fact that the functions of macrophages are closely related to their stage of maturation or development and to the fact that development of macrophages follows a complex and dynamic cascade of differentiation starting with bone marrow precursors (Adams and Marino, 1984; Adams and Hamilton, 1984). The effects of chemical or drug exposure are also often pleiotropic, so that a rational basis for understanding, studying, and characterizing dysfunction of the MPS has been difficult to establish.

The delicately balanced and regulated processes of development and activation are pivotal to understanding how xenobiotics interact with the MPS, since almost all macrophage functions can be modulated during activation (Adams and Marino, 1984). Derangement of this normal physiological process by chemicals and drugs could be deleterious to the host in several ways. On the one hand, activation of macrophages is a major mechanism of host defense to infectious agents and arising tumors. Deficiencies in macrophage activation could thus impair the host's defensive response to infectious agents. For example, macrophages from C3H/HeJ mice are extremely difficult to activate *in vivo*, and consequently these mice exhibit increased susceptibility to infection with rickettsia (Nacy *et al.*, 1981). On the other hand, increased or inappropriate macrophage reaction can damage normal host tissues. For example, macrophages exposed to a variety of particulate substances or stimulants can release large amounts of tissue-destructive substances such as proteases, hydrogen peroxide, and lysosomal hydrolases (Cohn, 1978). Macrophages containing silica represent an excellent example of how such a derangement can lead to massive host injury (Allison *et al.*, 1966; Kilroe-Smith *et al.*, 1973; Nourse *et al.*, 1975; see review by Bowden, 1973). These two forms of macrophage alteration are not necessarily mutually exclusive.

Studies from several laboratories have recently demonstrated that murine macrophages develop in stages (Hibbs *et al.*, 1977; Cohen, 1978; Meltzer, 1981) and that the stages of development can be clearly identified by quantifying certain objective biological and enzymatic markers, the expression of which characterizes each of the stages (Johnson *et al.*, 1983). This system of analysis has been used to characterize modulation of macrophage development, including that produced by agents of environmental concern (Adams and Dean, 1982; Dean *et al.*, 1984a,b). It is now clear that xenobiotics do alter macrophages by modulating their development.

Future progress in understanding the immunopharmacological effects of chemicals and drugs on the MPS can only be achieved if we systematically analyze macrophage activation following exposure to test compounds. We will need to define alterations in activation produced by xenobiotics at tbe cellular and molecular levels. Finally, we will need to devise sensitive methods for assessing the consequence of these alterations on host defense in experimental animals to allow better extrapolation of these effects to humans.

2. STAGING MACROPHAGE ACTIVATION USING BIOLOGICAL MARKERS

The MPS consists of blood monocytes and tissue macrophages whose development continues outside the marrow (van Furth, 1978). One culmination of this extramedullary developmental pathway is that macrophages are capable of destroying tumor cells and facultative obligate intracellular parasites. Macrophages possessing these characteristics are commonly referred to as being activated (Hibbs *et al.*, 1977; North, 1978; Adams and Marino, 1984).

Current evidence indicates that murine macrophages become activated through a sequence of operationally defined stages (Table 1) (Hibbs *et al.*, 1977; Meltzer *et al.*, 1979). In brief, these stages are defined by the inductive signals that must be applied to induce full activation (see top two rows of Table 1). Recently, a panel of objective markers characterizing these stages have been described as well (Johnson *et al.*, 1983). Young mononuclear phagocytes, when taken from sites of inflammation (i.e., responsive macrophages), express a variety of altered functions including increased phagocytic capacity, increased spreading and adherence to glass or plastic surfaces, secretion of neutral proteases, increased production of acid hydrolases, depressed levels of 5'-nucleotidase, and an increased capacity to generate O_2^- (Cohn, 1978). Responsive macrophages are closely akin to inflammatory macrophages as they display the

TABLE 1. STAGES OF MACROPHAGE ACTIVATION AND BIOLOGICAL CHANGES ASSOCIATED WITH EACH STAGE[a]

Source	Resident Mφ	Responsive Mφ	Primed Mφ	Activated Mφ
In vitro	Cultured monocytes	Resident peritoneal Mφ cultured for several days	Responsive Mφ exposed to lymphokine for 4–12 hr	Primed Mφ pulsed with LPS (ng amounts)
In vivo	Resident peritoneal Mφ	Inflammatory Mφ elicited by FCS, LPS, or thioglycollate broth	Mφ elicited by pyran copolymer	Mφ elicited by BCG and *C. parvum*
Function				
Spreading	±	+++	+++	+++
Phagocytosis via Fc receptors	++	++++	++++	++++
Phagocytosis via C3 receptors	−	++++	++++	++++
Secretion of plasminogen activator	−	++++	++++	++++
H_2O_2 production	±	±/++++	±/++++	±/++++
Cytostatic activity	−	+	++	++++
Selective binding of tumor cells	−	−	++++	++++
Cytolysis of tumor cells	−	−	−	++++
Secretion of cytolytic protease	−	−	−	++++
Enzyme markers				
5'-Nucleotidase	++++	+	+	+
Alkaline phosphodiesterase	++	++++	+	+
Leucine aminopeptidase	++	+++	+++	+++
Secretion of lysozyme	+	+++	++	++

[a]Adapted from Meltzer *et al.* (1979), Adams and Marino (1984), Morahan *et al.* (1980), and Dean *et al.* (1984b).

markers of increased spreading, increased phagocytosis of IgG-coated red cells, and increased secretion of plasminogen activator (Johnson *et al.*, 1983). Inflammatory macrophages can in turn be activated to kill tumor cells and facultative intracellular parasites by exposure to lymphokine and/or endotoxin. Primed macrophages continue to display these markers and now bind neoplastic targets selectively but do not kill them (Marino and Adams, 1980; Adams and Marino,

1984). Fully activated or cytotoxic macrophages, which share the properties of the primed macrophages, kill neoplastic or virally infected targets, and spontaneously secrete cytolytic protease (CP) (Johnson, et al., 1983; Adams and Marino, 1984).

Analysis of the capacity for secretion of reactive oxygen intermediates (ROI) such as H_2O_2 provides an additional and useful marker (Lewis and Adams, 1984). Macrophage competence for pharmacologically triggered release of H_2O_2 clearly marks macrophage activation in many systems (Nathan and Root, 1977; Murray, 1984), but the two can clearly be dissociated (Cohen et al., 1982). Additionally, certain populations of responsive macrophages, such as those elicited with casein, have increased competence for release of H_2O_2; others, such as those elicited by fetal bovine serum or peptone broth, do not (Nathan and Root, 1977; Johnson et al., 1983).

Certain ectoenzymes (Morahan et al., 1980), including leucine aminopeptidase, alkaline phosphodiesterase, and 5'-nucleotidase, may also be useful in characterizing stages in macrophage activation. Responsive macrophages contain increased amounts of leucine aminopeptidase and alkaline phosphodiesterase and markedly reduced amounts of 5'-nucleotidase compared to resident macrophages. Fully activated macrophages have increased levels of leucine aminopeptidase, but reduced levels of the other two enzymes (Morahan et al., 1980).

Thus, altered activation of mononuclear phagocytes, following chemical or drug exposure, should be examined in two ways. First, it should be determined whether resident tissue macrophages have any of the characteristics of macrophages in the latter stages of activation (i.e., whether or not the xenobiotic itself induces any activation). Second, it should be determined whether various activating stimuli of differing potencies induce the expected level of macrophage development (i.e., whether or not the xenobiotic blocks physiological activation of macrophages). Based on these considerations, it would appear that alterations in macrophage function should be assessed by examining the basal level of activation in resident cells and their capacity for activation in response to activational stimuli such as BCG or pyran copolymer.

3. EFFECTS OF POLLUTING GASES AND PARTICULATES ON THE MPS

The subject of the effect of environmental agents on lymphocytes or macrophages has been extensively reviewed (Bowden, 1973; Brain, 1980; Dean et al., 1982; Gardner, 1984). Emphasis in this section will be placed on summarizing the effects of polluting gases (e.g., NO_2, O_3, SO_4) and particulate matter (e.g., asbestos, silica, fly ash, and metallic dusts). The literature relating changes in macrophage function following exposure to polluting gases or particulates is summarized in Tables 2 and 3.

Since the respiratory tract is often a major route of exposure to many environmental agents, especially airborne pollutants, alveolar macrophages are potential cellular targets of airborne toxicants that elude the absorptive and

TABLE 2. EFFECT OF POLLUTING GASES ON CELLS OF THE MPS

Agent	Type of exposure	Source of macrophages[a]	Effect	References
Cigarette smoke	Inhalation	Human PA	Increased levels of aryl hydrocarbon hydroxylase in smokers	Cantrell et al. (1973), McLemore et al. (1977a,b)
			Increased elastase and protease levels in smokers	Harris et al. (1975)
			Increased O_2^- secretion and O_2 metabolism	Hoidal and Niewoehner (1982)
	Inhalation	Mouse PA	Increased number of lysosomes and β-glucuronidase	Matulionis and Traurig (1977)
			Decreased bacterial resistance	Green et al. (1977)
	Inhalation	Rat PA	Increased O_2 consumption and H_2O_2 release during phagocytosis	Drath et al. (1978)
Formaldehyde	Inhalation	Mouse PE	Increased H_2O_2 release	Dean et al. (1984a)
Ozone	Inhalation	Rat PA	Decreased mobility	McAllen et al. (1981)
		Mouse PA	Decreased phagocytosis	Coffin et al. (1968)
			Depressed bactericidal activity	Coffin and Gardner (1972)
Hydrogen sulfide	Inhalation	Rat PA	Decreased killing of Staphylococcus	Myrvik and Evans (1967)
	In vitro	Rabbit PA	Decreased phagocytosis and HMP shunt	Myrvik and Evans (1967)
Nitrogen dioxide	Inhalation	Rabbit PA	Decreased resistance to pox virus challenge and ability to produce interferon	Valand et al. (1970)
			Decreased resistance and phagocytosis	Acton and Myrvik (1972)
	Inhalation	Mouse PA	Impaired bactericidal activity	Ehrlich (1966)

[a]PA, pulmonary alveolar macrophages; PE, peritoneal exudate cells.

filtering action of the upper airway. The definitive role played by these pulmonary alveolar macrophages in protecting the lung against these agents is unknown. Not all toxic agents elicit an influx of macrophages into the lung and some including chrysotile asbestos (Harrington, 1976), quartz (Miller and Kagan, 1976), acrolein (Bouley et al., 1976), and O_3 (Coffin et al., 1968) even reduce the number of macrophages present through either direct cytolysis or inhibition of recruitment.

Direct cytotoxicity has often been observed in alveolar macrophages following inhalation of quartz and asbestos (Miller and Kagan, 1976, 1977). After ingestion of asbestos, macrophages develop large flattened pseudopodia, cytoplasmic blebbing, and asbestos bodies (McLemore et al., 1979). The cyto-

TABLE 3. EFFECT OF ENVIRONMENTAL PARTICULATES ON CELLS OF THE MPS

Agent	Type of exposure	Source of macrophages[a]	Effect	References
Asbestos	i.p. challenge	Mouse PE	Increased spreading, Fc receptor activity, and phagocytosis; secretion of plasminogen activator, neutral protease	Donaldson et al. (1982), Hamilton et al. (1976), Hamilton (1980)
	Inhalation	Mouse PA and PE	Increased phagocytosis and cytostasis	Boorman et al. (1984)
			Increased secretion of plasminogen activator	Hamilton (1980)
	In vitro	Mouse PE and PA	Toxicity of fibers variable; increased secretion of elastase, LDH, β-glucuronidase, and lysozyme	Davies et al. (1974), Kaw et al. (1982), White and Kuhn (1980)
Iron oxide	Inhalation	Hamster PA	Increased phagocytosis and macophage influx in lung	Kavet et al. (1978)
Silica	Inhalation	Guinea pig PA	Secretion of fibrogenic factor	Kilroe-Smith et al. (1973), Nourse et al. (1975)
	In vitro	Mouse PA and PE	Decreased viability; secretion of elastase, β-glucosaminidase, LDH, and lysosomal enzymes	Allison et al. (1966), Nadler and Goldfischer (1970), White and Kuhn (1980)
Nickel dust	Inhalation	Rabbit PA	Increased phagocytosis	Camner et al. (1978)
Quartz	Inhalation	Rat PA	Deterioration of plasma membrane	Miller et al. (1978a)
Fly ash	Inhalation	Mouse PA	Viability decreased	Aranyi et al. (1979)
Coal dust	Inhalation	Rat PA	Decreased phagocytosis, bactericidal activity, and lysosomal enzyme activity	Bingham et al. (1975)
Hay dust	In vitro	Mouse PE	Increased secretion of acetyl-β-glucosaminidase and β-galactosidase	Schorlemmer et al. (1977)

[a]PA, pulmonary alveolar macrophages; PE, peritoneal exudate cells.

plasm contains numerous lysosomes, free and aggregated ribosomes, mitochondria, and strands of rough endoplasmic reticulum (Miller et al., 1978b). In contrast, after ingestion of quartz, macrophages develop pronounced intracytoplasmic vacuolation, deterioration of the plasma membrane, and assume bizarre shapes (Miller et al., 1978a).

Fly ash particulates collected from coal-fired power plants, steel foundries, copper smelters, and aluminum smelters were also found to be directly cytotoxic for macrophages (see review by Gardner, 1984). The most toxic industrial samples released soluble cytotoxic substances into the medium that were shown to be responsible for a loss in cell viability. When fly ash was coated with various metals, exposed by inhalation, and the cytotoxicity of pulmonary alveolar macrophages determined, PbO-treated fly ash was found to be the most toxic, NiO- and MnO_2-treated particles had an intermediate effect, and untreated fly ash was the least toxic (Aranyi et al., 1979). In addition, as particle size increased, a significantly greater concentration was required to produce the same degree of toxicity.

Another macrophage function, critical to host resistance, that can be altered by exposure to particulates and gases is phagocytosis. For example, acute exposure of animals to O_3 or NO_2 produces a marked impairment of phagocytic activity (Acton and Myrvik, 1972; Coffin et al., 1968; Katz and Laskin, 1977). A variety of explanations have been suggested for this impairment. A priori, these gases could (1) affect macrophage mobility; (2) directly attack the cell membrane, causing loss of cell viability; or (3) alter some intracellular metabolic process necessary for phagocytosis. In contrast, exposure to agents such as nickel dust, SO_2, and formaldehyde can increase phagocytic activity (see Gardner, 1984). The precise causes of these alterations, however, remain to be established.

Impairment of phagocytic activity is frequently accompanied by changes in bacterial or viral resistance. Depressed resistance to bacterial challenge has been observed following exposure to high O_2 tension (Huber and LaForce, 1970) and the gases NO_2 (Ehrlich, 1966), O_3 (Coffin and Gardner, 1972; Goldstein, 1977), SO_2 (Fairchild et al., 1975), and cigarette smoke (Green et al., 1977). Particulates such as cadmium, alumina, and $PbCl_2$ (Dubreuil et al., 1979; Schlipkoter and Dolgner, 1981) have also been observed to depress bacterial resistance. Impairment of viral resistance was induced by exposure to environmental gases such as O_3, NO_2, and oxidants in automobile exhaust. This is believed to be associated with depressed interferon production by macrophages from exposed animals (Acton and Myrvik, 1972; Shingu et al., 1980). The observations of altered host resistance following exposure to the above xenobiotics may be important because of the ubiquitous and frequent nature of human exposure to these agents.

The mechanism(s) by which toxic gases and particulates are cytotoxic to or depress macrophage function is for the most part poorly characterized. Some particulate toxins such as silica and asbestos cause the release of lysosomal enzymes from mononuclear phagocytes (Davies et al., 1974; Harrington and Allison, 1965). The release of these tissue-destructive enzymes from macrophages may well account for much of the inflammation, tissue destruction, and fibrosis following exposure to these agents (Page et al., 1978). It has been proposed that substances such as silica and asbestos interact directly with the cell membrane (Allison, 1977). Silica could produce cytotoxicity by disrupting the phospholipid components of the cell membrane after forming hydrogen bond complexes with phenolic hydroxyl groups of silicic acid. In contrast, asbestos may alter membranes in a nonlytic fashion by the interaction of its magnesium groups with membrane glycoproteins (Gardner, 1984). Silica does not appear to cause the release of acid hydrolases from macrophages without cell death, while small amounts of asbestos fibers can apparently induce the selective release of lysosomal enzymes (Davies and Allison, 1976). However, many substances remain within the phagosome after ingestion without altering the phagosome membrane. For example, dusts like Carborundum and diamond fail to show toxicity (Luhr, 1958). Thus, these interactions are complex and remain poorly defined.

Gaseous pollutants such as O_3, NO_2, and SO_2 also produce marked alterations in macrophage enzyme activity. These oxidant gases significantly alter the levels of cytoplasmic lysozyme, β-glucuronidase, and acid phosphatase (Barry and Mawdesley-Thomas, 1970; Hurst et al., 1970). Oxidant gases may interact with the plasma and/or lysosomal membrane (Dowell et al., 1970). Any toxicant affecting the integrity of either membrane might be expected to result in enzyme leakage into extracellular fluids and produce extensive tissue damage. Increased secretion of lysosomal enzymes in macrophages from both humans and rodents exposed to cigarette smoke has been reported (Gee et al., 1979; Hinman et al., 1980). This increase is associated with the production of new lysosomal enzymes and not just an increase in enzyme content within the original lysosomes (Lewis et al., 1979). Macrophages from smokers also produce greater quantities of elastase (see review by Brain, 1980), which may lead to subsequent tissue damage and connective tissue degradation. These macrophages also release increased amounts of O_2^-, which may be a significant factor in the pathogenesis of emphysema. Studies have also shown that macrophages from smokers have significantly higher aryl hydrocarbon hydroxylase activity than found in macrophages from nonsmokers (Cantrell et al., 1973). This enzyme system is responsible for metabolizing polycyclic aromatic hydrocarbons to carcinogenic reactive electrophiles, which may contribute to the high lung cancer incidence among smokers.

Air pollutant dusts have been shown to activate oxidant production (H_2O_2 and O_2^-) in alveolar macrophages. All particles examined were found to stimulate the macrophage in a dose-dependent manner to different maximal levels of oxidant production (see Gardner, 1984). Three types of amphibole asbestos (anthophyllite, amosite, and crocidolite) were the most active of all the agents tested. Serpentine asbestos forms were about one-fourth as active. Silica, metal oxide-coated fly ash (PbO, NiO, and MnO_2), and polymethylmethacrylate beads had intermediate activity. The lowest activity was seen with exposure to uncoated fly ash, fiberglass, polybead carboxylate microspheres, and latex beads.

The release of oxidants may produce serious consequences when the oxidant and protease secretions reach levels that could contribute to chronic lung damage (Brain, 1980; Hinman et al., 1980). The amount of proteolytic enzymes released increases with increasing numbers of macrophages, the cytotoxic potential of the test substance, and the influx of other cells (e.g., PMNs) rich in similar hydrolytic enzymes (Janoff et al., 1977).

As is evident from Tables 2–4, a large number of studies have dealt with the effects of environmental agents interacting in vitro with various macrophage populations. These studies can provide useful information on the direct effects

TABLE 4. EFFECT OF CHEMICALS ON CELLS OF THE MPS

Agent	Type of exposure	Source of macrophages	Effect	References
Aflatoxin B$_1$	In vitro	Rabbit PA[a]	Decreased phagocytosis	Richard and Thurston (1975)
Aluminum	In vitro	Sheep PA	Decreased O$_2$ uptake during phagocytosis	Engelbrecht and DeKlerk (1972)
	In vivo	Guinea pig PE	Increased release of LDH	Badnoch-Jones et al. (1978)
Azathioprine	In vivo	Mouse PE	Decreased tumoricidal activity	Mantovani et al. (1980a)
Benz[a]anthracene	In vivo	Guinea pig and human PA and PE	Decreased aryl hydrocarbon hydroxylase (AHH) activity	McLemore et al. (1977a,b), Bast et al. (1976)
Benzo[a]pyrene	In vitro	Human PA	Increased AHH and metabolism of benzo[a]pyrene	Autrup et al. (1978)
Beryllium	In vitro	Human BM	Inhibited macrophage migration	Price et al. (1976)
Cadmium	In vivo	Mouse PE	Increased phagocytosis and acid phosphatase activity	Koller and Roan (1977)
	In vitro	Mouse PE	Decreased O$_2$ burst during phagocytosis	Loose et al. (1978)
	In vitro	Rabbit PA	Decreased cell viability, phagocytosis, and acid phosphatase	Graham et al. (1979), Waters et al. (1975)
Chromium	Inhalation	Rabbit PA	Increased phagocytosis	Johannsson et al. (1980b)
	In vitro	Rabbit PA	Decreased phagocytosis, acid phosphatase, and survival	Graham et al. (1979), Waters et al. (1975)
Cobalt	Inhalation	Rabbit PA	Increased phagocytosis	Johannsson et al. (1980b)
	In vivo	Mouse PE	Increased LDH release	Rae (1975)
Dieldrin	In vivo	Mouse PA and splenic	Decreased phagocytosis	Loose et al. (1981)
Diethylstilbestrol	In vivo	Mouse PE	Increased number, phagocytosis, and cytostasis; decreased H$_2$O$_2$ and ectoenzyme induction	Boorman et al. (1980), Dean et al. (1984b,c)

Compound		Cell type[a]	Effect	Reference
Dimethylbenz[a]anthracene	In vivo	Mouse PE	Altered stages of development	Hamilton et al. (1984)
Dimethyltriazenoimidazole carboxamide (DTIC)	In vivo	Mouse PE	Decreased tumoricidal activity	Mantovani et al. (1980a)
Ethanol	In vivo	Mouse PA	Decreased recruitment of macrophages	Guavneri and Laurenzi (1968)
Hexachlorobenzene	In vivo	Rat PA	Decreased Fc receptor expression	Ziprin and Fowler (1977)
Lead	In vivo	Mouse PA and PE	Decreased phagocytosis	Loose et al. (1981)
	In vivo	Mouse PE	Increased phagocytosis and acid phosphatase levels; decreased function during antibody induction	Koller and Roan (1977), Blakley and Archer (1981)
	In vitro	Rat PA	Decreased O_2^- release during phagocytosis	Castranova et al. (1980)
Lindane (γ-hexachlorocyclohexane)	In vitro	Mouse PE	Inhibited uridine uptake and incorporation and pinocytosis	Roux et al. (1978)
Mercury	In vitro	Rat PA	Decreased O_2^- release during phagocytosis	Castranova et al. (1980)
Nickel	In vitro	Rabbit PA	Decreased phagocytosis	Graham et al. (1979)
Paraquat and diaquat	In vitro	Rat PA	Reduced viability; inhibited O_2^- release through NADPH depletion	Forman et al. (1980)
Phorbol myristate acetate	In vivo	Mouse PE	Altered stages of development	Murray et al. (1984)
Polychlorinated biphenyls	In vivo	Mouse PA and splenic	Decreased phagocytosis	Loose et al. (1981)
Saccharin	In vitro	Rat and mouse PE	Tumoricidal activity unaltered	Mantovani et al. (1980b)
2,3,7,8- etrachlorodibenzo-p-dioxin	In vivo	Mouse PE	Numbers depressed; tumoricidal activity lysis	Mantovani et al. (1980c)
Vanadium	In vitro	Rabbit PA	Lysis	Graham et al. (1979)

[a]PA, pulmonary alveolar macrophages; PE, peritoneal exudate cells.

TABLE 5. EFFECT OF XENOBIOTICS ON STAGES OF MACROPHAGE ACTION[a]

Agent	Markers of responsive macrophages	Cytolysis of tumor cells and cytolytic potential	Secretion of H_2O_2	Conclusions
DES	Pushes resident Mφ to responsive Mφ	None by resident Mφ; decreased kill by primed plus LPS	No effect on resident Mφ; decreased secretion by primed and activated Mφ	Resident Mφ pushed to responsive, but development of primed Mφ activated is blocked. Development of capacity to secrete H_2O_2 suppressed
Formaldehyde	No changes in resident Mφ	No change in resident or primed Mφ	Increase secretion by primed Mφ	No changes in development of activation. Stimulated capacity for release of H_2O_2
Lead	No change (does increase phagocytosis)	No change	No change	No change except increased phagocytosis
Cadium	No change (does increase phagocytosis)	No change	No change	No change except increased phagocytosis
7,12-DMBA	Pushes resident Mφ to responsive Mφ	Resident Mφ pushed to responsive Mφ; primed Mφ pushed to activated Mφ	Capacity for secretion by resident Mφ increased	Resident Mφ pushed to responsive state, and primed Mφ pushed to activated. Stimulated H_2O_2 capacity by resident Mφ

[a]Adapted from Lewis and Adams (1984). Data from Dean et al. (1984a,b,c), Murray et al. (1984), and Hamilton et al. (1984).

of the pollutants under study on mononuclear phagocytes (Allison *et al.*, 1966; White and Kuhn, 1980). The *in vivo* significance of such studies, however, may be difficult to assess because the environmental agent in question (particularly organic compounds) may be metabolized (i.e., either activated or detoxified) *in vivo*. Thus, examination of the agent *in vitro* may not accurately reflect its *in vivo* effects. For example, the chrysotile form of asbestos is highly toxic *in vitro*, while the crocidolite form is not. Both, however, produce similar effects *in vivo* (Bey and Harrington, 1971).

The pleiotropic nature of the alterations induced in the MPS by environmental agents raises the distinct possibility that xenobiotic particles and gases derange the maturation of tissue macrophages. Save for studies on the effects of formaldehyde (see Table 5), this important possibility remains to be tested in depth.

4. EFFECTS OF ENVIRONMENTAL CHEMICALS ON THE MPS

The literature on the effects of environmental chemical exposure on macrophage function is summarized in Table 4. Environmental agents studied include: metals (e.g., aluminum, cadmium, nickel, and lead); aflatoxin B_1; hexachlorobenzene; diaquat and paraquat; formaldehyde; PCBs; lindane; diethylstilbestrol (DES); saccharin; TCDD: and polycyclic aromatic hydrocarbons.

Generalizations about the effects of environmental chemicals on macrophage function are not possible. Even for studies of one environmental agent, generalizations are difficult because various populations and functions of macrophages have been examined, usually without elicitation, and multiple routes of exposure have been tested (Table 4).

The effects of environmental chemicals on macrophages are quite pleiotropic. First, some chemicals may influence cell viability with or without causing cytolysis. When several trace metals (Mn^{2+}, Ni^{2+}, Cr^{2+}, and VO_3^-) were tested for cytotoxicity on macrophages *in vitro*, all produced a significant decrease in cell numbers at metal concentrations that caused cell death. Cd^{2+}, however, decreased cell viability without causing lysis. Second, environmental chemicals have been shown to alter functions such as phagocytosis without inducing cell death. Chemicals shown to increase phagocytosis include several metals and the environmental estrogen DES. In the case of DES, the actual number of mononuclear cells and the phagocytic activity are increased, whereas bactericidal and tumoricidal activity on a cellular basis are impaired (Boorman *et al.*, 1980; Dean *et al.*, 1984b,c). In contrast, a variety of chemicals can depress phagocytosis following *in vivo* or *in vitro* exposure including aflatoxin B_1, certain metals, dieldrin, hexachlorobenzene, and PCBs. Exposure of macrophages to some metals has also been associated with a reduced oxidative burst during phagocytosis, which at times has been correlated with increased susceptibility to bacterial challenge.

The mechanism(s) by which chemicals of environmental concern adversely effect the MPS is, for the most part, quite ill-defined. Nickel, which inhibits phagocytosis at concentrations below those that cause cell death, may reduce the energy available for phagocytosis by reducing the availability of ATP, since it forms a stable binary complex with ATP (Graham *et al.*, 1979). Alternatively, some metals are strong sulfhydryl alkylating agents and might act through SH on many targets throughout the cell, including microtubules, which are necessary for phagocytosis. It has been established that sulfhydryl reagents can alter phagocytosis in rabbit PMNs and disrupt the function of mouse peritoneal macrophages (Facchinetti *et al.*, 1978). Lindane-induced macrophage toxicity may be mediated by a similar mechanism, since it disrupts cytoskeletal structures and pinocytosis (Roux *et al.*, 1978). Other chemical-induced toxicity to the MPS may involve quite different mechanisms. For example, inhibition of the oxidative burst during phagocytosis by the herbicide paraquat appears to result from specific depletion of NADPH (Forman *et al.*, 1980).

It is now apparent, however, that xenobiotic chemicals can alter macrophage activation. To date, we have examined the effects of five xenobiotics on the MPS using the scheme described above. The results of these experiments are summarized in Table 5. *In vivo* exposure to the polycyclic aromatic hydrocarbon carcinogen 7,12-dimethylbenzanthracene (DMBA), for example, induced increased Fc-mediated phagocytosis and capacity for secretion of H_2O_2 in resident peritoneal macrophages. These peritoneal macrophages killed tumor cells when exposed to lymphokine plus LPS *in vitro*. Primed macrophages also kill tumor cells when exposed to lymphokine plus LPS *in vitro*. Primed macrophages elicited by pyran copolymer from these mice, furthermore, killed tumor cells without the need for stimulation with LPS. Taken together, we interpret these data to indicate that DMBA stimulates macrophage activation by pushing resident macrophages to the responsive state and primed macrophages to the fully activated state. DMBA also augments the capacity for secretion of H_2O_2 and does so at a very early stage of the developmental cascade. Exposure of animals to cadmium or lead increases the phagocytic capacity of macrophages but these cells are not responsive to lymphokines and LPS. This suggests that phagocytosis can be increased without an alteration in the state of activation (Table 5). In contrast, DES induces the development of resident to responsive macrophages but actually suppresses development of the later stages of activation (Table 5). Furthermore, DES suppresses the capacity of primed macrophages for release of H_2O_2. Finally, formaldehyde does not appear to effect activation at all but does prepare the macrophages for enhanced secretion of H_2O_2.

Study of these five xenobiotics indicates that certain environmental pollutants are fully capable of affecting the activation cascade of mononuclear phagocytes. Two general patterns of alteration in activation were observed: general induction of macrophage activation, and induction of early development of activation and the suppression of the later stages. The data, taken together, clearly support the hypothesis that xenobiotics can affect development of the MPS. Of more importance, they indicate that these developmental aberrations are induced systematically in the MPS. The effects on macrophage development are quite pleiotropic and appear to be quite precise, depending on the particular xenobiotic. It remains to be established whether the basic pattern of stimulation of the MPS by xenobiotics is a general property or results from the limited panel of agents tested to date. The data further document that control of H_2O_2 release is separate from control of the activation cascade.

5. CONCLUSIONS

At present, the effects of most environmental agents on macrophages are ill-defined, especially since each environmental agent can produce different and often pleiotropic effects. It is often unclear whether the agents acted directly on macrophages or on another cell regulating macrophage function. Furthermore, disparate observations of the same agent in increasing or decreasing certain functions of macrophages in different studies have been difficult to reconcile.

Evidence now exists that a number of chemicals and trace metals can alter either biochemical, physiological, morphological, or functional properties of the MPS and can cause a significant increase in susceptibility to infectious agents. Examples of agents that have been shown to enhance the incidence of bacterial pulmonary infection include: Ni^{2+}, Cd^{2+}, Zn^{2+}, Mg^{2+}, Pb^{2+}, H_2SO_4, and coal fly ash. Similarly, inhalation of a number of noxious gases and vapors has been shown to increase pulmonary infections in challenge models. The same gaseous pollutants also affected other macrophage functions. Individual gases such as O_3 and NO_2 as well as mixtures of NO_2 and O_3, H_2SO_4 and O_3, irradiated auto exhaust and diesel exhausts have all produced significant enhancement of bacterial infections in test animals. *In vivo* exposure to such chemicals as DES or phorbol diesters has been shown to alter the bactericidal and tumoricidal capacities of macrophage.

The widely diverse effects of environmental agents on the functions of the MPS *in vivo* and *in vitro* may be attributable to the fact that they induce developmental aberrations in this dynamic system of cells. It is of interest that of the five environmental chemicals we have examined to date, three have caused such changes.

Multiple reasons argue that such assessment of MPS function would be very useful. (1) Since xenobiotics affect macrophage activation, effects on numerous functions may be rationally predicted. For example, if an agent were shown to induce resident populations to the inflammatory state as measured by increased spreading in culture and Fc-mediated phagocytosis, then it would be resonable to hypothesize that these cells would also have increased C3-mediated phagocytosis plus increased secretion of O_2 and neutral proteases (e.g., elastase, collagenase, plasminogen activator). (2) This approach employs sensitive, quantitative assays, which objectively type macrophages as to their stage of activation. (3) Establishment of the developmental effects of a particular xenobiotic will allow for a broader prespective in evaluating biological relevance of the results. Specifically, one should be able to predict better which alterations will be important to the host. (4) By determining the exact stage(s) at which an agent exerts its effects, one will be in a better position to make accurate predictions and design rational experiments to investigate the molecular mechanisms by which xenobiotics act. For example, determining that an agent inhibits the development of primed macrophages would suggest two likely possibilities: (a) the xenobiotic reduces macrophage sensitivity to lymphokines, or (b) the xenobiotic diminishes production of lymphokines. Both of these possibilities are amenable to experimental verification. Thus, this approach should help us to begin to understand the fundamental cell biology of how xenobiotics alter the MPS. (5) The method outlined here appears to be sensitive and broadly applicable for assessing the impacts of xenobiotics on the MPS.

It is important to note that in many of these studies, dose–response data indicated that an affect could be produced with concentrations similar to those seen in the work environment. Several epidemiological studies have emphasized a relationship between increased concentrations of airborne pollutants and increased incidence of acute respiratory symptoms. An increased incidence of acute respiratory illness in humans has been associated with exposure to SO_2, suspended nitrates and sulfates, NO_2, cigarette smoke, and total suspended particles (Douglas and Waller, 1968; Finklea *et al.*, 1974; Levy *et al.*, 1977; Shy *et al.*, 1970).

Finally, if progress is to be made in our understanding of the effects of chemicals, gases, and particulates on the MPS and their role in immunotoxic manifestations, a more systematic approach will be required. Consideration must be given to more realistic routes of exposures; the use of relevant sources of macrophages in experimental studies; the use of human macrophages for confirmation; and subsequent alterations in macrophage function should be characterized in resident cells as well as in macrophages responding to an activational stimulus. Assays characterizing biological and enzymatic markers of macrophage activation are currently available for future studies.

REFERENCES

Acton, J. D., and Myrvik, Q. N., 1972, Nitrogen dioxide effects on alveolar macrophages, *Arch. Environ. Health* **24**:48.

Adams, D. O., 1976, The granulomatous inflammatory response: A review, *Am. J. Pathol.* **84**:164.

Adams, D. O., and Dean, J. H., 1982, Analysis of macrophage activation and biological response modifier effects by use of objective markers to characterize the stages of activation, in: *NK Cells and Other Natural Effector Cells* (R. B. Herberman, ed.), pp. 511–518, Academic Press, New York.

Adams, D. O., and Hamilton, T. A., 1984, The cell biology of macrophage activation, *Annu. Rev. Immunol.* **2**:283.

Adams, D. O., and Marino, P., 1984, Activation of mononuclear phagocytes for destruction of tumor cells as a model for study of macrophage development, in: *Contemporary Hematology-Oncology*, Volume III (A. S. Gordon, R. Silber, and J. LoBue, eds.), pp. 69–136, Plenum Press, New York.

Allison, A. C., 1977, Mechanisms of macrophage damage in relationship to the pathogenesis of some lung diseases, in: *Respiratory Defense Mechanisms* (J. D. Brain, D. F. Proctor, and L. M. Reid, eds.), Part II, pp. 1075–1102, Dekker, New York.

Allison, A. C., Harrington, J. S., and Birbeck, M., 1966, An examination of the cytotoxic effects of silica on macrophages, *J. Exp. Med.* **124**:141.

Aranyi, C., Miller, F. J., Andres, S., Ehrlich, R., Fenters, J., Gardner, D. E., and Waters, M. D., 1979, Cytotoxicity to alveolar macrophages of trace metals absorbed to fly ash, *Environ. Res.* **20**:14.

Aschoff, L., 1924. Das Reticulo-Endotheliale system, *Ergeb. Inn. Med. Kinderheilkd.* **26**:1.

Autrup, H., Harris, C. C., Stoner, G. D., Selkirk, J. K., Schafer, P. W., and Trump, B. F., 1978, Metabolism of [³H]benzo(a)pyrene by cultured human bronchus and cultured human pulmonary alveolar macrophages, *Lab. Invest.* **38**:217.

Badnoch-Jones, P., Turk, J. L., and Parker, D., 1978, The effects of some aluminum and zirconium compounds on guinea pig peritoneal macrophages and skin fibroblasts in culture, *J. Pathol.* **124**:51.

Barry, D. H., and Mawdesley-Thomas, L. E., 1970, Effect of sulfur dioxide on the enzyme activity of the alveolar macrophages of rats, *Thorax* **25**:612.

Bast, R. C., Okudra, T., Plotkin, E., Tarone, K., Rapp, H. J., and Gelboin, H. V., 1976, Development of an assay for aryl hydrocarbon hydroxylase in human peripheral blood monocytes, *Cancer Res.* **36**:1967.

Bey, E., and Harrington, J. S., 1971, Cytotoxic effects of some mineral dusts on Syrian hamster peritoneal macrophages, *J. Exp. Med.* **133**:1149.

Bingham, E., Barkley, W., Murthy, R., and Vassello, C., 1975, Investigation of alveolar macrophages from rats exposed to coal dusts, *Inhaled Part.* **4**(2):543.

Blakley, B. R., and Archer, D. L., 1981, The effect of lead acetate on the immune response in mice, *Toxicol. Appl. Pharmacol.* **61**:18.

Boorman, G. A., Luster, M. I., Dean, J. H., and Wilson, R. E., 1980, The effect of adult exposure to diethylstilbestrol in the mouse on macrophage function and numbers, *J. Reticuloendothel. Soc.* **28**:547.

Boorman, G. A., Dean, J. H., Luster, M. I., Adkins, B., Jr., Broady, A., and Hong, H. L., 1984, Bone marrow alterations induced in mice with inhalation of chrysotile asbestos, *Toxicol. Appl. Pharmacol.* **72**:148.

Bouley, G., Dubreuil, A., Godin, J., Boisset, M., and Boudene, C., 1976, Phenomena of adaptation in rats continuously exposed to low concentrations of acrolein, *Ann. Occup. Hyg.* **19**:27.

Bowden, D. H., 1973, The alveolar macrophage and its role in toxicology, *Crit. Rev. Toxicol.* **2**:95.

Brain, J. D., 1980, Macrophage damage in relation to the pathogenesis of lung disease, *Environ. Health Perspect.* **35**:21.

Camner, P., Johansson, A., and Lundborg, M., 1978, Alveolar macrophages in rabbits exposed to nickel dust, *Environ. Res.* **16**:226.

Cantrell, E., Warr, G. A., Busbee, D. C., and Martin, R. P., 1973, Induction of aryl hydrocarbon hydroxylase in human pulmonary alveolar macrophages by cigarette smoking, *J. Clin. Invest.* **32**:1881.

Castranova, V., Bowman, L., Reasoner, M. J., and Miles, P. R., 1980, Effects of heavy metal ions on selected oxidative metabolic processes in rat alveolar macrophages, *Toxicol. Appl. Pharmacol.* **53**:14.

Coffin, D. L., and Gardner, D. E., 1972, Interaction of biological agents and chemical air pollutants, *Ann. Occup. Hyg.* **15**:219.

Coffin, D. L., Gardner, D. E., Holzman, R. S., and Wolock, F. J., 1968, Influence of ozone on pulmonary cells, *Arch. Environ. Health* **16**:633.

Cohen, M. S., Taffet, S. M., and Adams, D. O., 1982, The relationship between secretion of H_2O_2 and completion of tumor cytotoxicity by BCG-elicited macrophages, *J. Immunol.* **128**:1781.

Cohn, Z. A., 1978, The activation of mononuclear phagocytes: Fact, fancy, and future, *J. Immunol.* **121**:813.

Davies, P., and Allison, A. C., 1976, Secretion of macrophage enzymes in relation to the pathogenesis of chronic inflammation, in: *Immunobiology of the Macrophage* (D. S. Nelson, ed.), pp. 427–461, Academic Press, New York.

Davies, P., Allison, A. C., Ackerman, J., Butterfield, A., and Williams, S., 1974, Asbestos induced selective release of lysosomal enzymes from mononuclear phagocytes, *Nature (London)* **251**:423.

Dean, J. H., Luster, M. I., and Boorman, G. A., 1982, Immunotoxicology, in: *Immunopharmacology* (P. Sirois and M. Rola-Pleszczynski, eds.), pp. 349–397, Elsevier, Amsterdam.

Dean, J. H., Lauer, L. D., House, R. V., Murray, M. J., Stillman, W. S., Irons, R. D., Steinhagen, W. H., Phelps, M. C., and Adams, D. O., 1984a, Studies of immune function and host resistance in B6C3F1 mice exposed to formaldehyde, *Toxicol. Appl. Pharmacol.* **72**:519.

Dean, J. H., Boorman, G. A., Luster, M. I., Adkins, B., Jr., Lauer, L. D., and Adams, D. O., 1984b, Effect of agents of environmental concern on macrophage function, in: *Mononuclear Phagocyte Biology* (A. Volkman, ed.), Dekker, New York (in press).

Dean, J. H., Lauer, L. D., Murray, M. J., Luster, M. I., Neptun, D., and Adams, D. O., 1984c, Studies of macrophage function using markers for stages of activation and resistance to *Listeria monocytogenes* in mice exposed to diethylstilbestrol, (submitted for publication).

Donaldson, K., Davis, J. M. G., and James, K., 1982, Characteristics of peritoneal macrophages induced by asbestos injection, *Environ. Res.* **29**:414.

Douglas, J. W. B., and Waller, R. E., 1968, Air pollution and respiratory infection in children, *Br. J. Prev. Soc. Med.* **20**:1.

Dowell, A. R., Lohrbauer, L. A., Hurst, D., and Lee, S. D., 1970, Rabbit alveolar macrophage damage caused by *in vivo* ozone inhalation, *Arch. Environ. Health* **21**:121.

Drath, D. B., Harper, A., Gharibian, J., Karnovsky, M. L., and Huber, G. K., 1978, The effect of tobacco smoke on the metabolism and function of rat alveolar macrophages, *J. Cell. Physiol.* **95**:105.

Ehrlich, R., 1966, Effects of nitrogen dioxide on resistance to respiratory infections, *Bacteriol. Rev.* **30**:604.

Engelbrecht, F. M., and DeKlerk, G., 1972, The oxygen uptake of alveolar and peritoneal macrophages during phagocytosis of toxic and non-toxic dust particles, *S.A. Med. J.* **46**:1791.

Facchinetti, T., Raz, A., and Goldman, R., 1978, A differential interaction of daunomycin, adriamycin, and trifluoroacetyl adriamycin 14-valerate with mouse peritoneal macrophages, *Cancer Res.* **38**:3944.

Fairchild, G. A., Kane, P., Adams, B., and Coffin, D., 1975, Sulfuric acid and streptococci clearance from respiratory tracts of mice, *Arch. Environ. Health* **30**:538.

Finklea, J. F., Hammer, D. I., House, D. E., Sharp, C. R., Nelson, W. C., Lowrimore, G. R., 1974, Frequency of acute lower respiratory disease in children: Retrospective survey of five Rocky Mountain communities, 1967–1970, in: *Health Consequences of Sulfur Oxides*: A Report from CHESS, 1970–1971", Volume 3, pp. 35–56, EPA 650/1-74-004. U.S. Environmental Protection Agency, Research Triangle Park, N.C.

Forman, H. J., Nelson, J., and Fisher, A. B., 1980, Rat alveolar macrophages require NADPH for superoxide production in the respiratory burst: The effect of NADPH depletion by paraquat, *J. Biol. Chem.* **255**:9879.

Gardner, D. E., 1984, Alterations in macrophage function by environmental chemicals, *Environ. Health Perspect.* (in press).

Gee, J. B. L., Boynton, B. R., Khandivala, A. S., and Smith, G. J., 1979, Pulmonary alveolar macrophage function: Some effects of cigarette smoke, in: *Assessing Toxic Effects of Environmental Pollutants* (S. D. Lee and J. B. Mudd, eds.), pp. 77–85, Ann Arbor Sciences, Ann Arbor, Mich.

Goldstein, E., 1977, The influence of environmental toxicity of the antibacterial activity of the alveolar macrophage, in: *Pulmonary Macrophage and Epithelial Cells* (C. L. Sanders, R. P. Schneider, G. E. Dagle, and H. A. Kagan, eds.), ERDA Symposium Series 43, CONF-760927, pp. 382–394.

Graham, J. A., Gardner, D. E., Waters, M. D., and Coffin, D. L., 1979, Effect of trace metals on phagocytosis by alveolar macrophage, *Infect. Immun.* **11**:1278.

Green, G. M., Jakab, G. J., Low, R. B., and Davis, G. E., 1977, Defense mechanisms of the respiratory membrane, *Am. Rev. Respir. Dis.* **115**:479.

Guavneri, J. J., and Laurenzi, A., 1968, Effect of alcohol on the mobilization of alveolar macrophages, *J. Lab. Clin. Med.* **72**:40.

Hamilton, J. A., 1980, Macrophage stimulation and the inflammatory response to asbestos, *Environ. Health Perspect.* **34**:69.

Hamilton, J., Vassalli, J. D., and Reich, E., 1976, Macrophage plasminogen activation: Induction by asbestos is blocked by anti-inflammatory steroid, *J. Exp. Med.* **144**:1689.

Hamilton, T. A., Dean, J. H., and Adams, D. O., 1984, Systemic administration of DMBA alters macrophage development, (in preparation).

Harrington, J. S., 1976, The biological effects of mineral fibers, especially asbestos, as seen from *in vitro* and *in vivo* studies, *Ann. Anat. Pathol.* **21**:155.

Harrington, J. S., and Allison, A. C., 1965, Lysosomal enzymes in relation to the toxicity of silica, *Med. Lav.* **56**:471.

Harris, J. O., Olsen, G. N., Castle, J. R., and Maloney, A. S., 1975, Comparison of proteolytic enzyme activity in pulmonary alveolar macrophages and blood leukocytes in smokers and non-smokers, *Am. Rev. Respir. Dis.* **5**:579.

Hibbs, J. B., Taintor, R. R., Chapman, H. A., and Weinberg, J. B., 1977, Macrophage tumor killing: Influence of the local environment, *Science* **197**:279.

Hinman, L. M., Stevens, C. A., Matthay, R. A., and Gee, J. B. L., 1980, Elastase and lysozyme activities in human alveolar macrophages, *Am. Rev. Respir. Dis.* **121**:263.

Hoidal, R., and Niewoehner, D. E., 1982, Lung phagocyte recruitment and metabolic alterations induced by cigarette smoke in humans and hamsters, *Amer. Rev. Respir. Dis.* **126**:548.

Huber, G. L., and LaForce, F. M., 1970, Comparative effects of ozone and oxygen on pulmonary antibacterial defense mechanisms, *Antimicrob. Agents Chemother.* **1**:129.

Hurst, D. J., Gardner, D. E., and Coffin, D. L., 1970, Effect of ozone on acid hydrolases of the pulmonary alveolar macrophage, *J. Reticuloendothel. Soc.* **8**:288.

Janoff, A., Sloan, B., Weinbaum, G., Damiano, V., Sandhaus, R. A., Elias, J., and Kimbel, P., 1977, Experimental emphysema induced with purified human neutrophil elastase: Tissue localization of the instilled protease, *Am. Rev. Respir. Dis.* **115**:461.

Johannsson, A., Lundborg, M., Hellstrom, P. A., Per-Ake, P., Camner, P., Keyser, T. R., Kirton, S. E., and Natusch, D. F. S., 1980b, Effect of iron, cobalt and chromium dust on rabbit alveolar macrophages: A comparison with the effects of nickel dust, *Environ. Res.* **21**:165.

Johnson, W. J., Marino, P. A., Schreiber, R. D. and Adams, D. O., 1983, Sequential activation of murine mononuclear phagocytes for tumor cytolysis: Differential expression of markers by macrophages in the several stages of development, *J. Immunol.* **131**:1038.

Katz, G. V., and Laskin, S., 1977, Effect of irritant atmospheres on macrophage behavior, in: *Pulmonary Macrophage and Epithelial Cells* (C. L. Sanders, R. P. Schneider, G. E. Dagle, and H. A. Kagan, eds.), ERDA Symposium Series 43, CONF-760927, pp. 358–373.

Kavet, R. I., Brain, J. D., and Levens, D. J., 1978, Characteristics of pulmonary macrophage lavaged from hamsters exposed to iron oxide aerosols, *Lab. Invest.* **38**:312.

Kaw, J. L., Tilks, F., and Beck, E. G., 1982, Reaction of cells cultured *in vitro* to different asbestos dusts of equal surface area but different fibre length, *Br. J. Exp. Pathol.* **63**:109.

Kilroe-Smith, T. A., Webster, L., Van Drummelen, M., and Marasas, L., 1973, An insoluble fibrogenic factor in macrophages from guinea pigs exposed to silica, *Environ. Res.* **6**:298.

Koller, L. D., and Roan, J. G., 1977, Effects of lead and cadmium on mouse peritoneal macrophages, *J. Reticuloendothel. Soc.* **21**:7.

Levy, D., Gent, M., and Newhouse, M. T., 1977, Relationship between acute respiratory illness and air pollution levels in an industrial city, *Am. Rev. Respir. Dis.* **116**:167.

Lewis, D. J., Braybrook, K. J., and Prentice, D. E., 1979, The measurement of ultrastructural changes induced by tobacco smoke in rat alveolar macrophages. A comparison of high and low tar cigarettes, *Toxicol. Lett.* **4**:175.

Lewis, J. G., and Adams, D. O., 1984, The mononuclear phagocyte system and its interactions with xenobiotics, in: *Toxicology of the Immune System* (J. H. Dean, A. E. Munson, M. I. Luster, and H. E. Amos, eds.), Raven Press, New York (in press).

Loose, L. D., Silkworth, J. B., and Simpson, D. W., 1978, Influence of cadmium on the phagocytic and microbicidal activity and murine peritoneal macrophages, pulmonary alveolar macrophages and polymorphonuclear neutrophils, *Infect. Immun.* **22**:378.

Loose, L. D., Silkworth, J. B., Charbonneau, T., and Blumenstock, F., 1981, Environmental chemical-induced macrophage dysfunction, *Environ. Health Perspect.* **39**:79.

Luhr, H. G., 1958, Comparative studies on phagocytosis of coal powders of various carbonification grades, also of quartz and diamond powders in tissue cultures, *Arch. Gewerbepathol. Gewerbehyg.* **16**:355.

McAllen, S. J., Chiu, S. P., Phalen, R. F., and Rasmussen, R. E., 1981, Effect of *in vivo* ozone exposure on *in vitro* pulmonary alveolar macrophage mobility, *J. Toxicol. Environ. Health* **7**:373.

McLemore, T. L., Martin, R. R., Toppell, K. L., Busbee, D. L., and Cantrell, E. T., 1977a, Comparison of aryl hydrocarbon hydroxylase induction in culture blood lymphocytes and pulmonary macrophages, *J. Clin. Invest.* **60**:1017.

McLemore, T. L., Warr, G. A., and Martin, R., 1977b, Induction of aryl hydrocarbon hydroxylase in human pulmonary alveolar macrophages and peripheral lymphocytes by cigarette tars, *Cancer Lett.* **2**:161.

McLemore, T., Corson, M., Mace, M., Arnott, M., Jenkins, T., Snodgrass, D., Martin, R., Wray, N., and Brinkley, B. R., 1979, Phagocytosis of asbestos fibers by human pulmonary alveolar macrophages, *Cancer Lett.* **6**:183.

Mantovani, A., Luini, W., Candiani, G. P., and Spreafico, F., 1980a, Effect of chemotherapeutic agents on natural and BCG stimulated macrophage cytotoxicity in mice, *Int. J. Immunopharmacol.* **2**:333.

Mantovani, A., Luini, W., Candiani, G. P., Salmona, M., Spreafico, F., and Garattini, S., 1980b, In vitro effects of saccharin on cell-mediated host defense mechanisms, *Toxicol. Lett.* **5**:287.

Mantovani, A., Vecchi, A., Luini, W., Sironi, M., Candiani, G. P., Spreafico, F., and Garattini, S., 1980c, Effect of 2,3,7,8-tetrachlorodibenzo-*p*-dioxin on macrophage and natural killer cell-mediated cytotoxicity in mice, *Biomedicine* **32**:200.

Marino, P. A., and Adams, D. O., 1980, Interactions of bacillus Calmette-Guerin activated macrophages and neoplastic cells in vitro. II. The relationship of selective binding to cytolysis, *Cell. Immunol.* **54**:26.

Matulionis, D. H., and Traurig, H. H., 1977, In situ response of lung macrophages and hydrolase activities to cigarette smoke, *Lab. Invest.* **37**:314.

Meltzer, M. S., 1981, Tumor cytotoxicity by lymphokine-activated macrophages: Development of macrophage tumoricidal activity requires a sequence of reactions, *Lymphokines* **3**:319.

Meltzer, M. S., Ruco, L. P., Boraschi, D., and Nacy, C. A., 1979, Macrophage activation for tumor cytotoxicity: Analysis of intermediary reactions, *J. Reticuloendothel. Soc.* **26**:403.

Metchnikoff, E., 1901, *L'immunité dans les maladies infectieuses*, Masson, Paris.

Miller, K., and Kagan, E., 1976, The in vivo effects of asbestos on macrophage membrane structures and population characteristics of macrophages: A scanning electron microscopy study, *J. Reticuloendothel. Soc.* **20**:159.

Miller, K., and Kagan, E., 1977, The in vivo effects of quartz on alveolar macrophages membrane topography and on the characteristics of the intrapulmonary cell population, *J. Reticuloendothel. Soc.* **21**:307.

Miller, K., Handfield, R. I. M., and Kagan, E., 1978a, The effect of different mineral dusts on the mechanism of phagocytosis: A scanning electron microscope study, *Environ. Res.* **15**:139.

Miller, K., Webster, I., Handfield, R. I. M., and Skikne, M. I., 1978b, Ultrastructure of the lung in the rat following exposure to crocidolite asbestos and quartz, *J. Pathol.* **124**:39.

Morahan, P. S., Edelson, P. J., and Gass, K., 1980, Changes in macrophage ectoenzymes associated with anti-tumor activity, *J. Immunol.* **125**:1312.

Murray, H. W., 1984, Activation of macrophages to display enhanced oxidative and antiprotozoal activity, *Contemp. Top. Immunobiol.* (in press).

Murray, M. J., Lauer, L. D., Luster, M. I., Leubke, R. W., Adams, D. O., and Dean, J. H., 1984, Correlation of murine susceptibility to tumor, parasite and bacterial challenge with altered cell-mediated immunity following systemic exposure to the tumor promoter phorbol myristate acetate, *Int. J. Immunopharmacol.* (in press).

Myrvik, M., and Evans, D. G., 1967, Metabolic and immunologic activities of alveolar macrophages, *Arch. Environ. Health* **14**:92.

Nacy, C. A., Leonard, E. J., and Meltzer, M. S., 1981, Macrophages in resistance to rickettsial infections: Characterization of lymphokines that induce rickettsiacidal activity in macrophages, *J. Immunol.* **126**:204.

Nadler, S., and Goldfischer, S. K., 1970, The intracellular release of lysosomal contents in macrophages that have ingested silica, *J. Histochem. Cytochem.* **18**:368.

Nathan, C. F., and Root, R. K., 1977, Hydrogen peroxide release from mouse peritoneal macrophages: Dependence on sequential activation and triggering, *J. Exp. Med.* **146**:1648.

North, R. J., 1978, The concept of the activated macrophage, *J. Immunol.* **121**:806.

Nourse, L. D., Nourse, P. N., Bates, H., and Schwartz, H. M., 1975, The effects of macrophages isolated from the lungs of guinea pigs dusted with silica on collagen biosynthesis by guinea pig fibroblasts in cell culture, *Environ. Res.* **9**:115.

Page, R. C., Davies, P., and Allison, A. C., 1978, The macrophage as a secretory cell, *Int. Rev. Cytol.* **52**:119.

Price, C. D., Pugh, A., Pioti, E. M., and Williams, W. J., 1976, Beryllium macrophage migration inhibition test, *Ann. N.Y. Acad. Sci.* **278**:204.

Rae, T., 1975, A study on the effects of particulate metals of orthopaedic interest on murine macrophages, *J. Bone J. Surg. Br. Vol.* **57**:444.

Richard, J. L., and Thurston, J. R., 1975, Effect of aflatoxin on phagocytosis of *Aspergillus fumigatus* spores by rabbit alveolar macrophages, *Appl. Microbiol.* **30**:44.

Roux, F., Puiseux-Dao, S., Treich, I., and Fournier, E., 1978, Effect of lindane on mouse peritoneal macrophages, *Toxicology* **11**:259.

Schlipkoter, H. W., and Dolgner, R., 1981, Air pollution and biological defense, *Zentralbl. Bakteriol. Parasitenkd. Infektionskr. Hyg. Abt. Orig. Reihe B* **172**:299.

Schorlemmer, H. U., Edwards, J. H., Davies, P., and Allison, A. C., 1977, Macrophage responses to mouldy hay dust, *Micropolyspora faeri* and zymosan, activators of complement by the alternate pathway, *Clin. Exp. Immunol.* **27**:198.

Shy, C. M., Creason, J. P., Pearlman, M. E., McClain, K. E., Benson, F. B., and Young, M. M., 1970, The Chattanooga School Study: Effects of community exposure to nitrogen dioxide. II. Incidence of acute respiratory illness, *J. Air Pollut. Control Assoc.* **20**:582.

Shingu, H., Sugiyama, M., Watanabe, M., and Nakajima, T., 1980, Effects of ozone and photochemical oxidants on interferon production by rabbit alveolar macrophages, *Bull. Environ. Contam. Toxicol.* **24**:433.

Valand, S. B., Acton, J. D., and Myrvik, Q. N., 1970, Nitrogen dioxide inhibition of viral-induced resistance in alveolar monocytes, *Arch. Environ. Health* **20**:303.

van Furth, R., 1978, Mononuclear phagocytes in inflammation, in: *Inflammation* (R. van Furth and S. H. Ferreria, eds.), p. 68, Springer-Verlag, Berlin.

Waters, M. D., Gardner, D. E., Aranyi, C., and Coffin, D. L., 1975, Metal toxicity for rabbit alveolar macrophages, *Environ. Res.* **9**:32.

White, R., and Kuhn, C., 1980, Effects of phagocytosis of mineral dusts on elastase secretion by alveolar and peritoneal exudative macrophages, *Arch. Environ. Health* **35**:106.

Ziprin, R. L., and Fowler, S. R., 1977, Rosette-forming ability of alveolar macrophages from rat lung: Inhibition of hexachlorobenzeine, *Toxicol. Appl. Pharmacol.* **39**:105.

15

Effects of Trace Elements on Immunoregulation

ARTHUR FLYNN

1. INTRODUCTION

In the past several decades there has been an increased awareness of the effects of "heavy" metals that act as pollutants of our environment. As greater technological advances in chemical detection and analysis of trace elements have been made, the more widespread has become the concern over exposure to these apparently ubiquitous metals (Chisolm, 1980). Since all elements are potentially toxic according to dose, almost all physiological systems are affected by pharmacological doses of trace elements, including the reticuloendothelial system.

Several examples of severe, high-dose exposures of adults and children to toxic levels of trace elements have provided the basis for concern. High-dose exposure to cadmium, lead, and mercury has provided information on the multitude of effects such toxic excesses can have in humans. The toxic effects of cadmium were first described clinically in the mid 1950s in Japan as a painful bone disease, "itai itai byo" or "ouch-ouch disease." Rice grown in water contaminated with cadmium from mine tailings was 10 times higher in cadmium than normal control rice. Consumption of the rice and shellfish from polluted waters was implicated in the development of this disease. The major manifestations of the chronic high-dose cadmium toxicity were hypochromic anemia, pigmentation of skin, renal osteomalacia, chronic nephropathy, and gastritis and enteropathy. All ages were affected by itai itai disease, but postmenopausal, multiparous women manifested the most marked symptoms and severe skeletal abnormalities of the femur, spine, and ribs (Friberg *et al.*, 1974). For well over 100 years, the toxic effects of lead have been recognized. Industrial exposures and inappropriate disposal of lead-containing products accounted for early descrip-

ARTHUR FLYNN • Department of Molecular and Cellular Biology, Research Division, Cleveland Clinic Foundation, Cleveland, Ohio 44106.

tions of lead intoxication. In the early 1930s, Williams (1933) reported severe acute lead poisoning in children and adults related to the use of lead battery casings as home heating fuel. Ataxia, stupor, convulsions, and coma are signs of acute severe lead poisoning in patients, particularly those with defective kidney function (Fanconi syndrome) (Anonymous, 1972). Mercury exposure and the related clinical problems were again found in Japan from the industrial dumping of mercury in Minamata Bay. Minamata disease demonstrated the neurotoxicological effects of mercury (Smith and Smith, 1975). In the early 1970s, methyl mercury poisoning was described in Iraq from the consumption of fungicide-treated wheat (methyl mercury) (Bakir, 1973). Some 6500 people were affected, with several hundred fatalities. Neurological, pulmonary, gastrointestinal, renal, cardiovascular, hormonal, and dermatological abnormalities were shown to be related to the mercury exposure. It was also noted that mercury was a potent fetotoxin. These three descriptions of the effects of trace elements generally considered nonessential demonstrate the basis for concern and interest in defining not only the acute severe exposure, but also the chronic low-dose exposure to toxic elements.

Low-dose exposure to cadmium and lead gives a very different profile of the pathological effects of toxic elements than acute poisoning with the same elements. Industrial exposure to cadmium is an obvious source, but natural water supplies and cigarette smoking have also been implicated as sources of the toxic element. Low levels of cadmium have been associated with hypertension, secondary to the destruction of distal tubules in the kidney (Schroeder and Vinton, 1962), a symptom not seen with high-dose exposure. Epidemiological studies of humans with active hypertension have related cadmium with the pathological condition (Perry, 1968). Cigarette smoking in particular has been correlated to significantly elevated kidney cadmium and tissue damage (Lewis et al., 1972). Low-dose lead intoxication has been implicated in faulty heme synthesis and oxygen transport in red blood cells and, in children, in mental retardation. Lead is known to interfere at several steps in the synthesis of heme by inhibiting four different enzymes (Bowen, 1979). Subtle, long-lasting impairment of nervous system activity has been described in preschool children with blood lead in excess of 50 µg/ml (Needleman et al., 1979). Whether lower blood leads in children, in the range of 30–50 µg/dl, are related to CNS defects is controversial (Chisolm, 1980). Low-level exposure to toxic elements has profound physiological effects and may not be easily related to the polluting source, but heightens concern on how this might affect the health of the public in general.

Underlying concerns for population exposures to toxic trace elements from the environment is the changing sensitization of the general population to irritants (including metals) and greater worker awareness. Epidemiological studies on contact dermatitis (North American Contact Dermatitis Group, 1973) have described the responsiveness of a population of 1200 people from 10 geographic areas of North America to 16 known allergens. Seventy-three percent of the white population and 67% of the black population tested had positive responses in the skin tests to at least one of these agents. The substance that elicited the greatest number of positive reactions was a trace metal compound, nickel sulfate. In the workplace, exposures to toxic substances are restricted by the regulations of the Occupational Safety and Health Act (OSHA). The potential for toxic exposure is great since the industrial usage of toxic metal compounds is in the millions of pounds each year (Chisolm, 1980). For example, beryllium is widely used in alloys and is known to cause dermatitis, acute pneumonitis, and chronic pulmonary granulomatosis (Reeves, 1976). The chronic effects of beryllium, also called berylliosis, have been generally associated with occupational inhalation of beryllium compounds. Strict safety precautions are now a part of the regulations governing the beryllium industry, with significant decreases in deleterious effects on workers (Lieben and Williams, 1969). This increased awareness of exposure to toxic elements has also led immunologists to more extensively investigate the impact of trace elements on a variety of immune responses.

2. TRACE ELEMENTS

2.1. CLASSIFICATION OF TRACE ELEMENTS

The vast majority of chemical elements are considered trace elements in that they represent less than 1/10,000th of the total mass of man (Bowen, 1979). Only about 12 elements are considered macroelements in concentration greater than trace (oxygen, carbon, hydrogen, nitrogen, calcium, phosphorus, sulfur, potassium, sodium, chlorine, magnesium, and perhaps silicon) (Underwood, 1977). The remaining 80 naturally occurring trace elements are divided into three categories: essential, potentially essential, and nonessential (Schwartz, 1974). *Essential*, although there is no consensus, has been defined as a five-point criterion:

1. Chemically suitable, transition element that forms organic chelates
2. Ubiquitous element, generally available to plants and animals
3. An element normally present in plants and animals
4. Orally nontoxic, except in astringent doses
5. Homeostatic mechanism exist for the element to maintain serum levels, excretion rates, and limit accumulation (Nielsen, 1974)

Twelve trace elements are generally accepted as essential in mammalian systems (vanadium, chromium, manganese, iron, cobalt, nickel, copper, zinc, selenium, molybdenum, tin, and iodine) (Schwartz, 1974). A series of other elements are being studied as potentially essential in mammalian systems: arsenic, boron, cadmium, lead, and lithium (Schwartz, 1974), but the evidence is yet to be verified. Each has been shown to relate to a specific biochemical mechanism, but not to meet all five of the points listed above. Some additional factors must also be considered as to the action of essential or potentially essential elements, which relate to limiting of availability. Valence state, the organic matrix, and element–element interaction that can occur, can significantly affect the action of a trace element (Davies, 1974).

Nonessential trace elements have no defined physiological action and are generally available as environmental pollutants. The more abundant nonessential trace elements generally fall short of the criterion for essentiality in not having homeostatic mechanisms to control accumulation. The less abundant elements are not usually chemically suitable for forming organic chelates and therefore are not normally present in plants and animals. Nonessential elements can be thought of as either potentially toxic at all levels or relatively nontoxic, with several elements standing out as very toxic: beryllium, cadmium, lead, and mercury (Wood, 1974).

2.2. DOSE RESPONSES OF ESSENTIAL AND NONESSENTIAL TRACE ELEMENTS

The dose–biological response curve generated for essential trace elements gives a broad range of action, with death being the result of absolute deficiency and excess. Oral intake of essential trace elements generally has a large plateau region of acceptable or optimal dietary intake (Smith, 1962). A typical dose–response curve for an essential trace element is shown in Fig. 1. A feature of the toxic effects of high-dose intake of essential metals is that at initially elevated levels the element acts as an irritant to actually increase the biological effect before the increasing dose suppresses biological activity. A similar curve cannot be generated for the nonessential elements since there are no deficiencies. The toxic response, however, to nonessential trace elements can generally be defined as a biphasic dose–response curve. Initially, there is a slow increase in toxic effects at lower levels, whereas at higher values dramatic toxic changes occur with minimal increases in the element intake (Bowen, 1979). The bimodal response curve for toxic effects is shown in Fig. 2. Part of the problem with the more toxic nonessential trace elements is that they have relatively long biological half-lives within the body [e.g., the nonessential element lead has a residence time in man of 35–40 days in soft tissue, but 25–30 years in bone (Underwood,

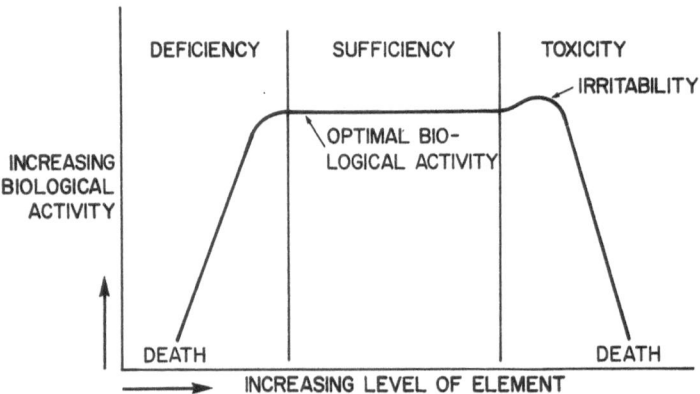

FIGURE 1. General scheme of relationship between increasing levels of an essential trace element and biological activity.

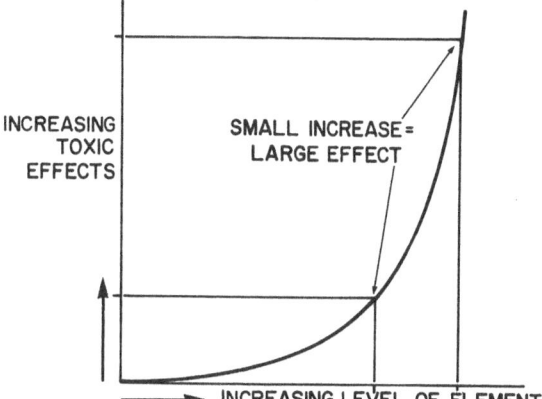

FIGURE 2. Dose–effect relationship between increasing levels of toxic nonessential trace element and toxic effects. Note that at higher levels of elements, small changes have significantly greater effects.

1977), whereas the essential metal zinc has a biological half-life of only 154 days (Halsted *et al.*, 1974)]. These long half-lives for nonessential elements indicate that even minimal exposure may be toxic and a long latency period between exposure and toxic response may exist.

2.3. ACTIONS OF ESSENTIAL AND NONESSENTIAL TRACE ELEMENTS

2.3.1. Essential Trace Elements

Trace elements are generally bound by proteins and the interactions of the metal ions with proteins fall within two general categories: metalloproteins and metal-activated proteins or metal–protein complexes (Frieden, 1978). The relationship between metal and protein is reciprocal; i.e., the trace element can affect the structure of the protein and so its reactivity, and the complex nature of the protein can result in unusual stereochemistries of the trace element. Trace elements in this biological setting with proteins, therefore, act in only a limited number of ways: (1) as templates for structural orientations in bioorganic synthesis; (2) as Lewis acids (electron acceptors); and (3) as catalysts in oxidation–reduction reactions (Hughes, 1972).

The simplest function for a trace element is to act as a template in organic synthesis to bring reacting groups into the proper orientation for reaction. The majority of trace elements have basic structures [tetrahedral (sp^3), square planar (dsp^3), or octahedral (d^2sp^3)] that contain a limited number of ligand sites (4 or 6) (Matrone, 1974).

Complex compounds, such as the porphyrin ring of heme or cobalamin, provide examples of such template effects of iron and cobalt. These structural functions are also the basis for understanding some of the interactions or competitions that can occur between trace elements. Trace elements have also been described as providing structural "stiffness" to certain biological structures, such as membranes, by bridging neighboring groups (Hughes, 1972).

Trace elements can accept electron pairs and thus act as Lewis acids (Steitz *et al.*, 1967). Strengths of the Lewis acid activity of trace elements appear to relate to the charge on the metal and to the ionic radius. The role of trace elements as Lewis acids, as catalysts, differs from proton acid catalysts in two ways: (1) the trace element can coordinate to multiple ligand sites at one time, and (2) metal ion catalysis can take place in physiological pH ranges where proton donor acid catalysis is ineffective. Zinc is a good example of a strong Lewis acid that is involved in hydrolytic enzymes, particularly phosphatases, peptidases, and esterases. Manganese is a much weaker Lewis acid and acts as a catalyst with enzymes whose substrates have weaker base centers (i.e., polyphosphates). The ability to replace one trace element with another, because of structured similarity yet different acid strength, has allowed the study of Lewis acid activity of trace elements in enzyme systems (Vallee *et al.*, 1971).

In oxidation–reduction reactions (redox), trace elements generally catalyze a change in valence state of the substrate (Hughes, 1972). The more important metals in redox reaction catalysis are iron, copper, and cobalt. The methods for catalysis vary from electron transfer, oxygen atom and hydroxyl group incorporation, to hydrogen atom and hybridge ion removal. A characteristic feature of metalloenzymes involved in redox behavior is an irregular stereochemistry of the metal's environment (Smith and Williams, 1970). Iron is an excellent example of a trace element involved in redox reactions. Iron is a component of cytochromes, peroxidases, and catalase, as well as respiratory processes of hemoglobin and myoglobin. Copper as blue hemocyanin is also involved in oxygen transport, but is also important in a number of oxidases. The major copper protein, ceruloplasmin, is capable of oxidizing a number of substrates: Fe(II), *p*-phenylenediamine derivatives, aminophenols, catecholamines, 5-hydroxyindoles, and phenothiazines (Frieden, 1980).

The essential trace elements, therefore, play a vital role in protein chemistry and the functioning of enzymes. The three distinct roles of essential trace element activity define areas for interaction between differing metal ions and differing potential ligands that may explain the toxic actions of trace elements and methods of detoxification.

2.3.2. Nonessential Trace Elements

The mode of nonessential trace elements in biological systems as toxicants is generally thought of in two ways: (1) the element displaces the normal catalytic metal ion from its binding site on the protein (enzyme) and thus disrupts activity (Chvapil, 1976); and (2) the toxic element disrupts membrane stability and transport properties of the cell (McLaughlin *et al.*, 1971). Both actions on the part of toxic elements could be said to mimic essential trace element binding or activity, as related in Table 1. An example of action of a toxic element can be seen in cadmium. Vallee *et al.* (1971) have reported that cadmium can replace zinc in several enzymes, but this replacement severely affects enzymatic activity. Cadmium interacts, in addition to zinc, with copper, iron, and selenium (Davies, 1974). Spivey-Fox (1978) reported that the interaction between cadmium and

TABLE 1. COMPARISON OF BIOLOGICAL ACTIONS OF ESSENTIAL AND NONESSENTIAL TRACE ELEMENTS

Actions of essential elements	Actions of nonessential elements
Structural—orient reacting groups for proper structure, act as template	Disrupt structure of membranes or transport systems
Lewis acids—electron acceptors, multiple ligand coordination, physiological pH range	Displace essential trace elements from binding sites on proteins (enzymes)
Catalyst in redox reactions—change valence state of substrate	

iron and zinc could be reversed by significantly increasing the availability of the two essential elements. Recognition that many effects of toxic nonessential trace elements came from the mimicking or displacement of essential trace elements may explain the specificity of some toxic responses.

2.4. IMMUNOLOGICAL POTENTIAL OF TRACE ELEMENTS

Immunological responses generally encompass proliferation (Wu *et al.*, 1975), membrane stability (Lafferty *et al.*, 1980), protein synthesis (Smith, 1980), and cell–cell interaction (contact) (Katz, 1979). The potential effects of trace elements on these leukocyte responses appear to be great. Sandstead and Rinaldi (1969) reported that DNA polymerase is zinc dependent and that deficiency can severely affect proliferation. Chvapil (1976) demonstrated that trace elements are critical to membrane function, and numerous studies have demonstrated that trace element lack decreases protein synthesis (Underwood, 1977). Studies on the effects of deficiencies of essential trace elements on immune reactivity have shown that a number of cell-mediated and humoral responses are depressed in the absence of an essential trace element. Fraker *et al.* (1977) first reported that zinc deficiency in mice, produced by feeding a deficient diet for 4 weeks, interfered with normal T-helper cell development. Subsequent studies have also shown that the rapid involution of the thymus accompanying zinc deficiency is associated with a depressed antibody response, depressed T-killer cell activity, and low NK cell activity (Fernandes *et al.*, 1979). In both B- and T-cell mitogenic responses, zinc deficiency was shown to depress proliferation (Gross *et al.*, 1979). Copper deficiency in mice has been reported to suppress the number of antibody-producing cells (Prohaska and Lukasewycz, 1981). *In vitro* studies on copper, magnesium, and zinc deficiencies have shown that rapid changes in lymphocytes can occur and are related to suppression of cytotoxic T-cell generation (Flynn and Yen, 1981). The potential of trace element changes, both decreases and increases from the norm, influencing immune responses is significant.

Elevated levels of trace elements have been shown to affect the basic components of immune reactions: proliferation, membrane stability, protein synthesis, and cellular interactions. Kirchner and Ruhl (1970) reported that elevated zinc levels were mitogenic for human peripheral blood lymphocytes, and Caron *et al.* (1970) showed that mercury had a mitogenic effect on lymphocytes. DNA synthesis was stimulated by increased levels of zinc and mercury (Berger and Skinner, 1974; Caron *et al.*, 1970), whereas elevated cadmium, cobalt, copper, manganese, and nickel inhibited DNA synthesis in lymphocytes *in vitro*. The integrity of membranes may be disrupted with elevated zinc displacing or inhibiting calcium uptake by the cell (Chvapil, 1976). At cadmium levels greater than 10^{-4} M, lymphocytes cultured *in vitro*, with and without mitogenic stimulation, had a significant depression of protein synthesis (Balter *et al.*, 1980). Thus, both deficient and elevated levels of trace elements may influence physiological mechanisms associated with the development of an immune response.

2.5. PHYSIOLOGICAL EFFECTS OF TRACE ELEMENTS

In order to provide an adequate overview of the differing effects trace elements may have on immune responses, eight elements shall be reviewed, three essential (copper, manganese, and zinc) and five nonessential trace elements (aluminum, beryllium, cadmium, mercury, and lead).

2.5.1. Aluminum

Recognized as a nonessential element, aluminum has a relatively low toxicity. Schroeder and Mitchener (1975) found that the addition of 5 ppm Al to the drinking water of rats did not effect median life span, longevity, tumorigenesis, serum cholesterol, glucose, or uric acid. At much higher levels (several orders of magnitude), Al is a gastrointestinal irritant and interferes with gut absorption of phosphate (Debold and Elvehjem, 1953). Neurological defects in Alzheimer's disease have also been linked with Al (Sorenson *et al.*, 1974). Exposures to aluminum sufficient to cause toxic effects are generally only available through industrial exposure (Sorenson *et al.*, 1974).

2.5.2. Beryllium

Beryllium, a nonessential trace element, can cause contact dermatitis, acute pneumonitis, and chronic pulmonary granulomatosis (Reeves, 1976). The dermatitis and pneumonitis are usually related to exposure to soluble salts of beryllium, but the chronic and more severe granulomatosis can also occur with insoluble beryllium compounds.

2.5.3. Cadmium

Cadmium is considered a toxic, nonessential trace element that appears to accumulate in man with age. At birth, the human body is almost completely lacking in cadmium, but with aging, up to 50 years of age, is retained, usually in the liver and kidney (Underwood, 1977). In low-dose-exposure experiments, Schroeder (1965) and Perry (1968) initially showed a significant increase in hypertension. Other studies have linked hemorrhagic necrosis of the testes and epididymis to cadmium exposure (Parizek and Zahor, 1956; Gunn et al., 1963). Similarly, hemorrhagic necrosis of the ovaries has been described (Parizek, 1964). Chronic high-dose exposure to cadmium (described in Section 1) is manifested in renal and gastrointestinal lesions and osteomalacia.

2.5.4. Copper

The essentiality of copper was recognized in 1928 when its relationship to iron utilization and anemia was first described (Hart et al., 1928). Homeostatic mechanisms in the liver generally maintain a proper balance of copper and limit its use and transport via a copper-containing glycoprotein, ceruloplasmin (Evans, 1973). In animal studies, diets containing copper levels 100 times normal did not result in toxic effects (Braunde et al., 1973), but only if there was a sufficiency of other essential metals (i.e., iron and zinc). Severe high-dose poisoning results in hemolytic anemia (Underwood, 1977).

Two genetically linked diseases, Wilson's disease and Menke's syndrome, are related to defects in copper metabolism and homeostasis. The defect in Wilson's disease is inherited in an autosomal recessive fashion resulting in toxic accumulations of copper in the liver and then the brain, kidneys, eyes, and erythrocytes (Sternlieb, 1982). The concentration and total amounts of copper excreted in the bile (the normal excretory pathway for copper) of Wilson's disease patients are significantly decreased (Frommer, 1974). The major metabolism of ceruloplasmin is also varied in Wilson's disease, being significantly reduced in 95% of patients with this genetic defect.

Menke's syndrome is an X-linked genetic defect that relates to malabsorption of copper from the gut (Camakaris et al., 1982). There are significant depressions in various copper-dependent enzymes and the disease usually results in death by 1 year of age. It appears that copper accumulates normally in the brain and kidneys of patients with this syndrome but its accumulation in the liver is disturbed and very low concentrations are found.

2.5.5. Lead

Mainly considered a nonessential toxic trace element, lead has been the topic of numerous studies to define its mode of toxicity. The impact of lead toxicity in young children has particularly been highlighted and is related to gut absorption, which is significantly higher in children than in adults (Chisolm, 1980). On a cellular basis, lead appears to accumulate in the cytosol and then the microsomes (Barltrop et al., 1971). Several vital enzymes in hemoglobin synthesis are affected by lead (Smith et al., 1976). Studies on the effects of chronic lead exposure demonstrate a general targeting of major effects on the central nervous system (encephalopathy and neuropathy), renal tubular dysfunction, and anemia (Flink, 1971). There has also been reported an increased susceptibility to bacterial infection (Hemphill *et al.*, 1971).

2.5.6. Manganese

An essential trace element with very low toxicity, manganese has been associated with a number of vital enzyme systems in mammals including the mitochondrial form of superoxide dismutase and glycosyltransferases (Utter, 1976). The average dietary intake of manganese in the United States is about 3.7 mg/day (North *et al.*, 1960), whereas the first toxic effects are seen with diets containing almost 500 times that level (Bowen, 1979). Only about 3–4% of orally ingested manganese is absorbed, with the liver playing an important role in homeostasis and excretion (Leach, 1976). In animal studies, toxic doses of manganese were related to decreased serum iron and hemoglobin (Matrone *et al.*, 1959). Occupational exposure of man to manganese oxide has been related to severe psychiatric problems (locura manganica) and a crippling neurological disorder similar to Parkinson's disease (Underwood, 1977). Attempts to treat these CNS-related manganese-caused syndromes with chelation therapy have been unsuccessful.

2.5.7. Mercury

Mercury, a very toxic element with no known biological function, is absorbed mainly in its organic form. The toxic accumulation of this element is dramatically related to its long half-life: inorganic forms have a half-life of 29–60 days, whereas the alkyl organic derivatives of mercury have a half-life of 70–100 days (Clarkson, 1972). The major toxic effects of mercury are related to the functioning of the CNS. The sequelae of mercury toxicity of the CNS comprise steps of progressive incoordination, then loss of hearing and sight with mental deterioration arising from neuroencephalopathy of the cerebral and cerebellar cortex (Smith and Smith, 1975).

2.5.8. Zinc

The essential qualities of zinc have been known for centuries and are currently related to some 80 different enzymes (Underwood, 1977). Zinc is relatively nontoxic, the recommended daily allowance of the USDA being 15 mg. No apparent adverse effects were seen with human diets containing 200–300 mg of zinc (Sandstead, 1973). Elevated dietary zinc levels do have an effect on the absorption of copper and iron, producing suboptimal levels of these two essential elements. Occupational exposures have been related to fume fever in welders (Underwood, 1977) and anemias (microcytic and hypochronic) (Witham, 1963).

A summary of the intake levels by humans of these eight elements is provided in Table 2 (Bowen, 1979).

TABLE 2. NORMAL, TOXIC, AND LETHAL ORAL INTAKE LEVELS
OF SELECTED TRACE ELEMENTS[a]

	Normal	Toxic	Lethal
Aluminum	2–45	5000	N.D.[b]
Beryllium	0.01	N.D.	N.D.
Cadmium	0.007–0.3	3–300	1500–9000
Copper	0.5–6	N.D.	175–250
Lead	0.06–0.5	1.0	10,000
Manganese	0.4–10	N.D.	N.D.
Mercury	0.004–0.02	0.4	150–300
Zinc	5–40	150–600	6000

[a]Milligrams of element in the diet for a reference man weighing 70 kg and eating 750 g/day.
[b]N.D., not determined.

3. LEUKOCYTE RESPONSES TO TRACE ELEMENTS

With this background on the effects of trace elements on biological systems or, more specifically, cellular mechanisms that could be associated with immune responses, we can now examine the responses of leukocytes. The studies and reports on immune reactivity relate to the general understanding that animals and humans exposed to toxic levels of trace elements are more susceptible to infectious disease. Trace element deficiencies have likewise been related to a greater susceptibility to bacterial and viral infections. Both excesses and deficiencies of trace elements can make normally sublethal infections lethal.

Historically, studies on the effects of toxic trace elements on leukocytes preceded studies on the effects of their deficiency. This may be due to at least two reasons: (1) the concern over environmental exposure to heavy metals in the 1960s, and (2) the simplicity of adding soluble salts of trace elements to well-defined *in vitro* immune systems. In addition, *in vivo* models of toxic metal effects appear to relate to physiological events more than do the extremely variable results of *in vitro* studies. Another interesting facet of trace element effects on leukocytes is that elevated levels may be both inhibitory and stimulatory according to which components of the immune response are monitored.

The following two sections on phagocytic cells and lymphocytes and their responses to trace element variations provide only an overview as to what type of responses can be expected.

3.1. PHAGOCYTIC CELL ACTIVITY AND TRACE ELEMENTS

Studies on phagocytic cells have focused on the two predominant cell types, macrophages and polymorphonuclear neutrophils (PMN), owing to the unique biochemical and physiological characteristics of these phagocytes. The effects of elevated levels of trace elements on macrophages and PMNs have been shown to mainly involve phagocytosis and lysosomal enzymes. *In vitro* studies by Koller and Roan (1977), using peritoneal exudate cells (PEC) from two strains of mice given cadmium or lead, demonstrated a significant increase in the phagocytic ability of the PEC. Cadmium was provided to the mice in their drinking water at levels of 3, 30, or 300 μg/ml for 70 days at which time PEC were removed, placed in normal media, and their phagocytic ability tested against SRBC. The phagocytic ability of the PEC was significantly increased in the group receiving 300 μg/ml in both strains of mice. Another group of mice was given lead at 13, 130, or 1300 μg/ml in their drinking water for the same period. The phagocytic ability of the PEC was increased at the two higher levels of lead. The viability of the PEC under both conditions was unchanged from control levels, and the only untoward effect of the high levels of either metal was that the animals given high-level cadmium had a significant decrease in body weight. Long-term studies by the same group focused on the effects of lead in the drinking water of mice over an 18-month period (Koller *et al.*, 1977). A significant decrease in the phagocytic ability of PEC against SRBC was noted at the lowest level given, 13 μg/ml. In the group given the highest level (1300 μg/ml), the phagocytic ability was comparable with controls. An important factor in the assessment of the effects of lead over an 18-month period is not only the lead being provided but also the aging process in the mice. These investigators demonstrated that a significant change in phagocytic ability of PEC against SRBC was noted just with the aging process. In contrast to these *in vivo* studies, *in vitro* studies with cadmium and manganese have demonstrated no change or a suppression of phagocytic ability by macrophages and PMN dosed in culture. Graham *et al.* (1975) studied the ability of alveolar macrophages from rabbits to phagocytize latex spheres in the presence of cadmium or manganese. The phagocytic ability in the presence of cadmium appeared to be unaffected by the 24-hr exposure. Studies with manganese (100 μg/ml) demonstrated that the phagocytic ability was suppressed by approximately 25% and the viability decreased to less than 70%. More recent studies by Loose *et al.* (1977) in alveolar macrophages, PEC, and PMN demonstrated that their phagocytic ability against heat-killed bacteria was also significantly affected by *in vitro* exposure to cadmium. Cadmium was given at levels from 3.6×10^{-3} to 36 meq/liter medium and oxygen consumption was monitored during phagocytosis as an indicator of activity. In all three cell types, activity at cadmium levels above 3.6×10^{-2} meq/liter was significantly decreased. In another study on alveolar macrophages, PEC, and PMN from mice, Loose *et al.* (1978) demonstrated that higher levels of cadmium added to the media significantly affected phagocytosis of yeast and the microbial activity of the cells. All three cell types had a significant decrease in phagocytic activity at the higher cadmium levels (8.0×10^{-2} to 8.0×10^{-1} meq/liter medium). Microbial activity was also depressed in the alveolar macrophages at the highest cadmium level.

The differences between the *in vivo* and the *in vitro* studies on the effects of cadmium on phagocytosis may relate to the actual levels of cadmium taken up by the macrophages. Neither group determined the level present in the cells. Hart (1978), studying the uptake of [109]Cd by alveolar macrophages over a 50-min period, found a linear increase in cadmium uptake at concentrations from 0.10 μg/ml to 1.50 μ/ml. Rate of uptake reached a plateau with cadmium concentrations of 1.0 μg/ml. Serum proteins in the medium interfered with cellular uptake, whereas added zinc potentiated cadmium uptake in a concentration-dependent manner. The zinc effect may relate to an increase in transport sites and an increased affinity of these sites for cadmium.

The ability of macrophages to produce lysosomal enzymes has been studied in response to the addition of aluminum or beryllium to *in vitro* cultures. Badenoch-Jones *et al.* (1978) and Badenoch-Jones (1978) initially studied the release of enzymes from guinea pig peritoneal macrophages in response to $Al(OH)_3$ and aluminum chlorhydrate. In 24-hr cultures with aluminum (1 μg/ml), LDH release was significantly increased 24 hr after the addition of aluminum to the cultures. The other hydrolases studied, N-acetyl-β-D-glucosaminidase, β-glycerophosphatase, cathepsin D, were not elevated with the addition of aluminum over an already high release of the enzymes under control conditions. Kang and Salvaggio (1978) studied the effects of aluminum chlorhydrate on rabbit alveolar macrophages at levels up to 500 μg/ml medium. Four fractions (enzyme content of the medium, whole cell homogenates, mitochondria, and supernatants) were studied over a 24-hr period for increased synthesis and/or release of enzymes. Significant increases in acid phosphatase, N-acetyl-β-D-glucosaminidase, and β-glucuronidase were noted in the mitochondrial fraction of the macrophages at all levels of aluminum exposure. The intracellular increase in the hydrolases was not detected outside of the cell for there was no significant release of enzymes into the medium. The phagocytic ability of the alveolar macrophages was not affected by the levels of aluminum used in this study. Kang *et al.* (1979), studying the effects of beryllium on rabbit alveolar macrophages, also noted changes in lysosomal enzymes. Alveolar macrophages were exposed to 3, 10, or 30 μg/ml beryllium sulfate *in vitro* over a 24-hr period. Viability at the highest level of beryllium was significantly depressed, being less than 50%. At 20–24 hr after the beginning of the cultures, significant increases in acid phosphatase were noted in the medium at the two higher levels and in the mitochondria at all levels. Increased activity of β-N-acetylglucosaminidase was reported in the mitochondria at all levels and at the two higher levels in the culture supernatants. Changes in β-glucuronidase were most widespread. Whole cell homogenate levels were significantly increased at the two higher levels, mitochondrial enzyme activity was increased at the lowest level, and culture supernatant activity was significantly increased at the two higher beryllium levels (Kang *et al.*, 1979).

The receptors on macrophages for the Fc portion of the immunoglobulin molecule were examined by their binding with erythrocyte–antibody (EA) complex and the formation of EA rosettes. Receptors for the C3 component of complement were also monitored by erythrocyte–antibody–complement (EAC) rosetting. Koller *et al.* (1977) found that the addition of 13 μg/ml Pb in the drinking water of mice for 18 months resulted in a slight elevation of both EA and EAC rosetting. Lead at 1300 μg/ml slightly suppressed the two rosetting responses. Since no significant changes in rosetting ability were noted, it has been concluded lead, even at a very high level for an extended period of time, does not change the membrane receptors for these two important immunological signals.

Two additional studies focused on the *in vitro* and *in vivo* effects of elevated zinc levels on macrophage and PMN responses. Chvapil (1976) found that O_2 consumption *in vitro* was markedly reduced in activated macrophages from rats by the addition of 0.4 mM zinc to cultures. Changes in macrophage shape were also noted with the addition of 0.1 and 0.5 mM zinc. The rounding up of the cells was reversible and directly related to the uptake and release of zinc by the macrophages. *In vitro* and *in vivo* effects of zinc on PMN were reported by Mapes *et al.* (1979). Very high levels of zinc in culture (2.0 mM) completely inhibited prostaglandin synthesis in PMN. There was also an inhibition of the production of endogenous pyrogen by macrophages, which has recently been equated with interleukin-1 (Flynn *et al.*, 1982). *In vivo* dietary zinc increases PMN and macrophage function. Rabbit febrile responses to endogenous pyrogen and theophylline were markedly altered by single injections of $ZnCl_2$ 1 hr before mediator or theophylline injection (Mapes *et al.*, 1979). Instead of the recognized monophasic response, the fever response was continuous during the 2 hr monitoring period with no diminution of fever with time.

One other report relating to macrophage function deals with macrophage migration inhibitory factor (MIF) in workers exposed to beryllium (Price *et al.*, 1977). Those workers who have developed responses to beryllium were shown to have significantly depressed MIF indices. The T-cell-produced factor, which is responsible for "holding" macrophages at the inflammatory site, appears to be either produced in lesser amounts or the macrophages do not have receptors for the factor.

3.2. LYMPHOCYTES AND THEIR ACTIVITIES IN RELATION TO TRACE ELEMENTS

3.2.1. B-Lymphocyte Responses and Trace Elements

The B-lymphocyte responses that have been reported to be associated with trace elements are (1) changes in immunoglobulin synthesis (or number of immunoglobulin-producing cells) and (2) cellular proliferation or cell number in response to B-cell mitogen or trace element deficiency/excess. The production of immunoglobulins is the most widely measured parameter of B-cell or humoral response and both stimulation and suppression of immunoglobulin synthesis are noted. Resnick *et al.* (1970) reported an altered immunoglobulin synthesis in human populations exposed to beryllium. In subjects with short-term beryllium exposure, IgG was slightly depressed. Chronic exposure and evidence of beryllium-related dermatitis, however, was related to hypergammaglobulinemia. Other long-term beryllium-exposed workers without any signs of beryllium toxicity also had increased IgG levels. In a clinical study on lead-exposed children with metabolic impairment, immunoglobulin levels and an anamnestic response to tetanus toxoid antigen were normal when compared with age-matched control children (Reigart and Graber, 1976).

Studies of antibody production against specific antigens in animals have demonstrated variable responses of toxic trace elements, with the majority of reports showing suppression of antibody synthesis. Two studies have focused on the effects of single-dose effects of cadmium and lead on immunoglobulin production. Koller *et al.* (1976) inoculated mice i.p. with either 4 mg lead or 0.15 mg cadmium and then challenged the mice with SRBC. The primary response was depressed with cadmium, but only delayed with lead, whereas the secondary response was depressed with lead and delayed with cadmium. These findings are unclear as to the specific effect of cadmium and lead on antibody production, especially when they are compared with the report of Graham *et al.* (1978). Using single i.m. injections of cadmium (between 1.5 and 12.0 μg/g body wt), the number of immunoglobulin-producing cells was unchanged when the animals were challenged with SRBC. Longer-term studies using oral dosing of mice and rats with cadmium or lead show a distinct supression of antibody synthesis. Koller *et al.* (1975) reported that antibody production in mice receiving 3 or 300 ppm cadmium in their drinking water for 10 weeks was significantly depressed in both groups when challenged with SRBC in both primary and secondary responses. Koller and Kovacic (1974) reported that in mice given oral lead acetate (13.75, 137.5, and 1375 ppm in water) for 8 weeks and then inoculated with SRBC, the primary immune response was suppressed in a dose-related manner. The secondary response was significantly depressed in all treated animals. The production of IgG, the secondary immune response, was much more affected than the primary response, reflecting perhaps the amplification of the degradation of this protein-producing system. Luster *et al.* (1978) conducted a somewhat similar study in rats receiving 25 or 50 ppm lead acetate in their drinking water for 7 weeks. Looking specifically at the classes of immunoglobulin produced, they showed that IgM was affected in a dose-related manner, whereas IgG was depressed to an equal degree with both 25 and 50 ppm lead. Cadmium and lead are generally suppressive to both primary and secondary immune responses.

The effects of mercury on antibody production are not as clear as for cadmium and lead. Koller (1979) concluded that methyl mercury can decrease antibody titers in response to virus or SRBC, but increases the memory response to SRBC. Prouvost-Danon *et al.* (1981) reported that mercuric chloride can induce a striking increase in serum IgE in rats. The IgE response was nonspecific and may represent a mechanism seen with some parasitic infections. Prolonged administration of mercuric chloride (0.15 mg/100 g body wt for 27 weeks) resulted in mesangial glomerulonephropathy with IgG and IgM deposition (Makker and Aikawa, 1979). Thus, although immunoglobulin stimulation can occur, this may be linked with pathological consequences.

Two other brief reports deal with exposure to manganese and aluminum and antibody production. Inhalation of manganese produced a twofold increase in IgG, but no differences in IgA or IgM in animals challenged with streptococcal infection (Adkins *et al.*, 1980). The absorption of antigen on aluminum oxide was linked to Ige production in a similar response as noted for mercuric chloride (Vijay *et al.*, 1979).

Transformation and proliferation of B lymphocytes may also be related to trace elements and their ability to synergize with mitogens. A series of reports in 1979 highlight the effects of cadmium and lead. Gallagher *et al.* (1979) reported that cadmium and lead (10^{-7} to 10^{-3} M) were mitogenic for splenocytes. Koller *et al.* (1979) found that cadmium potentiated blastogenesis by LPS, a B-cell mitogen, whereas lead tended to inhibit B-lymphocyte proliferation by LPS. Muller *et al.* (1979) reported similar findings in mice, i.e., the synergy of cadmium and mitogen. Cadmium treatment in rats was related to marked germinal center formation containing reactive B lymphocytes (Powell *et al.*, 1979). Mercuric chloride was earlier reported to be a nonspecific stimulant of lymphocyte transformation (Caron *et al.*, 1970). Normal karyotype blast cells are induced that, when treated with tetanus toxoid antigen, synthesize DNA and divide, but do not incorporate tritiated thymidine. Cunningham-Rundles *et al.* (1980) related a more specific response of B lymphocytes to zinc. Proliferation and a positive plaque-forming cell response were related to zinc levels in the medium. The general concept, with the exception of lead's interaction with mitogens, is that trace elements in elevated levels are mitogenic for B cells and can influence antibody production.

A deficiency of trace elements may also affect the production of antibody. The essential trace element copper is inportant in immunoglobulin production. In Menke's disease, Pedroni *et al.* (1975) reported that the mitogen responsiveness of peripheral blood lymphocytes was depressed. Sullivan and Ochs (1978) found that although T- and B-lymphocyte numbers were normal and total immunoglobulin levels were similar to controls, the secondary immune response was only 7% IgG compared with 56% IgG in controls. Studies on copper-deficient mice have demonstrated an impaired humoral response (Prohaska and Lukasewycz, 1981). Subsequent studies by the same group (Lukasewycz *et al.*, 1982) indicate that the numbers of B cells are actually elevated, but the T-helper cell is significantly depressed resulting perhaps in decreased immunoglobulin production.

3.2.2. T-Lymphocyte Activities Related to Trace Elements

The effects of trace elements on T lymphocytes concern mitogen responses and variations in cellular function in transformed cells, mixed lymphocyte response, and cell-mediated lysis. Koller (1979) reviewed the effects of cadmium and lead in relation to Con A, PHA, and PWM and found either no effect or a suppression of proliferation. In proliferative studies on T lymphocytes, cadmium, lead, and methyl mercury had no significant effect on the MLR (Koller and Roan, 1980). In this study, cadmium and mercury and the lower dose of lead produced a slight but insignificant response. Balter *et al.* (1980) reported that cadmium and lead did interfere with various components of transformation. Using human peripheral blood lymphocytes, cadmium and lead, at levels between 10^{-7} and 10^{-3} M, significantly affected cell viability and DNA, RNA, and protein synthesis. Higher levels of cadmium decreased cell viability and completely inhibited DNA, RNA, and protein synthesis. Lead, on the other hand, increased DNA synthesis, and slightly inhibited RNA and protein synthesis but only in the control cell population and not in the Con A-stimula lls. Proliferation and transformation of T lymphocytes appear to be influ nly to a minor degree by trace elements.

Two interesting studies on cytotoxic T lymphocytes examined the effects of trace element toxicity and deficiency on the generation of these lymphocytes. Gately and Martz (1981) reported that manganese inhibited the calcium-dependent programming necessary for target lysis. The manganese effect can be moderated with increased calcium levels, which may relate to competition between manganese and calcium. Flynn and Yen (1981) showed that the lack of the essential elements copper and zinc could also interfere with the generation of cytotoxic T cells. In an *in vitro* system, cell-mediated lympholysis was analyzed in an alloantigen-stimulated mixed lymphocyte culture using a ^{51}Cr-release assay. Lymphocytes cultured in copper-deficient medium failed to generate cytotoxic T-cell activity, whereas zinc-deficient medium supported reduced specific lysis. This study suggests that copper- and zinc-dependent steps are involved in the generation of cytotoxic T lymphocytes. In addition, under conditions of copper and zinc deficiency, helper factors (lymphokines) were not produced by the lymphocytes.

4. CONCLUSIONS

Both excesses and deficiencies of trace elements have profound effects on the immune response. All types of leukocytes, phagocytic cells (macrophages and PMN) and lymphocytes (B and T cells), appear to be influenced by any disturbance of trace elements from the "normal" biological range. Elevated levels of essential and nonessential elements have also been associated with proliferation and then decreased viability of leukocytes. Figure 3 is a schematic summary of the major cellular systems influenced by excesses and deficiencies of trace elements.

The variety of responses seem to vary with trace element alterations appear to be inclusive of all immune systems monitored to date. Table 3 summarizes the types of responses and the general direction of the responses noted for leukocytes related to trace element excesses and deficiencies. At present, the mechanisms for the interaction of trace elements with the majority of immune systems studied are not known, but further study using *in vitro* systems may explain the nature of these interactions.

One point for consideration in the development of future studies is the relevancy of the model used for determining immunoregulatory changes to the *in vivo* setting. A number of studies have utilized levels of trace elements *in vitro* that have not been reported to occur *in vivo*. For studies to define the impact of excesses and deficiencies of trace elements on developing and mature immune systems, the model must control for the appropriate dose, chemical form, and

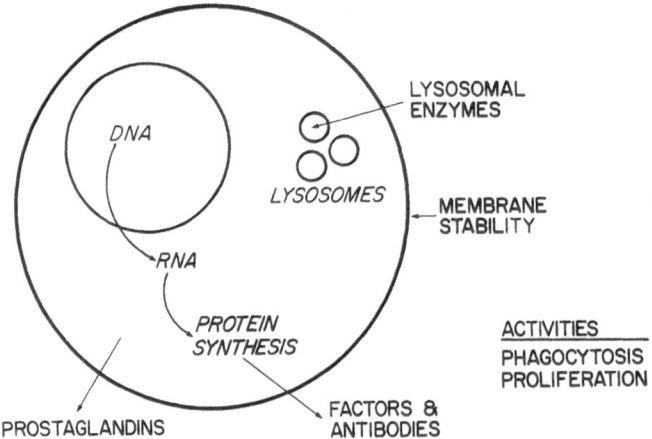

FIGURE 3. Leukocyte systems potentially affected by trace elements.

method of delivery of the element under study. A direct relationship should exist between the *in vitro* state and the physiological state with regard to the levels of trace element. *In vitro* studies appear to be the route for developing data on the cellular targets and on the biochemical mechanisms for the effects of trace elements.

Historically, the initial studies on trace elements and immunoregulation focused on the untoward effects of toxic nonessential trace elements. Only recently have studies on the effects of trace element deficiencies been reported. A combination of these studies in the future may define more clearly the important roles trace elements play in immunoregulation.

TABLE 3. GENERAL EFFECTS OF TRACE ELEMENT EXCESS AND DEFICIENCY ON PHAGOCYTIC CELLS AND LYMPHOCYTES[a]

Cell type/activity	Trace element excess	Trace element deficiency
Phagocytic cells		
Phagocytosis	↓, ↑	N.D.
Lysosomal enzymes	↑	N.D.
Prostaglandins	↑	N.D.
B lymphocytes		
Antibody synthesis	↓, ±, ↑	↓
Proliferation, mitogens	±, ↑	↓, ±
T lymphocytes		
Proliferation, mitogens	↑	↓, ±
Mixed lymphocyte response	±	±
Cytotoxic T-cell activity	↓	↓
Factor production	N.D.	↓

[a] ↓, Decreased response; ↑, increased response; ±, no change; N.D., not determined.

REFERENCES

Adkins, B., Jr., Luginbuhl, G. H., Miller, F. J., and Gardner, D. E., 1980, Increased pulmonary susceptibility to streptococcal infection following inhalation of manganese oxide, *Environ. Res.* **23**:110.

Anonymous, 1972, Lead, airborne lead, in: *National Academy of Sciences Perspective* p. 330.

Badenoch-Jones, P., 1978, Metal activation of macrophages, *Ann. Rev. R. Coll. Surgeons* **60**:211.

Badenoch-Jones, P., Turk, J. L., and Parker, D., 1978, The effects of some aluminum and zirconium compounds on guinea pig peritoneal macrophages and skin fibroblasts in culture, *J. Pathol.* **124**:51.

Bakir, F., 1973, Methylmercury poisoning in Iraq: An interuniversity report, *Science* **181**:230.

Balter, N. H., Matarazzo, W. J., Gallagher, K., Monos, D., Strasburg, S., and Gary, I., 1980, Modulation of human lymphocyte transformation by cadmium and lead, in: *Trace Substances in Environmental Health* (D. D. Hemphill, ed.), pp. 167–174, University of Missouri Press, Columbia.

Barltrop, D., Barrett, J. A., and Dingle, J. T., 1971, Subcellular distribution of lead in the rat, *J. Lab. Clin. Med.* **77**:705.

Berger, N. A., and Skinner, A. M., 1974, Characterization of lymphocyte transformation induced by zinc ions, *J. Cell Biol.* **61**:45.

Bowen, H. J. M., 1979, *Environmental Chemistry of the Elements,* Academic Press, New York.

Braude, R., Mitchell, K. G., and Pittman, R. J., 1973, A note on cuprous chloride as a feed additive for growing pigs, *Anim. Prod.* **17**:321.

Camakaris, J., Danks, M., Phillips, M., Herd, S., and Mann, J. R., 1982, Copper metabolism in Menke's syndrome and mottled mouse mutant, in: *Inflammatory Diseases and Copper* (J. R. J. Sorenson, ed.), pp. 85–96, Humana Press, Clifton, N.J.

Caron, G. A., Poutala, S., and Provost, T. T., 1970, Lymphocyte transformation induced by inorganic and organic mercury, *Int. Arch. Allergy Appl. Immunol.* **37**:76.

Chisolm, J. J., Jr., 1980, Poisoning from heavy metals (mercury, lead and cadmium), *Pediatr. Ann.* **9**:28.

Chvapil, M., 1976, Effects of zinc on cells on biomembranes, *Med. Clin. North Am.* **60**:799.

Clarkson, T. W., 1972, Recent advances in the toxicology of mercury with emphasis on alkylmercurials. *CRC Crit. Rev. Toxicol.* **1**:203.

Cunningham-Rundles, S., Cunningham-Rundles, C., Dupont, B., and Good, R. A., 1980, Zinc induced activation of human B lymphocytes, *Clin. Immunol. Immunopathol.* **16**:115.

Davies, N. T., 1974, Recent studies of antagonistic interactions in the aetiology of trace element deficiency and excess, *Proc. Nutr. Soc.* **33**:293.

Debold, H. J., and Elvehjem, C. A., 1953, The effect of feeding high amounts of soluble iron and aluminum salts, *Am. J. Physiol.* **111**:118.

Evans, G. W., 1973, Copper homeostasis in the mammalian system, *Physiol. Rev.* **53**:535.

Fernandes, G., Nair, M., Onone, K., Tanada, T., Floyd, R., and Good, R. A., 1979, Impairment of cell-mediated immunity functions by dietary zinc deficiency in mice, *Proc. Natl. Acad. Sci. USA* **76**:457.

Flink, E. B., 1971, Heavy metal poisoning, in: *Cecil–Loeb Textbook of Medicine* (C. B. Beeson and W. McDermott, eds.), 13th ed., p. 63, Saunders, Philadelphia.

Flynn, A., and Yen, B. R., 1981, Mineral deficiency effects on the generation of cytotoxic T-cells and T-helper cell factors in vitro, *J. Nutr.* **111**:907.

Flynn, A., Finke, J. H., and Hilfiker, M. L., 1982, Placental mononuclear phagocytes as a source of interleukin-1, *Science* **218**:475.

Fox, M. R., 1976, Protective effects of ascorbic acid against toxicity of heavy metals, *Ann. N.Y. Acad. Sci.* **258**:144.

Fraker, P. H., Hass, S. M., and Leucke, R. W., 1977, Effects of zinc deficiency on the immune response of the young adult A/J mouse, *J. Nutr.* **107**:1889.

Friberg, L., Piscator, M., Nordberg, G. F., and Kjellstrom, T., 1974, *Cadmium in the Environment,* 2nd ed., CRC Press, Cleveland, Ohio.

Frieden, E., 1978, Modes of metal metabolism in mammals, in: *Trace Element Metabolism in Animals* (M. Kirchgessner, ed.), pp. 8–14, ATW Freising-Weihenstephan.

Frieden, E., 1980, Ceruloplasmin: A multi-functional metalloprotein of vertebrate plasma, in: *Roles of Copper* (R. G. Feldman, R. R. Young, and W. P. Koella, eds.), pp. 93–124, Excerpta Medica, Amsterdam.

Frommer, D. J., 1974, Defective biliary excretion of copper in Wilson's disease, *Gut* **15**:125.

Gallagher, K., Matarazzo, W. J., and Gray, I., 1979, Trace metal modification of immunocompetence. II. Effect of Pb, Cd and Cr on RNA turnover, hemoxolkinase and blastogenesis during B lymphocyte transformation in vitro, *Clin. Immunol. Immunopathol.* **13**:369.

Gately, M. K., and Martz, E., 1981, Early steps in specific tumor cell lysis by sensitized mouse T lymphocytes. V. Evidence that manganese inhibits a calcium dependent step in programming lysis, *Cell. Immunol.* **61**:78.

Graham, J. A., Gardner, D. E., Waters, M. D., and Coffin, D. L., 1975, Effect of trace metals on phagocytosis by alveolar macrophages, *Infect. Immun.* **11**:1278.

Graham, J. A., Miller, F. J., Daniels, M. J., Payne, E. A., and Gardner, D. E., 1978, Influence of cadmium, nickel and chromium on primary immunity in mice, *Environ. Res.* **16**:77.

Gross, R. L., Osdin, N., Fong, L., and Newberne, P. M., 1979, Depressed immunological function in zinc deprived rats as measured by mitogen response of spleen, thymus and peripheral blood, *Am. J. Clin. Nutr.* **32**:1260.

Gunn, S. A., Gould, T. C., and Anderson, W. A. D., 1963, The selective injurious response of testicular and epididymal blood vessels to cadmium and its prevention by zinc, *Am. J. Pathol.* **42**:685.

Halsted, J. A., Smith, J. C., Jr., Irwin, M. J., 1974, A conspectus of research on zinc requirements of man, *J. Nutr.* **104**:345.

Hart, B. A., 1978, Transport of cadmium by the alveolar macrophage, *J. Reticuloendothel. Soc.* **24**:363.

Hart, E. B., Steenbock, H., Waddell, J., and Elvehjem, C. A., 1928, Iron in nutrition. VII. Copper as a supplement to iron for hemoglobin building in the rat, *J. Biol. Chem.* **77**:797.

Hemphill, F. E., Kaeberle, M. L., and Buck, W. B., 1971, Lead suppression of mouse resistance to *Salmonella typhimurium*, *Science* **172**:1031.

Hughes, M. H., 1972, *The Inorganic Chemistry of Biological Processes*, Wiley, New York.

Kang, K. Y., and Salvaggio, J., 1978, Effects of zirconium and aluminum salts on the alveolar macrophages, *Tohoku J. Exp. Med.* **126**:317.

Kang, K. Y., Bice, D., D'Amato, A., Ziskind, N., and Salvaggio, J., 1979, Effects of asbestos and beryllium on release of alveolar macrophage enzymes, *Arch. Environ. Health* **34**:133.

Katz, D. H., 1979, Adaptive differentiation of murine lymphocytes: Implications of mechanisms of cell–cell recognition and the regulation of immune responses, *Fed. Proc.* **38**:2065.

Kirchner, H., and Ruhl, H., 1970, Stimulation of human peripheral lymphocytes by Zn^{2+} in vitro, *Exp. Cell Res.* **61**:229.

Koller, L. D., 1979, Some immunological effects of lead, cadmium and methylmercury, *Drug Chem. Toxicol.* **2**:99.

Koller, L. D., and Kovacic, S., 1974, Decreased antibody formation in mice exposed to lead, *Nature (London)* **150**:148.

Koller, L. D., and Roan, J. G., 1977, Effects of lead and cadmium on mouse peritoneal macrophages, *J. Reticuloendothel. Soc.* **21**:7.

Koller, L. D., and Roan, J. G., 1980, Response of lymphocytes from lead, cadmium and methylmercury exposed mice in the mixed lymphocyte culture, *J. Environ. Pathol. Toxicol.* **4**:393.

Koller, L. D., Exon, J. H., and Roan, J. G., 1976, Humoral antibody response in mice after single dose exposure to lead or cadmium, *Proc. Soc. Exp. Biol. Med.* **151**:339.

Koller, L. D., Exon, J. H., and Roan, J. G., 1975, Antibody suppression by cadmium, *Arch. Environ. Health* **30**:598.

Koller, L. D., Roan, J. G., Brauner, J. A., and Exon, J. H., 1977, Immune response in aged mice exposed to lead, *J. Toxicol. Environ. Health* **3**:535.

Koller, L. D., Roan, J. G., and Kerkvliet, N. I., 1979, Mitogen stimulation of lymphocytes in CBA mice exposed to lead and cadmium, *Environ. Res.* **19**:177.

Lafferty, K. J., Andrus, L., and Prowse, S. J., 1980, Role of lymphokine and antigen in the control of specific T-cell response, *Immunol. Rev.* **51**:279.

Leach, R. M., Jr., 1976, Metabolism and function of manganese, in: *Trace Elements in Human Health and Disease II* (A. S. Prasad, ed.), pp. 235–247, Academic Press, New York.

Lewis, G. P., Jusko, W. J., and Coughlin, H., 1972, Cadmium accumulation in men: Influence of smoking, occupation, alcoholic habit and disease, *J. Chronic Dis.* **25**:717.

Lieben, J., and Williams, R. R., 1969, Respiratory disease associated with beryllium refining and alloy fabrication, . *J. Occup. Med.* **11**:480.

Loose, L. D., Silkworth, J. B., and Warrington, D., 1977, Cadmium induced depression of the respiratory burst in mouse pulmonary macrophages, peritoneal macrophages and poly-morphonuclear neutrophils, *Biochem. Biophys. Res. Commun.* **79**:326.

Loose, L. D., Silkworth, J. B., and Simpson, D. W., 1978, Influence of cadmium on the phagocytic and microbicial activity of murine peritoneal macrophages, pulmonary alveolar macrophages and polymorphonuclear neutrophils, *Infect. Immun.* **22**:378.

Lukasewycz, O. A., Prohaska, J. R., Schmidtke, J. R., Hatfield, S. M., Marder, P., and Meyer, S. B., 1982, Alterations in lymphoid subpopulations and mitogen reactivity in copper deficient mice, *Fed. Proc.* **41**:341.

Luster, M. I., Faith, R. E., and Kimmel, C. A., 1978, Depression of humoral immunity in rats following chronic developmental lead exposure, *J. Environ. Pathol. Toxicol.* **1**:397.

McLaughlin, S. G. A., Szabo, G., and Eisenman, G., 1971, Divalent ions and surface potential of charged phospholipid membranes, *J. Gen. Physiol.* **58**:667.

Makker, S. P., and Aikawa, M., 1979, Mesangial glomerulonephropathy with deposition of IgG, IgM and C3 induced by mercuric chloride, *Lab. Invest.* **41**:45.

Mapes, C. A., Bailey, P. T., Matson, C. F., Hauer, E. C., and Sobocinski, P. Z., 1978, *In vitro* and *in vivo* actions of zinc ion affecting cellular substances which influence host metabolic responses to inflammation, *J. Cell Physiol.* **95**:115.

Matrone, G., 1974, Chemical parameters in trace element antagonisms, in: *Trace Element Metabolism in Animals II* (W. G. Hoekstra, J. W. Suttie, H. E. Ganther, and W. Mertz, eds.), pp. 91–104, University Park Press, Baltimore.

Matrone, G., Harman, R. H., and Clawson, A. J., 1959, Studies of manganese iron antagonism in the nutrition of rabbits and baby pigs, *J. Nutr.* **67**:309.

Muller, S., Gillert, K. E., Krause, C., Jautzke, G., Gross, U., and Diamantstein, T., 1979, Effects of cadmium on the immune system of mice, *Experientia* **35**:909.

Needleman, H. L., Gunnoe, C., Leviton, A., Reed, R., Peresie, H., Mober, C., and Barrett, P., 1979, Psychological performance of children with elevated lead levels, *N. Engl. J. Med.* **300**:689.

Nielsen, F. H., 1974, Essentiality and function of nickel, in: *Trace Element Metabolism in Animals II* (W. G. Hoekstra, J. W. Suttie, H. E. Ganther, and W. Mertz, eds.), pp. 381–396, University Park Press, Baltimore.

North American Contact Dermatitis Group, 1973, Epidemiology of contact dermatitis in North America (1972), *Arch. Dermatol.* **108**:537.

North, B. B., Leichseuring, J. M., and Voris, L. M., 1960, Manganese metabolism in college women, *J. Nutr.* **72**:217.

Parizek, J., 1964, Vascular changes at sites of oestrogen biosynthesis produced by parenteral injections of cadmium salts: The destruction of placenta by cadmium salts, *J. Reprod. Fertil.* **7**:263.

Parizek, J., and Zahor, Z., 1956, Effect of cadmium salts on testicular tissue, *Nature (London)* **177**:1036.

Pedroni, E., Bianchi, E., Ugazio, A. G., and Burgio, G. R., 1975, Immunodeficiency and steely hair, *Lancet* **1**:1303.

Perry, H. M., Jr., 1968, Hypertension and trace metals, particularly cadmium, in: *Trace Elements in Environmental Health II* (D. D. Hemphill, ed.), pp. 101–125, University of Missouri Press, Columbia.

Powell, A. L., Joshi, B., Dwivedi, C., and Green, L., 1979, Immunopathological changes in cadmium treated rats, *Vet. Pathol.* **16**:116.

Price, C. D., Williams, W. J., Pugh, A., and Joynson, D. H., 1977, Role of in vitro and in vivo tests of hypersensitivity in beryllium workers, *J. Clin. Pathol.* **30**:24.

Prohaska, J. R., and Lukasewycz, O. A., 1981, Copper deficiency suppresses the immune response of mice, *Science* **213**:559.

Prourost-Danon, A., Abadie, A., Sapin, C., Bazin, H., and Druet, P., 1981, Induction of IgE synthesis and potentiation of anti-ovalbumin IgE antibody response by $HgCl_2$ in the rat, *J. Immunol.* **126**:699.

Reeves, A. L., 1976, Berylliosis as an autoimmune disorder, *Ann. Clin. Lab. Sci.* **6**:256.

Reigart, J. R., and Graber, C. D., 1976, Evaluation of the humoral immune response of children with low level lead exposure, *Bull. Environ. Contam. Toxicol.* **16**:112.

Resnick, H., Roche, M., and Morgan, W. K. C., 1970, Immunoglobulin concentrations in berylliosis, *Am. Rev. Respir. Dis.* **101**:504.

Sandstead, H. H., 1973, Zinc nutrition in the United States, *Am. J. Clin. Nutr.* **26**:1251.

Sandstead, H. H., and Rinaldi, R. S., 1969, Impairment of deoxyribonucleic acid synthesis by dietary zinc deficiency in the rat, *J. Cell. Physiol.* **73**:81.

Schroeder, H. A., 1965, Cadmium as a factor in hypertension, *J. Chronic Dis.* **18**:647.

Schroeder, H. A., and Mitchener, M., 1975, Life-term studies in rats: Effects of aluminum, barium, beryllium and tungsten, *J. Nutr.* **105**:421.

Schroeder, H. A., and Vinton, W. H., Jr., 1962, Hypertension induced in rats by small doses of cadmium, *Am. J. Physiol.* **202**:515.

Schwartz, K., 1974, New essential trace elements (Su, V, F, Si): Progress report and outlook, in: *Trace Element Metabolism in Animals II* (W. G. Hoekstra, J. W. Suttie, H. E. Ganther, and W. Mertz, eds.), pp. 355–380, University Park Press, Baltimore.

Smith, D. W., and Williams, R. J. P., 1970, *Structure and Bonding*, Volume 7, Springer-Verlag, Berlin.

Smith, K. A., 1980, T-cell growth factor, *Immunol. Rev.* **51**:337.

Smith, P. F., 1962, Animal intake of essential elements for various dietary sources, *Annu. Rev. Plant Physiol.* **13**:81.

Smith, T. J., Temple, A. R., and Reading, J. C., 1976, Cadmium, lead and copper blood levels in normal children, *Clin. Toxicol.* **9**:75.

Smith, W. E., and Smith, A. M., 1975, *Minamata*, Holt, Rinehart & Winston, New York.

Sorenson, J. R. J., Campbell, I. R., Tepper, L. B., and Lingg, R. D., 1974, Aluminum in the environment and human health, *Environ. Health Perspect.* **8**:3.

Steitz, T. A., Wiley, D. C., and Lipscomb, W. N., 1967, The structure of aspartate transcarbamylase. I. A molecular twofold axis in the complex with cytidine triphosphate, *Proc. Natl. Acad. Sci. USA* **64**:1859.

Sternlieb, I., 1982, Wilson's disease, in: *Inflammatory Diseases and Copper* (J. R. J. Sorenson, ed.), pp. 75–84, Humana Press, Clifton, N.J.

Sullivan, J. L., and Ochs, H. D., 1978, Copper deficiency and the immune system, *Lancet* **2**:686.

Underwood, E. J., 1977, *Trace Elements in Human and Animal Nutrition*, 4th ed., Academic Press, New York.

Utter, M. F., 1976, Biochemistry of manganese, *Med. Clin. North Am.* **60**:713.

Vallee, B. L., Riordan, J. F., Johansen, J. T., and Livingston, D. M., 1971, Spectro-chemical probes for protein conformation and function, *Cold Spring Harbor Symp. Quant. Biol.* **36**:517.

Spivey-Fox, M. R., 1978, Nutritional considerations in designing animal models of metal toxicity in man, *Environ. Health Physiol.* **25**:137.

Vijay, H. M., Lavergne, G., Huang, H., and Bernstein, I. L., 1979, Preferential synthesis of IgE reaginic antibodies in rats immunized with alum-absorbed antigens, *Int. Arch. Allergy Appl. Immunol.* **59**:227.

Williams, H., 1933, Lead poisoning from the burning of battery casings, *Am. Med. Assoc.* **100**:1485.

Witham, I. J., 1963, Depression of cytochrome oxidase activities in livers of zinc intoxicated rats, *Biochim. Biophys. Acta* **73**:509.

Wood, J. M., 1974, Biological cycles for toxic elements in the environment, *Science* **183**:1049.

Wu, S., Bach, F. H., and Auerbach, R., 1975, Cell-mediated immunity: Differential maturation of mixed lymphocyte reaction and cell-mediated lympholysis, *J. Exp. Med.* **142**:1301.

16

Drug Abuse
Effects on the Reticuloendothelial and Immune Systems

STANLEY S. LEFKOWITZ

1. INTRODUCTION

1.1. IMMUNOSUPPRESSION

Numerous references can be found in the literature concerning drugs that have immunosuppressive properties. Some of these substances are frequently abused, and have significant effects on bodily functions. There is an increased frequency of certain types of infections associated with the use and abuse of these drugs. It follows that the action of these substances could be through their effects on the immune system. Before attempting to discuss the drugs and substances that have immunosuppressive properties and are frequently abused, it is necessary to define what is meant by immunosuppressive. The latter can be defined as "substances depressing immune responses." This definition has considerable merit because of its simplicity. However, one problem with measuring immunosuppression is that there are various "arms" of the immune system, and immunosuppressive agents may suppress one or more types of immune reactions. It may be more correct to define immunosuppressive as any substance that inhibits at least one type of immune response.

Measurement of immunocompetence and/or immunosuppression can be done by a number of simple tests (Bach, 1975). These include (1) measurements of serum immunoglobulins and/or specific antibodies to naturally occurring antigens, (2) measurement of responses to immunization with new or "novel" antigens, (3) assessing circulating lymphocyte numbers or determining percentages of B, T, or null cells, (4) determining delayed hypersensitivity (a) using skin test antigens such as mumps, *Candida albicans*, etc., or (b) to other antigens to

STANLEY S. LEFKOWITZ • Department of Microbiology, Texas Tech University Health Science Center, Lubbock, Texas 79430.

which the host has not been previously sensitized, such as dinitrochlorobenzene (DNCB), (5) determining the ability of lymphocytes to respond to various mitogens *in vitro*, and (6) measurements of lymphokines produced after appropriate stimulation, etc.

At this point it is appropriate to consider various *in vitro* tests of lymphoid function, such as lymphocyte transformation, which measures the proliferative capacity of T and/or B cells. *In vitro* data obtained using these types of tests are interesting since they provide information on activity of lymphoid cells independent of their *in vivo* metabolism. However, there are a number of pitfalls with this approach since *in vitro* data do not necessarily correspond with *in vivo* activity. Furthermore, many products may only be active *in vivo*, needing some type of metabolic alteration or transformation. It is·also conceivable that many products may not act at a stage of the immune response that can be measured by an *in vitro* response, even using relatively complex immune reactions, such as the Mishell–Dutton (1967) technique, etc. Other substances may be immunosuppressive *in vitro* at nontoxic levels, but the active metabolite does not reach a sufficient serum level *in vivo* to have a significant effect. These types of approaches tend to make comparisons of immunosuppressive activity difficult between *in vivo* and *in vitro* responses.

In spite of the limitations of various methodologies to assess immunosuppression, as well as the combination of a number of factors that affect selected immune responses, a number of generalizations can be made relative to the effects of drugs on immunity: (1) A primary immune response is more readily inhibited than a secondary response. (2) The stages of the immune response differ in their susceptibility to drugs. Most immunosuppressive agents are effective if used immediately prior to antigen exposure during the "induction phase." They are much less effective once the immune reaction has entered the established phase. (3) Immunosuppressive substances frequently exert a differential toxicity for T or B lymphocytes, which would tend to affect either the cellular or the humoral arm of the immune system. (4) Under rare circumstances, augmentation of a particular immune response may occur. This augmentation may result from interference with, or toxicity to, suppressor lymphocytes. (5) Ability to inhibit the immune response may result from activities of nonspecific effectors, such as certain types of inflammatory cells that would be present at a site of infection. The numbers and functions of these effectors are not well understood.

1.2. DRUG ABUSE

Throughout history every society has relied on various drugs that produce effects on mood or feelings. There are always individuals who deviate from the "established" custom with respect to the amount, the time, or the circumstances in which these drugs were used. The term *drug abuse* refers to the self-administration of any substance in a manner that deviates from the approved social or medical patterns within a given society. Therefore, what would be acceptable drug use in a given society might be construed as drug abuse in another. Most abused drugs have their primary action on the central nervous system.

There are a number of patterns of drug abuse. Drugs may be used experimentally where the individual may ultimately reject its use. A second pattern is the social use of drugs, the most common examples of which are alcohol and cigarettes. Another pattern is the episodic abuse that occurs when a person abuses a drug for short periods of time. The most detrimental situation occurs with the compulsive abuser. A number of individuals have experimented with one drug or another and have reached a stage where they require and/or become dependent on a given drug either physiologically, psychologically, or both. It should be noted that there is a difference between drug abuse and drug dependence, since both of these states can exist independently.

There are a number of different ways to characterize and/or subdivide the various commonly abused drugs in our society. No attempts will be made to include all classes of substances that are abused, nor all types within a given class, but only to give the reader information on some of the major categories of abused drugs, along with an appreciation of their effects on immune parameters both in man and in animals. For a number of drugs, there are not sufficient data to include them in this review. The classes of drugs to be discussed in this review are as follows:

1. Narcotics (opiates): These include heroin, morphine, and other alkaloids that have a strong potential for compulsive abuse. In addition, synthetic compounds, such as methadone, are also considered in this class.
2. Major sympathetic stimulants: These include diet pills such as the amphetamines and methamphetamines. These drugs were prescribed originally some years ago as anorectic agents and are characterized as "speed." A "new" drug for the affluent is cocaine. It is generally inhaled or sniffed and is one of the strongest naturally occurring stimulants.
3. The minor stimulants (caffeine, tobacco): These include those socially acceptable minor stimulants that affect the nervous system, such as nicotine in cigarettes and caffeine in coffee. They will be discussed here even though they are socially acceptable drugs, since they have the potential for abuse, as well as a number of effects on biological systems.
4. The sedative hypnotic drugs: Probably the most important of these is alcohol, which is likely the most widely abused drug available. In addition to alcohol, other drugs included in this category are the barbiturates, methaqualone, meprobamate (Librium), and other sedatives.
5. Marijuana (cannabis): Marijuana is basically a sedative, but is frequently classified separately from other drugs having this effect. The most active ingredient is Δ^9-tetrahydrocannabinol (THC), which affects both the physiology and the behavior of users.
6. Hallucinogens: This group of compounds also fits under the category of sedative hypnotic drugs and are also termed psychedelic or psychotomimetic substances. These have very dramatic effects on perceptions, thoughts, and feelings. Representative drugs are lysergic acid diethylamide (LSD), mescaline, phencyclidine hydrochloride (PCP), etc.

Interest in the immunosuppressive activities of many of these abused drugs probably extends from recognition of the infectious complications of frequent drug abuse. This phenomenon was recognized in the 1960s when a number of infections were attributed to the use and abuse of certain drugs, particularly those administered parenterally. It follows that these substances may lower the host resistance to various infectious agents through their effects on the immune system. It is primarily to this area that this review is directed.

2. CLASSES OF ABUSED DRUGS

2.1. THE OPIATES (NARCOTICS)

The opiates or narcotics include the natural psychotropic alkaloids of the opium poppy, a number of semisynthetic derivatives, and some entirely synthetic compounds. Morphine is a naturally occurring alkaloid of the poppy plant. Heroin is an acetyl derivative of morphine. Methadone, which is used to treat addiction to the narcotics, is an entirely synthetic preparation.

There are numerous indications that these substances may affect host immunity. One effect of these substances is directly on lymphoid cell populations. It has been shown that there is atrophy of lymphoid germinal centers in mice injected with morphine (Lefkowitz and Chiang, 1975a). This could be mediated through a morphine-induced stress reaction (Munson, 1974). During the stress reaction, hypothalamic–pituitary function is altered. The stressing substance induces several reactions directly via the hypothalamus, which affect the physiological state of the organism. ACTH released from the pituitary gland initiates the secretion of corticosteroids from the adrenal cortex. Corticosteroids cause extensive destruction of small lymphocytes in mice. McDonough et al. (1980) have reported that opiate addiction results in a depression of the absolute number of T lymphocytes. Associated with this decrease is an increase in null cells with no effect on B-cell numbers.

Morphine has a number of other effects, including an induction of hypothermia. This has a number of significant effects on various physiological processes. At the cellular level, morphine is capable of inhibiting protein synthesis. Some of these effects were discussed by Hung et al. (1973).

A number of studies have been conducted on the medical sequelae, as well as the epidemiology of death from opioid addiction (Louria et al., 1967; Cherubin et al., 1972, Wetli et al., 1972). Addiction to narcotics is associated with extremely high mortality rates (Abelson, 1970; Cushman, 1978). It is estimated that perhaps as many as 1% of all addicts may die any given year. Many of these hazards result from the life-styles adapted by the addict rather than directly from the abused drug. Part of the problem may be caused by other drugs, alcoholism, violence, and, to a lesser extent, infectious diseases. Among the more frequent medical complications of heroin addicts is bacterial endocarditis (Banks et al., 1973; Curtis et al., 1974; Reiner et al., 1976; El-Khatib et al., 1976). In addition to increased frequencies of systemic infections, such as endocarditis, tetanus, etc., there are a number of other infections including abscesses, cellulitis, infections involving bone, muscle, joint, central nervous system, etc. (Cherubin, 1971;

Lewis, 1973; Goldin *et al.*, 1973; Light and Dunham, 1974; Louria, 1974; Lewis *et al.*, 1975).

Probably the disease most frequently associated as an epidemiological marker in the incidence of opiate abuse is hepatitis B. It is frequently found among those whose opiate abuses are of relatively recent onset. The association, therefore, of this disease with heroin use, as well as other types of "mainlining," has been adequately documented (Cherubin *et al.*, 1970; Rutherdale *et al.*, 1972; Nathenson *et al.*, 1974; Blanck *et al.*, 1979; Miller *et al.*, 1979).

In addition to the large numbers of infectious diseases associated with opiate abuse, there are also a number of abnormalities in immunoglobulin levels. The presence of abnormally high levels of IgM has been reported by a number of investigators (Nickerson *et al.*, 1970; Grieco and Chuang, 1973; Cushman, 1974; Brown *et al.*, 1974; Blanck *et al.*, 1980; Matsuyama *et al.*, 1980). A number of these investigators also reported other abnormalities in the immunoglobulin system including significant elevations of both IgA and IgG over nonusers. Treatment of heroin addicts with methadone could also contribute to abnormal immunoglobulin levels.

In addition to elevated immunoglobulins, there is evidence for an autoimmune component in heavy users. Narcotic abuse is associated with an increase in the rheumatoid factor (Spiera *et al.*, 1974), as well as antibody to smooth muscle (Husby *et al.*, 1975). The high incidence of various precipitins to certain microorganisms also may simply indicate the injection of various types of antigenic foreign microorganisms intravenously with subsequent antibody formation (Smith *et al.*, 1975). Direct effects of the narcotics on cell-mediated immunity are limited. Hung *et al.* (1973) demonstrated that narcotics inhibit production of interferon in mice. In a study of the effect of morphine addiction on Con A-stimulated blastogenesis in mice, Ho and Leung (1979) reported a decreased response in addicted mice, which could be reversed by naloxone. Güngör *et al.* (1980) reported that morphine exerted a dose-dependent inhibitory effect on the immune responses of mice, which was antagonized by naloxone. This suggested to the authors that the inhibitory effect of morphine was specific and possibly mediated by receptors. A review by Cushman (1980) has summarized the major medical sequelae of opioid addiction.

Methadone, a synthetic drug very similar to heroin, is the treatment of choice of the heroin addict. The use of this substance is not without medical complications (Kreek, 1978). Many of these complications may be due to concurrent drug abuse, particularly alcohol. However, it has been reported that there are abnormal percentages of rosette-forming cells in methadone patients (Cushman *et al.*, 1977). This indicates that there are alterations in the percentage of peripheral lymphocytes, particularly those with cell surface complement receptors, in methadone-treated narcotic addicts. Studies in mice have also indicated possible immunosuppressive effects of methadone (Nemeth-Lefkowitz *et al.*, 1980).

The direct and indirect effects of opiates on the immune system are multifactorial. In certain instances there is a direct injection of various infectious materials parenterally along with certain abused drugs. Yet it is also clear that the nonparenteral abuse of these substances also could affect many of the homeostatic mechanisms capable of regulating immunity and the immune response. The high frequencies of immunological disorders and diseases associated with these classes of substances are probably both direct and indirect consequences of opiate abuse.

2.2. THE MINOR STIMULANTS (TOBACCO AND CAFFEINE)

No discussion would be complete without some mention of the effects of tobacco and nicotine on the immune system. The consumption of cigarettes in the 1960s was more than 600 billion per year. The rate of increase has slowed down somewhat since then, but has not been reversed, despite the report by the Surgeon General of the association of cigarettes and lung cancer. In 1978 approximately 38% of the adult population of the United States were smokers (Jaffe, 1980).

About 4000 compounds are generated by the burning of tobacco. Smoke obtained from this source can be separated into a gaseous and a particulate phase. Of the compounds generated by smoking, two of the most important are nicotine and tar, both of which are present in the particulate phase. However, a number of gaseous compounds are also produced, including carbon monoxide, carbon dioxide, nitrogen oxide, nitrosamines, etc. (Jaffe, 1980). Because of the legion of compounds associated with smoke, it is not surprising that certain of these would have a detrimental effect on the immune system.

A number of studies have shown that immune responses of cigarette smokers (Finklea et al., 1971) and mice chronically exposed to fresh cigarette smoke (Thomas et al., 1974a,b,c) were impaired. Using the plaque-forming cell (PFC) response of the mouse as a measure of immunity, these investigators administered sheep erythrocytes either intravenously or intratracheally. They noted a progressive impairment of responses over the entire exposure period. This was evident using immune cells taken from blood, lymph nodes, and lung, all of which had a reduced ability to form plaques. More recently, Herscowitz and Cooper (1979) have shown that there is an effect of cigarette smoke on the maturation of the antibody response in spleens from newborn mice. These investigators showed that there was no effect on the PFC response of smoke-exposed animals immunized with sheep erythrocytes up to day 9 postpartum. However, by day 10 there was a statistically significant reduction in the number of splenic PFC. By 4 to 10 weeks, there was essentially a 90% reduction in the numbers of PFC. It was suggested that this inhibitory effect may be at the level of the macrophage or thymus-derived lymphocyte. Jacob et al. (1980) reported that there was an absolute decrease of T lymphocytes in spleens of mice exposed to water-soluble condensates of tobacco smoke. Furthermore, these T cells were unable to cooperate with B cells and macrophages. These authors noted a lesser suppression of B-cell activity.

A number of studies have indicated a direct effect of cigarette smoke on the macrophage. Some investigators reported that the phagocytosis of viable staphylococci and other inert particles was minimally, but consistently, depressed in rat lung macrophages (Drath *et al.*, 1979a); however, others (Demoulin and Demoulin-Brahy, 1979) suggested that the phagocytic properties of macrophages were not altered in lung washings from animals exposed to smoke, but rather the "germicidal" activity of the macrophages was reduced. A number of morphological changes of alveolar macrophages have been reported following exposure to tobacco smoke *in vitro*. These changes include decreased glass adherence, vacuolization of cytoplasm, alteration of phagocytic and germicidal activities, changes in oxidative metabolism, etc. (Ketkar *et al.*, 1977; Davies *et al.*, 1978; Drath *et al.*, 1978, 1979b; Lewis *et al.*, 1979). Changes in polymorphonuclear leukocyte function have also been reported (Corberand *et al.*, 1980). A review on the effects of tobacco smoke on alterations of lung structure and function has recently been published (Huber *et al.*, 1981).

In addition to effects on T and B lymphocytes, NK cell activity is also affected by smoking (Ferson *et al.*, 1979). It was shown that NK activity of blood leukocytes in smokers was significantly lower than that of nonsmokers. However, no differences in the percentages of T cells (rosettes) were detected.

In addition to effects on immune cells, a number of investigators have shown major alterations in immunoglobulin production. Some recent reports indicate that IgG, IgM, and IgA levels were significantly lower in smokers (Jedrychowski, 1978; Gerrard *et al.*, 1980). These results suggest that smoking also affects the B-cell system and its products. However, it is not known at what level the specific lesions occur. Another study indicated that there is an effect of cigarette smoke on the specificity of the secondary immune response. Mackenzie and Flower (1979) noted that in mice exposed to influenza virus, the secondary immune response was normal but was less specific than that elicited by the control mice. This suggests a qualitative, as well as a quantitative, effect on the immune system. Changes in splenic architecture associated with tobacco smoke also suggest major effects on the immune system (Ayre *et al.*, 1981).

Whatever the basic mechanism, it is clear that there is a relationship between cigarette smoking and a number of major diseases. The substances isolated from cigarette smoke contain a number of potentially dangerous substances that could have deleterious effects on the immune system. Human lymphocytes exposed to small quantities of tobacco smoke condensate have been reported to develop a number of DNA lesions that result in sister chromatid exchanges (Hopkin and Evans, 1979). It is clear that effects of cigarette smoke could be both direct and indirect through a number of products generated by metabolizing cells.

Excessive drinking of coffee frequently occurs in our society. The substance usually associated with the negative effects of coffee is caffeine. Using the estimate of approximately 80–120 mg of caffeine per cup of coffee, it is apparent that many heavy drinkers may imbibe large amounts of caffeine each day. There are a number of medical complications associated with so-called "caffeinism." Its use has been associated with insomnia, irritability, palpitations, weight loss, upset stomach, peptic ulcers, etc.

Caffeine has been shown to depress protein synthesis, as well as inhibit the primary immune response in mice (Laux and Klesius, 1973; Lefkowitz and Chiang, 1975a). At the present time the effect of caffeine on immunity in man is not known; however, there are some data regarding the effects of caffeine on human peripheral lymphocytes. A number of investigators have shown that caffeine inhibits both pre- and postreplication repair of DNA lesions in human lymphocytes (Ishi and Bender, 1978; Okoyama and Kitao, 1981). The significance of these reports relative to the immune response awaits further investigation.

It would be unfair to leave discussion of coffee and caffeine without alluding to the possibility that many other very commonly used substances could have an effect on immunity. Probably one of the most frequently used drugs in our society is aspirin. It has been shown (Opelz and Terasaki, 1973; Crout *et al.*, 1975) that lymphocyte transformation is markedly inhibited after ingestion of physiological doses of aspirin. The significance of these findings raises more questions than are answerable at the present time.

2.3. THE SEDATIVE HYPNOTIC DRUGS

2.3.1. Alcohol

In our society alcohol has the dubious distinction of being the only agent producing self-induced intoxication that is completely socially acceptable. It is estimated that perhaps 65% of all adults use alcohol occasionally, and perhaps as much as 12% can be considered heavy users. If one excludes smoking, the morbidity and mortality directly and indirectly due to alcoholism indicate that this is obviously the most serious drug problem in the United States and probably in most other Western countries (Jaffe, 1980).

Excessive use of alcohol has been shown to be associated with a number of adverse hematological effects, as well as infectious complications. This alteration of susceptibility to various infectious agents can be explained, in part at least, on the direct effect of alcohol on host defenses and the immune system (Straus and Berenyi, 1973; Lundy *et al.*, 1975; Johnson, 1975; Smith and Palmer, 1976; Leevy *et al.*, 1976; Steinberg and Hillman, 1980; Smith *et al.*, 1980). Infectious diseases particularly prevalent among alcoholics are pneumonia, tuberculosis, bacterial peritonitis, bacteremia, pyelonephritis, and acute bacterial endocarditis. In addition to these types of infectious agents, a prevalence of hepatitis B virus infection has been associated with heavy alcohol drinking (Naito *et al.*, 1977). This altered immunity in patients with alcohol-induced liver disease results in an alteration of immune regulation. It has been suggested that this may be related to the development of malignancy (Mihas and Doos, 1975; Lundy *et al.*, 1975). The increase in NK cell activity shown in alcoholism (Saxena *et al.*, 1980) would not correspond to an increased susceptibility to cancer. Other reports have not shown a direct correlation between alcoholism and diminished host cell defenses (Gluckman *et al.*, 1977; Ericsson *et al.*, 1980).

A function of the immune system that may be affected by frequent consumption of alcohol is the phagocytic capacity of the reticuloendothelial cells. It has been shown that the phagocytic function of fixed macrophages may be depressed in male alcoholic patients who do not have clinical evidence of cirrhosis (Liu, 1979). These data have been extended to animal studies. Rat liver macrophages isolated *in vitro* from ethanol-treated animals had slightly lower phagocytic activity than control animals, but were not able to kill phagocytized bacteria, suggesting an impairment of the bactericidal activities of hepatic macrophages (Galante *et al.*, 1980). Rimland and Hand (1980) have studied the effects of alcohol on rabbit alveolar macrophage adherence. They found a transient loss of adherence, as well as an alteration of phagocytosis of latex particles by macrophages exposed to ethanol. These authors discuss possible mechanisms for the effect of alcohol on macrophages.

A number of studies have shown a major effect of alcohol on granulocytes. There may be a transient granulocytopenia suggesting direct toxicity on the granulopoietic stem cell (Liu, 1980). Functional impairment of granulocytes, including adherence, motility, and chemotaxis, has also been reported (MacGregor *et al.*, 1978; Wozniak and Silverman, 1979).

A number of studies have shown the effects of alcohol on thymus-dependent lymphocytes (Bernstein *et al.*, 1974; Berenyi *et al.*, 1974; Ogunye *et al.*, 1978; Takagi, 1979; Lang *et al.*, 1980; Smith *et al.*, 1980). These investigators have shown that there is a reduction in the number of T cells in patients with alcoholic hepatitis and/or cirrhosis. In addition to cell number, there was also an associated decrease in autologous rosette-forming T lymphocytes.

In addition to the absolute number of lymphocytes, lymphocyte transformation is also affected by alcohol. There is an inhibition of lymphocyte stimulation by PHA using plasma from patients with advanced alcoholic cirrhosis (Hsu and Leevy, 1971; Young *et al.*, 1979a,b). These results suggest that serum inhibitory factors from alcoholics alter cell-mediated immunity and may contribute to development and/or perpetuation of liver damage. Because of the various lesions of the immune system associated with alcoholism, it is possible that delayed hypersensitivity may also be affected by chronic alcoholism. A number of studies have indicated that delayed hypersensitivity, i.e., cellular immunity as exemplified by responses to PPD, mumps antigens, sensitization to DNCB, etc., is not intact in cases of chronic alcoholism and/or chronic liver disease associated with acute alcoholism (Straus *et al.*, 1971; Berenyi *et al.*, 1974; Takagi, 1979; Bjorkholm, 1980). However, not all investigators have shown that skin testing with DNCB is impaired in alcoholic patients (Lundy *et al.*, 1975). These investigators reported that a number of the immunological defects associated with acute alcoholism are reversible.

Several papers have recently been published outlining the effects of ethanol on interferon production in mice (Tyring *et al.*, 1979, 1980). These investigators noted a severe reduction in interferon levels in mice injected with alcohol.

In addition to the effects on the cellular arm of immunity, there are major effects of alcohol on serum immunoglobulins. Transitory changes in the levels of IgG and IgM occur; however, there is a marked elevation of IgA in the serum of chronic alcoholics (Wilson *et al.*, 1969; Van Epps *et al.*, 1975; Bogdal *et al.*, 1976; Iturriaga *et al.*, 1977; Smith *et al.*, 1980).

In addition to many of the cellular/humoral aberrations induced by excessive consumption of alcohol and/or alcohol-associated liver disease, there may also be an effect of alcohol on possible development of autoimmune diseases, which in turn may contribute to the chronicity of liver disease (Zinneman, 1975; Zetterman and Leevy, 1975; Zetterman et al., 1976; Kakumu and Leevy, 1977; Van Thiel et al., 1977). This autoimmune process is exemplified by reduction of T cells as well as the increases in the specific serum immunoglobulins and may be manifested by lymphocyte cytotoxicity toward liver cells of patients with alcoholic hepatitis (Kakumu and Leevy, 1977) or autoantibodies to spermatozoa and to testicular antigens (Van Thiel et al., 1977), etc. The finding of increased chromosomal aberrations in peripheral lymphocytes of alcoholics further suggests the increased likelihood of disease (Obe et al., 1980).

2.3.2. Barbiturates

Among the drugs most frequently prescribed to induce sedation and sleep are the barbiturates. About 2500 derivatives of barbiturates have been synthesized; however, only about 15 are in widespread use. They represent another group of abused drugs shown to have effects on the immune system. Transformation of human lymphocytes is affected by the use of phenobarbital (Park and Brody, 1971). These investigators noted a reduction in the lymphocyte response to PHA following administration of phenobarbital. There are also reports indicating a depression of the immune response following surgery (Slade et al., 1975; Duncan and Cullen, 1976). A recent study using dogs anesthetized by phenobarbital (Formeister et al., 1980) indicated that 3 hrs after anesthesia, the ability of lymphocytes to respond to mitogens was less than 50% of their preanesthetic values. Recovery to normal capability occurred within several days. In a series of studies, Güttner et al. (1973a,b) noted the immunosuppressive effects of barbituric acid derivatives in mice. These effects were seen at several levels including phagocytosis, cell-mediated immunity through lymphocyte transformation, and through effects on antibody production. Lefkowitz and Nemeth (1976) have also shown the effects of these substances on other immune parameters, including the production of rosette-forming cells in mice.

2.4. MARIJUANA (CANNABINOIDS)

Cannabis is obtained from the flowering tops of hemp plants. The dried leaves and flowering shoots also contain small amounts of the active substance, which is primarily THC, although other substances present in lesser amounts may have pharmacological effects in animals.

The THC content of marijuana ranges from 0.5 to about 6%. It is estimated that when smoked with maximal efficiency, no more than 50% of the THC in a cigarette is actually absorbed. Therefore, a 1-g cigarette will deliver about 10–20 mg to the lungs. This level of THC is capable of causing alterations in mood, memory, coordination, sensorium, time–spatial relationships, self-perceptions, etc. These occur within minutes after exposure and may last several hours (Jaffe, 1980). It is estimated that there may be as many as 50 million or more sporadic users in the United States and at least four times that number throughout the world.

There is sufficient evidence indicating that marijuana in one or more forms probably interferes with the immune response in man. The effects of tobacco on a number of physiological processes have been discussed previously. Exposure to tobacco smoke has been shown to have an immunosuppressive effect on both humoral (Esber *et al.*, 1973; Thomas *et al.*, 1973a; Nulsen *et al.*, 1974) and cellular (Thomas *et al.*, 1973b, 1974a,b,c) immunity, as well as the reticuloendothelial system (Green and Carolin, 1967; Powell and Green, 1972). Various cannabinoids have been reported to suppress both humoral and cell-mediated immunity in animals. Findings in human subjects smoking marijuana have been inconsistent.

There does not seem to be a direct correlation between the psychotomimetic effect and their capacity to suppress immune responses. Huber *et al.* (1980) reported that intrapulmonary inactivation of aerosolized *Staphylococcus aureus* in rats was markedly affected by exposure to marijuana smoke. Bacterial inactivation was impaired in a dose-dependent manner. Toxicity of the smoke to the lung, which impaired antibacterial defenses, did not correlate with parenterally administered THC. Other studies in man also suggest that highly toxic effects relate directly to marijuana smoke (Vachon, 1976).

2.4.1. Effects in Man

Differences in the phagocytic capability of cells from smokers and nonsmokers have been reported (Mann *et al.*, 1971). Preparations from smokers contain fewer polymorphonuclear leukocytes capable of phagocytizing yeast cells (Petersen *et al.*, 1974). Suppression of *in vitro* migration of leukocytes obtained from both marijuana smokers and nonsmokers using both marijuana extracts and/or THC has also been reported (Schwartzfarb *et al.*, 1974). Marijuana extracts were more effective than THC in these studies.

Recent evaluation of cell-mediated and humoral immunity in chronic marijuana users has yielded contradictory results. Conditions and procedures that possibly contributed to these inconsistencies have been discussed by Maugh (1975). Serious concern about the possibility that cannabis may cause impairment of the immune system was first aroused when Nahas *et al.* (1974) reported that lymphocytes from regular users of cannabis showed an impaired capacity to proliferate in the presence of the mitogen PHA. In a similar study with chronic marijuana smokers and matched nonsmoker controls, the number of T cells with respect to the T/B cell ratio was lowered (Petersen *et al.*, 1974). Petersen *et al.* (1975) reported a statistically significant decrease in the response to mitogenic stimulation in a group of chronic marijuana smokers compared to a matched control group. There is little evidence that either marijuana or THC has a significant effect on humoral immunity in man (Gupta *et al.*, 1974; Rachelefsky *et al.*, 1976).

White *et al.* (1975), however, failed to demonstrate defects in thymidine uptake following PHA stimulation of lymphocytes from smokers. Silverstein and Lessin (1974, 1976) found no impairment in the responsiveness of chronic marijuana smokers to DNCB, which elicits a delayed-type hypersensitivity reaction. Other reports also failed to substantiate an association between chronic marijuana smoking and decreased cell-mediated immunity (Cushman and Khurana, 1976; Cushman *et al.*, 1976; Lau *et al.*, 1976; Rachelefsky *et al.*, 1976).

When the *in vitro* influence of cannabinoids on cellular immunity was tested, thymidine incorporation into lymphocytes was suppressed (Armand *et al.*, 1974; DeSoize *et al.*, 1975). Petersen *et al.* (1976) reported that the effects of marijuana on the response to mitogenic stimulation were transitory and variable.

The depressive effect of THC on the proliferation of neoplastic cells *in vivo* (Harris *et al.*, 1974, 1976) has been substantiated by various studies investigating drug-induced effects on the cellular division and biosynthesis of eukaryotic cells (Zimmerman *et al.*, 1977). The suppressed response of lymphocytes from marijuana smokers to mitogenic stimulation was believed to result from interference of DNA synthesis by THC (Nahas *et al.*, 1974). In subsequent studies, Nahas and co-workers suggested that cannabinoids not only interfere with DNA synthesis in lymphocytes, but also affect synthesis of other macromolecules possibly through effects on cell membranes (Nahas, 1975; Nahas *et al.*, 1976, 1977). Cytogenetic studies on mutagenesis and chromosomal changes are also in conflict. When leukocytes were cultured from humans given oral doses of THC, marijuana, or hashish extracts, no increase in chromosomal breakage was noted (Nichols *et al.*, 1974). *In vitro* exposure of human leukocyte cultures to THC resulted in a decrease in the mitotic index, but the number of breaks and/or gaps did not increase (Neu *et al.*, 1969, 1970). Similar results were demonstrated when THC was placed in tissue culture media after PHA had been added to leukocytes from healthy human donors (Stenchever and Allen, 1972; Stenchever *et al.*, 1976). Martin and co-workers (Martin, 1969; Martin *et al.*, 1974) exposed both rat and human leukocytes to cannabis resins *in vitro* and demonstrated a dose-related decrease in mitotic activity. Again, however, no alteration in the mutation rate was detected.

In a series of papers, it has been reported (Leuchtenberger and Leuchtenberger, 1971; Leuchtenberger *et al.*, 1973a,b, 1976) that smoke from marijuana cigarettes passed over cultures of human lung explants produced, in addition to some initial cytotoxicity, abnormalities of mitosis and impairment of contact inhibition, as well as variations of DNA content and chromosome number.

2.4.2. Animal Studies

A review of the effects of THC on the immune response in rodents has disclosed more consistent findings. Splenic lymphocytes prepared from mice treated with THC were found to be inhibited in their response to PHA and *E. coli* LPS (Levy *et al.*, 1975; Munson *et al.*, 1976). These results appear to indicate an effect on both cellular and humoral arms of the immune system. THC has also been shown to increase the graft survival time of mouse skin allografts (Levy *et al.*, 1974; Munson *et al.*, 1976).

In addition to inhibiting the proliferation of lymphocytes in the rodent immune system, investigators have suggested that other parameters could also be affected. In a study involving rats exposed to cannabis smoke, there was an observed suppression of circulating antibody (Munson *et al.*, 1976; Rosenkrantz, 1976). Spleen cells harvested from the same rats had a decreased capacity to produce antibodies when exposed to antigens (Rosenkrantz, 1976). Dose-dependent reduction in hemolytic PFC numbers has also been reported (Levy and Heppner, 1981). When administered orally, THC demonstrated immunosuppressive activity on both the inductive and the productive phase of the primary immune response (Rosenkrantz and Miller, 1975). Suppression of the antigenic response by THC was reflected as a reduction of splenic weight and a reduction in the percentage volume of splenic white pulp to total spleen volume (Zimmerman *et al.*, 1977). In a separate study, Munson *et al.* (1976) observed a decreased spleen size, as well as a depletion in the number of nucleated spleen cells and peripheral leukocytes. Lefkowitz and Chiang (1975b) also reported an impairment in the number of PFC in spleens from mice injected with THC.

The stimulation of immunocyte maturation and proliferation occurs only after the antigen is processed by macrophages. Cannabis possibly interferes with macrophage function by causing structural alterations, inhibiting biochemical pathways, or altering transport mechanisms. Mellors (1976) found that smaller doses of THC given to rats inhibited the production of migration inhibitory factor, a substance that prevents macrophages from leaving the site of interaction between a T cell and an antigen.

Several studies have reported that cannabinoids have an affinity for lung tissue (Fleischman *et al.*, 1975; Rosenkrantz *et al.*, 1975). Marijuana has been shown to affect the alveolar macrophages, which are the key host defense cells of the lung, by influencing their structure, function, and mobilization (Fleischman *et al.*, 1975; Chari-Bitron, 1976; McCarthy *et al.*, 1976). Studies involving both man and animals have yielded similar results. The cytoplasmic and morphological changes in mouse peritoneal macrophages are similar to those seen in alveolar macrophages of hashish smokers (Raz and Goldman, 1976).

More recently, Fleischman *et al.* (1979) have shown that a number of pathological changes occur in rat lungs exposed to marijuana smoke. After 1 year an alveolitis or pneumonitis is apparent including some pronounced inflammatory and proliferative changes of the lung tissue. Davies *et al.* (1979) indicated major alterations of the lipid biochemistry of alveolar macrophages of rats exposed to both marijuana and tobacco smoke. These changes in the lipid biochemistry of macrophages could reflect alterations in cell membranes, which in turn could relate to changes in immunological function. Not all investigators have obtained identical results, but some (Drath *et al.*, 1979a,b) indicated that despite metabolic alterations in response to marijuana and tobacco smoke, the alveolar macrophages were not compromised with respect to their ability to ingest various particles, including staphylococci.

With regard to cytogenetic studies, injections of marijuana extract into hamsters also did not result in chromosomal breakage (Nicholson *et al.*, 1973). In these experiments THC was present throughout the 72-hr culture period in a number of different concentrations. At the higher concentrations, there was a noticeable increase in cell death and a decreased mitotic activity, but no chromosomal breakage. Similarly, no chromosomal damage was found in rat cells after exposure to either THC or marijuana resins (Pace *et al.*, 1971).

Because marijuana is often used by young people (Marihuana and Health, 1972, 1974), pharmacological studies of THC in animals should obviously include chronic drug regimens in young, developing animals. The acute and chronic behavioral effects of THC in young mice have been described (Radouco-Thomas *et al.*, 1976), but few studies have involved the effect of THC on the immune response in young mice, as compared to that in older mice, with the exception of one by Pruess and Lefkowitz (1978).

Other studies have indicated that the injection of THC may directly affect host resistance. In a series of studies using resistance of mice to *Listeria monocytogenes* and herpes simplex virus, Morahan *et al.* (1979) showed a dramatic decrease in resistance to these agents following the administration of THC.

Cannabis use has also evoked a number of allergic reactions (Liskow *et al.*, 1971; Nahas *et al.*, 1973; Shapiro *et al.*, 1974, 1976) suggesting that marijuana and its components may serve as antigens. Cannabinoids have also been found to inhibit myelopoiesis in rat bone marrow (Johnson and Wiersema, 1974).

It is apparent that the many effects of marijuana on both man and animals are not clearly delineated. There is a general consensus that smoke from marijuana contains harmful and injurious agents that could affect macrophages and/or macrophage function. These effects could be mediated through alterations in lipid biochemistry. A number of other parameters of immunity may be affected by smoking marijuana. Several studies support the contention that there are effects on the immune system through the psychotropic agent in marijuana, i.e., THC. Throughout the literature, however, there is considerable inconsistency regarding these parameters. It is clear that further work is necessary to delineate the effects of this frequently abused substance on immunity.

2.5. HALLUCINOGENS

Of the hallucinogenic drugs available on the street, one of the most widely publicized over the years has been LSD. It is a semisynthetic compound produced from lysergic acid, a naturally occurring substance found in fungus of rye. A number of studies have suggested that this substance damages chromosomes and is mutagenic. Others have suggested that there is a teratogenic potential associated with this drug capable of causing chromosomal breaks, etc. However, not all investigators have been able to substantiate these effects of LSD (Dishotsky *et al.*, 1971; Maugh, 1973). A number of other reports found in the literature are also concerned with the teratogenic effects of LSD on developing embryos.

A number of studies have reported on the effect of LSD on immunoglobulin synthesis *in vitro* (Voss *et al.*, 1973a,b; Winkelhake *et al.*, 1974; Winkelhake and Voss, 1975). These workers showed that LSD interferes with tryptophan incorporation into antibody. These workers also showed that the interference in immunoglobulin synthesis by LSD could be reversed by the addition of exogenous tryptophan. The relationship of these studies to the possible immunosuppressive properties of LSD awaits further investigation. In addition to LSD, mescaline and peyote have been shown to affect the production of interferon in mice (Hung *et al.*, 1973). It would not be surprising if a number of drugs in this class had major effects on immunity and host resistance.

3. CONCLUSION

It is clear that many of the frequently abused drugs are detrimental to the host. The significance of the immunosuppressive properties of many of these drugs cannot be ascertained with the present information, but may represent another insult to normal homeostatic mechanisms that could result in altered immune responses.

A number of these studies indicate that certain of these drugs have major effects on the immune system. Some of these studies employ almost exclusively animal systems, whereas others utilize *in vitro* models. It is probable that in many of these systems, direct correlation between the effect of these drugs on animals to that of man is not applicable because of dosage, route, etc. This is also true with *in vitro* studies where it is sometimes difficult to assess the significance of the effects of many of these substances

It is also clear, however, that the effects of many of these substances on immunity may represent a very minor component of the overall picture. Furthermore, making direct correlations of drug usage to immunity is further complicated since drug abusers frequently abuse more than one substance at a given time. In addition, other factors, such as nutrition, life-styles, etc., which regulate and/or affect health, may also be compromised in an individual who is abusing drugs.

Note: Since this review was written the literature continues to contain frequent references to the immunological imbalance associated with chronic alcoholism as well as the frequency of infections in parenteral drug abusers, alcoholics, etc. A clinical disease not previously recognized has recently been described. It is referred to as acquired immune deficiency syndrome (AIDS). This disease is characterized by an inverse T-lymphocyte helper:suppressor ratio where the helper T-cell subpopulation is greatly depleted. These patients frequently develop opportunistic infections including Candida albicans, Pneumocystis carinii, etc. A high percentage of these patients also develop Kaposi's sarcoma. Patients at risk for developing this disease include homosexuals, intravenous drug abusers, Haitian immigrants, and hemophiliacs. The causes of this disease have been attributed to the use of amyl nitrite as well as certain herpesvirus infections. Current evidence strongly indicates a transmissible agent with the human T-cell leukemia virus (HTLV-III) as the primary suspect.

REFERENCES

Abelson, P. H., 1970, Death from heroin, *Science* **168**:1289.

Armand, J. P., Hsu, J. T., and Nahas, G. G., 1974, Inhibition of blastogenesis of T lymphocytes by delta-9-THC, *Fed. Proc.* **33**:539.

Ayre, D. J., Keast, D., and Papadimitriou, J. M., 1981, Effects of tobacco smoke exposure on splenic architecture and weight during the primary immune response of BALB/c mice, *J. Pathol.* **133**:53.

Bach, J. F., 1975, The mode of action of immunosuppressive agents, *Front. Biol.* **41**:1–20.

Banks, T., Fletcher, R., and Ali, N., 1973, Infective endocarditis in heroin addicts, *Am. J. Med.* **55**:444.

Berenyi, M. R., Straus, B., and Cruz, D., 1974, *In vitro* and *in vivo* studies of cellular immunity in alcoholic cirrhosis, *Dig. Dis.* **19**:199.

Bernstein, I. M., Webster, K. H., Williams, R. C., and Strickland, R. G., 1974, Reduction in circulating T lymphocytes in alcoholic liver disease, *Lancet* **2**:488.

Bjorkholm, M., 1980, Immunological and hematological abnormalities in chronic alcoholism, *Acta Med. Scand.* **207**:197.

Blanck, R. R., Ream, N., and Conrad, M., 1979, Hepatitis B antigen and antibody in heroin users, *Am. J. Gastroenterol.* **71**:164.

Blanck, R. R., Ream, N., and Deegan, M. J., 1980, Immunoglobulins in heroin users, *Am. J. Epidemiol.* **111**:81.

Bogdal, J., Cichecka, K., Kirchmayer, S., Mika, M., and Tarnawski, A., 1976, Immunoglobulins in chronic alcoholics, *Arch. Immunol. Ther. Exp. (Warsz)* **24**:799.

Brown, S. M., Stimmel, B., Taub, R. N., Kochwa, S., and Rosenfield, R. E., 1974, Immunologic dysfunction in heroin addicts, *Arch. Intern. Med.* **134**:1001.

Chari-Bitron, A., 1976, Effect of delta-9-tetrahydrocannabinol on red blood cell membranes and on alveolar macrophages, in: *Marihuana: Chemistry, Biochemistry and Cellular Effects* (G. G. Nahas, ed.), Springer-Verlag, Berlin.

Cherubin, C. E., 1971, Infectious disease problems of narcotic addicts, *Arch. Intern. Med.* **128**:309.

Cherubin, C. E., Hargrove, R. L., and Prince, A. M., 1970, The serum hepatitis related antigen (SH) in illicit drug users, *Am. J. Epidemiol.* **91**:510.

Cherubin, C. E., McCusker, J., Baden, M., Kavaler, F., and Amsel, Z., 1972, The epidemiology of death in narcotic addicts, *Am. J. Epidemiol.* **96**:11.

Corberand, J., Lahangne, P., Nguyen, F., Datau, G., Fontanilles, A. M., Gleizes, B., and Gyrard, E., 1980, *In vitro* effect of tobacco smoke components on the functions of normal human polymorphonuclear leukocytes, *Infect. Immun.* **30**:649.

Crout, J. E., Hepburn, B., and Ritts, R. E., 1975, Suppression of lymphocyte transformation after aspirin ingestion, *N. Engl. J. Med.* **292**:221.

Curtis, J., Richman, B. L., and Feinstein, M. A., 1974, Infective endocarditis in drug addicts, *South Med. J.* **67**:4.

Cushman, P., Jr., 1974, Hyperimmunoglobulinemia in heroin addiction: Some epidemiologic observations, including some possible effects of route of administration and multiple drug abuse, *Am. J. Epidemiol.* **99**:218.

Cushman, P., 1978, Methadone maintenance: Long-term follow-up of detoxified patients, *Ann. N.Y. Acad. Sci.* **311**:165.

Cushman, P., 1980, The major medical sequelae of opioid addiction, *Drug Alcohol Depend.* **5**:239.

Cushman, P., and Khurana, R., 1976, Marijuana and T lymphocyte rosettes, *Clin. Pharmacol. Ther.* **19**:310.

Cushman, P., Khurana, R., and Hashim, G., 1976, Tetrahydrocannabinol: Evidence for reduced rosette formation by normal T lymphocytes, in: *The Pharmacology of Marihuana*, Volume 1 (M. C. Braude and S. Szara, eds.), Raven Press, New York.

Cushman, P., Jr., Gupta, S., and Grieco, M. H., 1977, Immunological studies in methadone maintained patients, *Int. J. Addict.* **12:**241.

Davies, P., Sornberger, G. C., Engel, E. E., and Huber, G. L., 1978, Stereology of lavaged populations of alveolar macrophages: Effects of *in vivo* exposure to tobacco smoke, *Exp. Mol. Pathol.* **29:**170.

Davies, P., Sornberger, G. C., and Huber, G. L., 1979, Effects of experimental marijuana and tobacco smoke inhalation on alveolar macrophages: A comparative stereologic study, *Lab. Invest.* **41:**220.

Demoulin, A., and Demoulin-Brahy, L., 1979, Effect of tobacco smoke and gaseous atmospheric pollutants on the antimicrobial activity of alveolar macrophages, *Acta Clin. Belg.* **34:**88.

DeSoize, B., Hsu, J., Nahas, G. G., and Morishima, J., 1975, Inhibition of human lymphocyte transformation *in vitro* by natural cannabinoids and olivetol, *Fed. Proc.* **34:**783.

Dishotsky, N. I., Loughman, W. D., Mogar, R. E., and Lipscomb, W. R., 1971, LSD and genetic damage, *Science* **172:**431.

Drath, D. B., Harper, A., Gharibian, J., Karnovsky, M. L., and Huber, G. L., 1978, The effect of tobacco smoke on the metabolism and function of rat alveolar macrophages, *J. Cell. Physiol.* **95:**105.

Drath, D. B., Karnovsky, M. L., and Huber, G. L., 1979a, Tobacco smoke effects on pulmonary host defense, *Inflammation* **3:**281.

Drath, D. B., Karnovsky, M. L., and Huber, G. L., 1979b, The effects of experimental exposure to tobacco smoke on the oxidative metabolism of alveolar macrophages, *J. Reticuloendothel. Soc.* **25:**597.

Duncan, P. G., and Cullen, B. F., 1976, Anesthesia and immunology, *Anesthesiology* **45:**522.

El-Khatib, M. R., Wilson, F. M., and Lerner, A. M., 1976, Characteristics of bacterial endocarditis in heroin addicts in Detroit, *Am. J. Med. Sci.* **271:**197.

Ericsson, C. D., Kohl, S., Pickering, L. K., Davis, J., Glass, G., and Faillace, L. A., 1980, Mechanisms of host defense in well nourished patients with chronic alcoholism, *Alcholism: Clin. Exp. Res.* **4:**261.

Esber, H. J., Menninger, F. F., Jr., Bogden, A. E., and Mason, M. M., 1973, Immunological deficiency associated with cigarette smoke inhalation by mice: Primary and secondary hemagglutinin response, *Arch. Environ. Health* **27:**99.

Ferson, L., Edwards, A., Lind, A., Milton, G. W., and Hersey, P., 1979, Low natural killer-cell activity and immunoglobulin levels associated with smoking in human subjects, *Int. J. Cancer* **23:**603.

Finklea, J., Hasselblad, V., Riggan, W., Nelson, W., Hammer, D., and Newill, V., 1971, Cigarette smoking and hemagglutination inhibition response to influenza after natural disease immunization, *Am. Rev. Respir. Dis.* **104:**368.

Fleischman, R. W., Sprague, R. A., Hayden, D. W., Braude, M. C., and Rosenkrantz, H., 1975, Chronic marihuana-inhalation toxicity in rats, *Toxicol. Appl. Pharmacol.* **34:**467.

Fleischman, R. W., Baker, J. R., and Rosenkrantz, H., 1979, Pulmonary pathologic changes in rats exposed to marihuana smoke for one year, *Toxicol. Appl. Pharmacol.* **47:**557.

Formeister, J. F., MacDermott, R. P., Wickline, D., Locke, D., Nash, G. S., and Reynolds, D. G., 1980, Alteration of lymphocyte function due to anesthesia: *In vivo* and *in vitro* suppression of mitogen-induced blastogenesis by sodium pentobarbital, *Surgery* **87:**573.

Galante, D., Perna, P., Andreanna, A., Utili, R., and Ruggiero, G., 1980, Hepatic clearance of *Escherichia coli* during chronic ethanol intoxication, *Boll. Soc. Ital. Biol. Sper.* **56:**1007.

Gerrard, J. W., Heiner, D. C., Mink, J., Meyers, A., and Dosman, J. A., 1980, Immunoglobulin levels in smokers and non-smokers, *Ann. Allergy* **44:**261.

Gluckman, S. J., Dvork, V. C., and MacGregor, R. R., 1977, Host defenses during prolonged alcohol consumption in a controlled environment, *Arch. Intern. Med.* **137:**1539.

Goldin, R. H., Chow, A. W., Edwards, J. E., Jr., Louie, J. S., and Guze, L. B., 1973, Sternoarticular septic arthritis in heroin users, *N. Engl. J. Med.* **289:**616.

Green, G., and Carolin, D., 1967, The depressant effect of cigarette smoke on *in vitro* antibacterial activity of alveolar macrophages, *N. Engl. J. Med.* **276:**421.

Grieco, M. H., and Chuang, C. Y., 1973, Hypermacroglobulinemia associated with heroin use in adolescents. *J. Allergy Clin. Immunol.* **51:**152.

Güngör, M., Genc, E., Sağduyu, H., Eroğlu, L., and Koyuncuoğlu, H., 1980, Effect of chronic administration of morphine on primary immune response in mice, *Experientia* **36**:1309.

Gupta, S., Cushman, P., and Grieco, M. H., 1974, Impairment of rosette-forming T lymphocytes in chronic marijuana smokers, *N. Engl. J. Med.* **292**:104.

Güttner, J., Aschiesche, W., and Werner, W., 1973a, Immunosuppressive effects of barbituric acid derivatives. I. Influence on humoral antibody response and phagocytic activity in mice, *Chemotherapy* **19**:47.

Güttner, J., Heinecke, H., Kuchler, W., and Werner, W., 1973b, Immunosuppressive effects of barbituric acid derivatives. II. Effect of 1,3-bis (piperidinomethyl)-5-phenyl-barbituric acid on humoral and cell-mediated immunity in mice, *Chemotherapy* **19**:305.

Harris, L. S., Munson, A. E., Friedman, M. A., and Dewey, W. L., 1974, Retardation of tumor growth by Δ^9-tetrahydrocannabinol (Δ^9-THC), *Pharmacologist* **16**:259.

Harris, L. S., Munson, A. E., Friedman, M. A., and Dewey, W. L., 1976, Antitumor properties of cannabinoids, in: *The Pharmacology of Marihuana*, Vol. 1 (M. C. Braude and S. Szara, eds.), pp. 749–762, Raven Press, New York.

Herscowitz, H. B., and Cooper, R. B., 1979, Effect of cigarette smoke exposure on maturation of the antibody response in spleens of newborn mice, *Pediatr. Res.* **13**:987.

Ho, W. K. K., and Leung, A., 1979, The effect of morphine addiction on concanavalin A-mediated blastogenesis, *Pharmacol. Res. Commun.* **11**:413.

Hopkin, J. M., and Evans, H. J., 1979, Cigarette smoke condensates damage DNA in human lymphocytes, *Nature (London)* **279**:241.

Hsu, C. S., and Leevy, C. M., 1971, Inhibition of PHA-stimulated lymphocyte transformation by plasma from patients with advanced alcoholic cirrhosis, *Clin. Exp. Immunol.* **8**:749.

Huber, G. L., Pochay, V. E., Pereira, W., Shea, J. W., Hinds, W. C., First, M. W., and Sornberger, G. C., 1980, Marijuana, tetrahydrocannabinol, and pulmonary antibacterial defenses, *Chest* **77**:403.

Huber, G. L., Davies, P., Zwilling, G. R., Pochay, V. E., Hinds, W. C., Nicholas, H. A., Mahajan, V. K., Hayashi, M., and First, M. W., 1981, A morphologic and physiologic bioassay for quantifying alterations in the lung following experimental chronic inhalation of tobacco smoke, *Bull. Eur. Physiopathol. Respir.* **17**:269.

Hung, C. Y., Lefkowitz, S. S., and Geber, W. F., 1973, Interferon inhibition by narcotic analgesics, *Proc. Soc. Exp. Biol. Med.* **142**:106.

Husby, G., Pierce, P. E., and Williams, R. C., Jr., 1975, Smooth muscle antibody in heroin addicts, *Ann. Intern. Med.* **83**:801.

Ishi, Y., and Bender, M. A., 1978, Caffeine inhibition of prereplication repair of mitomycin C-induced DNA damage in human peripheral lymphocytes, *Mutat. Res.* **51**:419.

Iturriaga, H., Pereda, T., Estevea, A., and Ugarte, G., 1977, Serum immunoglobulin A changes in alcoholic patients, *Ann. Clin. Res.* **9**:39.

Jacob, C. V., Stelzer, G. T., and Wallace, J. H., 1980, The influence of cigarette tobacco smoke products on the immune response, *Immunology* **40**:621–627.

Jaffe, J. H., 1980, Drug addiction and drug abuse, in: *The Pharmacological Basis of Therapeutics* (L. Goodman and A. Gilman, eds.), pp. 535–584, Macmillan Co., New York.

Jedrychowski, W., 1978, Variability of IgG, IgA, and IgD levels witb relation to age and tobacco addiction in healthy men, *Patol. Pol.* **29**:153.

Johnson, R. J., and Wiersema, V., 1974, Effects of delta-9-tetrahydrocannabinol metabolite on bone marrow myelopoiesis, *Res. Commun. Chem. Pathol. Pharmacol.* **8**:393.

Johnson, W. D., Jr., 1975, Impaired defense mechanisms associated with acute alcoholism, *Ann. N.Y. Acad. Sci.* **252**:343.

Kakumu, S., and Leevy, C. M., 1977, Lymphocyte cytotoxicity in alcoholic hepatitis, *Gastroenterology* **72**:594.

Ketkar, M. D., Rexnik, G., and Mohr, U., 1977, Pathological alterations in Syrian golden hamster lungs after passive exposure to cigarette smoke, *Toxicology* **7**:265.

Kreek, M. J., 1978, Medical complications in methadone patients, *Ann. N.Y. Acad. Sci.* **311**:110.

Lang, J. M., Rushcer, H., Hasselmann, J., Granjean, P., Bigel, P., and Mayer, S., 1980, Decreased autologous rosette-forming T lymphocytes in alcoholic cirrhosis, *Int. Arch. Allergy Appl. Immunol.* **61**:337.

Lau, R. J., Tubergren, D. G., Barr, M., Jr., Domino, E. F., Benowitz, N., and Jones, R. T., 1976, Phytohemagglutinin-induced lymphocyte transformation in humans receiving delta-9-tetrahydrocannabinol, *Science* **192**:805.

Laux, D. C., and Klesius, P. H., 1973, Suppressive effects of caffeine on the immune response of the mouse to sheep erythrocytes, *Proc. Soc. Exp. Biol. Med.* **144**:633.

Leevy, C. M., Chen, T., Luisada-Opper, A., Kanagasundaram, N., and Zetterman, R., 1976, Liver disease of the alcoholic: Role of immunologic abnormalities in pathogenesis, recognition, and treatment, *Prog. Liver Dis.* **5**:516.

Lefkowitz, S. S., and Chiang, C. Y., 1975a, Effects of certain abused drugs on hemolysin forming cells, *Life Sci.* **17**:1763.

Lefkowitz, S. S., and Chiang, C. Y., 1975b, Effects of delta-9-tetrahydrocannabinol on mouse spleens, *Res. Commun. Chem. Pathol. Pharmacol.* **11**:659.

Lefkowitz, S. S., and Nemeth, D., 1976, Immunosuppression of rosette-forming cells, *Adv. Exp. Med. Biol.* **73**:269; and in: *The Reticuloendothelial System in Health and Disease* (H. Friedman, M. Escobar, and S. M. Reichard, eds.), p. 269, Plenum Press, New York.

Leuchtenberger, C., and Leuchtenberger, R., 1971, Morphological and cytochemical effects of marihuana cigarette smoke on epithelial lung explants from mice, *Nature (London)* **234**:227.

Leuchtenberger, C., Leuchtenberger, R., and Ritter, V., 1973a, Effects of marihuana and tobacco smoke on DNA and chromosomal complement in human lung explants, *Nature (London)* **242**:403.

Leuchtenberger, C., Leuchtenberger, R., and Schneider, A., 1973b, Effects of marihuana and tobacco smoke on human lung physiology, *Nature (London)* **241**:137.

Leuchtenberger, C., Leuchtenberger, R., Abinden, J., and Scheleh, E., 1976, Cytological and cytochemical effects of whole smoke and of the gas vapor phase from marihuana cigarettes on growth and DNA metabolism of cultured mammalian cells, in: *Marihuana: Chemistry, Biochemistry and Cellular Effects* (G. G. Nahas, ed.), pp. 243–256, Springer-Verlag, Berlin.

Levy, J. A., and Heppner, G. H., 1981, Alterations of immune reactivity by haloperidol and delta-9-tetrahydrocannabinol, *Int. J. Immunopharmacol.* **3**:93.

Levy, J. A., Munson, A. E., Harris, L. S., and Dewey, W. L., 1974, Effects of delta-8-tetrahydrocannabinol and delta-9-tetrahydrocannabinol on the immune response in mice, *Pharmacologist* **16**:259.

Levy, J. A., Munson, A. E., Harris, L. S., and Dewey, W. L., 1975, Effects of delta-9-tetrahydrocannabinol on the immune response of mice, *Fed. Proc.* **34**:782.

Lewis, D. J., Braybrook, K. J., and Prentice, D. E., 1979, The measurement of ultrastructural changes induced by tobacco smoke in rat alveolar macrophages: A comparison of high and low tar cigarettes, *Toxicol. Lett.* **4**:175.

Lewis, R. J., 1973, Infections in heroin addicts, *J. Am. Med. Assoc.* **223**:1036.

Lewis, R. J., Richmond, A. S., and McGrory, J. P., 1975, *Diplococcus pneumoniae* cellulitis in drug addicts, *J. Am. Med. Assoc.* **232**:54.

Light, R. W., and Dunham, T. R., 1974, Vertebral osteomyelitis due to *Pseudomonas* in the occasional heroin user, *J. Am. Med. Assoc.* **228**:1272.

Liskow, B., Liss, J. L., and Parker, C. W., 1971, Allergy to marihuana, *Ann. Intern. Med.* **75**:571.

Liu, Y. K., 1979, Phagocytic capacity of reticuloendothelial system in alcoholics, *J. Reticuloendothel. Soc.* **25**:605.

Liu, Y. K., 1980, Effects of alcohol on granulocytes and lymphocytes, *Semin. Hematol.* **17**:130.

Louria, D. B., 1974, Infectious complications of nonalcoholic drug abuse, *Annu. Rev. Med.* **25**:219.

Louria, D. B., Hensle, T., and Rose, J., 1967, The major medical complications of heroin addiction, *Ann. Intern. Med.* **67**:1.

Lundy, J., Raaf, J. H., Deakins, S., Wanebo, H. J., Jacobs, D. A., Lee, T., Jacobowitz, D., Spear, C., and Oettgen, H. F., 1975, The acute and chronic effects of alcohol on the human immune system, *Surg. Gynecol. Obstet.* **141**:212.

McCarthy, C. R., Cutting, M. B., Simmons, G. A., Pereira, W., Laguarda, R., and Huber, G. L., 1976, The effect of marihuana on the *in vitro* function of pulmonary alveolar macrophages, in: *The Pharmacology of Marihuana*, Volume 1 (M. C. Braude and S. Szara, eds.), Raven Press, New York.

McDonough, R. J., Madden, J. J., Falek, A., Shafer, D. A., Pline, M., Gordon, D., Bokos, P.,

Kuehnle, J. C., and Mendelson, J., 1980, Alteration of T and null lymphocyte frequencies in the peripheral blood of human opiate addicts: *In vivo* evidence for opiate receptor sites on T lymphocytes, *J. Immunol.* **125**:2539.

MacGregor, R. R., Gluckman, S. J., and Senior, J. R., 1978, Granulocyte function and levels of immunoglobulins and complement in patients admitted for withdrawal from alcohol, *J. Infect. Dis.* **138**:747.

Mackenzie, J. S., and Flower, R. L. P., 1979, The effect of long-term exposure to cigarette smoke on the height and specificity of the secondary immune response to influenza virus in a murine model system, *J. Hyg.* **83**:135.

Mann, P. E. G., Cohen, A. B., Finley, T. N., and Ladman, A. J., 1971, Alveolar macrophages: Structural and functional differences between nonsmokers and smokers of marihuana and tobacco, *Lab. Invest.* **25**:111.

Marihuana and Health, 1972, Second annual report to Congress, Publ. 72-0113, U.S. Government Printing Office, Washington, D.C.

Marihuana and Health, 1974, Fourth annual report to Congress, Publ. 75-181, U.S. Government Printing Office, Washington, D.C.

Martin, P. A., 1969, Cannabis and chromosomes, *Lancet* **1**:370.

Martin, P. A., Thorburn, M. J., and Bryant, S. A., 1974, *In vivo* and *in vitro* studies of the cytogenetic effects of *Cannabis sativa* in rats and man, *Teratology* **9**:81.

Matsuyama, S. S., Charuvastra, V. C., Ouren, J., Schwartz, J., and Jarvik, L., 1980, Immunoglobulin levels in heroin addicts after treatment with methadone and methadyl acetate, *Drug Alcohol Depend.* **6**:345.

Maugh, T., II, 1973, LSD and the drug culture: New evidence of hazard, *Science* **179**:1221.

Maugh, T. H., II, 1975, Marihuana: New support for immune and reproductive hazards, *Science* **190**:865.

Mellors, A., 1976, Cannabinoids: Effects on lysosomes and lymphocytes, in: *Marihuana: Chemistry, Biochemistry and Cellular Effects* (G. G. Nahas, ed.), pp. 283–298, Springer-Verlag, Berlin.

Mihas, A. A., and Doos, W. G., 1975, Multiple primary malignancies in patients with alcoholic liver disease, *Oncology* **31**:280.

Miller, D. J., Kleber, H., and Bloomer, J. R., 1979, Chronic hepatitis associated with drug abuse: Significance of hepatitis B virus, *Yale J. Biol. Med.* **52**:135.

Mishell, R. I., and Dutton, R. W., 1967, Immunization of dissociated spleen cell cultures from normal mice, *J. Exp. Med.* **126**:423.

Morahan, P. S., Klykken, P. C., Smith, S. H., Harris, L. S., and Munson, A. E., 1979, Effects of cannabinoids on host resistance to *Listeria monocytogenes* and herpes simplex virus, *Infect. Immun.* **23**:670.

Munson, A. E., Levy, J. A., Harris, L. S., and Dewey, W. L., 1976, Effects of Δ^9-tetrahydrocannabinol on the immune system, in: *The Pharmacology of Marihuana*, Volume 1 (M. C. Braude and S. Szara, eds.), pp. 187–197, Raven Press, New York.

Munson, P. L., 1974, Effects of morphine and related drugs on the corticotrophin (ACTH)—stress reaction, *Prog. Brain Res.* **39**:361.

Nahas, G. G., 1975, Effects of marijuana smoking and natural cannabinoids on the replication of human lymphocytes and the formation of hypodiploid cells, in: *Marijuana and Health Hazards* (J. R. Tinklenberg, ed.), Academic Press, New York.

Nahas, G. G., Azgury, D., and Schwarts, I. W., 1973, Evidence for the possible immunogenicity of delta-9-tetrahydrocannabinol (THC) in rodents, *Nature (London)* **243**:407.

Nahas, G. G., Suciu-Foca, N., Armand, J. P., and Morishima, J., 1974, Inhibition of cellular mediated immunity in marihuana smokers, *Science* **183**:419.

Nahas, G. G., DeSoize, B., Hsu, J., and Morishima, J., 1976, Inhibitory effects of Δ^9-tetrahydrocannabinol on nucleic acid synthesis and proteins in cultured lymphocytes, in: *Marihuana: Chemistry, Biochemistry, and Cellular Effects* (G. G. Nahas, ed.), pp. 299–312, Springer-Verlag, Berlin.

Nahas, G. G., Morishima, J., and DeSoize, B., 1977, Effects of cannabinoids on macromolecular synthesis and replication of cultured lymphocytes, *Fed. Proc.* **36**:1748.

Naito, K., Tsuji, T., Nozaki, H., and Nagashima, H., 1977, High prevalence of hepatitis B virus infection among heavy alcohol drinkers in Japan, *Microbiol. Immunol.* **21**:735.

Nathenson, G., Cohen, M. I., Millman, I., and Blumberg, B. S., 1974, Association of antibodies to Gm and antibodies to Australia antigen in adolescent drug addicts, *Proc. Soc. Exp. Biol. Med.* **145**:358.

Nemeth-Lefkowitz, D., Tyring, S. K., and Lefkowitz, S. S., 1980, Hematological and immunological effects of methadone administration in mice, *Res. Commun. Subst. Abuse* **1**:177.

Neu, R. L., Powers, H. O., King, S., and Gardner, L. I., 1969, Cannabis and chromosomes, *Lancet* **1**:675.

Neu, R. L., Powers, H. O., King, S., and Gardner, L. I., 1970, Delta-8- and delta-9-tetrahydrocannabinol: Effects on cultured human leukocytes, *J. Clin. Pharmacol.* **10**:228.

Nichols, W. W., Miller, R. C., Heneen, W., Bradt, C., Hollister, L., Kanter, S., 1974, Cytogenetic studies on human subjects receiving marijuana and delta-9-tetrahydrocannabinol, *Mutat. Res.* **26**:413.

Nicholson, M. T., Pace, H. B., and Davis, W. M., 1973, Effects of marihuana and lysergic acid diethylamide on leukocyte chromosomes of the golden hamster, *Res. Commun. Chem. Pathol. Pharmacol.* **6**:427.

Nickerson, D. S., Williams, R. C., Boxmeyer, M., and Quie, P. G., 1970, Increased opsonic capacity of serum in chronic heroin addiction, *Ann. Intern. Med.* **72**:671.

Nulsen, A., Holt, P. G., and Keast, D., 1974, Cigarette smoking, air pollution, and immunity. A model system, *Infect. Immun.* **10**:1226.

Obe, G., Gobel, D., Engeln, H., Herha, J., and Natarajan, A. T., 1980, Chromosomal aberrations in peripheral lymphocytes of alcoholics, *Mutat. Res.* **73**:377.

Ogunye, O. O., Sheagren, J. N., and McPherson, M., 1978, Effect of alcohol on thymus-dependent lymphocytes, *Br. J. Addict.* **73**:9.

Okoyama, S., and Kitao, Y., 1981, Inhibition of chromosome repair by caffeine or isonicotinic acid hydrazide on chromosome damage induced by mitomycin C in human lymphocytes, *Mutat. Res.* **81**:75.

Opelz, G., and Terasaki, P. I., 1973, Suppression of lymphocyte transformation by aspirin, *Lancet* **1**:478.

Pace, H. D., Davis, W. M., and Borgen, L. A., 1971, Teratogenesis and marihuana, *Ann. N.Y. Acad. Sci.* **191**:123.

Park, S. K., and Brody, J. I., 1971, Suppression of immunity by phenobarbital, *Nature New Biol.* **233**:181.

Petersen, B. H., Graham, J., Lemberger, L., and Dalton, B., 1974, Studies of the immune response in chronic marihuana smokers, *Pharmacologist* **16**:259.

Petersen, B. H., Lemberger, L., Graham, J., and Dalton, B., 1975, Alterations in the cellular-mediated immune responsiveness of chronic marihuana smokers, *Psychopharmacol. Commun.* **1**:67.

Petersen, B. H., Graham, J., and Lemberger, L., 1976, Marihuana, tetrahydrocannabinol and T-cell function, *Life Sci.* **19**:395.

Powell, B. M., and Green, G. M., 1972, Cigarette smoke—A proposed metabolic lesion in alveolar macrophages, *Biochem. Pharmacol.* **21**:1785.

Pruess, M. M., and Lefkowitz, S. S., 1978, Influence of maturity on immunosuppression by Δ^9-tetrahydrocannabinol, *Proc. Soc. Exp. Biol. Med.* **158**:350.

Rachelefsky, G. S., Opelz, G., Mickey, M. R., Lessin, P., Kiuchi, M., Silverstein, M. J. and Stiehm, E. R., 1976, Intact humoral and cell-mediated immunity in chronic marijuana smoking, *J. Allergy Clin. Immunol.* **58**:483.

Radouco-Thomas, S., Magnan, F., and Radouco-Thomas, C., 1976, Pharmacogenetic studies on cannabis and narcotics: Effects of Δ^1-tetrahydrocannabinol and morphine in developing mice, in: *Marihuana: Chemistry, Biochemistry and Cellular Effects* (G. G. Nahas, ed.), pp. 481–494, Springer-Verlag, Berlin.

Raz, A., and Goldman, R., 1976, Effect of hashish compounds on mouse peritoneal macrophages, *Lab. Invest.* **34**:69.

Reiner, N. E., Gopalakrishna, K. V., and Lerner, P. I., 1976, Enterococcal endocarditis in heroin addicts, *J. Am. Med. Assoc.* **235**:1861.

Rimland, D., and Hand, W. L., 1980, The effect of ethanol on adherence and phagocytosis by rabbit alveolar macrophages, *J. Lab. Clin. Med.* **95**:918.

Rosenkrantz, H., 1976, The immune response and marihuana, in: *Marihuana: Chemistry, Biochemistry and Cellular Effects* (G. G. Nahas, ed.), pp. 441–456, Springer-Verlag, Berlin.

Rosenkrantz, H., and Miller, A. J., 1975, Delta-9-tetrahydrocannabinol suppression of the primary immune response in rats, *J. Toxicol. Environ. Health* 1:119.

Rosenkrantz, H., Sprague, R. A., Fleischman, R. W., and Braude, M. C., 1975, Oral delta-9-tetrahydrocannabinol toxicity in rats treated for periods up to six months, *Toxicol. Appl. Pharmacol.* 32:399.

Rutherdale, J. A., Medline, A., Sinclair, J. C., Buchner, B., and Olin, J. S., 1972, Hepatitis in drug users, *Am. J. Gastroenterol.* 58:275.

Saxena, Q. B., Mezey, E., and Adler, W. H., 1980, Regulation of natural killer activity *in vivo*. II. The effect of alcohol consumption on human peripheral blood natural killer activity, *Int. J. Cancer* 26:413.

Schwartzfarb, L., Needle, M., and Chavaez-Chase, M., 1974, Dose-related inhibition of leukocyte migration by marihuana and delta-9-tetrahydrocannabinol (THC) *in vitro*, *J. Clin. Pharmacol.* 14:35.

Shapiro, C. M., Orlina, A. R., Unger, P., and Billings, A. A., 1974, Antibody response to cannabis, *J. Am. Med. Assoc.* 230:81.

Shapiro, C. M., Orlina, A. R., Unger, P., Telfer, M., and Billings, A. A., 1976, Marihuana induced antibody response, *J. Lab. Clin. Med.* 88:194.

Silverstein, M. J., and Lessin, P. J., 1974, Normal skin test response in chronic marihuana users, *Science* 186:740.

Silverstein, M. J., and Lessin, P. J., 1976, 2,4-Dinitrochlorobenzene skin testing in chronic marihuana users, in: *The Pharmacology of Marihuana*, Volume 1 (M. C. Braude and S. Szara, eds.), Raven Press, New York.

Slade, M. S., Simmons, R. L., Unis, E., and Greenburg, L. J., 1975, Immunodepression after major surgery in normal patients, *Surgery* 78:363.

Smith, F. E., and Palmer, D. L., 1976, Alcoholism, infection, and altered host defenses: A review of clinical and experimental observations, *J. Chronic Dis.* 29:35.

Smith, W. I., Jr., Van Thiel, D. H., Whiteside, T., Janoson, B., Magovern, J., Puet, T., and Rabin, B. S., 1980, Altered immunity in male patients with alcoholic liver disease: Evidence for defective immune regulation, *Alcoholism: Clin. Exp. Res.* 4:199.

Smith, W. R., Wells, I. D., Glauser, F. L., and Novey, H. S., 1975, High incidence of precipitins in sera of heroin addicts, *J. Am. Med. Assoc.* 232:1337.

Spiera, H., Oreskes, I., and Stimmel, B., 1974, Rheumatoid factor activity in heroin addicts on methadone maintenance, *Ann. Rheum. Dis.* 33:153.

Steinberg, S. E., and Hillman, R. S., 1980, Adverse hematologic effects of alcohol, *Postgrad. Med.* 67:139.

Stenchever, M. A., and Allen, M., 1972, The effect of delta-9-tetrahydrocannabinol on the chromosomes of human lymphocytes *in vitro*, *Am. J. Obstet. Gynecol.* 114:819.

Stenchever, M. A., Parks, K. J., and Stenchever, M. R., 1976, Effects of delta-8-tetrahydrocannabinol, delta-9-tetrahydrocannabinol and crude marijuana on human cells in tissue culture, in: *Marihuana: Chemistry, Biochemistry and Cellular Effects* (G. G. Nahas, ed.), pp. 257–263, Springer-Verlag, Berlin.

Straus, B., and Berenyi, M. R., 1973, Infection and immunity in alcoholic cirrhosis, *Mt. Sinai J. Med. N.Y.* 40:631.

Straus, B., Berenyi, M. R., Huang, J. M., and Straus, E., 1971, Delayed hypersensitivity in alcoholic cirrhosis, *Dig. Dis.* 16:509.

Takagi, S., 1979, Altered humoral and cell mediated immunity on chronic alcoholics, *Nippon Shokakibyo Gakkai Zasshi* 76:184.

Thomas, W. R., Holt, P. G., and Keast, D., 1973a, Cellular immunity in mice chronically exposed to fresh cigarette smoke, *Arch. Environ. Health* 27:372.

Thomas, W. R., Holt, P. G., and Keast, D., 1973b, Effect of cigarette smoking on the primary and secondary humoral responses in mice, *Nature (London)* 243:240.

Thomas, W. R., Holt, P. G., and Keast, D., 1974a, Development of alterations in the primary immune response of mice by exposure to fresh cigarette smoke, *Int. Arch. Allergy Appl. Immunol.* 46:481.

Thomas, W. R., Holt, P. G., and Keast, D., 1974b, Local and systemic immune response of mice after intratracheal and intravenous inoculations of sheep erythrocytes, *Int. Arch. Allergy Appl. Immunol.* **46**:487.

Thomas, W. R., Holt, P. G., and Keast, D., 1974c, Recovery of immune system after cigarette smoking, *Nature (London)* **248**:358.

Tyring, S., Klager, K., Luk, A., Messiha, F., and Lefkowitz, S. S., 1979, Ethanol, disulfiram, and pyrazole: Effects on interferon production in mice, *Immunopharmacology* **2**:63.

Tyring, S., Klager, K., Luk, A., Messiha, F., and Lefkowitz, S. S., 1980, The effect of acute and short-term ethanol administration on interferon production in mice, in: *Alcoholism: A Perspective* (F. Messiha, ed.), pp. 479–490, P. J. D. Publications, Westburg, N.J.

Vachon, L., 1976, The smoke in marijuana smoking, *N. Engl. J. Med.* **294**:160.

Van Epps, D. E., Strickland, R. G., and Williams, R. C., 1975, Inhibitors of leukocyte chemotaxis in alcoholic liver disease, *Am. J. Med.* **59**:200.

Van Thiel, D. H., Gavaler, J. S., Smith, W. I., and Rabin, B. S., 1977, Testicular and spermatozoal autoantibody in chronic alcoholic males with gonadal failure, *Clin. Immunol. Immunopathol.* **8**:311.

Voss, E. W., Jr., Babb, J. E., Metzel, P., and Winkelhake, J. L., 1973a, In vitro effects of *d*-lysergic acid diethylamide on immunoglobulin synthesis, *Biochem. Biophys. Res. Commun.* **50**:950.

Voss, E. W., Jr., Metzel, P., and Winkelhake, J. L., 1973b, Incorporation of a lysergic acid diethylamide intermediate into antibody protein in vitro, *Mol. Pharmacol.* **9**:421.

Wetli, C. V., Davis, J. H., and Blackbourne, B. D., 1972, Narcotic addiction in Dade County, Florida, *Arch. Pathol.* **93**:330.

White, S. C., Brin, S. C., and Jamiki, B. W., 1975, Mitogen-induced blastogenic responses of lymphocytes from marihuana smokers, *Science* **188**:71.

Wilson, D., Onstad, G., and Williams, R. C., Jr., 1969, Serum immunoglobulin concentrations in patients with alcoholic liver disease, *Gastroenterology* **57**:59.

Winkelhake, J. L., and Voss, E. W., Jr., 1975, Studies on the mechanism of covalent incorporation of a lysergyl derivative to immunoglobulin peptides in vitro, *J. Biol. Chem.* **250**:2164.

Winkelhake, J. L., Voss, E. W., Jr., and Lopatin, D. E., 1974, Comparative inhibitory action of D- and L-tryptophan on the effect of *d*-lysergic acid diethylamide in vitro, *Mol. Pharmacol.* **10**:68.

Wozniak, K. J., and Silverman, E. M., 1979, Granulocytic adherence in chronic alcoholism, *Am. J. Clin. Pathol.* **71**:269.

Young, G. P., Dudley, F. J., and Van Der Weyden, M. B., 1979a, Suppressive effect of alcoholic liver disease sera on lymphocyte transformation, *Gut* **20**:833.

Young, G. P., Van Der Weyden, M. B., Rose, I. S., and Dudley, F. J., 1979b, Lymphopenia and lymphocyte transformation in alcoholics, *Experientia* **35**:268.

Zetterman, R. K., and Leevy, C. M., 1975, Immunologic reactivity and alcoholic liver disease, *Bull. N.Y. Acad. Med.* **51**:533.

Zetterman, R., Chen, T., and Leevy, C. M., 1976, Autoimmunity and alcoholic liver disease, *Diseases of the Liver and Biliary Tract*, 5th Quadr. Meet., Int. Assoc. Study of the Liver, Acapulco pp. 27–31.

Zimmerman, A. M., and Zimmerman, S. B., 1976, The influence of marihuana on eukaryote cell growth and development, in *Marihuana: Chemistry, Biochemistry and Cellular Effects* (G. G. Nahas, ed.), pp. 195–205, Springer-Verlag, Berlin.

Zimmerman, S., Zimmerman, A. M., Cameron, I. L., and Laurence, H. I., 1977, Delta-1-tetrahydrocannabinol, cannabinol, and cannabidiol effects on the immune response of mice, *Pharmacology* **15**:10.

Zinneman, H. H., 1975, Autoimmune phenomena in alcoholic cirrhosis, *Dig. Dis.* **20**:337.

Index

Formaldehyde, 394
  macrophage function and, 400, 401
  phagocytosis and, 396
FPL 55712, 79
Frentizole, 270
Freund's complete adjuvant, 17, 160
  monooxygenase activity, 6
Fusarium equiseti, 223

Gallium hydroxide, 273
Gentamicin, 363, 364
Glass, 117
Glucagon, 29
Glucan, 220–221, 222
  antitumor activity, 221
  composition, 255
  mononuclear phagocytes and, 161–163
Glucorticoids, 374–376, see also Corticosteroids, inflammatory
Glycoproteins, 350
Graft-versus-host disease
  CDDP in, 362
  cyclophosphamide in, 351
  cytostipin in, 370–371
  methotrexate in, 353
  vermiculine in, 371
Granuloma
  lentinan-potentiated, 291
  trehalose diesters and formation of, 216
Granulopoiesis, 162
Guanosine monophosphate
  formation of, 58
  neutrophils and, 27
  platelet degranulation and, 27
Guanosine triphosphate, 58
Guanylate cyclase, 58

Hageman factor, 119
  inactivation of, 120
Hallucinogens, 446–447
Haptoglobin, 302
Hay dust, 395
Heme oxygenase, 5
Hemopexin, 302
Heparin, 52
  release from mast cell, 118
Hepatic microsomal enzyme system, 2
Hepatotoxicity, 3
Hexachlorobenzene, 399, 401
Hexobarbital
  endotoxin and, 11, 12
  lipopolysaccharides and pharmacokinetics of, 11
  sleep-time, 6

Histamine, 52
  adenylate cyclase activation by, 58
  basophil secretion and, 60
  colchicine inhibition of, 66
  hypersensitivity, 9
  macrophage activity and, 29, 30, 124
  oligomycin inhibition of, 65
  release from mast cell, 118
  vinblastine inhibition of, 66
Histamine-sensitizing factor, 9
Hodgkin's disease
  immunologic mechanisms in, 144
  procarbazine in, 372
  vinblastine in, 335
Hydrocortisone, 375
  lentinan inhibition by, 304
  macrophage cyclic nucleotides and, 30
Hydrogen sulfide, 394
Hydroxylamine, 30
Hypercholesteremia, 368
Hypersensitivity
  delayed-type, 157, 158, 200, 349
    in alcoholism, 441
    cyclophosphamide and, 312, 351
    desensitization model of, 106–107
    induction of, 160
    lentinan and, 296, 298
    methotrexate in, 350
    TEI-3096 and, 374
    tetracyclines and, 363
  immediate, 52–54, 157

Imidazole
  cyclic adenosine monophosphate and, 59
  cyclic guanosine monophosphate and, 38
  phosphodiesterase activity and, 58
Immune response
  carbohydrate derivatives and, 369
  cyclic nucleotides and, 27
  prostaglandins and, 143–144
Immunity, acquired, 158
Immunoglobulin(s), 121–122
  alcohol and, 441
  cigarette smoke and, 439
  6-mercaptopurine and biosynthesis of, 311
  narcotic abuse and, 437
Immunoglobulin E
  binding to mast cell, 52
  macrophage cyclic nucleotides and, 29
  receptor, 53–54
Immunoglobulin G
  auranofin and, 361
  macrophage cyclic nucleotides and, 29